Rhabdomyosarcoma and Related Tumors in Children and Adolescents

Editors
Harold M. Maurer
Professor and Chairman
Department of Pediatrics
Children's Medical Center
Virginia Commonwealth University
Richmond, Virginia

Frederick B. Ruymann
Director
Division of Hematology/Oncology
Children's Hospital
Professor, Department of Pediatrics
The Ohio State University
Columbus, Ohio

Carl Pochedly
Director
Pediatric Hematology/Oncology
King/Drew Medical Center
Los Angeles, California

CRC Press
Boca Raton Ann Arbor Boston London

Library of Congress Cataloging-in-Publication Data

Rhabdomyosarcoma and related tumors in children and adolescents/
  editors, Harold M. Maurer, Frederick B. Ruymann, Carl E. Pochedly.
    p. cm.
  Includes bibliographical references and index.
  ISBN 0-8493-6902-9
  1. Tumors in children. 2. Rhabdomyosarcoma. 3. Soft tissue
tumors. I. Maurer, Harold M. II. Ruymann, Frederick B.
III. Pochedly, Carl.
    [DNLM: 1. Rhabdomyosarcoma--in adolescence. 2. Rhabdomyosarcoma-
-in infancy & childhood. QZ 345 R468]
  RC281.C4R53 1991
  616.99′4—dc20
  DNLM/DLC
  for Library of Congress   91-20574
                                                        CIP

This book represents information obtained from authentic and highly regarded sources. Reprinted material is quoted with permission, and sources are indicated. A wide variety of references are listed. Every reasonable effort has been made to give reliable data and information, but the author and the publisher cannot assume responsibility for the validity of all materials or for the consequences of their use.

All rights reserved. This book, or any parts thereof, may not be reproduced in any form without written consent from the publisher.

Direct all inquiries to CRC Press, Inc., 2000 Corporate Blvd., N.W., Boca Raton, Florida 33431.

© 1991 by CRC Press, Inc.

International Standard Book Number 0-8493-6902-9

Library of Congress Card Number 91-20574

Printed in the United States of America   1 2 3 4 5 6 7 8 9 0

FOREWARD

Rhabdomyosarcoma, in several important respects, is the prototype cancer of children and adolescents. Rhabdomyosarcoma provides the model tumor system which best illustrates the multidisciplinary teamwork and the multimodality treatment and research, which have become the only acceptable mode for the management of children and adolescents with cancer in many parts of the world. This evolution has taken two decades. The major thrust behind the change has been cooperative clinical investigation in a multi-institutional setting by the Intergroup Rhabdomyosarcoma Study (IRS). The sophistication of the current team management and multimodality clinical investigation of rhabdomyosarcoma, which has been so largely responsible for advancing the understanding of these tumors and the cure rate of affected children, could not have been accomplished otherwise.

The IRS, which has been supported by the Cancer Therapy Evaluation Program of the National Cancer Institute for about 20 years, has provided such a body of research data and research collaboration that it now is considered an international resource. The estimate that 85% of children with rhabdomyosarcoma diagnosed in the United States are entered into the IRS is a clinical investigation statistic that probably is unequaled for any cancer of children or adults anywhere in the world. The IRS has not only fostered interdisciplinary teamwork within the institutions participating in the IRS, but also interdisciplinary collab oration and international cooperation among specialists in many nations in various fields of pediatric oncology care and research.

In 1968, I was elected chairman of the Children's Cancer Study Group (CCSG), which had been up to that time almost exclusively involved in clinical trials of chemotherapeutic agents. Chemotherapy was achieving successes in treating some tumors of children but needed to be used earlier in the course and in more effective combinations with surgery and radiation therapy. Several groups of experts in pediatric surgery, radiation therapy, and pediatric tumor pathology were requested to form committees in the CCSG to provide leadership in transforming the CCSG into a multidisciplinary cooperative group conducting clinical trials utilizing all appropriate therapeutic modalities. This was met with enthusiasm and early success.

The following year Dr. Larry Foye, chief of the Clinical Investigations Branch, DCT, NCI, agreed to fund a series of meetings of clinical investigators of childhood cancers to explore intergroup collaboration in clinical trials of therapy for children with solid tumors. These were proposed to be based upon the organization of the three existing NCI cooperative groups studying cancers of children. A small group of investigatiors from the CCSG and the pediatric divisions of the Acute Leukemia Group B and the Southwest Oncology Group were convened on two occasions that year. Participants represented the three principal therapeutic modalities of the era and also pediatric tumor pathology. Progress was slow but measurable. Dr. William Hammond, who succeeded Dr. Foye as chief of the Clinical Investigations Branch, agreed to continue to provide travel funds for these intergroup meetings and the effort was sustained.

By 1971, the design of intergroup clinical trials of rhabdomyosarcoma had been generally adopted by all three groups, and design of intergroup studies of Ewing's sarcoma were emerging. One of the principal contributors to the proposed therapeutic trials for rhabdomyosarcoma had been Dr. Harold Maurer and he was selected as chairman of the proposed IRS. The success of the multidisciplinary intergroup collaboration which has characterized the IRS is a tribute to his leadership of the effort. It has sustained the commitment of the current NCI cooperative groups studying childhood cancers, the CCSG, and the Pediatric Oncology Group.

For this volume, Dr. Maurer and his co-editors, Dr. Frederick B. Ruymann and Dr. Carl E. Pochedly, have wisely drawn upon the experience of the participants in the IRS and its collaborators and other experts throughout North America and Europe. This is the first definitive textbook on rhabdomyosarcoma and related tumors. It is destined to become the benchmark text in the field.

G. Denman Hammond, M.D.

PREFACE

A great deal has been learned about childhood rhabdomyosarcoma and related tumors in the past 25 years. Intensive clinical and laboratory research has led to impressive progress in elucidating the epidemiologic, biologic, and clinical characteristics of these malignancies while significantly improving the cure rate through the development of effective multimodality treatments. In this volume we have tried to provide a comprehensive source of information on most, if not all, aspects of rhabdomyosarcoma written by clinicians and scientists who are not only experts, but who have made central contributions to the field.

The Foreword is written by Dr. Denman Hammond who had the vision to form the Intergroup Rhabdomyosarcoma Study in 1970-71 and remains not only an active participant but an inspiration to the study committee. The first section of the book deals with the epidemiology, pathology, and tumor biology. The second part contains the clinical manifestations including staging and tumor imaging. It also includes a chapter on the prognostic factors which play a key role in treatment planning. This chapter serves as a lead into the next section which deals with multimodality treatment, including pharmacologic considerations in cancer chemotherapy, and patterns of treatment failure. Since certain primary sites of tumor origin require special consideration because of the clinical heterogeneity of rhabdomyosarcoma, the next section addresses specific sites of involvement. The book concludes with a section containing the growing body of information on nonrhabdomyosarcomatous soft tissue sarcomas, particularly the pathology which continues to evolve, the clinical manifestations and the current therapeutic considerations.

We have focused our effort on providing the latest information from leading U.S. and European experts in the field of childhood soft tissue sarcoma patient care and research. We hope this volume will consolidate information and clarify issues that up to now have been available or discussed only in diverse sources.

Finally, we would like to acknowledge the hundreds of individual investigators in the United States and international communities who have participated in local and regional cooperative trials over the past 25 years. Without their ongoing commitment to sound clinical trials this progress would not have occurred.

Harold M. Maurer, M.D.
Frederick B. Ruymann, M.D.
Carl Pochedly, M.D.

EDITORS

Harold M. Maurer, M.D., is the Jessie Ball duPont Professor and Chairman of the Department of Pediatrics, Children's Medical Center, Medical College of Virginia, Virginia Commonwealth University, Richmond, Virginia.

Dr. Maurer graduated in 1957 from New York University with a B.A. degree in Biology and earned his M.D. degree in 1961 from the State University of New York, Downstate Medical Center, Brooklyn. He interned in Pediatrics at Kings County Hospital, Brooklyn and served a pediatric residency and then fellowship in pediatric hematology and oncology at Babies Hospital, Columbia-Presbyterian Medical Center, New York.

Dr. Maurer has received the University Award of Excellence from Virginia Commonwealth University and the Dean's Award for Outstanding Contributions to the School of Medicine of the Medical College of Virginia. He has been extensively involved in University, State and National affairs, particularly as they pertain to Pediatrics and Oncology. He has served as Chairman of the Intergroup Rhabdomyosarcoma Study Committee since 1972 and as Chairman of the Soft Tissue Sarcoma Committee of the Pediatric Oncology Group since 1980. He has served on the Cancer Clinical Investigation Review Committee of the National Cancer Institute. Dr. Maurer chaired the Section of Oncology/Hematology of the American Academy of Pediatrics. He is currently Vice President, President-elect of the American Society of Pediatric Hematology/Oncology.

Dr. Maurer has been a major contributor to the literature, having published over 150 articles. He is editor of a textbook of Pediatrics and currently serves on the editorial board of *Medical & Pediatric Oncology*. His current major research interests relate to the diagnosis and treatment of rhabdomyosarcoma and other soft tissue sarcomas of childhood.

Frederick B. Ruymann, M.D., is the Director of the Division of Hematology/Oncology at Children's Hospital and Professor, Department of Pediatrics at the Ohio State University School of Medicine in Columbus, Ohio.

Dr. Ruymann graduated in 1958 from Stanford University with a B.A. in Biology and received his M.D. degree in 1962 from the University of Southern California School of Medicine in Los Angeles, California. He completed a rotating internship at Letterman Army Medical Center in San Francisco and a Pediatric Residency at Madagan Army Medical Center, Fort Lewis, Washington. After serving as the Chief of Pediatrics at Walson Army Hospital in Fort Dix, New Jersey, he completed a Research Fellowship at the Walter Reed Army Institute of Research in Washington DC, which was followed by a Pediatric Hematology/Oncology Fellowship at Water Reed Army Medical Center. Dr. Ruymann continued at Walter Reed as Director of Pediatric Hematology/Oncology and Assistant Chief, Department of Pediatrics. He established the Pediatric Hematology/Oncology Fellowship at Walter Reed. With support of the National Cancer Institute he founded the Uniform Services Onocology Consortium in the Pediatric Oncology Group which links major military hospitals in the United States in the coordinated care of military dependent children with cancer.

Dr. Ruymann was awarded the Legion of Merit from the Department of the Army in recognition of his contribution to Pediatric Medicine and Pediatric Hematology/Oncology within the Armed Forces when he retired from the Army Medical Corps with the rank of Colonel. He has also received the Outstanding Service Medal from the Uniformed Services University of Health Sciences for his work in establishing the Division of Hematology/Oncology at the Uniformed Services University of Health Sciences in Bethesda, Maryland.

In 1982, Dr. Ruymann moved to Ohio State University to be the Director of Hematology/Oncology at Children's Hospital. Since that time he and his staff have developed a major clinical and laboratory research program with excellence in teaching and patient care. He has been a member of the Intergroup Rhabdomyosarcoma Study Committee since 1976. He is Vice Chairman of the Solid Tumor Committee and a Principal Investigator in the Children's Cancer Study Group.

Dr. Ruymann has contributed extensively to the pediatric literature and published over one hundred and thirty articles and abstracts. His major oncology research interests relate to the treatment of childhood soft tissue sarcomas and acute myleocytic leukemia.

Carl Pochedly, M.D., is Director of Pediatric Hematology/Oncology at the Martin Luther King, Jr./Charles R. Drew Medical Center in Los Angeles, California. He is a former member of the Section of Pediatric Hematology/Oncology at the Wyler Children's Hospital and Professor of Clinical Pediatrics at the University of Chicago in Chicago, Illinois.

Dr. Pochedly graduated in 1952 from Hiram College in Hiram, Ohio, and earned his M.D. degree in 1956 from Case Western Reserve University in Cleveland. He trained in Pediatrics at the Children's Hospital National Medical Center and served a fellowship in pediatric hematology at New York Medical College.

Dr. Pochedly is a member of the American Academy of Pediatrics, the American Society of Hematology, and the American Society of Clinical Oncology. He is Secretary/Treasurer of the American Society of Pediatric Hematology/Oncology which he helped to found in 1981. He was given the Turner Award for Significant Achievement in Biology and Medicine by Hiram College in 1986.

Dr. Pochedly is author or co-arthur of over 150 articles and book chapters and he has written or edited 29 books dealing with various aspects of cancer and blood diseases in children. He is the founder and editor of the *American Journal of Pediatric Hematology/ Oncology* which has been published since 1979.

CONTRIBUTORS

Marija Auersperg, M.D.
Onkoloski Institut
Ljubljana, Yugoslavia

Modesto Carli, M.D.
Associate Professor
Division of Hematology/Oncology
Department of Pediatrics
University of Padova
Padua, Italy

Dominique Couanet, M.D.
Department of Radiology
Institut Gustave-Roussy
Villejuif, France

William Crist, M.D.
Member and Chairman
Department of Hematology/Oncology
St. Jude Children's Research Hospital
Professor of Pediatrics
University of Tennessee School of
  Medicine
Memphis, Tennessee

Lakshmana Das Narla, M.D.
Assistant Professor
Department of Radiology
Medical College of Virginia
Virginia Commonwealth University
Richmond, Virginia

Louis P. Dehner, M.D.
Professor and Director
Lauren V. Ackerman Laboratory of
  Surgical Pathology
Department of Pathology
Washington University School of
  Medicine
St. Louis, Missouri

Paul S. Dickman, M.D.
Associate Professor
Department of Pathology
Children's Hospital of Pittsburgh
University of Pittsburgh
Pittsburgh, Pennsylvania

Francoise Flamant, M.D.
Chairman
Malignant Mensenchymal Tumor Group
  of the International Society of Pediatric
  Oncology
Department of Pediatric Oncology
Institut Gustave-Roussy
Villejuif, France

Lisa A. Garnsey, M.S.
Applications Analyst
Pediatric Intergroup Statistical Center
Department of Biomathematics
M. D. Anderson Cancer Center
University of Texas
Houston, Texas

Edmund A. Gehan, Ph.D.
Kathryn O'Connor Professor
Department of Biomathematics
M. D. Anderson Cancer Center
University of Texas
Houston, Texas

Fereshteh Ghavimi, M.D.
Department of Pediatrics
Memorial Sloan-Kettering Cancer Center
Associate Professor of Clinical Pediatrics
Cornell University Medical College
New York, New York

W. Gohde, M.D.
Institute of Radiotherapy
University of Münster
Münster, Germany

Seymour Grufferman, M.D.
Professor and Chairman
Department of Clinical Epidemiology and
  Preventive Medicine
University of Pittsburgh School of
  Medicine
Pittsburgh, Pennsylvania

G. Denman Hammond, M.D.
Associate Vice President, Health Affairs
University of Southern California
Professor of Pediatrics
U.S.C. School of Medicine
Chairman, Children's Cancer Study
  Group
Arcadia, California

Ala Hamoudi, M.D.
Clinical Professor
Department of Pathology
Children's Hospital
The Ohio State University
Columbus, Ohio

Daniel M. Hays, M.D.
Professor
Department of Surgery
Children's Hospital of Los Angeles
University of Southern California School
  of Medicine
Los Angeles, California

Ruth M. Heyn, M.D.
Professor Emeritus
Department of Pediatrics
University of Michigan Medical School
Ann Arbor, Michigan

Julie K. Horton
Medicine Branch
National Cancer Institute
Bethesda, Maryland

Janet A. Houghton
Laboratories for Developmental
  Therapeutics
Department of Biochemical and Clinical
  Pharmacology
St. Jude Children's Research Hospital
Memphis, Tennessee

Peter J. Houghton
Laboratories for Developmental
  Therapeutics
Department of Biochemical and Clinical
  Pharmacology
St. Jude Children's Research Hospital
Memphis, Tennessee

Norman Jaffe, M.D.
Professor
Department of Pediatrics
M. D. Anderson Cancer Center
University of Texas
Houston, Texas

Janez Lanovec, M.D.
Onkoloski Institut
Ljubljana, Yugoslavia

Walter Lawrence, Jr., M.D.
Professor and Director Emeritus
Division of Surgical Oncology
Massey Cancer Center
Medical College of Virginia
Richmond, Virginia

Ya-Yen Lee
Division of Diagnostic Radiology
M. D. Anderson Cancer Center
Houston, Texas

Bernard Luboinski, M.D.
Chief
Department of Head and Neck Tumors
Institut Gustave-Roussy
Villejuif, France

Marcio Malogolowkin, M.D.
Visiting Assistant
Department of Pediatrics
Children's Hospital of Los Angeles
University of Southern California School
  of Medicine
Los Angeles, California

Harold M. Maurer, M.D.
Jessie Ball duPont Professor and Chairman
Department of Pediatrics
Children's Medical Center
Medical College of Virginia
Virginia Commonwealth University
Richmond, Virginia

Heither McDowell, M.D.
Department of Pediatric Oncology
Institut Gustave-Roussy
Villejuif, France

James S. Miser, M.D.
Associate Professor
Division of Pediatric Hematology/
  Oncology
Department of Pediatrics
University of Washington
Seattle, Washington

William A. Newton, Jr., M.D.
Professor Emeritus
Departments of Pathology and Pediatrics
Children's Hospital
The Ohio State University
Columbus, Ohio

Jorge A. Ortega, M.D.
Section Head
Clinical Oncology
Children's Hospital of Los Angeles
Professor of Pediatrics
University of Southern California Medical
  School
Los Angeles, California

Ray C. Pais, M.D.
Director
Division of Hematology/Oncology
East Tennessee Children's Hospital
Knoxville, Tennessee

Giorgio Perilongo, M.D.
Division of Hematology/Oncology
Department of Pediatrics
University of Padova
Padua, Italy

Carl Pochedly, M.D.
Director, Pediatric Hematology/Oncology
King/Drew Medical Center
Los Angeles, California

Olga Porenta, M.D.
Onkoloski Institut
Ljubljana, Yugoslavia

Charles B. Pratt
Member
Department of Hematology/Oncology
St. Jude Children's Research Hospital
Professor
Department of Pediatrics
University of Tennessee
College of Medicine
Memphis, Tennessee

Abdelsalam H. Ragab, M.D.
Director
Pediatric Hematology/Oncology
Professor
Department of Pediatrics
Emory University School of Medicine
Atlanta, Georgia

R. Beverly Raney, Jr., M.D.
Deputy Director
Department of Pediatrics
M. D. Anderson Cancer Center
University of Texas
Houston, Texas

Frederick B. Ruymann, M.D.
Director
Division of Hematology/Oncology
Children's Hospital
Professor, Department of Pediatrics
The Ohio State University
Columbus, Ohio

Robert L. Saylors, III, M.D.
Edward Mallinckrodt Department of
  Pediatrics
Washington University School of
  Medicine
St. Louis, Missouri

Paul E. Swanson, M.D.
Assistant Professor
Lauren V. Ackerman Laboratory of
  Surgical Pathology
Department of Pathology
Washington University School of
  Medicine
St. Louis, Missouri

Melvin Tefft, M.D.
Department of Radiation Therapy
The Cleveland Clinic Foundation
Cleveland, Ohio

Paul Thomas, M.D.
Associate Clinical Professor
Department of Pediatrics
Santa Rosa Children's Hospital
University of Texas Health Science
 Center
San Antonio, Texas

Timothy J. Triche, M.D., Ph.D.
Professor
Department of Pathology
Children's Hospital of Los Angeles
University of Southern California
Los Angeles, California

Joern Treuner, M.D.
Professor
Department of Oncology/Hematology
Pediatric Center
Olga Hospital
Stuttgart, Germany

Maria Tsokos, M.D.
Chief
Ultrastructural Pathology Section
Laboratory of Pathology
National Cancer Institute
Bethesda, Maryland

Marija Us-Krasovec, M.D.
Onkoloski Institut
Ljubljana, Yugoslavia

Teresa J. Vietti
Professor
Edward Mallinckrodt Department of
 Pediatrics
Washington University School of
 Medicine
Chairman, Pediatric Oncology Group
St. Louis, Missouri

James W. Walsh, M.D.
Professor
Department of Radiology
University of Minnesota
Minneapolis, Minnesota

Bruce Webber, M.D.
Department of Pathology
Baptist Memorial Hospital
Memphis, Tennessee

Eugene S. Wiener, M.D.
Assistant Professor
Department of Surgery
Children's Hospital of Pittsburgh
University of Pittsburgh School of
 Medicine
Pittsburgh, Pennsylvania

TABLE OF CONTENTS

Section I
Tumor Biology and Histology

Chapter 1

INTRODUCTION AND EPIDEMIOLOGY OF SOFT TISSUE SARCOMAS

Frederick B. Ruymann and Seymour Grufferman

TABLE OF CONTENTS

I. THE CHALLENGE OF SOFT TISSUE SARCOMAS

Soft tissue sarcomas in children and adolescents constitute a diverse group of malignancies which have been treated most successfully by a multimodality approach. Rhabdomyosarcoma (RMS) is the prototype of soft tissue sarcomas, constituting 55% of this group. This tumor has been under investigation by members and colleagues of the Intergroup Rhabdomyosarcoma Study (IRS) Committee since 1972.[1-4]

The diverse interest of RMS and soft tissue sarcomas involves many disciplines. First, for clinicians, soft tissue sarcomas have great variability in their presentation, being able to mimic acute leukemia,[5] Hodgkin's disease,[6,7] neuroblastoma,[5] hepatitis,[8] and many benign tumors. This deceptive presentation can lead to delays in diagnosis and definitive therapy, which can increase the intensity of therapy necessary to cure the malignancy and change the prognosis. Second, soft tissue sarcomas are associated with a growing number of congenital syndromes,[9-13] congenital anomalies,[14,15] familial cancer syndromes which entail an increased risk for breast cancer,[16-19] and environmental exposures.[20] Third, although striated muscle differentiation suggests the primordial roots of RMS,[21,22] the origins of undifferentiated sarcomas[22] and extraosseous Ewing's sarcoma[23-25] remain unclear. An international team of pathologists have made great progress in the development of an international classification of childhood soft tissue sarcomas.[26]

Fourth, surgeons working with sarcomas feel the challenge of tumors arising in diverse sites, the need for adequate tissue to establish the proper histopathological diagnosis, the preservation of function while attempting to resect the tumor,[27] the timing of second look operations,[28,29] and the role of planned reexcision strategies.[30] Fifth, radiotherapists have been challenged by the difficulty of local and regional control.[31-33] The use of radiotherapy is restrained by the need to respect the tissue tolerance of vital structures, to avoid injury to growing bones in small children,[34,35] to minimize bone marrow suppression with irradiation of large pelvic fields,[36] and to prevent intracranial extension in parameningeal primaries.[37,38] The increased risk for second malignant neoplasms in irradiated fields is well known.[39] Sixth, pediatric oncologists, although achieving great progress with use of multiagent chemotherapy for clinical group III patients,[2-4] remain challenged by patients with metastatic disease[5,40] as well as the increasing limitations imposed by myelotoxicity and risks of septicemia.[41-44]

Finally, basic scientists investigating the biology and molecular biology of RMS have found a plethora of homologous chromosomal deletions,[45] translocations,[46,47] abnormalities in ploidy analysis[48] and *ras* gene mutations.[49] These observations require pathological and prognostic correlations which will chart new directions in the biology and management of RMS.

In summary, soft tissue sarcomas, and rhabdomyosarcoma in particular, have been the subject of intense multidisciplinary and international investigation for 20 years. These studies have yielded a wealth of clinical and scientific information on the origin, differentiation, diagnosis, and management of RMS in children and adolescents. In many ways, it can be said that there is something for every medical discipline in this challenging malignancy. Most importantly, and gratefully, with these multidisciplinary efforts, the survival of children with RMS has been greatly improved in the past 20 years.[1-4]

II. HISTORICAL DESCRIPTION

RMSs are highly malignant tumors of mesenchymal origin which can occur anywhere in the body. The classical striated muscle differentiation is best seen in botryoid, embryonal, and alveolar RMSs. The original distinction of soft tissue sarcomas and bone sarcomas from epithelial and hematopoietic tumors is attributed to Virchow who, in the middle 1850s, propounded his theory of "cellular pathology" which ascribed the origin of tumors to specific types of cells.[50] The first description of RMS was by Weber in 1854 who reported a 21-year-old man with a recurrent tumor of the tongue muscle.[51] The first description in the English literature was in 1937 by Rakov who described 15 cases from the Oncology Institute in Leningrad.[52] Only two of these cases were in individuals less than 20 years of age.

In 1946, Stout described 14 new cases and reviewed 107 previously reported cases.[21] Twenty-three (19%) of these 121 cases were under 20 years of age. Stout's seminal description of RMS is credited with stimulating further studies on this malignancy. The pathologic and clinical diversity of soft tissue sarcomas was emphasized by Pack in several articles.[53,54] The common embryonal histology of RMS occurring in children and adolescents was described by Stobbe and Dargeon in 1950.[55] Riopelle and Theriault were the first to describe the "alveolar" variant of RMS in 1956. The term alveolar was used because of the similarity in appearance of the tumor to lung parenchyma.[56] The association of alveolar RMS with extremity and trunk sites was emphasized by Enzinger and Shiraki's review of RMSs with alveolar histology, in which 89 out of 110 (81%) arose from these unfavorable sites.[57]

In 1958, Horn and Enterline delineated the four classical forms of RMS as being embryonal, botryoid, alveolar, and pleomorphic.[58] These investigators noted the presence of rhabdomyoblasts in all types of RMSs, thus unifying the origins of this soft tissue sarcoma. The botryoid RMS presenting in the external auditory canal, nasopharynx, and oropharynx share a common botryoid histology with RMSs of the urogenital tract.[59] The distinctive grape-like appearance of the botryoid variant of embryonal RMS has been attributed to its origin under a mucosal surface, whereas tumors with the classical embryonal histology occur in deeper sites.

Tefft, Vawter, and Mitus described a paravertebral tumor morphologically similar to Ewing's sarcoma but arising in soft tissue.[60] Subsequently, these tumors were found to be comparable to the special cell type I and II of the early IRS.[24] These tumors are now known as extraosseous Ewing's sarcomas.[23,25] By agreement with investigators on the original Intergroup Ewing's Sarcoma Study Committee, these soft tissue sarcomas have been treated up to 1991 according to IRS protocols. A recent review has shown extraosseous Ewing's sarcomas to have an intermediate prognosis, similar to that of embryonal RMSs.[25]

The present classifications of RMS tumors includes the four classical categories of embryonal, botryoid alveolar, and pleomorphic. Undifferentiated sarcomas are considered eligible for the IRS. Undifferentiated RMSs have recently been shown to have as poor a prognosis as alveolar RMS.[22] Finally, the extraosseous Ewing's sarcoma constitutes the sixth category of tumor eligible for the IRS-III study. The possible origins and classification of extraosseous Ewing's sarcoma with respect to other small round cell tumors of childhood have been reviewed.[61]

III. EARLY PROGRESS IN THERAPY

The sensitivity of embryonal RMS to radiotherapy was noted by Stobbe and Dargeon in 1950.[55] Orbital RMSs were observed by several investigators to have a high cure rate when treated with limited surgery and radiotherapy.[62,63] The combined complete and partial response rates for dactinomycin,[64-66] cyclophosphamide,[67,68] vincristine,[69-71] and anthracyclines[72-75] are shown in Table 1. Overall, a complete and partial response rate of 33% was observed using these single agents in treatment of RMS.

In 1961, Pinkel and Pinkren proposed a multimodality approach to childhood RMS.[76] Studies done by single or small groups of institutions were initiated utilizing combination chemotherapy with specified radiotherapy following attempts at complete surgical removal. In a summary of 15 early independent trials, 823 patients had an overall survival rate of

TABLE 1
Summary of Early Single Drug Studies in Children
with Rhabdomyosarcoma

Drug	Total number	CR + PR (%)	Ref.
Dactinomycin	14	43	Pinkel, 1959
			Tan, 1959
			Shaw, 1960
Cyclophosphamide	26	35	Haddy, 1967
			Sutow, 1967
Vincristine	42	31	Sutow, 1966
			Sutow, 1968
			Selawry, 1968
Anthracyclines	40	30	Bonadonna, 1970
			O'Bryan, 1973
			Sutow, 1972
			Tan, 1973
TOTAL	122	33%	

54% at 2 to 5 years from diagnosis.[77] The leadership of the three U.S. cooperative pediatric cancer research groups, (The Children's Cancer Study Group, the pediatric sections of Cancer and Leukemia Group B, and the Southwest Oncology Group) in concert with the National Cancer Institute (NCI), formed the IRS Committee in 1972.

IV. INCIDENCE, GENDER, AGE, HISTOLOGY, AND SITE

A. INCIDENCE

The Surveillance, Epidemiology, and End Results (SEER) program of the NCI monitors about 12% of all new cases of malignancy in the U.S.[78] Based on this study, the annual incidence of soft tissue sarcoma from 1973 through 1982 in children under 15 years of age is estimated to be 8 per million white children and 7.7 per million black children. In 1985, there were an estimated 420 cases of soft tissue sarcomas including 230 cases of RMS in children under 15 years of age in the U.S.[78]

Of 1002 patients studied in protocol IRS-II, 128 (12.7%) were between 15 and 21 years of age. The calculated number of cases of RMS per year in the U.S. for this group is, therefore, 260 (1.13 × 230). The accrual of new cases from the U.S. on the IRS study in 1988 was about 18.5 per month with an annual accrual of 222 new cases per year. Overall, 85% (222 of the 260 cases) of the annual number of RMS cases under 21 years of age in the U.S. were placed on the IRS-III study in 1988.

In the period from 1958 to 1977, RMS was slightly less frequent than either neuroblastoma or Wilms' tumor according to the World Cancer Registry.[79] In the five continents surveyed, RMS showed no significant geographic predilection or change in incidence over a 20-year-period.

B. GENDER

A male predominance similar to that in childhood acute leukemia is characteristic of RMS. The male/female ratio of the 121 cases reviewed by Stout was 1.2 (62/52). Among patients included in the IRS-II, the overall male/female ratio was 1.4 for 1002 eligible patients, but the ratio was substantially higher (3.3) for tumors arising in the genitourinary/ bladder prostate (GU/BP), and (2.1) for genitourinary/nonbladder prostate (GU/non-BP). The male/female ratio was less than 1 for orbital (0.79) and extremity (0.88) primaries. The distribution of primary sites by gender is found in Table 2A. Statistically, these results are

TABLE 2A
Distribution of Sex of RMS by Primary Site[a]

Sex	Orbit	GU/BP	GU/nonBP	EXT	PM	H&N	Other	Total
Male	37	85	83	81	109	46	135	576
Female	47	26	40	92	69	34	118	426
TOTAL	84	111	123	173	178	80	253	1,002

$\chi^2 = 38.62$ df = 6 $p < 0.001$

TABLE 2B
Distribution of Age of RMS by Primary Site[a]

Age Distribution	Orbit	GU/BP	GU/nonBP	EXT	PM	H&N	Other	Total
<1	5	21	11	12	8	8	22	87
1—4	30	60	34	52	67	26	77	346
5—9	35	14	24	44	52	17	58	244
10—14	10	5	17	39	34	19	60	184
15+ . . .	4	10	33	25	16	8	32	128
Missing	—	1	4	1	1	2	4	13
TOTAL	84	111	123	173	178	80	253	1,002

$\chi^2 = 104.51$ df = 24 $p < 0.001$

Note: To calculate the chi-square test, the missing age group was excluded.

[a] In 1002 cases from the IRS-II.

highly significant ($p < 0.001$) indicating a strong relationship between primary site and gender.

C. AGE GROUPS

The distribution of primary sites by age groups (Table 2B) was significantly different ($p < 0.001$). The main reasons for the significant findings of the chi-square test are the relatively high percentage of GU/BP primaries in children under age 5 years (73%) and the increased numbers of GU/non-BP primaries in those over age 15 (27%). There is also a high percentage of orbital primaries (42%) in the age group 5 to 9 years.

D. HISTOLOGIC TYPES

Table 2C shows that the distribution of histologic types differs significantly ($p < 0.001$) by primary site. The key reasons for the significant chi-square findings were the relatively high percentage (54%) of alveolar histology among patients with extremity primaries and the increased percentage of botryoid histology in the genitourinary primary sites: bladder/prostate (23%) and nonbladder/prostate (68%). In addition, a relatively high percentage of the orbital primaries (81%) were shown to have embryonal histology.

E. DISTRIBUTION OF SEX AND HISTOLOGY BY AGE

Tables 3A and 3B give the distribution of sex and histology by age group. In Table 3A, the male/female ratio does not differ significantly ($p = 0.82$) by age group. Table 3B shows that there is a statistically significant relationship ($p < 0.001$) between age distribution and histologic types. Children less than 5 years of age have a high percentage of tumors with botryoid histology (10.6%) compared to the overall percentage of botryoid tumors (5.5%).

TABLE 2C
Distribution of Histologic Types of RMS[a]

Histology	Orbit	GU/BP	GU/nonBP	EXT	PM	H&N	Other	Total
EMB	68	69	84	39	117	45	88	510
ALV	7	2	3	94	20	19	63	208
BOT	—	26	20	—	6	1	2	55
PLEO	—	—	2	3	—	—	2	7
EOE	1	1	—	10	5	3	28	48
UND	2	1	—	16	8	5	34	66
Other[b]	6	12	14	11	22	7	36	108
TOTAL	84	111	123	173	178	80	253	1,002

$\chi^2 = 390.17$ df = 18 $p < 0.001$

Note: To calculate the chi-square test, some grouping of histologic types was done. The following types were grouped PLEO, EOE, UND, and Other

Abbreviations: EMB = embryonal; ALV = alveolar; BOT = botryoid; PLEO = pleomorphic; EOE = extraosseous Ewing's; UND = undifferentiated sarcoma; EXT = extremity; PM = parameningeal; H&N = head and neck.

[a] In 1002 cases in IRS-II.
[b] Other includes not classified and wrong.

TABLE 3A
Distribution of Sex of RMS by Age Distribution[a]

Sex	<1	1—4	5—9	10—14	15±	Missing	Total
Male	50	209	138	102	75	2	576
Females	37	137	106	82	53	11	426
TOTAL	87	346	244	184	128	13	1002

$\chi^2 = 1.56$ df = 4   P = 0.82

TABLE 3B
Distribution of Histologic Types of RMS by Age Distribution[a]

Histology	<1	1—4	5—9	10—14	15±	Missing	Total
EMB	37	194	148	70	60	1	510
ALV	11	65	55	53	24	—	208
BOT	13	33	2	2	5	—	55
PLEO	—	3	1	2	1	—	7
EOE	2	6	8	22	10	—	48
UND	13	17	12	15	9	—	66
Other	11	28	18	20	19	12	108
TOTAL	87	346	244	184	128	13	1002

$\chi^2 = 89.69$ df = 12 $p < 0.001$

Note: To calculate the chi-square test, the missing age group was not included and some histologic types were grouped. The following types were grouped PLEO, EOE, UND and Other. For abbreviations see Table 2.

[a] In 1002 cases from the IRS-II.

TABLE 4
A Comparison of the Rates of Congenital Anomalies per 1000 Persons in RMS and Wilms' Tumor with the Findings of the Collaborative Perinatal Project

Anomaly or organ system	Congenital anomalies/1000 persons		
	IRS rhabdomyosarcoma (n = 115)	NWTS Wilms' tumor (n = 1905)	Collaborative perinatal project (n = 53,257)
Genitourinary	86.9	73.9	27.7
Central nervous system	78.2	4.7	4.2
Upper alimentary tract/digestive systems	52.2	6.8	7.4
Cardiopulmonary	43.5	15.2	10.2
Accessory spleens	43.5	6.3	0.2
Musculoskeletal[a]	8.7	22.6	28.0
Aniridia	—	8.4	0.01
Hemihypertrophy	8.7	24.7	0.2

[a] Excluding clubfoot.

V. EPIDEMIOLOGY

A. CONGENITAL ANOMALIES AND SYNDROMES

Early reviews of a series of 20 and 43 children with RMS showed the presence of congenital anomalies in 4 out of 20 (20%)[14] and 7 out of 43 (16%).[80] An expanded autopsy review of 115 children and adolescents with RMS then showed 37 (32%) to have at least one congenital anomaly.[15]

Both RMS and Wilms' tumor share an increased incidence of genitourinary anomalies.[15] RMS, however, is unique in its association with anomalies of the central nervous system. Table 4 compares the anomalies associated with RMS and Wilms' tumor with those in the Collaborative Perinatal Project.[15] Of the 45 identified anomalies, 14 (12%) were major and 31 were minor. The review found 9 central nervous system anomalies, 10 genitourinary anomalies, 13 gastrointestinal anomalies, and 4 cardiovascular anomalies. One child with each of the following was observed: Rubinstein-Taybi syndrome, neurofibromatosis, single horseshoe kidney, hemihypertrophy, and Arnold-Chiari malformation. One of us is aware of two additional children with the Arnold-Chiari anomaly and RMS. An earlier report of Rubinstein-Taybi syndrome in association with RMS was published in 1981.[12] Two cases of Gorlin's nevoid basal cell carcinoma syndrome were observed in association with rhabdomyosarcoma.[10,13] A child with Down's syndrome had both acute leukemia and RMS.[81] In two cases, RMS arose within congenital cysts of the lung.[82,83]

In a controlled study of 43 cases of soft tissue sarcomas and 30 cases of bone sarcomas, there was a slight excess of congenital malformations in children and an increase in benign tumors and tumors of borderline malignancy in older mothers of the children who had sarcomas.[84] There was a suggestion of reduced fertility in cases of soft tissue sarcoma where a significant excess of the mothers had no other pregnancies. These findings are consistent with a genetic predisposition in the development of the sarcomas in this series.

Multiple neurofibromatosis is the best-known hereditary syndrome to be associated with RMS.[11,85] The risk for malignancy in patients with von Recklinghausen neurofibromatosis has been estimated at 4.4 to 5.2%.[86] In addition to RMS, neurofibromatosis is associated with childhood leukemia, Wilms' tumor, and multiple sarcomas.

The Li-Fraumeni familial cancer syndrome, first reported in 1969, includes soft tissue sarcomas occurring in siblings and cousins, with parents and other relatives having a variety of malignancies including RMS, adrenocortical carcinoma, glioblastoma, breast cancer, and lung cancer.[16,17] The occurrence of six cases of germ cell tumors in relatives of children with bone or soft tissue sarcomas suggests that germ cell tumors may also be associated with the Li-Fraumeni familial cancer syndrome.[87]

Twenty-four kindred, in the Cancer Family Registry of the NCI, having the syndrome of sarcoma, breast carcinoma, and other neoplasms were reviewed.[88] Cancer developed in an autosomal dominant pattern in 151 blood relatives, 119 (79%) of whom were affected before 45 years of age. The malignancies included 50 bone and soft tissue sarcomas, 28 breast cancers, 14 brain tumors, 9 leukemias, 4 adrenocortical carcinomas, and 6 second malignant neoplasms associated with radiotherapy. In Italy, a national survey of the living status or cause of death in 2223 close relatives of 195 children with soft tissue sarcomas revealed a significantly increased death rate from cancer among siblings.[89] In grandmothers, the number of cases of breast cancer was also increased over the expected number.[92]

In the fall of 1990, a germ cell line mutant p53 tumor suppressor gene was identified in kindreds with the Li-Fraumeni familial cancer syndrome.[90] As predicted earlier, the inheritance was autosomal dominant.[113] Originally described in 1984, p53 was thought to promote transformation. Additional studies showed that the wild-type p53 in its unsullied state functioned as a tumor suppressor gene. Mutant versions of p53 have been found in a great variety of human tumors and recently reviewed.[91] Additional investigators have confirmed the presence of mutant p53 germlines in patients with sarcoma. Studies are underway to confirm the incidence of the p53 germline mutation in a variety of malignancies.

The importance of having a reliable clinical marker in candidates for another familial concern syndrome, Gardner's colorectal polyposis, has recently been demonstrated.[92] Patients who have inherited the autosomal dominant variant of Gardner's familial colorectal polyposis have been shown to have congenital hypertrophy of the retinal pigment epithelium.

A predictible clinical association in the Li-Fraumeni syndrome is yet to be described. Such a phenotypic manifestation in the Li-Fraumeni syndrome would be invaluable in identifying those individuals at risk. The Li-Fraumeni syndrome has been described as an example of the expression of a cancer in a child before it is expressed in the parent who carries the putative gene.[93]

The awareness of pediatricians must be raised so their family histories will include the types of malignancy in near relatives of the child. It has become increasingly recognized that the occurrence of specific pediatric malignancies may be associated with increased risk for malignancy among other family members in both adults and children. In a review of 14 cases of adrenal cortical carcinoma, at least four of the families appeared to belong to the Li-Fraumeni family cancer syndrome.[94] The occurrence of this relatively rare malignancy should promote a search for additional cancers in the family.

Breast cancer in mothers has been shown to be the major associated malignancy in families of children with soft tissue malignancy. A review of the mothers of 143 children with RMS showed a 3 to 13.5 times increased risk for breast cancer over controls.[18] In a review of parental malignancy in 326 children referred to a single center, the incidence of breast cancer in mothers of children with solid tumors was increased 8.9-fold over expected.[95] No such increased incidence of cancer was found in mothers of children with leukemia or in fathers of children with leukemia or solid tumors.

Breast cancers in the mothers of children with osteosarcoma and chondrosarcoma were three times over the number expected.[96] The risk was highest in the mothers of boys who were under the median age of diagnosis. The increased risk for breast cancer in mothers of younger children with RMS supports a genetically determined syndrome. The incidence of malignant neoplasms in mothers of 62 children with Ewing's sarcoma was not in excess of the number expected.[97] Ewing's sarcoma of bone has not been associated with an increased familial risk for breast cancer. Thus, it will be of great interest to see whether extraosseous

Ewing's sarcoma, a tumor not of skeletal muscle origin, has an increased familial risk for breast cancer.

B. ENVIRONMENTAL FACTORS

The association of embryonal RMS of the bladder in a 17-month-old boy with fetal alcohol syndrome suggested the importance of intrauterine environmental factors.[98] Four additional malignancies associated with fetal alcohol syndrome were reviewed, including two neural crest tumors and one hepatoblastoma. Another study addressed the combined teratogenesis and presumed fetal oncogenesis of the fetal alcohol-hydantoin syndrome.[99] The organ predilection in adults with hydantoin-induced malignancy appears to be different from that in children. However, Hodgkin's disease was reported in a child with the fetal alcohol-hydantoin syndrome.[100] These weak associations with the fetal alcohol and hydantoin syndromes need further investigation.[101]

A case control study of 33 children in North Carolina showed an increased relative risk for rhabdomyosarcoma in association with paternal cigarette smoking, ingestion of organ meats, and exposure to chemicals.[20] Because fathers', but not mothers' cigarette smoking appeared to be a risk factor for RMS, they hypothesized that this is due, perhaps, to a direct effect of cigarette smoking on spermatogenesis.[102] This is supported by observations of sperm abnormalities in male cigarette smokers.[103] Interestingly, children born to fathers who were heavy cigarette smokers were found to have a two-fold increase in major congenital anomalies.[104] Except for a significantly decreased incidence of being immunized, a review of 555 children with malignancy failed to show any significant associations with past medical procedures or treatments.[105]

The finding that immunizations appeared protective against childhood RMS[105] was recently retested in a case-control study of 322 childhood RMS cases from IRS-III which utilized random digit dialing to identify control selection.[106] The study in IRS-III patients suggests that immunizations are selectively not given in young children with RMS because of therapy related immunocompromise.[107] This is in keeping with sound pediatric practices as recommended by the American Academy of Pediatrics.[108] The same group of investigators have shown that paternal smoking during gestation and organ meat ingeston, in contrast to their earlier study in North Carolina, was not a risk factor for RMS.[109] On the other hand *in utero* X-ray exposure of a child is associated with an increased risk of RMS.[110] Case mothers and control mothers had a 13.2 and 7.1% rate of X-ray exposure, respectively. Occupational exposure as a health diagnosing techician in case mothers had a 4.5 odds ratio with 95% confidence intervals of 1.0 to 20.8. The most striking outcome of the IRS-III case-control study was that the use of recreational drugs such as marijuana and cocaine appeared increased in parents of children with RMS over controls obtained by random digit dialing.[111] The odds ratio was 4.5 for the maternal use of cocaine with a 95% confidence interval of 1.0 to 20.8. The mothers use of recreational drugs was correlated significantly with that of the father's use.

Recently, investigators in England have combined the use of a machine for geographical analysis and advanced computer technology in uncovering five clusters of leukemia, four of which were heretofore unsuspected.[112] Such a technique applied to RMS may identify areas where environmental factors should be investigated.

Soft tissue sarcomas in adults have been associated with exposure to herbicides,[113-116] chloramphenicol,[117] and smokeless tobacco.[117] Four of 133 adult cases had prior radiotherapy to the same anatomic area where the sarcoma arose.[117] No instances of the Li-Fraumeni syndrome were identified in this case control study among kindred of the adults with sarcoma. Table 5 summarizes the reported anomalies, syndromes, and environmental factors associated with rhabdomyosarcoma.

TABLE 5
Associated Anomalies, Syndromes and Environmental Factors in RMS

	Familial			Environmental associations	
Anomalies	Syndromes	Cancer syndromes	Therapeutic factors	Children	Adults
Congenital Cyst of the lung	Gorlin's basal cell nevus	Neurofibromatosis	Radiation therapy	Fetal-Alcohol/hydantoin syndromes	Herbicide
GU — Similar to Wilms' tumor	Rubenstein-Taybi	Li-Fraumeni	Alkylating agents	In utero X-rays	Chloramphenicol
CNS — unique to RMS				Paternal use of marijuana and cocaine	Smokeless tobacco
				Exposure to chemicals	Woodworking

C. INTERACTIONS BETWEEN HEREDITARY AND ENVIRONMENTAL FACTORS

Both radiotherapy and chemotherapy with alkylating agents for treatment of childhood malignancies increase the risk for a subsequent bone sarcoma.[118] Second malignant neoplasms following the treatment of children with RMS have also been associated with prior administration of alkylating agents and radiotherapy in ongoing studies by the IRS.[39] *In vitro* testing of cell lines from individuals with Gorlin's nevoid basal cell carcinoma syndrome failed to show increased cytotoxicity or clastogenicity with radiation when they were compared to nonaffected relatives or cell bank controls.[119] Both retinoblastoma and RMS have been highlighted as models for examining the etiology of genetic effects and defining the risk for a second malignant neoplasm.[120]

The relatives of children with a soft tissue sarcoma and second malignant neoplasm have been found to have a markedly increased risk for cancer.[121] These studies suggest that a familial predisposition to cancer, as in the Li-Fraumeni syndrome, may increase the risk for a second tumor in a child who has survived a soft tissue sarcoma. If the presence of a familial cancer syndrome is suggested by the family history in a child with a soft tissue sarcoma, care should be taken to minimize the use of radiotherapy and alkylating agent chemotherapy without compromising the cure rate. In a patient at high risk for a second malignant neoplasm, a more aggressive surgical approach utilizing planned reexcision and second-look surgery might improve survival and minimize the risk for a second malignant neoplasm in later years.

VI. SUMMARY

RMSs constitute 55% of soft tissue sarcomas occurring in children and adolescents. The clinical presentations, pathology, treatment, molecular biology, and epidemiology of RMS have provided diverse motivations for clinical- and laboratory-based investigators. The multidisciplinary effort started in 1972 with the formation of the IRS Committee has been catalytic in improving the management and survival of children and adolescents with RMS.

The epidemiology of RMS was given impetus by the 1969 description by Li and Fraumeni of the familial associations of soft tissue sarcomas, breast cancer, and other malignancies. To date, the applicability of occupational and herbicide exposure with subsequent increased risk for sarcomas in adults has not been applicable to children. The identification of a cancer syndrome in a child with familial RMS may lead to cancer control strategies involving the entire family.

ACKNOWLEDGMENT

The authors are grateful to Miss Dawn Anderson for her assistance in preparing this manuscript.

REFERENCES

1. **Maurer, H. M., Beltangady, M., Gehan, E. A., et al.,** The Intergroup Rhabdomyosarcoma Study-I; a final report, *Cancer* 61, 209, 1988.
2. **Maurer, H. M., Gehan, E. A., Beltangady, M., et al.,** The Intergroup Rhabdomyosarcoma Study-II, *Cancer,* in press.
3. **Maurer, H., Gehan, E., Crist, W., et al.,** Intergroup Rhabdomyosarcoma Study (IRS)-III; a preliminary report of overall outcome, *(Abstr. 1154), Proc. Am. Soc. Clin. Oncol.* 8, 296, 1989.

4. **Ruymann, F.,** Rhabdomyosarcoma in children and adolescents; a review, in *Hematology/Oncology Clinics of North America,* Vol. 1(4), W. B. Saunders, Philadelphia, 1987.

5. **Ruymann, F. B., Newton, W. A., Ragab, A., et al.,** Bone marrow metastases at diagnosis in children and adolescents with rhabdomyosarcoma; a report from the Intergroup Rhabdomyosarcoma Study, *Cancer,* 53, 368, 1984.

6. **Raney, B., Ragab, A., Ruymann, F., et al.,** Soft tissue sarcoma of the trunk in childhood; results of the Intergroup Rhabdomyosarcoma Study (IRS), 1972—1976, *Cancer,* 49, 2612, 1982.

7. **Crist, W., Raney, B., Newton, W., et al.,** Intrathoracic soft tissue sarcomas in children, *Cancer,* 50, 598, 1982.

8. **Ruymann, F., Raney, R. B., Crist, W., et al.,** Rhabdomyosarcoma of the biliary tree in children; a report from the Intergroup Rhabdomyosarcoma Study, *Cancer,* 56, 575, 1985.

9. **D'Agostino, A. N., Soule, E. H., and Miller, R. H.,** Sarcomas of the peripheral nerves and somatic soft tissues associated with multiple neurofibromatosis (Von Recklinghausen's disease), *Cancer,* 16, 1015, 1963.

10. **Schweisguth, O., Gerard-Marchant, R., and Lemerle, J.,** Basal cell nevus syndrome; association with congenital rhabdomyosarcoma, *Arch. Fr. Pediatr.,* 25, 1083, 1968.

11. **McKeen, E. A., Bodurtha, J., and Meadows, A. T., et al.,** Rhabdomyosarcoma complicating multiple neurofibromatosis, *J. Pediatr.,* 93, 992, 1978.

12. **Sobel, R. A. and Woerner, S.,** Rubinstein-Taybi syndrome and nasopharyngeal rhabdomyosarcoma, *J. Pediatr.,* 99, 1000, 1981.

13. **Beddis, I. R., Mott, M. G., and Bullimore, J.,** Case reports; nasopharyngeal rhabdomyosarcoma and Gorlin's naevoid basal cell carcinoma syndrome, *Med. Pediatr. Oncol.,* 11, 178, 1983.

14. **Sloane, J. A. and Hubbel, M. M.,** Soft tissue sarcomas in children associated with congenital anomalies, *Cancer,* 23, 175, 1969.

15. **Ruymann, F., Maddux, H., Ragab, A., et al.,** Congenital anomalies associated with rhabdomyosarcoma; a report from the Intergroup Rhabdomyosarcoma Study, *Med. Pediatr. Oncol.,* 16, 33, 1988.

16. **Li, F. B. and Fraumeni, J. F., Jr.,** Rhabdomyosarcoma in children; epidemiologic study and identification of a familial cancer syndrome, *J. Natl. Cancer Inst.,* 43, 1365, 1969.

17. **Li, F. B. and Fraumeni, J. F., Jr.,** Prospective study of a family cancer syndrome, *JAMA,* 247, 2692, 1982.

18. **Birch, J. M., Hartley, A. L., Marsden, H. B., et al.,** Excess risk of breast cancer in the mothers of children with soft tissue sarcomas, *Br. J. Cancer,* 49, 325, 1984.

19. **Lynch, H. T., Katz, D. A., Bogard, P. J., et al.,** The sarcoma, breast cancer, lung cancer and adrenocortical carcinoma syndrome revisited, *Am. J. Dis. Child.,* 139, 134, 1985.

20. **Grufferman, S., Wang, H. W., DeLong, E. R., et al.,** Environmental factors in the etiology of rhabdomyosarcoma of childhood, *J. Natl. Cancer Inst.,* 68, 107, 1982.

21. **Stout, A. P.,** Rhabdomyosarcoma of the skeletal muscle, *Ann. Surg.,* 123, 447, 1946.

22. **Newton, W., Soule, E. H., Hamoudi, A., et al.,** Histopathology of childhood sarcomas, Intergroup Rhabdomyosarcoma Studies I and II; clinicopathologic correlation, *J. Clin. Oncol.,* 6, 67, 1988.

23. **Angervall, L. and Enzinger, F. M.,** Extraskeletal neoplasm resembling Ewing's sarcoma, *Cancer,* 36, 240, 1975.

24. **Soule, E. H., Newton, W., and Moon, T. E.,** Extraskeletal Ewing's sarcoma; a preliminary review of 26 cases encountered in the Intergroup Rhabdomyosarcoma Study, *Cancer,* 42, 259, 1978.

25. **Shimada, H., Newton, W., Soule, E., et al.,** Pathological features of extraosseous Ewing's sarcoma; a report from the Intergroup Rhabdomyosarcoma Study, *Hum. Pathol.,* 442, 1988.

26. **Newton, W., Triche, T., Marsden, H., et al.,** International Childhood Soft Tissue Sarcoma Pathology Classification Study; Design and Implementation Utilizing Intergroup Rhabdomyosarcoma Study II Clinical and Pathology Data, in *Soc. Pediatr. Path. Meet.,* February 27-28, 1988, Washington, D.C.

27. **Hays, D., Lawrence, W., Crist, W., et al.,** Partial cystectomy in the management of rhabdomyosarcoma of the bladder; a report from the Intergroup Rhabdomyosarcoma Study (IRS), *J. Pediatr. Surg.,* 25, 7, 719, 1990.

28. **Weiner, E. S., Hays, D., Lawrence, W., et al.,** Second-look operations in children in groups III and IV rhabdomyosarcoma (RMS), *(Abstr. 1183), Proc. Am. Soc. Clin. Oncol.,* 8, 304, 1989.

29. **Hays, D. M., Raney, R. B., Crist, W. M., et al.,** Second surgical procedures to evaluate primary tumor status in patients with chemotherapy responsive stage III-IV sarcomas, *J. Pediatr. Surg.,* 25, 10, 1100, 1990.

30. **Hays, D. M., Lawrence, W., Wharam, M., et al.,** Primary re-excision for patients with "microscopic residual" following initial excision of sarcomas of trunk and extremity sites, *J. Pediatr. Surg.,* 24(1), 5, 1988.

31. **Tefft, M., Lindberg, R., and Gehan, E.,** Radiation of rhabdomyosarcoma in children combined with systemic chemotherapy; local control in patients enrolled into the Intergroup Rhabdomyosarcoma Study (IRS), *NCI Monogr.,* 56, 75, 1981.

32. **Tefft, M., Wharam, M., Ruymann, F., et al.,** Radiotherapy (RT) for rhabdomyosarcoma (RMS) in children; a report from the Intergroup Rhabdomyosarcoma Study (IRS-II), *Proc. Am. Soc. Clin. Oncol.,* 4, 234, 1985.

33. **Tefft, M., Wharam, M., and Gehan, E.,** Local and regional control by radiation of rhabdomyosarcoma in IRS-II, *(Abstr. 1005), Proc. Am. Soc. Clin. Oncol.,* 7, 259, 1988.

34. **Heyn, R.,** Late effects of therapy in rhabdomyosarcoma, *Clinics Oncol.,* 4, 287, 1985.

35. **Heyn, R., Ragab, A., Raney, R. B., et al.,** Late effects of therapy in orbital rhabdomyosarcoma in children, *Cancer,* 57, 1738, 1986.

36. **Tefft, M., Hays, D., Raney, B., et al.,** Radiation to regional nodes for RMS of the genitourinary tract in children: Is it necessary? A report from the IRS-1, *Cancer,* 45(12), 3065, 1979.

37. **Tefft, M., Fernandez, C., Donaldson, M., et al.,** Incidence of meningeal involvement by rhabdomyosarcoma of the head and neck in children; a report of the Intergroup Rhabdomyosarcoma Study (IRS), *Cancer,* 42, 253, 1978.

38. **Raney, R. B., Tefft, M., Newton, W. A., et al.,** Improved prognosis with intensive treatment of children with cranial sarcoma arising in non-orbital parameningeal sites; a report from the Intergroup Rhabdomyosarcoma Study, *Cancer,* 59, 147, 1987.

39. **Heyn, R., Newton, W. A., Jr., Ragab, A., et al.,** Second neoplasms in patients treated for soft tissue sarcomas on the Intergroup Rhabdomyosarcoma Study I-II (IRS I-II), *(Abstr. 1090), Proc. Am. Soc. Clin. Oncol.,* 10, 310, 1991.

40. **Raney, R. B., Tefft, M., Maurer, H. M., et al.,** Disease pattern and survival rate in children with metastatic soft tissue sarcoma; a report from the Intergroup Rhabdomyosarcoma Study (IRS-I), *Cancer,* 62, 1257, 1988.

41. **Raney, R. B., Jr., Gehan, E. A., Maurer, H. M., et al.,** Evaluation of intensified chemotherapy in children with advanced rhabdomyosarcoma (Clinical Groups III and IV), *Clinical Cancer Trials,* Spring, 1979, p. 19.

42. **Hays, D., Raney, R. B., Wharam, M., et al.,** Subsets of pediatric patients with particular chemotherapy sensitivity in the Intergroup Rhabdomyosarcoma Study (IRS), Br. Assoc. Pediatr. Surg. XXXII Ann. Int. Congr. Vienna, July 1985. *J. Clin. Oncol.,* 9, 159, 1991.

43. **Ragab, A., Heyn, R., Tefft, M., et al.,** Infants younger than one year of age with rhabdomyosarcoma; a report of the Intergroup Rhabdomyosarcoma Study, *Cancer,* 58, 2606, 1986.

44. **Crist, W., Raney, B., Ragab, A., et al.,** Intensive chemotherapy including cis-platinum (CPDD) or CPDD and VP-16 improves the response rate for children with soft tissue sarcomas (STS), *Med. Pediatr. Oncol.,* 15, 51, 1987.

45. **Koufos, A., Hansen, M. F., Copeland, N. G., et al.,** Loss of heterozygosity in three embryonal tumors suggests a common pathogenetic mechanism, *Nature,* 316, 330, 1985.

46. **Seidal, T., Mark, J., Hagmar, B., and Angervall, J.,** Alveolar rhabdomyosarcoma; a cytogenetic and correlated cytological and histological study, *Acta Pathol. Microbial. Immunol. Scand. (A)* 90, 345, 1982.

47. **Turc-Carel, C., Lizard-Nacol, S., Justrabo, E., et al.,** Consistent chromosome translocation in alveolar rhabdomyosarcoma, *Cancer Genet. Cytogenet.,* 19, 361, 1986.

48. **Shapiro, D. N., Parham, D. M., Douglas, E. C., et al.,** Relationship of tumor cell ploidy to histologic subtype and treatment outcome in children and adolescents with unresectable rhabdomyosarcoma, *J. Clin. Oncol.,* 9, 159. 1991

49. **Stratten, M. R., Fisher, C., Gusterson, B. A., and Cooper, C. S.,** Detection of point mutations in N-*ras* and K-*ras* genes of human embryonal rhabdomyosarcoma using oligonucleotide probes and the polymerase chain reaction, *Cancer Res.,* 49, 6324, 1989.

50. **Peltier, L. F.,** Historical note on bone and soft tissue sarcoma, *J. Surg. Oncol.,* 30, 201, 1985.

51. **Weber, C. O.,** Anatomische Untersuchung einer Hypertrophische Zunge Nebst Bemerkungen Ueber die Neubildung Quergestreifter Muskelfasern, *Virchow. Arch. Pathol. Anat.,* 7, 115, 1854.

52. **Rakov, A. I.,** Malignant rhabdomyosarcomas of skeletal musculature, *Am. J. Cancer,* 30, 455, 1937.

53. **Pack, G. T. and Eberhart, W. F.,** Rhabdomyosarcoma of skeletal; report of 100 cases, *Surgery,* 32, 1023, 1952.

54. **Pack, G. T. and Ariel, I. M.,** Sarcomas of the soft somatic tissues in infants and children, *Surg. Gynecol. Obstet.,* 98, 765, 1954.

55. **Stobbe, G. D. and Dargeon, H. W.,** Embryonal rhabdomyosarcoma of the head and neck in children and adolescents, *Cancer,* 3, 826, 1950.

56. **Riopelle, J. L. and Theriault, J. P.,** Sur une forme meconnue de sarcome des parties molles; le rhabdomyosarcome alveolaire, *Ann. Anat. Path.,* 1, 88, 1956.

57. **Enzinger, F. M. and Shiraki, M.,** Alveolar rhabdomyosarcoma; an analysis of 110 cases, *Cancer,* 24, 18, 1969.

58. **Horn, R. C. Jr. and Enterline, H. T.,** Rhabdomyosarcoma; a clinicopathologic study and classification of 39 cases, *Cancer,* 11, 181, 1958.

59. **Mackenzie, A. R., Whitemore, W. F., Jr., and Melamed, M. R.,** Myosarcomas of the bladder and prostate, *Cancer,* 22, 833, 1968.
60. **Tefft, M., Vawter, G. F., and Mitus, A.,** Paravertebral "round cell" tumors in children, *Radiology,* 92, 1501, 1969.
61. **Triche, T. J., Askin, F. B., and Kissane, J. M.,** Neuroblastoma, Ewing's sarcoma and the differential diagnosis of small-round-blue-cell tumors, in *Pathology of Neoplasia in Children and Adolescents,* W. B. Saunders, Philadelphia, 1986, 145.
62. **Sagerman, R. N., Tretter, P., and Ellsworth, R. M.,** The treatment of orbital rhabdomyosarcoma of children with primary radiation therapy, *Am. J. Roentgenol. Radium Ther. Nucl. Med.,* 114, 31, 1972.
63. **Flamant, F., Bloch-Michel, E., and Lemaistre, O., et al.,** Les possibilites actuelles de traitment du rhabdomyosarcoma de l'orbite chez l'enfant; a propos de 20 cas observes a l'Institut Gustave Roussy (1960—1975), *J. Fr. Ophthalmol.,* 1, 451, 1978.
64. **Pinkel, D.,** Actinomycin D in childhood cancer; a preliminary report, *Pediatrics,* 23, 342, 1959.
65. **Tan, C., Dargeon, H. W., and Burchenal, J. H.,** The effect of actinomycin D on cancer in childhood, *Pediatrics,* 24, 544, 1959.
66. **Shaw, R. K., Moore, E. W., Mueller, P. S., et al.,** The effect of actinomycin D on childhood neoplasms, *Am. J. Dis. Child,* 99, 635, 1960.
67. **Haddy, T. B., Nora, A. H., Sutow, W. W., and Vietti, T. J.,** Cyclophosphamide treatment for metastatic soft tissue sarcoma; intermittent large doses in the treatment of children, *Am. J. Dis. Child,* 114, 301, 1967.
68. **Sutow, W. W.,** Cyclophosphamide (NSC-26271) in Wilms' tumor and rhabdomyosarcoma, *Cancer Chemother. Rep.,* 51, 407, 1967.
69. **Sutow, W. W., Berry, D. H., Haddy, T. B., et al.,** Vincristine sulfate therapy in children with metastatic soft tissue sarcoma, *Pediatrics,* 38, 465, 1966.
70. **Sutow, W. W.,** Vincristine (NSC-67574) therapy for malignant solid tumors in children (except Wilms' tumor), *Cancer Chemother. Rep.,* 52, 485, 1968.
71. **Selawry, O. S., Holland, J. R., and Wolman, I. J.,** Effect of vincristine (NSC-67574) on malignant solid tumors in children, *Cancer Chemother. Rep.,* 52, 497, 1968.
72. **Bonadonna, G., Monfardini, S., DeLena, M., et al.,** Phase I and preliminary phase II evaluation of adriamycin (NSC-123127), *Cancer Res.,* 30, 2572, 1970.
73. **O'Bryan, R. M., Luce, J. K., Talley, R. W., et al.,** Phase II evaluation of adriamycin in human neoplasia, *Cancer,* 32, 1, 1973.
74. **Sutow, W. W., Vietti, T. J., Lonsdale, D., Talley, R. W.,** Daunomycin in the treatment of metastatic soft tissue sarcoma in children. *Cancer,* 29, 1293, 1972.
75. **Tan, C., Etcubanas, E., Wollner, N., et al.,** Adriamycin; an anti-tumor antibiotic in the treatment of neoplastic diseases, *Cancer,* 32, 9, 1973.
76. **Pinkel, D. and Pinkren, J.,** Rhabdomyosarcoma in children, *JAMA,* 175, 293, 1961.
77. **Raney, R. B., Jr., Hays, D. M., Tefft, M., et al.,** Rhabdomyosarcoma and the undifferentiated sarcomas, in *Principles and Practice of Pediatric Oncology,* Pizzo, P. A. and Poplack, D. G., Eds., J. B. Lippincott, Philadelphia, 1988, 649.
78. **Young, J. L., Jr., Ries, L. G., Silverberg, E., et al.,** Cancer incidence, survival and mortality for children younger than 15 years, *Cancer,* 58, 598, 1986.
79. **Breslow, N. E. and Langholz, B.,** Childhood cancer incidence; geographical and temporal variations, *Int. J. Cancer,* 32, 703, 1983.
80. **Ruymann, F. B., Gaiger, A. M., and Newton, W. A., Jr.,** Congenital Anomalies in Children with Rhabdomyosarcoma (Abstr.). Birth Defects Conference, Memphis, TN, June 8-10, 1977.
81. **Wang, N., Leung, J., and Warrier, R. P., et al.,** Nonrandom chromosomal observations and clonal chromosomal evolution in acute leukemia associated with Down's syndrome, *Cancer Genet. Cytogenet.,* 28, 155, 1987.
82. **Ueda, K., Gruppo, R., Unger, F., et al.,** Rhabdomyosarcoma of lung arising in congenital cystic adenomatoid malformation, *Cancer,* 40, 383, 1977.
83. **Krous, H. F. and Sexauer, C. L.,** Embryonal rhabdomyosarcoma arising within a congenital bronchiogenic cyst in a child, *J. Pediatr. Surg.,* 16, 506, 1981.
84. **Hartley, A. L., Birch, J. M., McKinney, P. A., et al.,** The Inter-Regional Epidemiological Study of Childhood Cancer (IRESCC); case control study of children with bone and soft tissue sarcomas, *Br. J. Cancer.,* 58, 838, 1988.
85. **Hope, D. G. and Mulvihill, J. J.,** Malignancy in neurofibromatosis, in, *Advances in Neurology,* Vol 29 *Neurofibromatosis (Von Recklinghausen's Disease).* Riccardi, V. M. and Mulvihill, J. J., Eds., Raven Press, New York, 1981.
86. **Huson, S. M., Compston, D. A., and Harper, P. S.,** A genetic study of Von Recklinghausen neurofibromatosis in South East Wales. II. Guidelines for genetic counseling, *J. Med. Genet.,* 26, 712, 1989.

87. **Hartley, A. L., Birch, J. M., Kelsey, A. M., et al.,** Are germ cell tumors part of the Li-Fraumeni cancer family syndrome?, *Cancer Genet. Cytogenet.,* 42, 221, 1989.
88. **Li, F. P., Fraumeni, J. R., Jr., Mulvihill, J. J., et al.,** A cancer family syndrome in 24 kindred, *Cancer Res.,* 48, 5358, 1988.
89. **Pastore, G., Mosso, M. L., Carli, M., et al.,** Cancer mortality among relatives of children with soft tissue sarcomas; a national survey in Italy, *Cancer Litt.,* 37, 17, 1987.
90. **Malkin, D., Li, F. P., Strong, L. C., et al.,** Germ-line p53 mutations in a familial syndrome of breast cancer, sarcomas and other neoplasms, *Science* 250, 1233, 1990.
91. **Fields, S. and Jang, S. K.,** Presence of a potent transcription activating sequence in the p53 protien, *Science,* 249, 1046, 1990.
92. **Lyons, L. A., Lewis, R. A., Strong, L. C., et al.,** A genetic study of Gardner syndrome and congenital hypertrophy of the retinal pigment epithelium, *Am. J. Hum. Genet.,* 42, 290, 1988.
93. **Lynch, H. T., Katz, D. A., Bogard, P. J., et al.,** The sarcoma, breast cancer, lung cancer and adrenocortical carcinoma syndrome revisited; childhood cancer, *Am. J. Dis. Child.,* 139, 134, 1985.
94. **Hartley, A. L., Birch, J. M., Marsden, H. B., et al.,** Adrenal cortical tumors; epidemiological and familial aspects, *Arch. Dis. Child.,* 62, 683, 1987.
95. **Thompson, E. N., Dallimore, N. S., and Brook, D. L.,** Parental cancer in an unselected cohort of children with cancer referred to a single center, *Br. J. Cancer,* 57, 127, 1988.
96. **Hartley, A. L., Birch, J. M., Marsden, H. B., et al.,** Breast cancer risk in mothers of children with osteosarcoma and chondrosarcoma, *Br. J. Cancer,* 54, 819, 1986.
97. **Hartley, A. L., Birch, J. M., Marsden, H. B., et al.,** Malignant disease in mothers of children with Ewing's tumor, *Med. Pediatr. Oncol.,* 16, 95, 1988.
98. **Becker, H., Zaunschirm, A., Muntean, J., et al.,** Fetal alcohol syndrome and malignant tumors, *Wien. Klin. Wochenschr.,* 94, 364, 1982.
99. **Cohen, M. M., Jr.,** Neoplasia and the fetal alcohol and hydantoin syndromes, *Neurobehav. Toxicol. Teratol.,* 3, 161, 1981.
100. **Bostrom, B. and Nesbit, M. E.,** Hodgkin's disease in a child with fetal alcohol-hydantoin syndrome, *J. Pediatr.,* 103, 760, 1983.
101. **Florey, C. D.,** Weak associations in epidemiological research; some examples and their interpretation. *Int. J. Epidemiol.,* 17, 950, 1988.
102. **Grufferman, S., Delzell, E. S., Maile, M. C., and Michalopoulos, G.,** Parents' cigarette smoking and childhood cancer, *Med. Hypoth.,* 12, 17, 1983.
103. **Evans, H. J., Fletcher, J., Torrance, M., Hargraeve, T. B.,** Sperm abnormalities and cigarette smoking, *Lancet,* 1, 627, 1981.
104. **Mau, G. and Netter, P.,** Die Auswirkungen des Vaterlichen Zigaretlenkonsums auf die Perinatale Sterblichkeit und die Missbildungshaufigkeit, *Dtsch. Med. Wochenschr.,* 99, 1113, 1974.
105. **Hartley, A. L., Birch, J. M., and McKinney, P. A., et al.,** The Inter-Regional Epidemiological Study of Childhood Cancer (IRESCC); past medical history in children with cancer, *J. Epidemiol. Community Health,* 42, 235, 1988.
106. **Grufferman, S., Gula, M. J., Olshan, A., et al.,** Experience with random digit telephone dialing for control selection in a case-control study of children, *Paediatr. Perinat. Epidemiol.,* in press.
107. **Grufferman, S., Olshan, A., Gula, M. J., et al.,** The role of active immunization in the etiology of childhood cancer: protective or simply prescribed?, *Am. J. Epidemiol.,* 132, 758, 1990.
108. **Peter, G., Ed.,** *Report of the Committee on Infectious Diseases,* Committee on Infectious Diseases, American Academy of Pediatrics, 47, 1991.
109. **Grufferman, S., Gula, M. J., Olshan, A., et al.,** Absence of an association between parents' cigarette smoking and risk of rhabdomyosarcoma in their children, *Paediatr. Perinat. Epidemiol.,* in press.
110. **Grufferman, S., Gula, M. J., Olshan, A., et al.,** *In utero* X-ray exposure and risk of childhood rhabdomyosarcoma, *Paediatr. Perinat. Epidemiol.,* in press.
111. **Grufferman, S., Gula, M. J., Olshan, A., et al.,** Parents' use of recreational drugs and risk of rhabdomyosarcoma in their children, *Am. J. Epidemiol.,* in press.
112. **Openshaw, S., Craft, A. W., Charlton, M., and Birch, J. M.,** Investigation of leukemia clusters by use of a geographical analysis machine, *Lancet,* 8580, 272, 1988.
113. **Hoar, S. K., Blair, A., Holmes, F. F., et al.,** Agricultural herbicide use and risk of lymphoma and soft tissue sarcoma, *JAMA,* 256, 1141, 1986.
114. **Woods, J. S., Polissar, L., Severson, R. K., et al.,** Soft tissue sarcoma and non-Hodgkin's lymphoma in relation to phenoxy herbicide and chlorinated phenol exposure in western Washington, *J. Natl. Cancer Inst.,* 78, 899, 1987.
115. **Kang, H., Enzinger, F., Breslin, P., et al.,** Soft tissue sarcomas and military service in Viet Nam; a case control study, *J. Natl. Cancer Inst.,* 79, 693, 1987.

116. **Zahm, S. H., Blair, A., Holmes, F. F., et al.,** A case control study of soft tissue sarcoma and Hodgkin's disease; farming and insecticide use, *Scand. J. Work. Environ. Health,* 14, 224, 1988.
117. **Zahm, S. H., Blair, A., Holmes, F. F., et al.,** A case control study of soft tissue sarcoma, *Am. J. Epidemiol.,* 130, 665, 1989.
118. **Tucker, M. A., D'Angio, G. J., Boice, J. D. Jr., et al.,** Bone sarcomas linked to radiotherapy and chemotherapy in children, *N. Engl. J. Med.,* 317, 588, 1987.
119. **Little, J. B., Nichols, W. W., Troilo, P., et al.,** Radiation sensitivity of cell strains from families with genetic disorders predisposing to radiation-induced cancer, *Cancer Res.,* 49, 4705, 1989.
120. **Strong, L. C. and Williams, W. R.,** The genetic implications of long term survival of childhood cancer; a conceptual framework, *Am. J. Pediatr. Hematol. Oncol.,* 9, 99, 1987.
121. **Strong, L. C., Stine, M., and Norsted, T. L.,** Cancer survivors of childhood soft tissue sarcoma and their relatives, *J. Natl. Cancer Inst.,* 79, 1213, 1987.

Chapter 2

PATHOLOGY OF RHABDOMYOSARCOMA AND RELATED TUMORS: EXPERIENCE OF THE INTERGROUP RHABDOMYOSARCOMA STUDIES

William A. Newton, Jr., Ala Hamoudi, Bruce Webber, and Paul S. Dickman

TABLE OF CONTENTS

I. INTRODUCTION

This chapter will not present an encyclopedic review of the pathology of this very complex tumor system. (See Chapter 23 as well as other sources.[1-3]) Instead, this chapter will reflect the experience of the authors since 1972 as members of the Pathology Study Committee of the Intergroup Rhabdomyosarcoma Study (IRS). The IRS database is nonumental and represents a unique opportunity to examine this complex neoplasm with a great deal more precision than that available through the usual sources.

At the outset, it would be appropriate to begin with a historical review. This tumor has not been well understood by pathologists; it continues to be a problem for many with respect to its exact nature, its histogenesis, and its differentiation from other primitive soft tissue tumors of childhood. To quote Arthur Purdy Stout in his original description of rhabdomyosarcoma (RMS) in 1946, "The differential diagnosis of peripheral soft part tumors is always a challenge to the diagnostic acumen of the pathologist."[4] In his careful scrutiny of the literature at that time, Stout found only 107 cases that he would accept as RMS. Of that number, about one fifth were in children. The pendulum has swung quite far since that time. RMS is now diagnosed primarily in children and adolescents. In adults, malignant fibrous histiocytoma is more often the primary diagnosis than RMS. Stout emphasized the presence of cross striations in the cytoplasm of the tumor cells as confirming the diagnosis. At present, this criterion is seldom used since only the more obvious and differentiated tumors consistently show these striations.

Subtyping of RMS began in 1958 when Horn and Enterline proposed the first subclassification system. This system was based on only a very few cases, when compared to the large number available for study today.[5] Despite this limitation, the early classification system has held up well except for the pleomorphic subtype. The diagnosis of this subtype is rarely made now in children or adults. In children, tumors that would have been so classified in the past are now usually diagnosed as the embryonal subtype. The pleomorphic subtype previously diagnosed in adults is now classified as malignant fibrous histiocytoma in most instances. In Horn and Enterline's series, 11 of the 12 pleomorphic subtypes were in patients older than 20 years of age, and the majority were over 30 years of age. They properly included the alveolar subtype described two years earlier by Riopelle and Theriault.[6]

One limitation of Horn and Enterline's classification is that it did not include undifferentiated sarcomas which cannot be classified as to a specific cell type of origin or extent of differentiation. In addition, there are a number of types of soft tissue tumors which have had a poor survival rate and need to be included in the same group. Up until the mid-1960s, most children with RMS were considered to have a very aggressive, usually fatal, disease. It is only with the advent of very aggressive multimodal therapy that survival rates have been greatly improved in recent years. The same kind of therapeutic approach is now being tried in other variants of soft tissue sarcomas. There is increasing evidence that many of the lesions previously thought to be uniformly fatal, or very likely so, are now responding in a similar fashion to RMS.[7,8]

Fortunately, it was decided early to include patients with undifferentiated sarcoma as eligible for entry in the IRS. This decision was based in part on results from a Children's Cancer Study Group in which patients with undifferentiated sarcomas appeared to fare as well as those with other subtypes of RMS.[9] Similarly, the cases reported from the Mayo Clinic experience included a sizeable number, about one seventh, that had undifferentiated sarcomas.[10] Clinical findings were not available from that series to indicate prognosis of patients with these tumors. The patients in IRS-I and -II with undifferentiated sarcoma have had unfavorable survival with present therapy and are of particular interest. Their survival rate appears to be similar to that of patients with the alveolar subtype. Tumors such as synovial sarcoma, fibrosarcoma, etc., need to be evaluated in a large series so that we can better understand the behavior of these lesions in response to modern therapy.

It should be stated at the outset that the modern techniques for examining these primitive small cell tumors in children still lack definitive, absolute criteria for classification purposes. The traditional classification systems based on light microscopy of hematoxylin and eosin stained sections are only moderately successful in determining the biological nature and subtypes of these tumors. The addition of electron microscopy has been of some assistance. Unfortunately, however, many of the lesions that can be readily classified as embryonal RMS with light microscopy do not have characteristic features of myogenesis by electron microscopy. Moreover, cases which are difficult to classify by light microscopy are, for the most part, not further classified by electron microscopy. Immunohistochemistry is of some help in the identification of muscle differentiation in tumors, but the usefulness of this technique has limitations since sensitivity and specificity of the technique are still in question.

Continued utilization of the newer methods are needed in order to better define the biological nature of these tumors. Whether a separate schema based upon immunohisto-chemistry will be useful is yet to be determined. It is conceivable that in the future tumors will no longer be classified utilizing the conventional modified system of Horn and Enterline. Instead, antigen identification by immunohistochemistry combined with electron microscopy and molecular biologic markers might be used to more precisely determine the nature of these cells. It is still not possible to withhold aggressive therapy from any soft tissue sarcoma in a child on the basis of morphology alone.

Present practices of tumor therapy are based on limited case information on many subtypes of soft tissue sarcomas, as well as the obvious bias that is associated with personal experiences and limited information of the practicing physician. A nationwide or international study of childhood sarcomas should not restrict itself to diagnosis of traditional RMSs. Rather, such a study should include all sarcomas, with guidelines for identifying the recognizable subtypes that are known to exist as well as for recognizing those that traditionally have not been included. Patients with these latter tumors would be similarly treated and studied so that their true survival could be determined.

II. CLASSIFICATION OF RMS AND RELATED TUMORS

Soft tissue tumors in children present a difficult problem for the diagnostic pathologist. Most of these tumors consist of very primitive cellular elements which often defy definition as to histogenesis or cell type when examined by conventional light microscopy. It is not surprising that this problem is a confusing one and the proper classification of these tumors is still an unresolved issue. Stout's classification was the first for RMS. He did not subdivide them further.[4] Stobbe and Dargeon added the subtype of embryonal,[11] which was a logical term since most of these tumors consist of very primitive cells strongly resembling developing muscle cells in embryos. The term alveolar was first suggested by Riopelle and Theriault.[6]

The current popular classification that was proposed in 1958 by Horn and Enterline continues to be the most commonly used system.[12,13] Even so, the use of this system has varied, since many pathologists and clinicians have felt that the subtypes were simply not helpful with respect to prediction of behavior of the neoplasm.[14] These early guidelines are still in use today in many centers.[3,15] Of paramount importance is the decision regarding the subclassification of a given tumor so that the patient is included in a therapeutic regimen that is optimal for his or her tumor type. Survival of most children with soft tissue sarcomas was notoriously poor until the mid-1960s when therapy began to show a beneficial effect. It has become evident, as our experience has increased, that the subtypes within the Horn and Enterline classification do have prognostic significance.

It is also clear that tumors which may not express myogenesis, nevertheless, respond in a similar fashion to therapy effective for the treatment of RMS. This includes a significant number of tumors which are so primitive that one can only call them undifferentiated sarcomas. This is a meaningful diagnosis even though it would appear at first glance to be a diagnosis of exclusion. Pathologists in general are reluctant to be nonspecific in indicating histogenesis of a given tumor, that is, indicating whether the tumor arose from muscle, synovia, fibrous tissue, or another source of cell line. But we must realize that there is a sizable group of tumors in which identification of histogenesis is simply not yet possible with the available technology. This deficiency was emphasized by a review of the present classification of childhood RMS in 1979.[16] The early series of soft tissue sarcomas listed by Soule[17] included a significant number of tumors which were classified as "undifferentiated sarcomas" and, as indicated above, the experience at Columbus Children's Hospital included a significant proportion of these tumors which lack specific identity as to histogenesis.[18]

The problem is solvable but requires that progress be made with respect to our ability to detect features which can then be used in a subclassifying system. This problem has been well summarized in a recent discussion on current concepts in the diagnosis of human soft tissue sarcomas.[19] It was emphasized that conventional light microscopy must be used as well as ultrastructural and immunohistochemistry studies. In addition other features, such as the type of collagen present within the neoplasm may be used as a feature for subclassifying the tumor.

It has been proposed that soft tissue tumors should be classified on the basis of histogenesis.[20] These tumors have stem cells which can be multipotent, and thus may be quite heterogeneous in composition. Thus, the behavior of a given tumor may not be predicted by the apparent cellular differentiation pattern seen by light microscopy. Future classification systems may need to depend on identifying the specific cytological elements present in a given tumor in order to determine the proper therapy.

The classification system utilized by the IRS Pathology Committee when it began its studies in 1972 consisted of the four subtypes of Horn and Enterline. In addition, it included the category then designated as "small round cell sarcoma, type indeterminate". This was a somewhat redundant term to indicate "undifferentiated sarcoma" or sarcoma type indeterminate. It became apparent that there was a significant subset of tumors within this category which could be identified regularly as a distinct subtype of undifferentiated tumor. This subtype was initially called "undifferentiated sarcoma, type I and type II" because of the presence of certain varying features. These two types were later considered to be equivalent to the small and large cell types of Ewing's sarcoma of soft tissue, and have subsequently been classified as "extraosseous Ewing's sarcoma".[21]

It became clear that the pleomorphic subtype was quite uncommon and, in fact, as the study proceeded, this subtype became quite rare. The IRS Pathology Committee has now decided that pleomorphic RMS is not seen in soft tissue sarcomas in children often enough to warrant designation as a specific subtype. Even in adults, many pathologists believe that this subtype does not exist and the majority of the tumors are of nonmuscle origin, such as malignant fibrous histiocytoma.[22]

When a case is to be classified, the first step is to decide whether the tissue available for histologic examination warrants the diagnosis of sarcoma. At times, the lesion has the appearance of a sarcoma but, because of poor preservation or inadequate amount of tumor tissue, the diagnosis of sarcoma NOS (not otherwise specified) is made (Figure 1). The next step is to determine whether the cells present in the tumor show differentiation or myogenesis. If the tumor consists of very primitive cells, not showing cytoplasmic differentiation, then the tumor is classified as "undifferentiated sarcoma" or "extraosseous Ewing's" (EOE) as appropriate. Undifferentiated lesions other than the EOE type are quite variable in appearance. These tumors are currently under study to attempt further subclassification.

A. EMBRYONAL

The most common subtype of childhood RMS is embryonal. These tumors show evidence of maturation of both cytoplasm and nucleus to varying degrees, but most importantly for

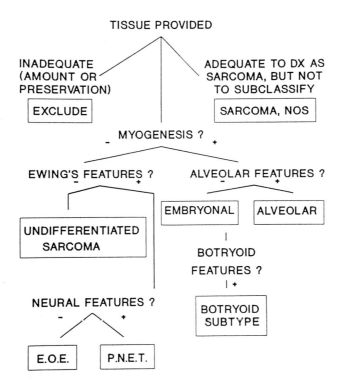

FIGURE 1.   Diagnosis decision tree used in classifying and subclassifying
lesions by the Intergroup Rhabdomyosarcoma Study Pathology Committee
for IRS I-III.

H&E diagnosis is the presence of evidence of maturation in the cytoplasm. The degree of
myogenesis varies from scanty to advanced, with formation of strap cells with cross striations.
The cellularity varies as well from sparse to densely cellular, sometimes with mixtures of
both. The nuclei show invagination of cell membranes, the chromatin is more coarse and
often stranded. Nucleoli are not prominent. If the lesion occurs in an open space, such as
the vagina, it tends to produce the unique picture of the botryoid variant. If the tumor occurs
in a paratesticular area, the lesion often has an almost specific morphology. This tendency
will be discussed below.

B. BOTRYOID

The subtype of RMS with the most favorable survival is botryoid. This fact has been
obscured because most studies have included this type with the embryonal type. The central
mass of a botryoid RMS is usually very loosely cellular, somewhat myxoid in appearance.
The diagnosis of botryoid has been applied regardless of whether the cambium layer is
present. However, in most instances there is a condensation of the loose cellular tumor cells
below the epithelial surface which forms the cambium layer in that area. Individual tumor
cells usually show evidence of myogenesis in their cytoplasm. On occasion, the tumor cells
appear to have the appearance of small miniature strap cells, or myotubes with identifiable
cross striations. One feature of the botryoid lesion is the almost uniform presence of eosin-
ophils within the loose stroma.

C. ALVEOLAR

One of the most difficult tumors to separate from the embryonal RMS is the alveolar
type. The typical alveolar type is not difficult to identify, but there is a histopathological

continuity from the typical alveolar structure as classically described[6] to a tumor which is simply a sheet of cells without any obvious lumen or alveolar-like spaces. The *sine qua non* for the identification of the alveolar type is the presence of tumor cells lined up along membranes, which in some areas are delicate in nature but in other areas appear as broad collagen bands. This pattern can be seen even though there is no obvious alveolar-like lumen adjacent to the pattern.

It has been shown that some alveolar lesions lack any identifiable alveolar structures, consisting mainly of mononuclear cells with only minimal nuclear and cytoplasmic differentiation, resembling those of the cells of typical alveolar RMS.[55] The nuclei show coarsely granular chromatin and membrane infolding and the cytoplasm shows some identifiable myogenesis. This picture is compared with the illustrations published by Riopelle and Theriault,[6] which show alveolar-like changes in parts of the tumor, but also show areas without any such features and having a more solid growth pattern. The cells appear similar to those designated as monomorphous round cell tumor by Palmer.[23] Patients in a large combined study who had this alveolar variant showed a very poor survival rate.[24]

The diagnostic criteria used currently by the IRS Pathology Committee requires that over one half of the tumor being classified needs to have an alveolar pattern before it can be called alveolar. This requirement has been used since the inception of the IRS pathology studies. However, this situation will change in the IRS-IV study. The presence of any alveolar features will then be adequate to classify the lesion as alveolar RMS.

D. UNDIFFERENTIATED SARCOMA

This category of tumor is as yet poorly defined. It consists of tumors whose cells show no evidence of myogenesis or other differentiation. The pattern is generally diffuse with no specific features. The tumor cells are round, larger than mature lymphocytes, and have a scanty or moderate amount of cytoplasm. The nuclear chromatin is finely dispersed giving a vesicular appearance and there are a few prominent nucleoli. The cells show some degree of pleomorphism or irregularity of nuclear contour. No immunochemical muscle markers can be detected in these cells. The cells are sufficiently variable so that further study may show the group to be heterogeneous.

E. EXTRAOSSEOUS EWING'S SARCOMA

Another tumor subtype included in the IRS-I and -II studies and continuing on in IRS-III has been the entity of EOE. This lesion was identified and defined during the early IRS studies and has constituted about 5% of all patients studied. This unusual subtype was first recognized in 1969[25] and was followed by a report of 50 extraskeletal tumors similar to Ewing's sarcoma in 1974.[26] The unique histologic appearance was identified early in the IRS studies, and these tumors were separated from the undifferentiated sarcoma and the small round-cell type indeterminate category.[27]

The term extraosseous Ewing's sarcoma was first coined by Angervall and Enzinger in 1975.[28] Studies of the ultrastructure, immunochemistry, and histology of this lesion over the ensuing years has convinced many investigators that the bone and soft tissue types of Ewing's sarcoma are the same from a morphologic point of view, differing only in their sites of origin. Study of sites observed in cases from IRS-I and -II showed that the main distribution of these tumors was in the trunk in 32%, extremity 26%, retroperitoneum 15%, and parameningeal areas 9%. There were lesser numbers of these tumors in the genitourinary tract, in the head and neck generally, orbit, intrathoracic, pelvic, and other sites. There was a slight male preponderance of 54% to 46%. The vast majority occurred in patients over 6 years of age, being mainly in the 11 to 15 year age group. In 91% there were no metastases at the time of diagnosis, compared to absence of metastases in 82% of all patients eligible for IRS-I and -II.

Since Ewing's sarcoma of bone has plagued those interested in its histogenesis for many years, it was hoped that study of extraosseous Ewing's might give additional clues as to its origin. Ultrastructural studies by many investigators have shown that the cells of this tumor are quite primitive in their nature. There are two components: a predominant principle cell and a lesser component of a smaller and darker cell. Also, presence of evidence of development of cytoplasmic dendritic processes and the presence of small, dense-core granules suggested neural differentiation.[29] While most investigators considered that the histogenesis was still unknown, some suggested that angiosarcoma must be considered.[30,31] Further evidence for the similar nature of the bone and soft tissue tumors was supported by the finding in both tumors of a similar cytogenetic abnormality with reciprocal translocation of chromosomes 11 and 22.[32]

In a study of 11 tumors, both classic Ewing's sarcoma and extraskeletal Ewing's, it was found that they both showed expression of intermediate filaments and cell junction proteins when examined by immunofluorescence and by immunoelectron microscopy and gel electrophoresis.[33-35] All 11 of these cases showed abundant vimentin filaments. True desmosomes were found in all in varying proportions. Some junctions were associated with vimentin intermediate filaments, nine showed simple epithelium-like cytokeratins 8 and 18; three showed neurofilament production. Because of these multicell-type constituents, it was suggested that the term Ewing's sarcoma would be best changed to Ewing's blastoma. Since there was minimal evidence of a neural constituent, Ewing's sarcoma could be differentiated from primitive peripheral neuroectodermal tumor. It was suggested that both EOE and Ewing's sarcoma of bone may constitute a specialized category of malignant neoplasm, with variable expression of mesenchymal, epithelial, and neural markers reflecting the multidirectional potential of their cell version.

Pathological analysis was performed on the 84 patients with extraosseous Ewing's that were treated on IRS-I and -II.[21] This study included light microscopy, immunohistochemistry, and ultrastructural studies of 14 cases of EOE sarcoma. The group was divided into three categories. The first type showed a combination of both neuronal and Schwannian cell markers, suggesting the potential for two lines of development. The second type showed only neuron specific enolase markers indicating monodirectional differentiation. Finally, a single case showed negative staining for all markers. Eighteen of 74 extraosseous Ewing's tumors had the appearance of Homer-Wright-type rosettes, which were abortive in most cases. The appearance of neural markers as detected immunohistochemically or by ultrastructure were found in selective cases irrespective of the finding of rosette formation by light microscopy.

An attempt is underway to establish an acceptable international histopathological classification of RMS. Once completed, this may be in use for only a short time, depending upon newer insight into this tumor system. Such a classification will be a major advance in the sense that we would then be able to use similar histopathological categories worldwide when placing children with these types of tumors on protocol studies. This will allow better comparison of study results. This classification system might need to be modified at an early date if immunohistochemistry becomes an important aspect of the diagnostic criteria of subtyping these tumors. Clinical and immunohistochemical data need to be accumulated which would be correlated to actual survival. Such a study is to be carried out during the IRS-IV.

III. IMMUNOHISTOCHEMISTRY

Immunohistochemistry (IHC) is now becoming a part of the day-to-day activities of pathology departments dealing with the diagnosis of cancer. The exact role of IHC is still in the developmental stage, but has obviously made a significant contribution to the practice

TABLE 1
Primary Antibodies used for Immunohistochemistry

Antibody	Clonality[a]	Clone	Source	Dilution	Digestion
Vimentin	M	V9	DAKO	1:10	−
Keratin — wide spectrum	P	—	DAKO	1:200	+
Keratin — epidermal	P	—	DAKO	1:200	+
EMA	M	E-29	DAKO	1:200	+
Desmin	P	—	DAKO	1:500	+
Desmin	M	DE-R-11	DAKO	1:25	+
Actin anti-muscle specific	M	HHF35	ENZO	1:3000	+
Myoglobin	P	—	DAKO	1:400	+
CKMM	P	—	Cambridge Medical Diagnostic	1:50	+
Neurofilaments	M	2F11	DAKO	1:800	+
GFAP	P	—	DAKO	1:500	+
S-100	P	—	DAKO	1:300	−
NSE	P	—	DAKO	1:50	−
LCA	M	PD7	DAKO	1:500	+
Alpha-1-antitrypsin	P	—	DAKO	1:500	+
Lysozyme	P	—	DAKO	1:500	+
Alpha-1-feto-protein	P	—	DAKO	1:400	+
Alpha-1-chymo-trypsin	P	—	DAKO	1:400	−

[a]   Monoclonal (M) or polyclonal (P).

of pathology. Immunohistochemical testing has been carried out on a fraction of the cases sent for review on the IRS-III. In general, these specialized techniques have been applied to the more difficult diagnostic cases in the hope that additional support for or against a particular diagnosis could be obtained.

A recent summary of our experience on IRS-III has shown that 159 cases have been studied out of a total of 950 classified by the IRS Pathology Committee. The antibodies used in studying these cases and their relationship to the final diagnosis and classification are listed in Table 1. The stains were carried out on formalin-fixed paraffin embedded tissue. Obviously, the tests were used most often for undifferentiated tumors and those lesions where there was concern about the diagnosis being appropriate for study purposes. For lesions classified as RMS (embryonal, alveolar, and botryoid), muscle specific actin seemed to be the most consistent reaction, being positive $3/4$ of the time, as opposed to less than half of the cases being positive using desmin and a $1/5$ with myoglobin. S-100 was positive in 9 out of 41 and neurone specific enolase (NSE) was positive in 10 out of 33 cases in which it was tried.

Lesions classified as undifferentiated sarcoma showed positive reactions with actin and myoglobin infrequently but were positive in a small sample using desmin and CK-MM. S-100 was positive in about $1/10$ and NSE was positive in 9 out of 21. EOE lesions generally showed no muscle antigen reactivity but significant numbers were positive for NSE and S-100. (Table 2). Patients whose diagnoses were considered to be ineligible for the IRS studies were perhaps the most useful subjects for use of IHC. The details as to the findings on histochemistry of these excluded cases are indicated in Table 3.

In general, IHC has not been consistently reliable enough to warrant making a diagnosis primarily on the basis of positive or negative reactions. Cross-reactions, nonspecificity, altered status of the tumor, (such as varying degrees of vitality) and perhaps suboptimum type of fixation, are all suspected reasons for a lack of confidence in this methodology. In the final analysis, conventional histology is still the most reliable method for establishing a

TABLE 2

Immunohistochemistry Findings in RMS and Related Tumors in Intergroup Rhabdomyosarcoma Study III (IRS-III)

Tumor Type	Total cases	Cases tested	Biological markers													
			Actin	Desmin	MGB	CK-MM	Myosin	8-100	NSE	VIM	LCA	Keratin	EMA	A1AT	AFP	NF
Embryonal	528	42	11/15[a]	16/41	3/14	5/8	—	4/28	3/19	1/3	1/5	1/7	1/8	3/3	—	—
Alveolar	186	23	6/8	12/22	2/10	—	—	5/13	7/14	1/2	—	1/4	0/4	1/1	0/13	0/1
Botryoid	45	1	1/1	—	—	—	—	—	—	—	—	—	—	—	—	—
Undifferentiated sarcoma	65	38	1/5	2/3	1/19	2/3	—	3/25	9/21	1/2	0/5	2/12	2/9	1/2	—	0/3
Sarcoma NOS[b]	36	5	0/1	0/5	0/2	—	—	0/3	0/5	0/1	—	0/1	0/1	—	—	—
EOE	35	14	0/6	0/12	0/3	0/1	—	5/11	7/13	0/2	0/2	—	—	—	—	0/1
Wrong dx	55	36	1/8	6/34	1/20	1/4	0/1	14/25	6/12	0/1	1/3	8/17	10/17	4/8	—	0/1
TOTAL	950	159														

[a] Number positive/number tested.

[b] NOS = not otherwise specified.

TABLE 3
Immunohistochemsitry of Cases Excluded From IRS-III

Type of tumor	n	Actin	Desmin	MGB	CK-MM	S-100	NSE	Lysozyme	LCA	Keratin	EMA	A1AT	A1ACT	NF
Extrarenal rhabdoid	8	0/1[a]	1/7	0/4	—	2/5	0/1	—	—	4/7	6/7	1/1	—	0/1
MFH	4	0/1	0/4	0/1	1/1	2/3	—	1/4	—	—	0/1	2/4	1/1	—
Ectomesenchymoma	3	0/1	3/3	0/1	0/1	3/3	3/3	—	—	0/2	0/2	—	3/3	0/1
Malignant mesenchymoma	2	—	0/2	0/2	—	1/2	—	—	—	—	—	—	—	—
Fibrosarcoma	1	—	0/1	0/1	—	0/1	0/1	—	—	—	—	—	—	—
Malignant lymphoma	3	0/1	0/3	—	0/1	0/1	0/1	—	1/3	—	—	—	—	—
Epithelioid sarcoma	3	—	0/3	0/1	—	2/2	—	0/1	—	2/3	2/3	1/1	—	—
Melanoma	1	—	0/1	0/1	—	1/1	1/1	—	—	—	—	—	—	—
Angiosarcoma	1	0/1	0/1	0/1	—	—	—	—	—	—	—	—	—	—
Pulmoblastoma	1	—	0/1	0/1	—	—	1/1	—	—	0/1	0/1	0/1	—	—
Malignant triton tumor	1	—	1/1	1/1	—	1/1	1/1	0/1	—	—	—	0/1	—	—
Leiomyosarcoma	1	1/1	—	—	—	1/1	0/1	—	—	—	—	—	—	—
Neurofibrosarcoma	1	0/1	—	—	—	1/1	0/1	—	—	—	—	—	—	—
Neurogenic sarcoma	1	0/1	0/1	—	—	0/1	—	1/1	—	—	—	—	—	—
Malignant schwannoma	1	—	0/1	0/1	—	0/1	—	—	—	1/1	1/1	—	—	—
Synovial sarcoma	1	—	0/1	0/1	—	0/1	0/1	—	—	0/1	0/1	—	—	—
Aggressive fibromatosis	1	—	0/1	0/1	—	—	—	—	—	0/1	1/1	—	—	—
Pseudosarcoma	1	—	0/1	0/1	—	—	—	—	—	—	—	—	—	—

Note: MFH = malignant fibrous histiocytoma.

[a] Number positive/number tested.

diagnosis. If histological findings are supported by the right immunospecific antigen, so much the better. All too often the diagnosis by H & E histology is clear, but is not supported by the immunohistochemical data, because of either inappropriate negative or positive staining.

When tissues are available, a systematic appraisal of the common muscle antigen antibodies will be carried out on all cases registered on IRS-IV. This will be done on alcohol-fixed material utilizing actin, desmin, myoglobin, CK-MM, and vimentin as the initial screen of antibodies. These findings will give a more extensive and detailed database so that issues such as survival can be studied with respect to the immunohistochemical subtypes of RMS. In addition, we may be able to establish more clearly, in a significant number of cases, the role of IHC in the diagnosis of these primitive cell tumors. Other antibodies will be used as well, to permit evaluation of maturity of the tumor cells and correlation of maturity with morphology at the ultrastructural level. The present study mainly utilizes tissues fixed with formalin, which is considered to be less than optimum for obtaining positive stains using muscle specific antibodies.

IV. ULTRASTRUCTURAL FEATURES OF RMS AND RELATED NEOPLASMS

The role of electron microscopy (EM) in the diagnosis of suspected RMS consists largely in resolving the classification of difficult cases. By and large, the majority of RMSs can be diagnosed accurately using a combination of light microscopy and IHC, but a small percentage of cases remain which are classifiable only as undifferentiated sarcoma or sarcoma, NOS (not otherwise specified) by light microscopy and may yield equivocal results by IHC. For these lesions, and other tumors in the differential diagnosis of rhabdomyosarcoma, such as EOE/primitive peripheral neuroectodermal tumor (PNET) and malignant rhabdoid tumor, EM is sometimes helpful in achieving more precise classification.

The classic ultrastructural features of RMS have been well described, and are valid regardless of the subtype of a given tumor.[16,37-44] These EM features are: (1) cytoplasmic arrangements of thin/actin and thick/myosin filaments with Z-band material, forming portions of sarcomeres; (2) amorphous masses of Z-band material with thin, intermediate, or thick filaments radiating from them; (3) thick filaments lined by ribosomes; or (4) some combination of these features. In addition, in tumors which lack any of the above features, it is possible to distinguish poorly differentiated, primitive RMS from EOE sarcoma ultrastructurally.[42] The tumor cells of primitive RMS tend to have oblong or spindled nuclei, accumulations of thin and intermediate filaments, focal cytoplasmic densities, occasional phagocytosed collagen, abundant extracellular collagenous matrix, and occasional basal lamina material. On the other hand, EOE sarcoma tends to have round nuclei and lacks the other features. Many primitive tumors with these features will also be identifiable as RMS by IHC, while others lack myogenous antigens and are true undifferentiated or primitive sarcomas as determined by these methods.

Ultrastructural studies of RMS have shown that EM is able to identify definitive muscle structures in about half of the tumors.[43] This makes is a less sensitive technique to identify a tumor as RMS than light microscopy or IHC.[44] The cells vary widely as to their degree of differentiation but follow a pattern similar to that seen in normal myogenesis. Those tumors that do not contain myoblastic features appear as undifferentiated embryonic cells without other identifying features. Those with specific myofilaments and/or Z-band material show a wide range of differentiation, from less than 1% of cells to a majority showing differentiation. The most advanced state of differentiation is at the myotube level. Ultrastructural features do not separate embryonal from alveolar subtypes.[44] One study assessed the relative value of EM vs. IHC in identifying a primitive round cell tumor such as RMS.[36]

TABLE 4
Review of Tumors from IRS-I to -III; diagnoses
Excluded from Study

Type of tumor	IRS-I	IRS-II	Total
Neuroblastoma	6	4	10
Malignant lymphoma	4	15	19
Fibrosarcoma	6	6	12
Malignant fibrous histiocytoma	9	4	13
Bone sarcoma	3	3	6
Miscellaneous sarcomas	11	11	22
Miscellaneous carcinomas	1	5	6
Benign tumors	2	1	3
Other	—	11	11
TOTAL	42	60	102

It was found that EM was a more sensitive method than using myoglobin and desmin immunostains. This conclusion was confirmed by one study[40] but not by others.[3,45]

Another category of neoplasm which may resemble RMS clinically or pathologically is malignant rhabdoid tumor of soft tissues.[41,42,46,47] This tumor is characterized ultrastructurally by dense whorls of intermediate filaments forming spherical cytoplasmic inclusions, which result in an eosinophilic, hyaline cytoplasm by light microscopy. IHC studies have demonstrated that the intermediate filaments may be positive for vimentin, keratin, desmin, or a combination of these proteins. Pure rhabdoid tumors, in which the vast majority of the cells contain these intermediate filament whorls, are regarded as entities distinct from RMS and are notable for their extremely aggressive course and poor prognosis. However, bona fide RMSs may harbor areas resembling the rhabdoid phenotype, with more of the usual features of RMS found in other regions of the tumor.[48,49] These rhabdoid areas may only be apparent by EM, and are not sufficient evidence for diagnosis of rhabdoid tumor in the face of other light microscopic, IHC, or EM features of RMS.

In recent ultrastructural studies of tumors of patients enrolled in the IRS-III, it was found that tumors could be divided into three groups by EM. The tumors were divided according to the degree of skeletal myogenesis as defined by the classical criteria described above.[48] In the first group were tumors showing extensive myogenic differentiation in almost every cell. The second group consisted of cases with only occasional differentiated cells, and in the third group no myogenesis was observed. Survival was associated with the degree of myogenesis. Thus, patients in the first group had a 90% 4-year survival, while patients whose tumors expressed little or no differentiation had a survival of only 60% at 4 years. Other reports tend to confirm this association between prognosis and differentiation in RMS.[47-53] Thus, for the purpose of classification as RMS, the degree of differentiation as a correlate of survival may have significance apart from the simple observation of the presence or absence of differentiation. This would be true whether the differentiation was assessed by light microscopy, EM, IHC, or even Myo D-1 expression.

V. DIFFERENTIAL DIAGNOSIS

One of the important reasons to conduct a review of pathologic findings in cases entered on the IRS is to advise the study committee when the institutional and review pathologists disagree. If the review diagnosis does not include one of the above eligible categories, then a recommendation is made to exclude the case from analysis in the study. This accounted for about 6% of all cases registered on IRS-I and -II.[53] Table 4 lists the general categories of diagnoses recommended for exclusion. The ''other'' category was nonmorphologic. The list of these diagnoses of exclusion goes from the obvious to ones for which exclusion from the study would be questionable. Diagnoses such as neuroblastoma, malignant lymphoma, fibrosarcoma, and miscellaneous carcinomas would, by anyone's standards, be appropriate for exclusion from the study. Likewise, bone sarcomas were excluded from study for obvious reasons. A few patients were registered with a diagnosis of fibrosarcoma, or at least interpreted by the study committee to be that. Other patients had malignant fibrous histiocytoma along with a variety of miscellaneous sarcomas of the more rare types including liposarcoma, neurofibrosarcoma, leiomyosarcoma, angiosarcoma, synovial sarcoma, epitheliod sarcoma, etc. During this study the entity of rhabdoid tumor of the kidney and subsequently, rhabdoid tumor of soft tissues was developed. Categorically, these patients were all considered to be ineligible for the study. Neural tumors, such as malignant schwanoma, malignant triton tumors, and ectomesenchymoma, were excluded as well as occasional patients with malignant peripheral neuroectodermal tumor.

Another reason for exclusion of patients from study analysis was the occurrence of lesions that would ordinarily be eligible for study except that they occurred in the kidney, lung, liver, brain, or heart. The reason for excluding these sites was that tumors of these areas frequently show multiple cell lines as seen in tumors of the liver, kidney, and brain. Therefore, the biology of their tumors could be significantly different and should not be put into the study with other more common types of RMS. The second reason for excluding these patients was that the number of patients with tumors in these sites was small.

Nonrenal rhabdoid tumor is not specifically named in Table 4. This lesion was not known to exist at the outset of IRS-I, and even now remains a somewhat controversial diagnosis. A recent review of all cases on IRS I-III identified 26 examples of this lesion.[54] It was concluded that there are cases whose morphology is similar to renal rhabdoid tumors by light microscopy, IHC, and ultrastructure. The patients often were infants under one year of age. The tumors predominantly affected soft tissues of the proximal extremities, trunk, retroperitoneum, and pelvis/abdomen. Nineteen died within an interval of 1 to 82 months (median 8 months) from the start of therapy. This survival data is in sharp contrast to patients with RMS.

During this study, 27 RMSs were identified which showed abundant cells with rhabdoid features.[49] They were shown to be RMS and not rhabdoid tumors of soft tissue because of the presence of a more coarse pattern of nuclear chromatin and positive immunocytochemical stains for muscle antigens. The survival of this group was better than that of patients with soft tissue rhabdoid tumors and was similar to comparable patients with RMS.

A number of newly described tumors have appeared during the period of time that the IRS studies were being carried out. One of the earliest newly described tumors was EOE sarcoma which was separated from the group of undifferentiated sarcomas. Others were the nonrenal rhabdoid tumor and PNET. This latter tumor has stimulated considerable interest and controversy. In order to better understand this controversy, it is appropriate that we review some of the historical basis for this diagnosis and the concepts that now exist.

The first description of PNET was by Stout in 1918,[56] who called attention to an ulnar nerve tumor made up of small rounded cells forming rosettes which grew axons in tissue culture, thus confirming their neuroblastic nature.

In retrospect, the tumor described by Askin in 1979[57] appears to be the first reference to a clinically important group of tumors in childhood developing in the thoracopulmonary region. It was not called a PNET because of the fact that the cases were frequently devoid of or contained little glycogen, which is one of the common features of PNET. Subsequently, many otherwise identical cases have been shown to contain abundant glycogen. The other features are consistent with PNET, with a uniform cellular proliferation of poorly differentiated cells which only occasionally showed structures suggestive of Homer-Wright pseudorosettes. Ultrastructurally, there was evidence of narrow to broad cytoplasmic processes and infrequent membrane bound, electron dense granules of neurosecretory type.

A review of the primary chest wall tumors of children collected in one study[58] identified a series of similar patients in which 3 out of 12 showed features suggestive of neuroectodermal differentiation. EM and immunohistologic findings further strengthened this interpretation. Neuroectodermal tumors were also observed to occur in bone.[59] The diagnosis was based strongly on the presence of NSE reactions in the tissue sections and in the long-term cultures. In addition, the tissue culture cells put out moderately long beaded processes in serum free medium, suggesting the neural nature of the cells. Ultrastructurally, there was only a rare neurosecretory granule. These findings were confirmed and neural histogenesis was demonstrated in tumor cell lines obtained from Ewing's tumor of bone.[60]

Subsequently, a number of reports have confirmed these findings and have prompted a number of nosologic discussions concerning the nature of these tumors and their interrelationship with other neoplasms.[61,62] From a clinical point of view, it was shown that peripheral neuroepithelioma is a tumor responsive to both chemotherapy and radiotherapy.[63]

When studying the series of patients with EOE sarcoma from the IRS-I and -II it was demonstrated that about 1 out of 7 patients with EOE sarcoma had features suggestive of PNET, with the presence of Homer-Wright-type rosettes and presence of positive staining to NSE and S-100 antibodies in a small number of cases.[21] Analysis of this phenomenon suggested that there is a continuum from EOE into other tumors. EOE tumor may be composed of a mixture of primitive undifferentiated neuroblastic and Schwannian cells, as represented by positive NSE staining for neuroblastic and positive S-100 staining for Schwannian cells. It has been suggested that EOE lesions, which do not show these neural features, represent a more undifferentiated state of a tumor which may differentiate into a variety of patterns based on the activation of one of these components.

Another review of this group of tumors has shown similar findings,[64] which indicated the need for an extended analysis, utilizing modern molecular biological technology to better understand the interrelationship of these tumors. It was noted that with combined modality therapy, the group designated PNET type did less well and survived a substantially shorter time than did patients with disseminated Ewing's sarcoma or disseminated neuroblastoma. Because of the relatively small number of children with EOE tumor, that tumor was not compared with PNET. It is clear from survival data from IRS-I and -II that EOE sarcoma patients respond to therapy in a fashion similar to those children with embryonal RMS. Thus, EOE tumors are considered as favorable morphology at the present time.

Additional evidence to support the interrelationship of PNET to Ewing's sarcoma of bone and EOE sarcoma is the demonstration of a reciprocal chromosomal translocation t(11;22) (q24;q12).[34,40,65,66] This finding suggests that Ewing's sarcoma may be derived from primitive and pleuripotential cells differentiating into mesenchymal, epithelial, and neural features in variable proportions. In a recent report,[67] a Japanese boy was born with a soft tissue mass in his right temporal facial region that had the morphology of primitive neuroectodermal tumor and contained glial proliferation. This finding supports the concept that PNET originates from pleuripotential cells.[68]

A committee of pathologists is developing an international classification for soft tissue sarcomas of children. Because of the current lack of ways to definitively separate EOE tumor from primitive neuroectodermal tumor, the committee recommended that for the near future these tumors should be considered jointly and not be separated for study purposes. All cases with a review diagnosis of PNET have been excluded from IRS I-III, but will be included in IRS-IV.

VI. PROGNOSTIC FACTORS

A. SITE

IRS-I patients with tumors in certain sites including extremity, parameningeal, trunk, and retroperitoneal, showed a poor survival.[69] The parameningeal site owes its poor outcome to the unique tendency of RMSs to extend locally.[70] Patients with extremity and trunk lesions had an unusually high incidence of alveolar morphology. Patients with retroperitoneal primary sites had the worst outcome, but this was not associated with alveolar histology. It is postulated that occurrence of tumors in this remote site makes early diagnosis difficult.

1. Extremity

It became clear early in the IRS-I study that children with extremity RMSs were experiencing a poor survival and the patients with alveolar histology were doing less well than those with embryonal histology.[71] Patients entered on IRS-I from 1972 until 1978 showed a mortality rate of 63% for those who had alveolar morphology, as compared with a mortality of 39% among patients with all other (nonalveolar) types combined. The predominant sites for these alveolar lesions were perianal, extremities, and trunk. The extremity as a site was associated with a poor survival in IRS-I, with a 5 year survival rate of only 47%, compared with a survival rate of 89% in all primary sites. This prompted an amendment to IRS-II shortly after the study opened. Intensified therapy was given to patients with extremity tumors in clinical groups I and II[71] and these patients were to be compared to the IRS-I control group. Patients given the more intensive therapy had a longer 3 year disease-free survival of marginal significance, T = 0.06 (69% vs. 57%). Clinicopathologic studies from IRS-I and -II showed that alveolar morphology in all sites was associated with a poor outcome. In addition, sites showing a particularly high incidence of alveolar subtype included the extremities as well as the perineum and anal area.[53]

2. Parameningeal

One of the sites associated with poor survival is that generally designated as cranial parameningeal. This was clinically identified during IRS-I.[69] It was reported that lesions located in sites adjacent to meninges including nasopharynx-nasal cavity, the middle ear-mastoid region, the paranasal sinuses (maxillary, ethmoid, and sphenoid), the pterygo-palatine-infratemporal fossa, and the parapharyngeal region, developed extension through the cranial bone into the meningeal spaces in 35% of the cases. (Figure 1). Once established, this extension of tumor led to death in 90% of these patients.[69] Another report described the sequence of events of tumor extension by review of IRS autopsy data on these patients.[70] Local extension led to cerebrospinal fluid dissemination of tumor to the brain, and in some cases there was invasion of the spinal meninges.[73] Figure 2 shows tumor cell infiltration of the meninges and Virchow-Robin spaces. IRS-II patients with parameningeal tumors were given an intensified treatment with a widened field of radiation together with cerebrospinal radiation and intrathecal chemotherapy. This proved to be successful in reducing the incidence of tumor extension to 6%, and the 3 year survival was 90%, compared to 57% in patients not give this intensified therapy.[78] This significant advance was a major factor in the improved survival of patients with group III tumors (having gross residual disease) in IRS-II.

3. Orbit

On the other hand, application of multimodal therapy has resulted in a very improved survival for patients with tumors in certain sites, notably the orbit and in the paratesticular area, and to a lesser extent, for the nonparameningeal head and neck lesions. Before the advent of modern chemotherapy, survival of patients with orbital RMS was only 20%. With the addition of aggressive management with chemotherapy and radiotherapy and, to a lesser extent, surgery, the 3 year survival rate for these tumors in IRS-I and -II was 93%. The reasons for this superior survival rate are not clear. The predominant histology is embryonal. Tumors in the majority of the patients were not surgically excised but given post-biopsy radiation and systemic chemotherapy. Although the incidence by sex was about equal at diagnosis, almost all of the relapsed patients were female and 3 of the 5 children who died were under the age of 12 months.[72]

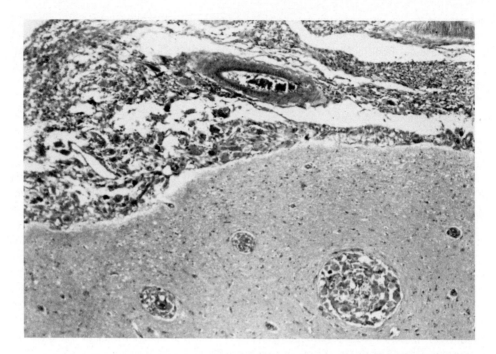

A

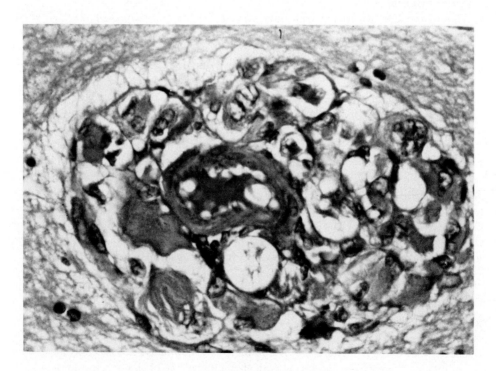

B

FIGURE 2.   (A) Infiltration of the meninges by RMS (H&E stain, magnification × 100) and (B) invasion of Virchow-Robin spaces (magnification × 500) in a patient with parameningeal sarcoma with extension.

4. Paratesticular

The paratesticular site was shown to be one having a favorable outcome in the early analysis of IRS-I.[73] This finding was further confirmed in the analysis of patients with tumors of that site in IRS-I and -II.[74] The overall survival of this group was 89% at 3 years compared to the survival rate of 63% for the entire IRS series. The tumor was typed as embryonal in 97% of these cases. It was noted earlier that, in patients treated on IRS-I, this site was associated with a subtype of embryonal RMS. This subtype, called type A, was associated with a survival rate as high as 85.2%. This observation was made while conducting a cytohistologic study of all lesions of IRS-I patients.[23].

This site has been subjected to a detailed analysis of its histology and will be reported separately. In brief, there is a high incidence of a spindle cell type lesion in paratesticular tumors which have a more favorable outcome than classical RMS.[76] With rare exceptions, this different pattern seen in the paratesticular site is not seen elsewhere in the body.

B. STAGE

Another important prognostic factor in RMS patients is the extent of disease at diagnosis. From the beginning of the IRS studies, the classification of the extent of tumors has been on the basis of the post-surgical grouping of patients rather than by traditional presurgical staging. This has been a very workable concept. The system, as first devised, was quite effective in separating patients on the basis of their expected outcome, particularly in IRS-I.[77] However, as therapy changed, the grouping system became less predictive because of the improvement of survival of patients in groups II and III.[78] This was largely due to a shift of patients previously classified as tumors of lesser extent to include those with gross residual disease, as well as due to improvements in therapy. This system is not completely satisfactory in that it limits the opportunity to do a study involving a surgical question. There was considerable interest in the development of an internationally acceptable staging system as well. Thus, patients being entered on IRS-IV will undergo staging presurgically and this information will be combined with the traditional grouping system for study purposes.

This new system will take into account the fact that certain sites are associated with a favorable survival rate while others have unfavorable survival. It also considers tumor size, tumor invasiveness, presence or absence of lymph node metastases regionally, and the presence or absence of distant metastases. It has been shown that tumors with diameters of 5 cm or more have a significantly less favorable outcome than smaller tumors, as do tumors showing invasiveness.[79] While the morphology of the tumors will be classified by committee review, the treatment design is not based on morphologic subtypes as it was to some extent in IRS-III.

C. HISTOLOGY

The question as to whether histologic subtype is a predictor of outcome has been very controversial. Histologic subtype was shown to be a predictor of survival in the analysis of data from IRS-I and -II. (Figure 3). This study was based upon survival data for 1628 patients who were eligible for analysis. Patients with botryoid histology fared the best, those with the alveolar type and undifferentiated sarcoma fared the worst, while those with embryonal rhabdomyosarcoma and EOE sarcoma had an intermediate survival rate. Even prior to the advent of the IRS studies, patients with the alveolar subtype were considered to have a less favorable outcome.

In IRS-I it was clearly shown that the alveolar histologic subtype is associated with a number of unfavorable prognostic features.[71] First of all, there was a higher mortality rate among those patients with alveolar histology, with a mortality rate of 63% compared to 39% for all other histologic subtypes. This subtype was seen in less than 20% of the patients but accounted for more than 29% of death ($p < 0.001$). It was also observed that patients with alveolar RMS showed increased local, regional, and distant metastases, which was partic-

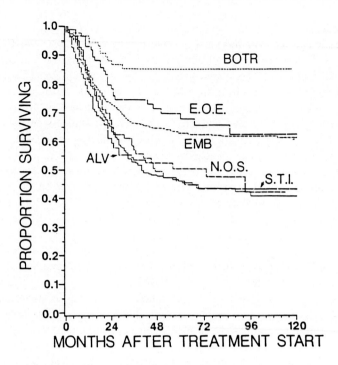

FIGURE 3.   Kaplan-Meier survival estimates by histologic subtype for
1626 patients in IRS-I and IRS-II.

ularly evident in those with tumors classified in clinical groups I and II. In patients with
grossly resected tumor (groups I and II), there was a 44% mortality rate in those with alveolar
morphology, compared to a mortality rate of 16% for all other patients. When the mortality
of patients with the alveolar type was compared to that of other subtypes of RMS according
to clinical group, group I patients with alveolar tumors showed a 38.5% mortality rate
compared to a mortality rate of only 4.8% for all other group I patients. In group II, the
mortality rate was 45.7% (alveolar) vs. 22.5% (all others), group III, 60.6% (alveolar) vs.
44.6% (all others), and in group IV 90.6% (alveolar) vs. 74.4% (all others).

   This finding of increased mortality was also observed when comparing according to site
the mortality rate of patients having alveolar lesions with the mortality of those with tumors,
of other histologies. The mortality rate was twice as high in the patients with alveolar RMSs
in the orbit, the mortality rate was about the same in head and neck overall. In the trunk it
was 65% (alveolar) vs. 39% (all others), extremities 60% (alveolar) vs. 50% (all others),
GU 75% (alveolar) vs. 21% (all others), intrathoracic 100% (alveolar) vs. 66% (all others),
perineum 66% (alveolar) vs. 75% (all others), retroperineum 88.9% (alveolar) vs. 54% (all
others), and GI tract 100% (alveolar) vs. 75% (all others). While one would have expected
that there would be an increased incidence of alveolar subtypes in patients with advanced
disease, this was not the case. The proportion of patients with the alveolar subtype was
actually about the same in all of the sites.

   From a review of the pathology of cases of fatal RMS from IRS-I and IRS-II, there
appeared to be a difference in the biological behavior of alveolar tumors.[80] This subtype
showed the highest rate of distant metastases and the lowest rate of local recurrence. In
patients with alveolar tumors, there were three times as many distant metastases, with or
without local progressive disease, as compared to local progression alone. In alveolar RMSs
of extremities, the proportion of distant metastases without local progression was considerably higher than with any other histologic type of this tumor.

   Because of the findings of IRS-I, the IRS-II study was designed to give increased intensity of therapy to patients with alveolar RMS of the extremities classified in clinical groups I and II. This resulted in an increase in the percentage of 3-year disease-free survival and overall survival of 69% (IRS-II) vs. 43% (IRS-I) and 77% (IRS-II) vs. 57% (IRS-I).[78] One conclusion of the IRS-II study was that repetitive pulse VAC (chemotherapy with vincristine, actinomycin D, and cyclophosphamide) increases disease-free survival in groups I and II patients with extremity alveolar lesions. Because of this finding, portions of IRS-III were designed to treat lesions with alveolar histology as an unfavorable predictor of outcome. These lesions were, therefore, given more intensive therapy. The final analysis of this data is not complete, but the overall survival rate for patients in IRS-III shows a significant improvement compared to those in IRS-I and -II. This is the case for all groups combined, being most marked in group I and III, with little change seen in patients in group IV.

A study was done to determine whether a presurgical staging system would be appropriate for future protocols. Patients selected for that study had been treated on IRS-II and had received more intensive therapy for extremity tumors with alveolar histology classified in clinical groups I and II.[81] When an analysis for histology as a prognostic factor was done, the lesions diagnosed as alveolar were added to those lesions predicted to be unfavorable, namely the monomorphous and anaplastic types.[23] Thus, the study did not evaluate alveolar morphology as a separate entity. It was shown by multivariate analysis that histology was not a prominent predictor of outcome in this group of patients. Site of primary tumor and extent of disease were found to be more predictive of outcome.

Although IRS-III was based upon the principle that alveolar morphology is associated with an unfavorable outcome, the study was designed to compensate for this behavior by increased intensity of therapy. The results of the study are not yet available. As with IRS-II, because of improved therapy, patients with alveolar RMS who had a relatively unfavorable outcome in the past may now show a survival rate similar to other histologic subtypes. It will be important to make sure that patients with alveolar histology are watched carefully in future studies, so that this apparent biological difference does not re-emerge as a significant factor when similar therapy is given to all histologic subtypes.

One of the histologic categories associated with poor survival in the cytohistologic study by Palmer was his group called anaplastic tumors.[23] The definition for this subgroup was the presence of abnormal multipolar mitotic figures in large cells, those about three times normal diameter. These cells were usually seen in tumors with many cells showing enlarged hyperchromatic nuclei. His analysis of survival was done by combining this group of patients with those of his second unfavorable category, the monomorphous round cell tumor. In another study of the tumors of 63 patients with RMS or undifferentiated sarcoma, seen since 1964, the most significant feature associated with poor survival was the presence of cellular anaplasia. This anaplasia was defined as nuclear enlargement, and the presence of hyperchromasia and abnormal mitoses.[82] Out of 47 patients in which sufficient clinical data was available for correlation, 12 patients with these features died on an average of about 2 years from diagnosis and only 10 of the remaining 33 died.

In an attempt to define the category of pleomorphic subtype of RMS, a study was performed on cases from IRS-I to -III.[83] This study showed that the presence of large hyperchromatic nuclei, either in single scattered cells, in groups of cells, or in cells diffusely situated throughout the tumor, was associated with a less favorable outcome.

D. BIOLOGIC FACTORS

Not only are embryonal and alveolar subtypes separable on histologic grounds, but a number of studies of the biologic nature of these two tumors have shown that there are significant molecular differences as well. Table 5 lists some reported changes in chromosomal structure and number, DNA content, and oncogene expression found in these two subtypes.[84-90] Deletion of the RBI gene is now being reported in a number of tumors other than

TABLE 5
Biological Differences in Subtypes of RMS

Molecular biology	Subtype of RMS			Ref.
	Alveolar	Embryonal	Pleomorphic	
Oncogenes				
C-Myc	Increased			84
N-Myc	5—20× increased	Not increased		86
	Not increased			84
N-ras and K-ras		Mutations seen in 35%		
Cytogenetics				
T(2,13)(q37;q14)		Trisomy 2		88
		Loss of constitutional heterozygosity for 11p		46
			Heterozygous loss of RB, gene	91
DNA content				
	Near tetraploid	Hyperdiploid		90
Muscle gene expression	Myo D, present	Myo D, present		46

retinoblastoma, including heterozygous deletion in a case of the so-called pleomorphic RMS.[89] In light of our current concepts of the nature of this histologic category, this case was probably an embryonal RMS. Clearly, there are significant differences between the embryonal and alveolar subtypes. These molecular differences support our continued study of the significant behavioral differences of these variants. As these types of studies continue, the finding of additional differences and similarities of genes may lead us to improved understanding of etiologic mechanisms for the pathogenesis of these neoplasms.

E. DIFFERENTIATION

It was suggested that the extent of differentiation of embryonal RMS, as determined by light microscopy and IHC, is related to the response to therapy.[50] Histologically, three subgroups were identified: primitive (containing less than 10% rhabdomyoblasts); intermediates (10 to 50% rhabdomyoblasts); and differentiated (more than 50% rhabdomyoblasts). Vimentin-positive cells predominated in the primitive tumors, a mixture of vimentin and desmin positive cells predominated in the intermediate stage, and myoglobin was predominant in the well-differentiated tumors. The sites of the three levels of differentiation also were different, with the primative and well-differentiated tumors occurring in the head and neck, and tumors with intermediate differentiation being in the abdomen. In another study of 47 cases, it was also observed that patients with well-differentiated tumors were more likely to survive.[82] However, a study using EM and IHC did show a correlation between degrees of tumor differentiation and survival rate.[41]

These studies were based on a limited number of cases, with response to therapy used as an indication of expected long-term behavior of the tumor.[50] When a similar study was carried out on 645 patients entered on IRS-II, with tumors having either embryonal or alveolar histology, the differences in survival rates of the patients with poor, intermediate, and well-differentiated tumors were not prognostically significant. This study is still in progress.[92]

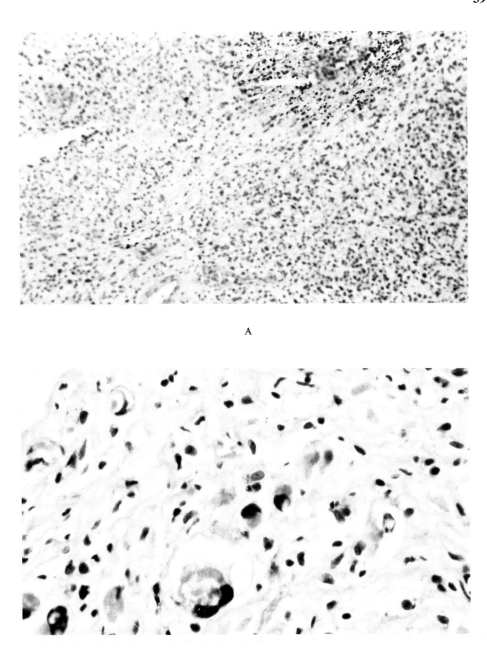

FIGURE 4. (A) Embryonal RMS pretherapy (H&E stain, magnification $\times$ 100). (B) The same lesion post-therapy showing maturation of the tumor cells (H&E stain, magnification $\times$ 500).

Therapy of RMS of certain pelvic sites in IRS-III consisted of initial chemotherapy followed by surgical excision of any residual tumor. In those patients whose tumors at initial surgery had not been totally excised, the remaining tumor cells removed at the second operation almost always showed considerable maturation when compared to the initial biopsy[93] (Figure 4). The biological activity of these cells is not known. At present these cells are considered to have malignant behavior.

VII. EPIDEMIOLOGY

A limited search of the literature has been carried out to determine the expected incidence of various childhood sarcomas (Table 6). The data from Harms are taken from the Pediatric Tumor Registry of the German Society of Pediatric Oncology located in Kiel.[94] The classification techniques in this series used the most recent advances in histopathological methodology. This collection represents most of the cases seen in Germany and all cases were studied in recent years.

Marsden's data represents the closest definition of the true incidence of these tumors in a defined geographic area. This is a collection of tumors from a well-defined population of children over an extended period of years, and all of the tumors were pathologically reviewed by an expert pediatric pathologist with particular interest in childhood cancer. This data was derived from the Manchester University Children's Tumor Registry in England.

Soule's data need to be considered to be nonincidence in type because they are derived from the total experience of the Mayo Clinic over a 16-year-period, 1950 through 1965.[17] This data was the first to show the importance of a group of tumors of unknown histogenesis.

The data from the Department of Pathology of Kyushu University are another series that were classified by use of the newest histologic methods. The data were collected from a Japanese population by a single university center, from children up to 15 years of age.[96]

The data from the Tumor Registry of Columbus (Ohio) Children's Hospital include the accumulated experience of over 35 years at a single pediatric institution located in the midwestern United States.[97] This hospital is a referral center and sees almost all children with cancer within the geographic area of service. The pathologic review has been consistent, carried out by a continuum of similar observers over this period.

The report of Strong lists children at M. D. Anderson Cancer Center who survived 3 years or more during a study extending 32 years.[98] This is the only study in which patients who died early were excluded. Obviously, this could influence the mix of tumor subtypes. However, since the ability of clinicians to cure patients with these types of tumors has been achieved in relatively recent times, and since the most recent of these cases was in 1976, the list would probably not have been much different if the entire series (including those cases who survived less than 3 years) had been given.

The last set of epidemiologic data was derived from the Third National Cancer Survey of the National Cancer Institute as reported initially by Silverberg in 1977.

A. LI-FRAUMENI SYNDROME

In this syndrome, mothers of children with RMS develop breast cancer at an early age and there is an increased incidence of a variety of other tumors in the family.[99] While the complete extent of this genetic syndrome has not been completely determined, it is clear that RMS is an important element. The Li-Fraumeni syndrome represents one of the few conditions in which clinical genetic factors are likely to play a role in the production of RMS. It is important that we examine the individuals in these pedigrees and study the morphology of any tumors for possible clues as to the etiology of their cancers. Unfortunately, the data available are still limited. The morphologic subtype of the RMSs in those cases where this information is known does not suggest that a particular tumor subtype is involved. (Table 7).

B. SECOND MALIGNANT TUMORS

A total of 378 children who developed a second primary cancer have been registered on an international protocol study.[100] The histopathology of this group of patients is under review. Diagnoses of the types of soft tissue tumors at present are a mixture of central review and institutional opinions, based upon H & E stained slides only. No attempt has been made in this analysis to separate those patients who have predisposing genetic factors, such as history of retinoblastoma.

TABLE 6
Incidence of Soft Tissue Sarcoma; types in Various Reported Series

Type of soft tissue sarcoma	Incidence (%) in various series							
	Harms	Marsden	Soule	Enjoji	Columbus	Strong	N.C.I.	Average
RMS	64.5	63.0	55.0	57.5	62.4	40.4	51.4	55.4
Undifferentiated or NOS	0.0	0.0	18.0	10.2	12.4	28.2	10.6	11.3
Fibrosarcoma	4.6	12.0	4.4	19.3	2.8	10.4	10.8	9.2
Synovial sarcoma	9.1	6.0	7.4	4.3	2.3	0.0	5.6	4.9
Malignant schwannoma or neurofibrosarcoma	5.0	2.4	3.7	4.5	3.7	5.0	3.4	3.6
Leiomyosarcoma	5.0	2.6	2.0	0.0	0.0	0.0	0.0	1.4
Malignant fibrous histiocytoma	1.5	2.0	0.0	0.0	8.2	0.0	0.0	1.7
PNET	1.5	0.0	0.0	3.4	0.0	0.0	0.0	0.7
EOE	0.0	0.0	0.0	0.0	3.2	0.0	0.0	0.5
Liposarcoma	0.0	1.5	1.5	0.0	0.0	0.0	4.5	1.0
Other	5.7	10.6	7.4	6.8	5.0	15.9	13.5	9.3
Total cases	262	150	135	88	215	163	UNK	

Note: NOS = sarcoma not otherwise specified; EOE = extraosseous Ewing's sarcoma.

TABLE 7
Soft Tissue Sarcomas Reported in the Li-Fraumeni Syndrome

Type of soft tissue sarcoma	Number	Percent
RMS, all types	9	39.0
Undifferentiated sarcoma	4	17.0
Leiomyosarcoma	3	13.0
Fibrosarcoma	2	9.0
Malignant fibrous histiocytoma	1	4.0
Other	4	17.0
TOTAL	23	

Forty-nine of the 378 primary and 66 second tumors were considered to be of soft tissue origin. RMS was the most common type of primary tumor (41%) but comprised only 9% of the second tumors. Malignant neural and fibrous tumors were uncommon primary tumors (6% and 4%), but more commonly occurred as second tumors (18% and 14%). Malignant fibrous histiocytoma, a relatively recently identified category of tumor, accounted for 10% of primary and 14% of second tumors. Perhaps more definitive differences will emerge as this study reveals distinctions allowing more precise diagnoses on these patients.

C. MALFORMATIONS AND RMS

There may be a common basis for pathogenesis of childhood cancer and birth defects. Thus, the available autopsy data regarding the incidence of malformations in children registered on IRS-I and -II was reviewed with a focus on the histology of the tumors in the children with birth defects.[75]

Congenital anomalies were identified in 37 out of 115 (32%) children and adolescents. Of the 45 identified anomalies, 14 were considered major and 31 minor. The distribution of the anomalies by system included central nervous system (9), genitourinary tract (10), gastrointestinal tract (13), and cardiovascular system (4). Ten patients had complex or miscellaneous anomalies. There was one child with each of the following: Rubinstein-Taybi syndrome; neurofibromatosis; single horseshoe kidney; hemihypertrophy; and Arnold-Chiari malformation. Aniridia was not noted in any cases of RMS.

The histologic types of RMS in children with congenital anomalies when compared to the total group of patients studied on IRS-I and -II show that the embryonal and alveolar types in children with congenital anomalies have a distribution similar to that of the group as a whole. In contrast, tumors of the undifferentiated type are significantly more common in children with congenital anomalies.

VIII. CASES OF INTEREST

Two unusual family histories illustrate familial cancer in siblings. In one, a brother developed an embryonal orbital RMS early in life which was cured, only to develop an osteosarcoma in the site of radiation therapy. His brother developed an osteosarcoma not in bone, but in an extraosseous site 10 years after his brother was first diagnosed. Their mother remains free of tumors.

In the second family, RMS occurred in two brothers. The first had an inoperable retroperitoneal embryonal tumor which led to death in 15 months. The second brother developed a laryngeal embryonal RMS which was excised but he died a few weeks later because of bleeding from the tracheostomy site. Their mother is living and well. However their father died from multiple myeloma.

Two other patients are of interest. The first of these is a black female who was first seen in June 1973, at the age of 19 years for a tumor of her right ethmoid-maxillary area. The tumor showed nasopharyngeal extension and metastases to the right cervical nodes and right parotid gland. The diagnosis by biopsy was embryonal RMS. She was given radiotherapy at a dose of 5800 cGy to the right maxillary-ethmoid areas, and chemotherapy consisted of VAC. Her local tumor mass and the regional metastases were well controlled and have never recurred. A nodule which was a similar type RMS was removed from her right breast 2 years later. The breast was radiated and additional chemotherapy was given. In December 1976, a lump was removed from her left breast, which was also a similar RMS. Repeated chest X-rays have been consistently negative throughout her course to date. She delivered a healthy daughter in January, 1981. She was last seen by her physician in December 1987 and was well.

The sequence of events in this patient would appear to be clear early in the course of the tumor, with the primary site being in the head and neck, with extension of the tumor locally, and metastasis to cervical nodes. From that point on, however, the sequence of events is not clear.

A histologically similar embryonal tumor was found in one breast two years later, and a similar tumor in the second breast 18 months after that. There was no evidence of tumor activity elsewhere at that time, or until this date almost 15 years later. One likely possibility is that this patient developed the breast tumors as second and third primary neoplasms.

The breast is an uncommon primary or secondary site of RMS. Only 14 patients registered on IRS-I, -II or -III have tumors that involved this site, 5 as the primary tumor, 9 as metastatic sites. Three of the five patients with breast as primary site of involvement are living after 69 to 256 weeks of followup. Their tumor was either fully excised or there was only microscopic residual. The other two patients had tumors that were metastatic at the time of diagnosis; one had metastases to the axillary lymph nodes, the other had metastases to bone marrow with development of a paravertebral mass which extended to the meninges. Their ages at diagnosis were 12 to 16 years; the histology was alveolar in three of the four that could be classified. Data on the patients whose breast involvement was considered a metastatic site are not yet completely analyzed.

The possibility that there can be more than one primary site of RMS in the same patient is further illustrated in a second patient. This 8 $\frac{1}{2}$-year-old white girl had radical resection of an alveolar RMS from her left vastus lateralis and vastus intermedius muscles. This was followed by radiation therapy of at a dose of 7000 cGy to the left thigh. She remained free of disease until 16 months later when she developed an alveolar RMS near her left scapula, which was excised followed by radiation and chemotherapy. There was no other evidence of tumor at that time or subsequently. She was doing well and without evidence of tumor at 30 years of age. She is married and is now pregnant. Her maternal grandmother had breast cancer diagnosed at age 40; she lived for more than 20 years, dying from heart disease. Her mother has been free of cancer, but her mother's sister had an endometrial cancer.

IX. CONCLUSIONS

This chapter has been an overview of the importance of morphology in the diagnosis and treatment of RMS. This information may also contribute to understanding the behavior of one of the most complex and diversely manifested groups of tumors, which account for about one tenth of all childhood neoplasms. Since these tumors are not seen in great numbers in any one institution, it would not have been possible to compile the data summarized in this chapter without the development of cooperative cancer therapy and research as sponsored by the IRS Group. It has been a privilege to have had the opportunity to be involved with this effort and to have this unprecedented amount of material to study.

This chapter of information on this complicated tumor is just a beginning. With the unfolding of the field of molecular pathology and biology, the next few years promise to yield exciting advances. Dissection of the gene structure of these tumors, along with the determination of exact paths of carcinogenesis may lead to the cure and perhaps prevention of these devastating tumors.

ACKNOWLEDGMENTS

We want to thank all who made this study possible. We include the hundreds of clinicians from all over the U.S. and parts of Europe who participated in clinical studies, the pathologists who were willing to share their case material, the many data managers both at the various institutions and in the IRS statistical center, as well as the National Institutes of Health for financial support. We are also grateful to our families for their patience and understanding.

In addition, we are indebted to the staff at the IRS Pathology Center, particularly Nancy Sachs and Jean Bowers, as well as Drs. Gaiger, Shimada, Leuschner, and Kodet. Dr. Edmund Gehan and his staff at the IRS Statistical Center were of continuous help in providing data and statistical analyses. Finally, we are grateful to Dr. E. H. Soule for the opportunity for sharing his lifelong expertise in soft tissue sarcomas over the early years of this effort.

REFERENCES

1. **Enzinger, F. M. and Weiss, S. W.**, Rhabdomyosarcoma, in *Soft Tissue Tumors,* Enzinger, F. M., Weiss, S. W., Eds., C. V. Mosby, St. Louis, 1983, 338.
2. **Raney, R. B., Hays, D. M., Tefft, M., and Triche, T. J.**, Rhabdomyosarcoma and the undifferentiated sarcomas, in *Principles and Practices of Pediatric Oncology,* Prizzo, P. A., Poplack, D. G., Eds., J. B. Lippincott, Philadelphia, 1989, 635.
3. **Bale, P. M., Parsons, R. E., and Stevens, M. M.**, Pathology and behavior of juvenile rhabdomyosarcoma, in *Pathology of Neoplasia in Children and Adolescents,* Finegold, M., Ed., W. B. Saunders Company, Philadelphia, 1986, 196.
4. **Stout, A. P. and Lattes, R.**, Rhabdomyosarcoma, in *Tumors of Soft Tissues,* Armed Forces Institute of Pathology, Washington, D.C., 1967, F5/89.
5. **Horn, R. C., Jr. and Enterline, H. T.**, Rhabdomyosarcoma; a clinicopathological study and classification of 39 cases, *Cancer,* 11, 181, 1958.
6. **Riopelle, J. L. and Theriault, J. P.**, Sur une forme meconnue de sarcome des parties molles; Le rhabdomyosarcome alveolaire, *Ann. d'Anat. Pathol.,* 1, 88, 1956.
7. **Brizel, D. M., Weinstein, H., and Hunt, M.**, Failure patterns and survival in pediatric soft tissue sarcoma, *Int. J. Radiat. Oncol. Biol. Phys.,* 15, 37, 1988.
8. **Treuner, J., Kaatsch, P., Anger, Y., et al.**, Ergebnisse der Behandlung von Rhabdomyosarkomen (RMS) bei Kindern. Ein Bericht der Cooperativen Weichteilsarkomstudie (CWS-81) der Gesellschaft fur Padiatrische Onkologie, *Klin. Padiatr.,* 198, 208, 1986.
9. **Heyn, R. M., Holland, R., Newton, W. A., Jr., et al.**, The role of combined chemotherapy in the treatment of rhabdomyosarcoma in children, *Cancer,* 34, 2128, 1974.
10. **Hossein-Mahour, G., Soule, E. H., Mills, S. D., and Lynn, H. B.**, Rhabdomyosarcoma in infants and children; a clinicopathologic study of 75 cases, *J. Pediatr. Surg.,* 2, 402, 1967.
11. **Stobbe, G. D. and Dargeon, H. W.**, Embryonal rhabdomyosarcoma of the head and neck in children and adolescents, *Cancer,* 3, 826, 1950.
12. **Enterline, H. T. and Horn, R. C.**, Alveolar rhabdomyosarcoma; a distinctive tumor type, *Am. J. Clin. Pathol.,* 29, 356, 1958.
13. **Patton, R. B. and Horn, R. C., Jr.**, Rhabdomyosarcoma; clinical and pathological features and comparison with human fetal and embryonal skeletal muscle, *Surgery,* 52, 572, 1963.
14. **Lattes, R. and Stout, A. P.**, Rhabdomyosarcoma, in *Tumors of the Soft Tissues,* Hartmann, W. H., Ed., Armed Forces Institute of Pathology, Washington, D.C., 1982, 169.
15. **Hajdu, S. I.**, Tumors of muscle, in *Pathology of Soft Tissue Tumors,* Hajdu, S. I., Ed., Lea & Febiger, Philadelphia, 1979, 325.
16. **Gonzalez-Crussi, F. and Black-Schaffer, S.**, Rhabdomyosarcoma of infancy and childhood; problems of morphologic classification, *Am. J. Surg. Pathol.,* 3, 157, 1979.
17. **Soule, H., Mahour, G. H., Mills, D., and Lynn, H. B.**, Soft-tissue sarcomas of infants and children; a clinicopathologic study of 135 cases, *Mayo Clinic. Proc.,* 43, 313, 1968.
18. **Newton, W. A.**, unpublished observation.
19. **Stern, R.**, Current concepts in the diagnosis of human soft tissue sarcomas, *Hum. Pathol.,* 12, 777, 1981.
20. **Katenkamp, D. and Raikhlin, N. T.**, Stem cell concept and heterogeneity of malignant soft tissue tumor; a challenge to reconsider diagnostics and therapy?, *Exp. Path.,* 28, 3, 1985.
21. **Shimada, H., Newton, W. A., Soule, E. H., et al.**, Pathological features of extraosseous Ewing's sarcoma; a report from the Intergroup Rhabdomyosarcoma Study, *Hum. Pathol.,* 19, 442, 1988.
22. **Seidal, T., Kindblom, L. G., and Angerval, L.**, Rhabdomyosarcoma in middle-aged and elderly individuals, *Acta Pathol. Microbiol. Immunol. Scand.,* 97, 236, 1989.
23. **Palmer, N. F., Sachs, N., and Foulkes, M.**, Histopathology and prognosis in rhabdomyosarcoma, *Abstr., Proc. Int. Soc. Pediatr. Oncol.,* 113, 1981.
24. **Tsokos, M.**, Unpublished observations, 1990.

25. **Tefft, M., Vawter, G. F., and Mitus, A.,** Paravertebral "round cell" tumors in children, *Radiology,* 92, 1501, 1969.
26. **Szakacs, J. E., Carta, M., and Szakacs, M. R.,** Ewing's sarcoma, extraskeletal and of bone; case report with ultrastructural analysis, *Ann. Clin. Lab. Sci.,* 4, 306, 1974.
27. **Soule, E. H., Newton, W. A., Moon, T. E., and Tefft, M.,** Extraskeletal Ewing's sarcoma; a preliminary review of 26 cases encountered in the Intergroup Rhabdomyosarcoma Study, *Cancer,* 42, 259, 1978.
28. **Angervall, L. and Enzinger, F. M.,** Extraskeletal neoplasm resembling Ewing's sarcoma, *Cancer,* 36, 240, 1975.
29. **Schmidt, D., Mackay, B., and Ayala, A. G.,** Ewing's sarcoma with neuroblastoma-like features, *Ultrastruct. Pathol.,* 3, 143, 1982.
30. **Bednar, B.,** Solid dendritic cell angiosarcoma; reinterpretation of extraskeletal sarcoma resembling Ewing's sarcoma, *J. Pathol.,* 30, 217, 1980.
31. **Llombart-Bosch, A., Blache, R., and Peydro-Olaya, A.,** Round-cell sarcomas of bone and their differential diagnosis (with particular emphasis on Ewing's sarcoma and reticulosarcoma), *Pathol. Annu.,* 17, 113, 1982.
32. **Aurias, A., Rimbaut, C., Buff, D., et al.,** Chromosomal translocation in Ewing's sarcoma, *N. Engl. J. Med.,* 309, 496, 1983.
33. **Turc-Carel, C., Philip, I., Berger, M.-P., et al.,** Chromosomal translocation in Ewing's sarcoma, *N. Engl. J. Med.,* 309, 497, 1983.
34. **Becroft, D. M. O., Pearson, A., Shaw, R. L., and Zwi, L. J.,** Chromosome translocation in extraskeletal Ewing's tumor, *Lancet,* 3, 400, 1984.
35. **Moll, R., Lee, I., Gould, V. E., et al.,** Immunocytochemical analysis of Ewing's tumors; patterns of expression of intermediate filaments and desmosomal proteins indicate cell type, *Am. J. Pathol.,* 127, 288, 1987.
36. **Raney, R., Tefft, M., Newton, W. A., et al.,** Improved prognosis with intensive treatment of children with cranial soft tissue sarcomas arising in nonorbital parameningeal sites, *Cancer,* 59, 147, 1987.
37. **Bundtzen, J. L. and Norback, D. H.,** The ultrastructure of poorly differentiated rhabdomyosarcomas, *Hum. Pathol.,* 13, 301, 1982.
38. **Triche, T.,** Pathology of cancer in the young, in *Cancer in the Young,* Levine, A. S., Ed., Masson Publishing, New York, 1982, 119.
39. **Kahn, H. J., Yeger, H., Kassim, O., et al.,** Immunohistochemical and electron microscopic assessment of childhood rhabdomyosarcoma, *Cancer,* 43, 1897, 1983.
40. **Seidal, T. and Kindblom, L. G.,** The ultrastructure of alveolar and embryonal rhabdomyosarcoma; a correlative light and electron microscopic study of 17 cases, *Acta Pathol. Microbiol. Immunol. Scand.,* 92, 231, 1984.
41. **Dickman, P. S.,** Electron microscopy for diagnosis of tumors in children, *Perspect. Pediatr. Pathol.,* 9, 171, 1987.
42. **Dickman, P. S. and Triche, T. J.,** Extraosseous Ewing's sarcoma versus primitive rhabdomyosarcoma, *Hum. Pathol.,* 17, 881, 1986.
43. **Mierau, G. W. and Favara, B. E.,** Rhabdomyosarcoma in children, *Cancer,* 46, 2035, 1980.
44. **Seidal, T., Kindbloom, L.-G., and Angervall, L.,** Alveolar and poorly differentiated rhabdomyosarcoma; a clinico-pathologic, light-microscopic, ultrastructural and immuno-histochemical analysis, *Acta Pathol. Microbiol. Immunol. Scand.,* 96, 825, 1988.
45. **Bale, P. M., Parsons, R. E., and Stevens, M. M.,** Diagnosis and behavior of juvenile rhabdomyosarcoma, *Hum. Pathol.,* 14, 596, 1983.
46. **Scrable, H., Witte, D., Shimada, H., et al.,** Molecular differential pathology of rhabdomyosarcoma, *Genes, Chromosomes and Cancer,* 1989; 1:23-35.
47. **Tsokos, M., Kouraklis, G., Chandra, R. S., et al.,** Malignant rhabdoid tumor of the kidney and soft tissues, *Arch. Pathol. Lab. Med.,* 113, 115, 1989.
48. **Dickman, P. S., Bodner, S., Salahi, W., et al.,** Electron microscopy (EM) and immunohistochemistry (IHC) of rhabdomyosarcoma (RMS); diagnosis and prognosis, *Lab. Invest.,* 62, 27A, 1990.
49. **Kodet, R. and Newton, W. A.,** Rhabdomyosarcomas with intermediate filament inclusions and features of rhabdoid tumors, *Am. J. Surg. Pathol.,* 15, 257, 1991.
50. **Schmidt, D., Reimann, O., Treuner, J., and Harms, D.,** Cellular differentiation and prognosis in embryonal rhabdomyosarcoma, *Virchows. Arch. (Pathol. Anat.),* 409, 183, 1986.
51. **Caillaud, J. M., Gerard-Marchant, R., Marsden, H. B., et al.,** Histopathological classification of childhood rhabdomyosarcoma, *Med. Pediatr. Oncol.,* 17, 391, 1989.
52. **Dickman, P. S. and Triche, T. J.,** Immunocytochemistry and prognosis in pediatric soft tissue sarcomas, unpublished observations, 1990.
53. **Newton, W. A., Jr., Soule, E. H., Hamoudi, A. B., et al.,** Histopathology of childhood sarcomas, Intergroup Rhabdomyosarcoma Studies I and II: Clinicopathologic correlation, *J. Clin. Oncol.,* 6, 67, 1988.

54. **Kodet, R., Newton, W. A., Jr., Sachs, N., et al.,** (for the Intergroup Rhabdomyosarcoma Committee). Rhabdoid Tumors of Soft Tissues; a clinicopathologic study of 26 cases enrolled on the Intergroup Rhabdomyosarcoma Study, *Human Pathology,* 22, 674, 1991.
55. **Tsokos, M. and Triche, T. J.,** Primative "solid variant" rhabdomyosarcoma, *Lab. Invest.,* 54, 65A, 1986.
56. **Stout, A. P.,** Tumor of the ulnar nerve, *Proc. New York Pathol. Soc.,* 18, 2, 1918.
57. **Askin, F. B., Rosai, J., Sibley, R. K., et al.,** Malignant small cell tumor of the thoracopulmonary region in childhood; a distinctive clinicopathologic entity of uncertain histogenesis, *Cancer,* 43, 2438, 1979.
58. **Gonzalez-Crussi, F., Wolfson, S. L., Misugi, K., and Nakajima, T.,** Peripheral neuroectodermal tumors of the chest wall in childhood, *Cancer,* 54, 2519, 1984.
59. **Jaffe, R., Santamaria, M., Yunis, E. J., et al.,** The neuroectodermal tumor of bone, *Am. J. Surg. Pathol.,* 8, 885, 1984.
60. **Cavazzana, A. O., Miser, J. S., and Jefferson, H. T. L.,** Experimental evidence for neural origin of Ewing's Sarcoma of bone, *Am. J. Pathol.,* 127, 507, 1987.
61. **Dehner, L. P.,** Peripheral and central primitive neuroectodermal tumors; A nosologic concept seeking a consensus, *Arch. Pathol. Lab. Med.,* 110, 997, 1986.
62. **Triche, T. J.,** Neuroblastoma; biology confronts nosology, *Arch. Pathol. Lab. Med.,* 110, 994, 1986.
63. **Miser, J. S., Kinsella, T. J., Triche, T. J., et al.,** Treatment of peripheral neuroepithelioma in children and young adults, *J. Clin. Oncol.,* 5, 1752, 1987.
64. **Marina, N. M., Etcubanas, E., Parham, D. M., et al.,** Peripheral primitive neuroectodermal tumor (peripheral neuroepithelioma) in children, *Cancer,* 64, 1952, 1989.
65. **Lopez-Gines, C., Pellin, A., and Llombart-Bosch, A.,** Two new cases of primary peripheral neuroepithelioma of soft tissue with translocation t(11;22) (q24;q12), *Cancer Genet. Cytogenet.,* 33, 291, 1988.
66. **Turc-Carel, C., Aurias, A., Mugneret, F., et al.,** Chromosomes in Ewing's sarcoma. I. An evaluation of 85 cases and remarkable consistency of t(11;22) (q24;q12), *Cancer Genet. Cytogenet.,* 32, 229, 1988.
67. **Hachitanda, Y., Tsuneyoshi, M., Enjoji, M., et al.,** Congenital primitive neuroectodermal tumor with epithelial and glial differentiation; an ultrastructural and immunohistochemical study, *Arch. Pathol. Lab. Med.,* 114, 101, 1990.
68. **Dehner, L. P.,** Whence the primitive neuroectodermal tumor?, *Arch. Pathol. Lab. Med.,* 114, 16, 1990.
69. **Tefft, M., Fernandez, C., Donaldson, M., et al.,** Incidence of meningeal involvement by rhabdomyosarcoma of the head and neck in children, *Cancer,* 42, 253, 1978.
70. **Gaiger, A. M., Soule, E. H., and Newton, W. A.,** Pathology of rhabdomyosarcoma; experience of the Intergroup Rhabdomyosarcoma Study, 1972—1978, *Natl. Cancer Inst. Monogr.,* 56, 19, 1981.
71. **Hays, D. M., Newton, W. A., Soule, E. H., et al.,** Mortality among children with rhabdomyosarcoma of the alveolar histologic subtype, *J. Pediatr. Surg.,* 18, 412, 1983.
72. **Wharam, M., Beltangady, M., Hays, D., et al.,** Localized orbital rhabdomyosarcoma, *Ophthalmology,* 94 (Abstr.), 251, 1987.
73. **Raney, R. B., Hays, D. M., Lawrence, W., Jr., et al.,** Paratesticular rhabdomyosarcoma in childhood, *Cancer,* 42, 729, 1978.
74. **Raney, R. B., Tefft, M., Lawrence, W., et al.,** Paratesticular sarcoma in childhood and adolescence. A report from the Intergroup Rhabdomyosarcoma Studies I and II, 1973-1983, *Cancer,* 60, 2337, 1987.
75. **Ruymann, F., Maddox, H., Ragab, A., et al.,** Congenital anomalies associated with rhabdomyosarcoma; an autopsy study of 115 cases. A report from the Intergroup Rhabdomyosarcoma Study Group, the Pediatric Oncology Group, the United Kingdom Children's Cancer Study Group, the Childrens Cancer Study Group, and the Pediatric Intergroup Statistical Center, *Med. Pediatr. Oncol.,* 1988; 16, 33, 1988.
76. **Carli, M., Grotto, P., Cavazzana, A., et al.,** (For the Italian Cooperative Group). Prognostic significance of histology in childhood RMS; improved survival with a new histological leiomyomatous subtype, unpublished observations, 1990.
77. **Maurer, H. M., Beltangady, M., Gehan, E. A., et al.,** The Intergroup Rhabdomyosarcoma Study-I, *Cancer,* 61, 209, 1988.
78. **Maurer, H. M., Gehan, E. A., Beltangady, M., et al.,** The Intergroup Rhabdomyosarcoma Study-II, *Cancer,* in press.
79. **Gehan, E. A., Glover, F. N., Maurer, H. M., et al.,** Prognostic factors in children with rhabdomyosarcoma, *Natl. Cancer Inst. Monogr.,* 56, 83, 1981.
80. **Shimada, H., Newton, W. A., Soule, E. H., et al.,** Pathology of fatal rhabdomyosarcoma, Report from Intergroup Rhabdomyosarcoma Study (IRS-I and IRS-II), *Cancer,* 59, 459, 1987
81. **Lawrence, W., Gehan, E. A., Hays, D. M., et al.,** Prognostic significance of staging factors of the UICC staging system in childhood rhabdomyosarcoma; a report from the Intergroup Rhabdomyosarcoma Study (IRS-II), *J. Clin. Oncol.,* 5, 46, 1987.
82. **Hawkins, H. K. and Camacho-Velasquez, J. V.,** Rhabdomyosarcoma in children. Correlation of form and prognosis in one institution's experience, *Am. J. Surg. Pathol.,* 11, 531, 1987.
83. **Kodet, R.,** Personal communication of unpublished data, 1990.

84. **Kelsey, A.,** C-myc and N-myc expression in childhood rhabdomyosarcoma — does it correlate with other prognostic features?, unpublished observations, 1990.
85. **Tsuda, H., Shimosato, Y., Upton, M. P., et al.,** Retrospective study on amplification of N-myc and c-myc genes in pediatric solid tumors and its association with prognosis and tumor differentiation, *Lab. Invest.,* 59, 321, 1988.
86. **Dias, P., Kuma, P., Marsden, H. B., et al.,** N- and c-myc oncogenes in childhood rhabdomyosarcoma, *J. Natl. Cancer Inst.,* 82, 151, 1990.
87. **Stratton, M. R., Fisher, C., Gusterson, B. A., and Cooper, C. S.,** Detection of point mutations in N-ras and K-ras genes of human embryonal rhabdomyosarcomas using oligonucleotide probes and the polymerase chain reaction, *Cancer Res.,* 49, 6324, 1989.
88. **Wang-Wuu, S., Soukup, S., Ballard, E., et al.,** Chromosomal analysis of 16 human rhabdomyosarcomas, *Cancer Res.,* 48, 983, 1988.
89. **Stratton, M. R., Williams, S., Fisher, C., et al.,** Structural alterations of the RB1 gene in human soft tissue tumors, *Br. J. Cancer,* 60, 202, 1989.
90. **Look, A. T., Shapiro, D. N., Parham, D., et al.,** Tumor specific genetic abnormalities correlate with histologic subtype and outcome in childhood rhabdomyosarcoma, unpublished observations, 1989.
91. **Stratton, M. R., Williams, S., Fisher, C., et al.,** Structural alterations of the RB1 gene in human soft tissue tumors, *Br. J. Cancer,* 60, 202, 1989.
92. **Leuschner, I.,** Unpublished data, 1990.
93. **Molenaar, W. M., Oosterhuis, J. W., and Kamps, W. A.,** Cytologic "differentiation" in childhood rhabdomyosarcomas following polychemotherapy, *Hum. Pathol.,* 15, 973, 1984.
94. **Harms, D., Schmidt, D., and Treuner, J.,** Solf-tissue sarcomas in childhood; a study of 262 cases including 169 cases of rhabdomyosarcoma, *Z. Kinderchir.,* 40, 140, 1985.
95. **Marsden, H. B.,** The pathology of soft-tissue sarcomas with emphasis on childhood tumors, in *Bone Tumors and Soft Tissue Sarcomas,* D'Angio, G. J. and Evans, A. E., Eds., Arnold Publishing, Baltimore, MD, 1985, 14.
96. **Enjoji, M. and Hashimoto, H.,** Diagnosis of soft tissue sarcomas, *Pathol. Res. Pract.,* 178, 215, 1984.
97. **Newton, W. A.,** Children's Hospital of Columbus Tumor Registry, unpublished data, 1990.
98. **Strong, L. C., Stine, M., and Norsted, T. L.,** Cancer in survivors of childhood soft tissue sarcoma and their relatives, *J. Natl. Cancer Inst.,* 79, 1213, 1987.
99. **Li, F. P. and Fraumeni, J. F., Jr.,** Prospective study of a family cancer syndrome, *JAMA,* 247, 2692, 1982.
100. **Meadows, A. T., Baum, E., Fossati-Bellani, F., et al.,** Second malignant neoplasms in children; an update from the Late Effects Study Group, *J. Clin. Oncol.,* 3, 532, 1985.

Chapter 3

BIOLOGY OF RHABDOMYOSARCOMA: CELL CULTURE, XENOGRAFTS, AND ANIMAL MODELS*

Paul S. Dickman, Maria Tsokos, and Timothy J. Triche

TABLE OF CONTENTS

* Partial funding of this work has been provided by the Pathology Education and Research Foundation, Pittsburgh, PA.

I. INTRODUCTION

Experimental models of human neoplasms have provided valuable tools for exploring numerous biological and clinical features of tumors. Rhabdomyosarcoma (RMS) has been studied using tumors induced in experimental animals, in cell lines derived from such tumors, in cell lines developed from human tumors, and in xenografts in athymic or nude mice using both human primary tumors and tumor cell lines. In this chapter the authors will describe these models, and information derived from the various tumor systems will be reviewed. Special emphasis is placed on biological and molecular biological findings, as well as using clinical or therapeutic relevance of studies of human cell lines and xenografts.

II. ANIMAL MODELS OF RMS

Malignant neoplasms similar to human RMS have been induced in rats, mice, and, in at least one instance, Syrian hamsters. The most common method used to induce RMS is the subcutaneous or intramuscular injection of nickel, either elemental or as nickel sulfide,[1-4] or by injection of a carcinogenic aromatic hydrocarbon, generally methylcholanthrene (MCA) or dimethylbenzanthracene (DMBA). In addition, a Moloney murine sarcoma virus-induced model of RMS has been used for several studies, and many studies have been done using cell lines developed from a tumor which arose in an irradiated rat. There are several spontaneously appearing RMSs in laboratory animals which have no known inciting factor. In none of these instances is it known why RMS, in particular, arose as a result of carcinogenic stimulation by these agents, although there have been many studies on the general mechanisms of carcinogenicity of nickel compounds and aromatic hydrocarbons.[1-5] Specific tumors induced in animals, and cell lines derived from them, are summarized in Tables 1 and 2.

Findings from studies of animal tumors and cell lines can be divided into two general areas: (1) biology and (2) treatment applications. Biology includes patterns of proliferation and metastasis, cytogenetics, histologic and ultrastructural morphology, and immunohistochemistry, as well as properties of adhesion, receptors, uptake, and production of various molecules. Treatment applications include radiotherapy, chemotherapy, and the use of differentiating or ''normalizing'' agents.

A. BIOLOGY

Growth patterns have been described in RMSs induced in rats by nickel or nickel compounds or DMBA, and in the R1 cell line derived from the BA1112 tumor which arose in an irradiated rat.

Early studies of proliferation of cells in the BA1112 tumor revealed that patterns of growth and proliferation correspond to the site in the primary tumor in which the cells reside, with a much more rapid growth rate among cells at the periphery of the tumor than in cells at the tumor's center.[6] This finding corresponds to observations in a variety of human tumors indicating that hypoxia and poor perfusion contribute to disadvantageous growth in the center of a tumor mass compared to the well-nourished periphery.

Cell lines derived from a tumor induced by intramuscular injection of metallic nickel have been designated 9-4.[2,3] A series of experiments showed that various lines cloned from the same original tumor have differing growth and metastatic capabilities.[7-9] Cell lines varied with respect to numbers of metastases, cell numbers necessary to induce new tumors, and growth rate as measured by doubling time *in vitro*. These biological features also varied according to the method of reinjection of cells into animals, that is, tumors with a high metastatic rate following subcutaneous injection might have a low rate of metastasis following intravenous injection, and vice versa. Comparisons of metastatic potential and chromosome number showed no relationship. One line was immunogenic with respect to its ability to

TABLE 1
Animal Rhabdomyosarcomas and Cell Lines Induced by Nickel and Nickel Compounds

Tumor	Cell line	Species	Ref.
9-4	9-4/0	WAG rat	7
Unnamed	NS-A	C3H mouse	25
	OVC-FRT	Fisher rat	23
	Unnamed	Fisher rat	27
Unnamed; ? transplantable	None	Sprague-Dawley rat	48
Unnamed	None	Sprague-Dawley rat	49
	Unnamed	Fischer, hooded rats	24
	None	Wistar rat, rabbit	29, 30
	None	Wistar rat	28
	None	Lewis, Fisher 344, Sprague-Dawley, Wistar rats	31

TABLE 2
Animal Rhabdomyosarcomas and Cell Lines Induced by Various Agents

Induction method	Tumor	Cell line	Species	Ref.
Methyl cholanthrene	MC-62; MC-III A7; MC-53; transplantable	Unnamed (from A-7)	CC57W mouse	378
	Unnamed; transplantable	None	NMRI mouse	32
Dimethyl benzanthrene	Unnamed	BA-HAN-1	Lewis rat	39
	Unnamed	None	BALB/c mouse	53
Moloney Sarcoma virus	Unnamed	None	BALB/c, C57BL mice	43
	Unnamed; transplantable	R2	BALB/c mouse	45
	Unnamed	None	Wistar/Furth rat	46
	Unnamed	None	BALB/c mouse	53
Radiation-associated	BA 1112; transplantable	R1 and progeny	Wistar rat	6,57
Spontaneous	Unnamed; transplantable	Unnamed	BALB/cAnN mouse	47
Unspecified	Unnamed; transplantable	None	C_3H mouse	379
	BW10139 transplantable	Unnamed	CE/J mouse	73

resist formation of subsequent tumors by injection of immunized rats, but immunization did not protect the animals from metastasis once tumors were established.[8] It is noteworthy that resistance of a cell line to natural killer (NK) cell lysis was associated with a high metastatic rate, although tumor cells which were sensitive to NK attack had variously high and low metastatic rates.[10] The mechanisms by which these influences on the various patterns of growth and metastasis of RMS cells affect the actual behavior of RMS have not yet been elucidated.

In a cell line derived from a tumor induced by injection of DMBA, there were two distinct cell types which differed in morphology and also varied in proliferative potential.[11] In a pattern similar to that observed in human RMS, this cultured line consistently contained both undifferentiated mononuclear cells which could proliferate and incorporate tritiated thymidine, and multinucleated, myotube-like cells which were amitotic and which may well have derived from the mononuclear myoblasts. This system is an important model for differentiation in RMS.

The adhesion properties of cell lines derived from a nickel-induced tumor in rats have been examined in a series of investigations, especially with respect to laminin.[12-14] A relationship was found between early attachment to endothelial cell layers, mediated by laminin in the extracellular matrix, and the potential for a given cell line to produce lung metastasis following reinjection. This finding supports the hypothesis that ability to attach to basement membrane components is a key indicator of a tumor's potential for invasion and metastasis.[15,16] The result is also consonant with data from related studies of cell surface proteoglycan metabolism and metastatic potential.[17-20] Weakly metastatic RMS cell lines have far more sulfated glycoproteins and glycosaminoglycans, especially chondroitin sulfate, on the cell surface than cells from strongly metastatic lines. Decreased amounts of cell surface glycosaminoglycans may be involved in enhancement of metastatic potential by mechanisms related to diminution of cell detachment from extracellular matrix elements such as laminin, reduction of contact inhibition, or both.

Another aspect of the biology of RMS in animal models which has been investigated is the uptake by tumor cells of α-fetoprotein (AFP). This has been studied in cell line 9-4/0.[21,22] All clones studied were found to bind AFP, and all but one internalized the molecule, as determined immunohistochemically. AFP localized in the cytoplasm and eventually was incorporated into lipid droplets. The mechanism of uptake was via coated pits on the cell surface, from which the AFP was transferred to receptosomes and then to the Golgi apparatus before localizing in lipid droplets; AFP receptors may recycle to the cell surface. This transport of AFP is also accompanied by AFP binding of polyunsaturated fatty acids, and AFP may play a role in intracellular delivery of these molecules. Of interest is the observation that AFP is not only present in fetal and neonatal skeletal muscle in rats, but it is accumulated by muscle after injection. Thus, the AFP uptake found in the cultured RMS cells appears to mimic a property of developing and mature skeletal muscle, a theme observed again in ultrastructural and immunohistochemical studies.

Cytogenetic information has been obtained on a number of animal RMS models, principally in nickel-induced tumors. In the 9-4 rat tumor and related cell lines, the model chromosome numbers (mean number of chromosomes per metaphase examined) were simliar in all sublines examined, being 70 to 80 (in the normal rat, $2N = 42$). However, the ranges of chromosome numbers varied widely, although no relationship was observed between chromosome numbers and tumorigenicity, defined as injected cell dose for tumor formation.[8] Only minor abnormalities were observed but not illustrated. In a cell line derived from another nickel-induced tumor, chromosome studies revealed both near-diploid (41 to 47 chromosomes) and near-tetraploid (75 to 86 chromosomes) cells with several markers, particularly a submetacentric aberrant chromosome.[23]

In a study of the cytogenetics of primary nickel sulfide-induced tumors, multiple abnormalities were found in a setting of predominantly diploid cells.[24] More recent studies of tumors in mice, induced by either nickel sulfide or MCA, found somewhat more consistent abnormalities, in particular minichromosomes (smaller than the smallest mouse chromosome, number 19) and marker chromosomes involving chromosome 4.[25,26] No relationship was found between chromosomal abnormalities and rearrangement or activation of either c-*mos* or c-*myc*. It is noteworthy that no consistent observations of chromosomal abnormalities, such as the t(2;13) translocation of human alveolar RMS, have been made in any of the animal systems.

Patterns of growth, metastasis, and cytogenetics in animal models tend to be peculiar to the particular system of laboratory study used. Therefore, the findings are of limited applicability to human neoplasms. In contrast, the morphology, histochemistry, and immunohistochemistry of tumors and cell lines in laboratory animals provide criteria for identification and degree of differentiation which can be directly compared to the extensive experience with human tumors.

In general, the light microscopic histology of RMSs induced in animals most closely resembles the pleomorphic type of human tumor, rather than the more common embryonal or alveolar types seen in children. Tumors induced by injection of nickel compounds are composed of spindled cells, with numerous strap cells exhibiting cross striations, sometimes resembling mature myotubes.[1,5,24,27-31] Pleomorphic cells are frequently described. Some tumors contain round cells,[1,5,28-31] with an appearance somewhat similar to that of human "solid alveolar" or undifferentiated RMS, but the tumors are not composed exclusively of such cells. RMSs induced by either MCA or DMBA have similar patterns.[11,32-41] In the BA1112 tumor and its derived cell lines, there is a pattern so pleomorphic as to suggest malignant fibrous histiocytoma (MFH).[35] However, in these tumors and cultured cells, strap cells showing cross striations and probable myotubes are also seen.[9,42] Tumors induced by the Moloney virus are similar in appearance to the nickel-associated RMS, being composed of spindled, pleomorphic, and true strap cells,[43-45] although there may be small cells as well.[46] In one report of a spontaneous RMS, the tumor contained only strap cells.[47]

The ultrastructure of RMS in animals is more similar to that of human tumors. A common finding is the presence of cells exhibiting various degrees of skeletal muscle differentiation. Four cell types have been described.

1. There are small, poorly differentiated cells with simple organelles and no specific evidence of rhabdomyogenesis. These cells correspond to the small or round cells seen histologically and they are generally the cells in which mitosis is observed.
2. There are also immature myoblasts, in an early stage of differentiation, which contain thin (actin) filaments or intermediate filaments.
3. There are better differentiated myoblasts which contain actin, myosin, and Z-bands forming incomplete sarcomeres, or there may be Z-band material with radiating thin or intermediate filaments, which fulfill the standard ultrastructural criteria for identifying skeletal muscle differentiation.
4. There may be mature myotubes containing well-formed, oriented sarcomeres. The latter cell types do not seem to undergo mitosis, as befits their mature status.

In a study of cells in a nickel-induced tumor, so-called cylindrical laminated bodies, composed of 4-nm fibrils, were found in various tumor cells and interpreted as being abnormal, paracrystalline collections of contractile filaments. However, the composition of the bodies was not determined.[30] Other studies of cell lines derived from DMBA-induced tumors[11,39-41] suggest that the more primitive cells give rise to mature myoblasts, since both cell types (primitive cells and myoblasts) always appear after recloning. This finding suggests that these tumors, in culture, recapitulate normal skeletal myogenesis.

The variety of cells present in nickel-induced,[29-31,48,49] DMBA-induced,[11,36-41,50-52] and Moloney virus-associated tumors[43-45,53] is similar to that observed in human RMSs, regardless of histologic classification. Thus, in this respect the resemblance of the animal tumors to human RMS is quite close.

In view of the similarity of cell types found by electron microscopy in animal tumors and in cell lines of human RMS, it is not surprising that the immunohistochemical profile of the tumors and the cell lines studied is also reminiscent of that found in the human tumor. The range of cellular differentiation seen ultrastructurally corresponds to a similar range defined by immunoreactivity for cytoskeletal proteins. In particular, better differentiated cells contain desmin, the late-appearing, muscle-specific intermediate filament protein, while vimentin predominantes in more primitive cells.[11,28,39-41] Myoglobin is seen only in well-differentiated strap cells or myotubes.[33,34]

Myosin and myosin subtypes (isoforms) have been examined in Moloney virus-induced tumors.[46,53] A study of myosin types, defined by reactivity to monoclonal antibodies, showed that although myosin in general was expressed much less often than desmin, embryonic and neonatal myosin isoforms were predominant. Only rarely did cells react exclusively to the antibody specific for adult myosin isoforms. Occasionally, single cells expressed both adult and embryonic types of myosin.

Other proteins have been studied. Immunoreactivity of tumor cells was determined for α-sarcomeric actin, an actin subtype found normally only in skeletal muscle. This protein was identified in myoblasts with other evidence of rhabdomyogenesis as well as in myotube-like tumor cells,[11,31,39-41] the stage of rhabdomyogenesis roughly corresponding to the degree of desmin positivity. Sarcomeric and smooth muscle types of actin were studied in a nickel-induced tumor. Surprisingly, RMS cells expressed the smooth muscle protein, and often the same cells expressed both types of actin.[31] Thus, the animal RMS cells are capable of exhibiting phenotypes of actin not seen in normal skeletal muscle. If these data are found to be applicable in the human tumor, it casts doubt on the ability to classify RMSs according to immunoreactivity of actin subtypes.

Another confounding observation is the immunoreactivity of murine RMS cells for antibodies to cytokeratin (especially types 8, 19, and 18), a finding ordinarily expected in epithelial cells but not in mesenchymal cells.[34] The intermediate filaments, once thought to be quite tissue-specific in the distribution of their subtypes, have now been observed in numerous cell types different from their assumed category. Again, this means that use of immunohistochemical methods for diagnosis of tumors must be viewed with caution.

One study of lectin histochemistry has been reported in a RMS induced by MCA. Three lectin phenotypes were found to decrease in histochemical positivity as desmin immunoreactivity increased. These phenotypes were WGA (binding β-D-Glc Nac and sialic acid), RCA-1 (binding α,β-Gal[β1,4]-Glc Nac), and LCA (binding α-D-Man and Glc Nac). Reactivity to these lectins decreased to zero in myoglobin-positive cells. These findings document another way in which experimental RMS mimics normal muscle development, in which decreasing reactivity for these lectins is observed as embryonic skeletal muscle matures.[33]

B. TREATMENT APPLICATIONS

Areas of investigation of animal models of RMS with respect to treatment fall into three areas: (1) response to chemotherapy, principally with chlorozotocin (CZT), and induction of drug resistance; (2) response to radiation; and (3) induction of differentiation or "normalization" of tumor cells.

Treatment of cultured cells derived from a nickel-induced mouse tumor with CZT, a nitrosourea compound, increases the ability of the cells to form colonies in soft agar. When mice were treated with the drug and then injected with the RMS cells, there was an enhancement of lung metastasis.[54] This is in contrast to the usual toxic effect of nitrosoureas on neoplastic cells. This effect may be due to depression of the mouse immune response or due to an increase in vascular permeability caused by the drug. Further studies of this system resulted in the acquisition of multidrug resistance, including resistance to adriamycin and cisplatin in CZT resistant cells after repeated cloning in soft agar.[55,56] The cells were also able to proliferate *in vitro* without serum (with transferrin and insulin). The presence of the multidrug resistance gene (*mdr*-1) in these cells has not yet been determined, but such studies would be of great importance in relating this phenomenon to human tumors expressing this gene.

The rat RMS BA1112[57,58] and cell lines derived from it, R1 and its progeny, have been used extensively in the study of response to irradiation.[59-64] Recent studies have examined the effects of administration of oxygenating compounds, such as fluosol and carbogen, on irradiation response of the tumor. These oxygenating agents, administered in combination, enhance radiosensitivity as a function of the dose of fluosol.[65] Another recent investigation found that there was little interaction between treatment with neon ion radiation and X-rays. It was concluded that the time interval between sequential treatments using these two types of radiation could be shortened without increasing damage to normal tissue.[66]

The ability of various compounds to induce differentiation or "normalization" in tumor cells has been intriguing. This approach has only recently been applied successfully to pediatric solid tumor patients with malignancies, such as neuroblastoma.[67,68] Early studies examined the effect of the planar-polar compounds, the prototype being dimethylsulfoxide, on Friend erythroleukemia cells[69,70] as well as in various human tumor systems.[71,72] In experimental RMS, these compounds, as well as retinoic acid and butyrate, have been examined for their effect on cultured cells. Various studies of the DMBA-induced cell line, BA-HAN-1 and its derivatives, have utilized retinoic acid, dimethylsulfoxide, hexamethylene bisacetamide, sodium butyrate, N-methylformamide, and dimethylformamide.[11,39-41,50,51]

In general, these compounds had the greatest effect on cell line BA-HAN-1C. This line is composed predominantly of primitive round cells which show no morphologic differentiation, but the cells are capable of fusing to form multinucleated differentiated myoblasts. When the BA-HAN-1C cell line was treated with one of the above agents, there was an inhibition of proliferation, an increase in the number of multinucleated myotube-like cells, and an increased production of creatine kinase. There was also the appearance in the mononuclear cells of actin and myosin filaments detectable by electron microscopy, a finding which was never observed in untreated cells. Thus, differentiation could be enhanced by these agents, although the tumor lines never proceeded beyond partial or incomplete differentiation; mature skeletal muscle did not appear.

Similar results were obtained in a transplantable mouse RMS treated with dimethylformamide or butyrate.[73,74] In these experiments, it was found that no tumors occurred after reinjection of treated cells, and growth of tumor cells in soft agar was blocked. Amounts of creatine kinase produced rose to levels observed in normal chick myoblasts prior to fusion. Thus, although differentiation was stimulated, it only occurred to a point equivalent to an early (prefusion) stage of skeletal myogenesis.[75] Again, multinucleated tumor cells appeared in these cultures, but there were no actual myotubes, emphasizing the incomplete nature of this normalization.

III. HUMAN RMS CELL LINES AND XENOGRAFTS

Cultured cell lines and xenografts derived from human RMS provide experimental models of this tumor, which can be expected to resemble the native tumors to a degree greater than the animal models described above. It is likely that many of the findings observed in these human cell lines will provide information that is closely related to, and predictive of, at least some features relevant to clinical manifestation and diagnosis of human RMS. In the following section, various aspects of the biology and therapeutic applications are discussed, followed by review of additional recent developments in the study of human RMS *in vitro*.

A. BIOLOGY
Human RMS cell lines and xenograft models have been developed in approximately the same numbers as the animal systems. Several venerable cell lines, such as RD[76] and A204,[77] have been utilized with great frequency since they were originally described, as have the xenograft models in athymic mice, described elsewhere in this book (see Chapter 10). Characteristics of the cell lines discussed here are summarized in Table 3.

The tumor from which the RD cell line was derived as a pelvic mass in a 7-year-old girl who had been treated with cyclophosphamide and radiation therapy. This tumor was described as an embryonal RMS, containing spindle cells and occasional giant cells (Figure 1, top panel). The RD cell line contained similar cell types, but no cross striations were found. Myoglobin, detected by a hemagglutination inhibition method, was present in the cultured cells, but the ultrastructural findings were not specific for RMS. Tumor cells were remarkable only for the presence of cytoplasmic intermediate filaments, as were seen in several of the animal models and in numerous native human RMSs. Nonetheless, the myoglobin production and the findings in subsequent immunohistochemical and immunoblotting

TABLE 3
A Current List of Human Rhabdomyosarcoma Cell Lines and Xenografts

Cell line	Xenograft	Original tumor	Ref.
A204	—	RMS; 1.1-year F	77
Birch	Nude mice	ERMS; 15-year M, paratesticular	Unpublished
CCA	Nude mice	ERMS; 8-year M, vesicorectal recurrence	88
CCI-136	—	RMS	107
HS-57	—	ERMS; lung met	380
HUS 2	—	Probable ERMS; 80-year M, chest wall	81
HX170c	Nude mice	ERMS; 5-year M, paratesticular	91
JR-1	—	ERMS; 7-year F, lung met; 1° in L broad ligament	85
KYM-1	ATS treated Syrian golden hamsters	ARMS; 9-month M, neck	82
RD	Nude mice	ERMS; 7-year F, pelvis	76, 87
Rh 10, 18, 28	HxRh 6, 7, 8, 10, 12, 14, 18; immune deprived (T − B +) mice	ERMS; ARMS; Ascites, bladder, groin, perineum, buttock, inguinal region	100, 103
RMZ	—	ARMS; 2-year M, bone marrow met of L thigh 1°	89
SMS-CTR	—	ERMS	67
TC-147	—	Unclassified RMS	94
TC-206	Nude mice	ARMS; 5-month M, arm	192
TC-212	Nude mice	Solid ARMS; 16-year M, testis met	192
TC-280	Nude mice	ARMS; ?12-year F, lymph node met	192
TU-442	—	ERMS; 10-year M, liver	Unpublished
TU-487 (CHLA 37)	—	ARMS; 1-year M, 1° submandib, L thigh met	Unpublished
TU-516	—	ERMS; 12-year M, prostate	Unpublished
TU-547	—	Solid ARMS; 13-year F, pelvis	Unpublished
YN	YNNu, nude mice	ERMS; 15-year M, paratesticular	86
Unnamed	—	RMS; 3-year F, L face	381
Unnamed	Nude mice	RMS; subcut breast met	98
Unnamed	—	(Not given)	106
Unnamed	—	ARMS; 2-year M, bone marrow met	90
Unnamed	Nude mice	Undiff RMS (?ARMS); 14-year F, R chest wall	83, 84
Unnamed	Nude mice	ERMS; 42-year F, nasal cavity	99

Abbreviations: RMS — rhabdomyosarcoma, ERMS — embryonal RMS, ARMS — alveolar RMS, undiff — undifferentiated, ATS — antithymocyte serum, M — male, F — female, 1° — primary, met — metastasis.

studies confirmed that the RD cell line does express skeletal myogenesis in culture.[78] This line was initially used in heterologous transplantation experiments[76,79,80] in which the histology and ultrastructure of the resulting tumors were similar to those of the initial human tumor. More recently, the RD cell line has been studied in various other settings.

The ultrastructural study of other human RMS lines has resulted in descriptions of tumors showing a range of differentiation, from the appearance of nonspecific features or the presence of intermediate filament bundles only,[81-84] to full-blown rhabdomyogenic differentiation, with thin and thick filaments and Z-bands or focal densities.[83,84,86] Particularly notable is a cell line derived from a chest wall tumor in a 14-year-old girl.[83,84] The original neoplasm was poorly differentiated when examined by light and electron microscopy, resembling extraosseous Ewing's sarcoma or solid alveolar RMS, and initially cultured cells were similar in morphology. After growth in serum-free media, however, the tumor cells expressed well-

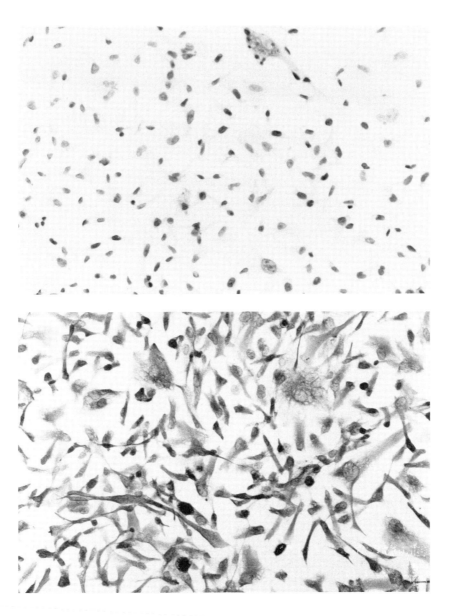

FIGURE 1. Top panel: RD rhabdomyosarcoma cells. Most cells are spindle-shaped or angular. Note multinucleated giant cell at top. Hematoxylin. (Original magnification × 64: final magnification × 210.) Bottom panel: RD rhabdomyosarcoma cells. Immunohistochemistry using monoclonal antibody to desmin. Dark filamentous staining is seen in cytoplasm, indicating rhabdomyogenic differentiation. Avidin-biotin-peroxidase method, hematoxylin counterstain. (Original magnification × 64; final magnification × 210.)

developed myogenic features by electron microscopy. They produced increasing amounts of creatine kinase MM, an effect similar to that observed in the animal tumors and lines treated with differentiating agents, as described earlier.

The immunohistochemical profile of cultured human RMS is also somewhat variable, but immunostaining for the myogenic proteins desmin, embryonic myosin, actin, creatine kinase MM, myoglobin, and vimentin, has been observed (Figures 1 [bottom panel] and 2).[82,85-91] Different cell lines have different proportions of positive cells in various degrees for these proteins as detected immunohistochemically. In one instance, desmin and myo-

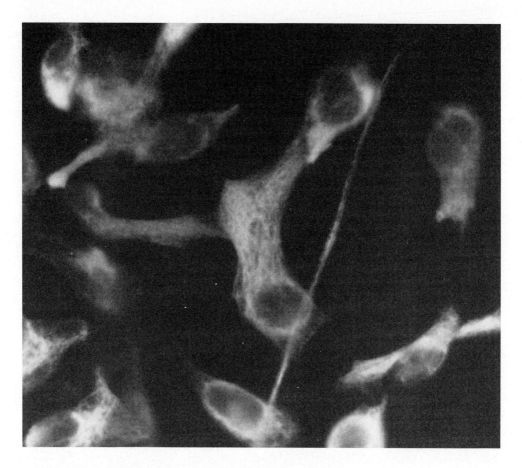

FIGURE 2.   RD rhabdomyosarcoma cells. Immunofluorescence using monoclonal antibody to desmin. Cyto-plasmic filaments are markedly positive. Indirect immunofluorescence. (Original magnification × 200; final magnification × 980.)

globin were detected immunohistochemically in more cells after the tumor was grown in nude mice.[86] A set of monoclonal antibodies has been used to define cell membrane markers found in various small round cell tumors of childhood, including leukemias, neuroblastoma, RMS, Ewing's sarcoma, and neuroectodermal tumors. These monoclonal antibodies were applied to RMS cell lines, including RD and A204.[92] None of the monoclonal antibodies were specific for RMS, but several (BA-1 and Pl153/3), which were never positive in RMS cells, were positive in neuroblastoma cells and leukemic lymphoblasts. These antibody-defined markers may thus prove to be useful in excluding RMS from consideration in a diagnostic setting.

Various cell lines have been studied with regard to the production of extracellular matrix, and possible characteristic patterns have been detected. Cells of cell line A204 were found to produce type V collagen[93,94] and a subunit of laminin,[94] while RD cells make type IV collagen, a basal lamina component, and fibronectin.[94,95] A cell line derived from an un-classifiable RMS (TC147) expresses interstitial collagens I and III as well as type IV collagen and fibronectin.[94] The findings in RD cells, derived from an embryonal RMS, are similar to those observed in an immunohistochemical study of childhood tumors. In this study, embryonal RMS contained type IV collagen, laminin, and fibronectin, while alveolar RMS rarely produced any of these elements.[96]

The production of matrix elements and proteases is of interest because of its possible relationship to the ability of cells to invade and metastasize. The KYM-1 cell line[82] produces large amounts of the glycosaminoglycan hyaluronic acid as well as tissue plasminogen activator. While the hyaluronic acid in animal RMS cell lines was found to correlate with a low metastatic rate,[17-19] the production of tissue plasminogen activator might be expected to be related to invasive potential; but this has not yet been examined. In other studies, when the metastatic potential of human RMS cell lines RMZ, RD, and CCA was assessed in nude mice, none of the animals developed metastases when the cultured cells were injected subcutaneously or intramuscularly.[87,88] However, in animals pretreated with cyclophosphamide, injection of RD cells produced pulmonary and renal metastases quite efficiently.

B. THERAPEUTIC APPLICATIONS

Human RMS models have been used to study cancer therapy in the form of explants,[97] cultured cells, and as xenografts in nude or immune-deprived mice.[98,99] Extensive studies of chemotherapeutic agents in the RMS xenograft model[100-105] are described in Chapter 10.

Unlike the situation in the animal RMS BA1112 and cell line R1, the radiation response in human RMS models has not been extensively studied. A study of the effect of cobalt-60 gamma irradiation on cultured tumor cells showed that the RMS line Hx170c is exquisitely radiosensitive.[91] The surviving cells also had a very poor ability to recover from radiation damage.

Studies on the effects of chemotherapy on human RMSs *in vitro* are more plentiful. Uptake, metabolism, and cytotoxicity of adriamycin have been studied in human RMS.[106] As expected, cytotoxicity was proportional to concentration of the drug in the culture media. Another cell line has been examined with respect to the effect of numerous chemotherapeutic agents, including several drugs used clinically in RMS, such as etoposide and vincristine.[107] Treatment of cells with any of the drugs studied was associated with extensive DNA methylation, when the drugs were used at a dose high enough to kill 90 to 100% of the cells. It was postulated that this drug-induced effect, which was also observed in several leukemic patients, may be related to the induction of drug resistance in the treated tumor cell populations. However, the specific connection between methylation and drug resistance was not determined.

Finally, several studies have been conducted in which tumor cells reverted to normal. An early study of the effects of dibutryryl cyclic AMP on RD cells showed growth inhibition and decreased ability to form colonies in soft agar.[108] In a study of differentiation of human RMS cells, it was found that treatment of cells of the RMZ-RC2 line with various chemotherapeutic agents resulted in enhanced myogenesis, as shown by a nearly doubled proportion of cells which express myosin, as well as by an increase in the numbers of multinucleated, myotube-like cells.

IV. RECENT DEVELOPMENTS IN MOLECULAR BIOLOGY OF RMS

Various aspects of human RMS *in vitro* merit special consideration because of the rapid advances in these areas. In this section, the authors will discuss recent findings in the areas of cytogenetics, molecular cytogenetics, cytoskeletal differentiation, and oncogenes. The next section will be devoted to tumor suppressor genes. The following section will review growth factors, the genetic basis of myogenesis, and neural differentiation in RMS.

A. CYTOGENETICS

Cytogenetic analysis, performed on tumors in short-term culture, offers an alternative approach to the differential diagnosis and contributes to the understanding of tumor biology.[109] In RMS, aneuploidy appears to be the rule. In one study, all of 11 desmin-positive tumors were noted to be markedly aneuploid in metastatic tumors, whereas other pediatric malignant tumors were generally diploid or near diploid.[110] There appears to be a specific clonal chromosomal rearrangement, t(2;13)(q37;q14), in some tumors of the alveolar subtype.[84,104,111-117] Opinions vary as to whether this chromosomal abnormality is specific for all alveolar RMSs, since the same translocation has also been detected in some embryonal and undifferentiated RMSs.[114,116] Therefore, this rearrangement might identify disease progression, as opposed to tumor subtype. Since this abnormality was not identified in more than 100 cases of other pediatric solid tumors studied, or in more than 50 tumors in another study,[118] it appears to be specific for RMS. Two cases of embryonal RMS showed a t(2;8)(q37;q13)[119] or t(2;5)(q37;q31) translocation,[120] suggesting that the critical breakpoint in the tumor chromosomes is probably at 2q37.[119]

Other abnormalities reported in RMS are the presence of double minute chromosomes, small ring chromosomes, abnormalities in chromosome 1p, and trisomy 8.[114]

B. MOLECULAR CYTOGENETICS

Conventional cytogenetic analysis of cultured embryonal RMS has identified abnormalities of chromosome segment 2q37. However, various recombinant DNA probes of chromosome 11p 13-15 have shown a loss of constitutional heterozygosity in embryonal but not in alveolar RMS,[121] suggesting a different etiology in the genesis of these two subtypes. Furthermore, a similar or identical chromosomal locus appears to be involved in two other histologically unrelated embryonal tumors, Wilms' tumor and hepatoblastoma.[121] Probing of the 11p 15.4-15.5 segment with multiple known probes (CAT, CALC, PTH, HBBC, D11S12, INS IGF2, HRAS1, centromeric to telemeric, respectively,[122] and D11S24[123]) has demonstrated uniform loss of heterozygosity in all embryonal, but in none of the alveolar RMSs.[122,123] This embryonal RMS specific locus at 11p 15.5 has been termed RdL.[124] The exact identity of the functional gene or genes in the RdL locus is still unknown, but efforts to clone the gene or genes in question are actively underway.[124a]

An important observation in both normal and neoplastic myogenesis is recognition of the apparently central role of a single gene called MyoD1.[125] This gene is largely responsible for initiating the cascade of gene expression that ultimately results in terminal differentiation of myoblasts.[126] With use of a cDNA clone of the human MyoD1 gene and a variety of human/murine hybrid cells lacking various portions, or all, of 11p, the MyoD1 gene has been mapped to 11p 15.4, which is close to, but physically separate from, the RdL locus.[124] Thus, it is unlikely that MyoD1 participates in tumorigenesis per se in RMS.

In the above observations, it is assumed that an inactivating event affecting the gene or genes causative in malignant transformation leading to the genesis of a RMS must affect both alleles. The concept of genome imprinting[127-130] proposes an alternative mechanism whereby only one allele need be genetically inactivated. In this model, it is proposed that a gamete-dependent epigenetic effect functionally inactivates the gene or even chromosomal segment on either the maternally or paternally inherited chromosome. Striking evidence for this mechanism in RMS[131] and other tumors[132] has implicated paternal inheritance of genetic predisposition to this tumor. In eight cases of embryonal RMS studied (six sporadic, two familial), all cases were isodisomic for alleles on 11p, and these alleles were of paternal origin.[131] The maternal alleles were lost, presumably by genomic alteration (that is, by mutation, deletion, translocation, or otherwise).

The mechanism for gene inactivation by genome imprinting is unknown, but known gene-inactivating factors such as DNA methylation and heterochromatin formation appear to be involved.[127,129] A possible mechanism suggested by studies on control of gene expression in yeast invokes the gamete-dependent expression of a helix-loop-helix (HLH) protein. This is a class of protein which includes MyoD1 and is already known to regulate some forms of gene expression, such as creatine kinase. This hypothetical factor could then potentially suppress gene expression over broad areas of a chromosome or in multiple chromosomes.

Regardless of the specific nature of the gene-inactivating event, the result indicates that Knudson's two-hit model of tumorigenesis[133-135] may not always apply. Rather, the first event in the genesis of a RMS may be the less precise, epigenetic phenomenon of genomic imprinting involving the locus in question, namely, 11p. In this case, only a single additional gene alteration would be required for oncogenesis to occur. At the same time, this mechanism offers an explanation for the observed maternal or paternal pattern of inheritance observed in certain cancer-prone families, such as in the Li-Fraumeni syndrome.[136-138] Moreover, it helps to explain the observed "mosaicism" in tissue susceptibility to oncogenesis, as seen in the Beckwith-Wiedemann syndrome, in Wilms' tumor, and in embryonal RMS.[129,131,132] The abnormal chromosomal loci in all of these neoplastic diseases appear to be on chromosome 11p.

C. CYTOSKELETAL DIFFERENTIATION

In both animal models and human RMS *in vitro,*, it has been noted that the tumor cells express various proteins characteristic of normal adult or embryonic skeletal muscle. Within a given tumor system, there is often morphologic, ultrastructural, immunohistochemical, or enzymatic expression consistent with either a given stage of muscle differentiation or a range of such stages. The degree of muscle differentiation of various cell lines has been modified by drug treatment or changes in culture conditions. It has been noted that the particular pattern of expression of myogenic proteins, as detected biochemically or immunohisto-chemically, may constitute evidence that a tumor corresponds to early or late skeletal myogenesis.

Both muscle and nonmuscle myosin have been documented in embryonal RMS, on the basis of both unique myosin light chain (LC) molecular weights on SDS-polyacrylamide gel electrophoresis, as well as differential light chain phosphorylation by platelet myosin kinase.[139] Immunoreactivity of cells of the line RMZ to antibodies against embryonic myosin, in both humans and rats, is expressed during fetal life but not in adults.[140-142] In one study, it was noted that while most cells apparently contain desmin, embryonic myosin is often present as well and may represent a marker of a somewhat larger stage of differentiation.[87,89,90] Similarly, in another human RMS line, CCA, it was observed that while all the cells expressed vimentin, only 40% expressed desmin and only 5% were embryonic myosin-positive. Thus, the CCA cell line may correspond to an earlier, vimentin-dominant stage of myogenesis.

More recent studies suggest that it is possible to classify cultured human RMS lines in a fairly precise manner. Cell lines have been classified according to their position on the time line of muscle development, as determined by expression of two sets of cytoskeletal proteins, the intermediate filament proteins and the spectrins. During muscle development, these sets of proteins change phenotype at the time of myoblast fusion, and thus can be used as markers along the developmental time line. Early in myoblast differentiation, vimentin is produced exclusively. At the time of fusion, vimentin production gradually decreases, and this protein is largely replaced in the intermediate filament structures by desmin. For a time, filaments are present containing both proteins (vimentin and desmin), but once myotubes are mature and sarcomeres form, desmin is the predominant intermediate filament protein. Thus, the presence and quantity of these two structural proteins, which surround the Z-bands and connect them to one another and to the cell membrane, can be used to date muscle development.[143-146] Similarly, spectrin, which assists in binding the sarcomeres to the cell membrane at the level of the Z-band, has phenotypes that also switch at fusion, from α-γ to α-β. Thus, spectrins can similarly serve as markers of the stage of myoblastic differentiation.[75,147]

In the RD and A204 cell lines, these intermediate filament and spectrin phenotypes were studied by immunocytochemistry and immunoblotting.[78] It was found that in RD cells, protein production fit a pattern of late myoblast development; that is, desmin, some vimentin, and α-β spectrin were detected. In contrast, the pattern in A204 cells was that of early myoblasts: vimentin, but not desmin, and α-spectrin (which is present in both early and late myoblasts), but not β-spectrin, were found. Thus, these two RMS cell lines correspond to two distinct stages in myoblast development: early stage, before myoblast fusion (in the A204 cell line), and late stage, after myoblast fusion (in the RD cell line).

The therapeutic implications of classifying RMSs *in vitro* according to stage of myogenesis are intriguing. There is some evidence that undifferentiated sarcomas and poorly differentiated RMSs have a worse prognosis than that of more differentiated tumors.[148-150] There is also the possibility that the ability to enhance differentiation or "normalization" of RMSs in patients, as described above in various animal and human cell lines, might result in the formation of tumors which are less aggressive and therefore somewhat easier to cure. While this possibility remains hypothetical in RMS, agents such as retinoic acid may turn out to be capable of inducing such changes without causing unacceptable toxicity.

D. ONCOGENES

It is now well established that the viral genes that cause cancer in many animals are in part composed of normal cellular genes, or proto-oncogenes.[151-155] These normal cellular genes play a critical role in fetal development and in later events, such as wound healing, but are otherwise expressed at low levels or not at all. In human tumors, and especially in malignant tumors, more than 20 of these genes have been implicated in various roles. Although there is not a one-to-one correlation between a specific oncogene and a specific tumor, there are certain patterns of proto-oncogene expression that are characteristic of specific tumors.[156,157]

The search for relevant oncogenes in RMS started in 1972.[158] Successful transformation of human fibroblasts with DNA isolated from human RMS cell lines suggested the presence of transforming DNA sequences, which was interpreted as being an unknown C-type virus[159,160] or an unknown gene.[161,162] Further studies, using high molecular weight DNA isolated directly from tumors, revealed the same dominant transforming gene in various carcinomas and a childhood RMS. This gene was shown to possess sequence homology with the Kirsten strain of murine sarcoma virus, called Ki-*ras* in current terminology.[163] Such a gene was subsequently identified in the RD cell line. It was found to be an activated N-*ras* gene with an alteration in the second exon, resulting in substitution of histidine for glutamine at the 61st amino acid position of the encoded p21 protein.[164] However, N-*ras* alone is insufficient to maintain the malignant phenotype; multiple oncogenes are typically involved, often in complementary pairs.[165]

Studies of developmental regulation of cellular oncogenes during normal muscle differentiation have shown conflicting findings regarding the expression of N-*ras*. High levels of expression were observed in fusion-defective subclones of muscle cells, and paradoxically high levels were observed at the myotube stage of a differentiating muscle cell line.[166] In normal myogenesis, activated N-*ras* was found to have an inhibitory effect when transfected into myoblastic cell lines,[167,168] but it had no effect at the myotube stage of differentiation.[169,170] These findings suggested that *ras* probably acts earlier in myogenesis than the transitional stages that confer irreversibility on differentiated cells.[170]

Research over the past decade has delineated seven classes of activity into which oncogenes may be categorized.[171] These activities are outlined in Figure 3. The *ras* family of oncogenes (H−, Ki−, and N−) are members of the class of membrane-associated guanine nucleotide-binding proteins. The next three classes of oncogenes (growth factors, growth factor receptors, and membrane-associated tyrosine kinases) are more proximal in the signal-transduction pathway. Two more distal categories of oncogenes include the cytoplasmic threonine kinases and the cytoplasmic hormone receptor, *erb*A. The seventh and perhaps most intensively studied class is the nuclear oncogenes, of which there are at least eight

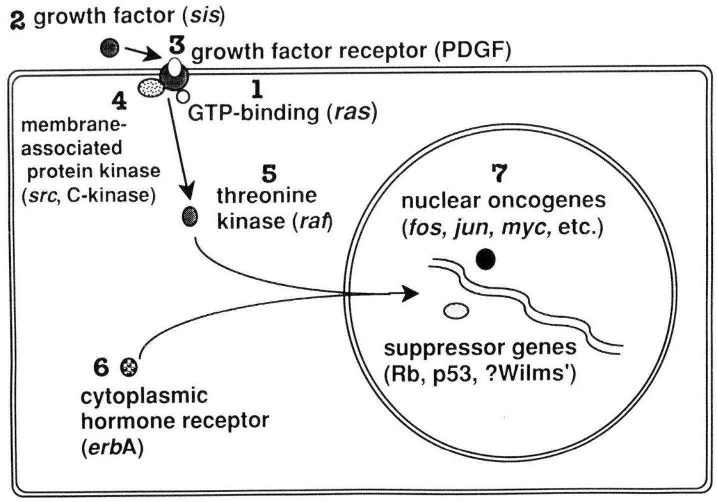

FIGURE 3.   Schema showing classes of oncogenes, arranged according to major site of activity in the cell.

members currently characterized. The foremost member of the group is *myc* with three well-documented human forms: c-*myc*, L-*myc*, and N-*myc*.

The first has been shown to be routinely overexpressed in human malignancy[172] and is often amplified or rearranged as well.[165,173,174] Expression of a c-*myc* shows no tissue or tumor specificity; RMS is known to overexpress c-*myc*.[174-176] However, *myc* expression is tightly linked to proliferation. This may present a problem in studies of cultured cell lines as opposed to original tumors. Routine overexpression of c-*myc* (among others) has been found in both malignant and normal breast epithelium *in vitro*, for example, but not in the original tissue.[177] Nonetheless, deregulated expression of c-*myc* has been observed in too many malignancies, both *in vivo* and *in vitro,* to believe that elevated levels of expression are artifacts of culture conditions.[178-182] For this reason, levels of c-*myc* expression may, if all other factors are equal, correlate with clinical aggressiveness in RMS.

Two other members of the *myc* family are well known: L-*myc* for small cell lung cancer and N-*myc* for neuroblastoma. N-*myc* was first identified in childhood neuroblastoma[183-186] and was quickly recognized to correlate strongly with clinical outcome.[185-188] Although amplication and expression of the N-*myc* gene are uniquely associated with neuroblastoma, it has occasionally been found to be amplified or expressed in RMS as well.[83,84,189-191] One of these cases was an undifferentiated tumor which subsequently differentiated *in vitro,*[83,84] and another was a RMS with bone metastases,[190] which is an unusual finding for this tumor. A third case may have been a malignant ectomesenchymoma.[189,189a] The most recent case, a well-characterized embryonal RMS, appears to be solely RMS, as opposed to the complex or ill-characterized tumors mentioned above. Nonetheless, expression or amplification of the N-*myc* oncogene in RMS is a very uncommon event. N-*myc* aplification or expression was not detected in 6 other RMS cell lines,[192] or in 25 such tumors on dot blot hybridization studies.[174] Certainly there is no clinical correlation between N-*myc* expression and prognosis in RMS, such as that seen in neuroblastoma.

Marked down-regulation of the c-*myc* gene is associated with a differentiating phenotype in normal muscle cells *in vitro*.[193] This finding led to the hypothesis that c-*myc* may function as a negative regulator of myogenesis.[166,194] However, it is known that reinduction of the c-*myc* gene at the myotube stage does not suppress muscle-specific genes,[195] and the autonomous expression of c-*myc* in transgenic mice does not inhibit normal muscle development.[178] Thus, introduction of a deregulated c-*myc* oncogene into mammalian muscle cells may not be sufficient to prevent myogenic differentiation.[170] Instead, there is evidence to suggest that the impact of c-*myc* on the differentiation process is indirect, through altered cell proliferation. This conclusion has been derived from experiments that show two features of c-*myc* activity. First, in cells which express tissue specific properties, independent of cell cycle withdrawal, c-*myc* transfection has no influence on these properties.[196,197] Second, erythroleukemia cells require growth arrest to express a differentiated phenotype, like muscle cells, in which transfection of erythroleukemia cells with c-*myc* blocks the differentiation process[179,182] by enhancing the cells' proliferative capacity.[181]

However, c-*myc* activation is not always related to the cell cycle[198-200] and tumors do not necessarily follow the rules for cell proliferation of their normal counterparts. To evaluate the role of c-*myc* oncogene as a molecular marker in human RMS, six cell lines were studied.[192] Elevated levels of c-*myc* expression were observed in all six lines. More importantly, all three embryonal RMSs showed lower levels of expression when compared with the three tumors of the alveolar type. This difference may merely reflect variable differentiation stages in the studied cell lines. However, if c-*myc* is consistently expressed at high levels in the more aggressive alveolar RMS, assays of c-*myc* expression may be used as a marker of aggressiveness in this tumor. The levels of c-*myc* expression in this study were independent of rates of cell proliferation and also correlated with tumor aggressiveness in the nude mouse model. High levels of c-*myc* expression were observed in a case of canine RMS.[201] C-*myc* amplification, on the other hand, was detected in some RMS cell lines in the previous study, and in 1 out of 25 such tumors in another study,[174] but c-*myc* amplification did not correlate with histologic subtype or biologic aggressiveness.

V. TUMOR SUPPRESSOR GENES ("ANTI-ONCOGENES")

Prior to the recognition of any known tumor suppressor gene, Knudson hypothesized the existence of an entire class of recessive, regulatory genes important in oncogenesis, which he termed "anti-oncogenes".[202,203] Evidence for their existence was based on observations on two other childhood tumors, Wilms' tumor and retinoblastoma. In both cases, constitutional deletion of chromosomal segments on 11p[204,205] and 13q, respectively, indicated that the loss of a gene or gene cluster could result in cancer. This was a striking departure from the situation with oncogenes described above. With oncogenes, overexpression, mediated by translocation, mutation, or other events resulting in loss of regulation, is the fundamental defect resulting in oncogenesis.

It has now become clear that the chromosomal segments in question harbor defined suppressor genes, and that this phenomenon is not limited to Wilms' tumor and retinoblastoma. Using loss of heterozygosity of the alleles in question as an index, it is now evident that many human malignancies are associated with reduction to homozygosity in informative alleles. Tumors with chromosomes harboring suppressor or putative suppressor genes include neuroblastoma with chromosome 1p, renal cell carcinoma with chromosome 3p, colorectal carcinoma with chromosome 5q, and a number of childhood tumors (Wilms', hepatoblastoma, and embryonal RMS) and adult tumors (bladder carcinoma, breast carcinoma, and cervical carcinoma) with chromosome 11p. In addition, retinoblastoma, osteosarcoma, breast carcinoma, small cell carcinoma of lung, and gastric carcinoma are associated with a suppressor gene on chromosome 13q. Also, chromosomes 17p and 18q harbor suppressor genes and are associated with colon carcinoma.[206] The list of chromosomes harboring suppressor genes will undoubtedly grow with continued research in this field.

The function of the suppressor genes is yet to be worked out in detail, but several areas of investigation have shed light on their interaction with both oncogenes and normal cellular genes. It has been recognized for years that malignant transformation is a multistep process, and that no one gene alone is responsible for the malignant phenotype.[155,207] Furthermore, recent studies on colorectal carcinoma have demonstrated specific genetic defects associated with the progressive stages of malignant transformation of colonic epithelium from hyperplastic adenoma to full-fledged, invasive, and metastatic colonic carcinoma.[208-211] It is noteworthy that the genetic defects in question include both oncogenes and known suppressor genes.[210-212] There is also a new suppressor gene, DCC, encoding an N-CAM-like, presumed cell-adhesive protein that appears to be important in invasion of the extracellular matrix leading to metastasis.[212]

These findings clearly indicate that both classes of defects (oncogenes and suppressor genes) are important in the development of cancer, but their mechanisms of action need to be elucidated. Mechanistic information for human tumor suppressor genes is largely limited to the two suppressor genes noted earlier, those of retinoblastoma and Wilms' tumor. In Wilms' tumor, information is still extremely limited, since the putative gene involved has only recently been cloned.[209,213-215]

The gene in question, LK15[216] or WT33,[214] is located in one of two known sites of allele loss in Wilms' tumor,[215] probably on chromosome 11p13. This gene is as yet incompletely cloned, but certain characteristics strongly suggest that it is a Wilms' tumor specific gene.[217] In particular, the gene encodes a 2.9- or 3.0-kb mRNA with four zinc-finger motifs, commonly found in transcription factors. This region is similar to the early growth response gene (EGR2), a known transcription regulator. However, ubiquitous expression of the gene was found in virtually all Wilms' tumor specimens examined. Thus, simple absence of the gene fails to account for development of Wilms' tumor, and a more complex mechanism is surely involved.

Furthermore, this gene and locus (11p13) are not associated with the Beckwith-Wiedemann syndrome, which includes predisposition to development of Wilms' tumor and embryonal RMS. This gene is localized to chromosome 11p15, indicating that there probably are multiple suppressor genes involved in the genesis of Wilms' tumor. The suppressor effect of such a candidate gene for Wilms' tumor, and perhaps for embryonal RMS as well, has been amply demonstrated by somatic-cell hybrid experiments. In these experiments, retention of a normal chromosome 11 by the hybrid cell results in suppression of tumorigenicity.[213] Thus, the Wilms' tumor model may eventually have great relevance to RMS, but there are insufficient data to document this at present.

A. RETINOBLASTOMA GENE PRODUCT

Compared to the putative Wilms' tumor gene, the cloning of the retinoblastoma (RB) gene is farther along, and there are extensive data on its direct and singular role in the development of retinoblastoma. Research on this gene is important, not only for its implication in retinoblastoma but also for the broad implications for tumor suppression in general. The gene appears to be active in a wide variety of malignancies in addition to retinoblastoma.

Earlier studies documented that the tumor cells of patients with familial retinoblastoma had defects on chromosome 13q14[218-220] and in an enzyme localized to chromosome 13q14, esterase D (ESD).[221] Thus, it was proposed that the suppressor gene responsible for tumor formation was closely linked to this locus. Subsequent studies with probes for additional loci on chromosome 13q14, as well as in ESD, showed deletions or partial homozygosity in 10 to 75% of retinoblastoma patients, even in those with seemingly normal chromosomes 13.[222-225] The actual gene involved was cloned[226,227] and eventually was shown to be complex. The gene consists of 27 exons, spanning over 200 kbp of genomic DNA and producing a 4.7-kb mRNA that encodes a 928-amino acid, 110-kDa nuclear phosphoprotein.[227-230] The gene lacks an upstream TATA box, but possesses a small upstream promoter region, like many "housekeeping" genes.[231] It has also been suggested that a smaller, 98-kDa RB protein may be translated from a smaller mRNA transcribed from a second AUG start codon 3' of the usual start codon.[232]

Early reports suggested expression of the RB gene was absent in retinoblastomas.[233] However, subsequent studies have documented that the majority of retinoblastomas in fact, express seemingly normal 4.7-kb RB mRNA.[234,235] More recently, polymerase chain reaction (PCR) amplification of both genomic DNA and mRNA has revealed subtle abnormalities in the majority of[236] or all[237] retinoblastoma patients; most of these abnormalities were point mutations leading to deletion of one or more exons in the mRNA. There is universal or nearly universal incidence of mutations in the RB gene in tumor cells, as opposed to normal cells from the same patient (in nonheriditary retinoblastoma). Thus, detection of the RB gene promises to be a means of separating familial from simplex retinoblastoma, and thereby provides an estimate of risk that may be useful for genetic counseling.[238] It is interesting also that the paternal chromosome appears to preferentially undergo germline mutation.[239] This is true not only for retinoblastoma[240] but for osteosarcoma as well.[241]

The normal function of the RB gene is still somewhat unclear, but a great deal of information has become available in the past few years. It was first noted that the RB protein binds to DNA-cellulose columns, which suggested a similar role *in vivo*.[242] Later, this DNA binding ability was localized to the carboxyl terminal region of the gene, from aa 612 to 928 carboxyl terminus.[231] Moreover, c-terminal truncation of the product in osteosarcoma was noted to lead to functional inactivation.[241] It was also noted that this region contains multiple phosphorylation sites, and that the c-terminal truncated protein is nonphosphorylated.[242] The ability to bind DNA would suggest that the RB gene can function as a *trans*-acting transcription factor, like a host of other proteins such as certain viral oncoproteins (adenovirus E1a, SV40 large T antigen, and human papilloma virus E7) and the c-*myc* oncogene.[243-245] Thus, a simple interpretation of the functional role of the RB gene would be that it somehow competes with c-*myc* and virally encoded oncoproteins, such as E1a, for a DNA binding site important in the regulation of cell proliferation.[244,245] Unfortunately, this model fails to explain several additional observations.

The first problem relates to a second property of the RB protein, namely, its documented ability to bind adenovirus E1a, SV40 large T antigen, and human papilloma virus E7, the same DNA binding transcription factors noted above.[244-251] This property is mediated by other portions of the c terminal region of the RB protein than that required for DNA binding,[250] and this complex formation is required for cell transformation mediated by adenovirus E1a.[249]

These loci are also frequent sites of inactivating mutations of the RB gene in naturally occurring tumors.[252,253] Thus, interactions between these viral oncoproteins and the RB protein seem to inactivate the normal growth-suppressive effects of this protein in a manner indistinguishable from the effect seen when RB protein is completely absent or inactivated by deletional mutations. This observation suggests a more complicated scheme involving DNA binding sites, RB protein, c-*myc* oncogene or similar promiscuous activator, and viral oncoproteins or cellular equivalent. The exact relationships between these various factors are still unclear.

Although details of the function of the RB gene are unknown, it has a definite role in regulation of the cell cycle. An early clue as to its function was the observation that viral oncoproteins, like SV40 large T, bind preferentially to RB protein or bind only to its underphosphorylated form.[245,250] Second, RB protein was noted to undergo dramatic changes in phosphorylation, which are synchronized with the cell cycle.[253-258] Furthermore, phosphorylation of RB protein is associated with dissociation of RB and SV40 large T complexes.[259,260] Moreover, this phosphorylation appears to be mediated by a known cell division cycle (cdc) kinase, histone H1 kinase (composed of cdc2 kinase and cyclin), that can phosphorylate six separate sites on the RB protein.[261] Considered together, this information overwhelmingly implicates RB protein in some facet of cell cycle regulation. This would be an appropriate role for a putative tumor suppressor gene that appears to antagonize the effects of dominant oncogenes such as c-*myc*.[262] This interpretation is further substantiated by recent findings indicating that the potent polypeptide growth inhibitor, transforming growth factor-beta (TGF-β), inhibits phosphorylation of RB protein and inhibits c-*myc* transcription. This inhibition of phosphorylation blocks cells in late G1 phase of the cell cycle, thereby causing growth arrest.[263,264] Clearly, the exact mechanism of the action of RB protein in tumor cell suppression remains to be elucidated, but its importance as a suppressor of the malignant phenotype is equally clear. It is for that reason that the possible role of RB protein in a variety of human tumors has been extensively pursued, and why RB would be expected to play a role in the genesis of RMS.

B. ROLE OF THE RB GENE IN HUMAN CANCER

A pivotal role for the RB gene in retinoblastoma is now unequivocal. This conclusion is based not only on the observations discussed above, but also on experimental studies. These studies show that reintroduction of a functional RB gene by a retroviral vector into retinoblastoma or osteosarcoma cells suppresses the neoplastic phenotype *in vitro* and suppresses tumorigenicity in immunodeficient mice.[265,266] This finding clearly indicates that the RB gene suppresses malignancy, as would be expected of a putative tumor suppressor gene, even if the exact mechanism of action remains unclear.

Since most retinoblastomas still express some form of RB protein, and since osteosarcoma has been implicated as another tumor in which the RB plays a pivotal role, it is not surprising that the RB protein is suspected to have a broader role in human cancer. This suspicion has been vindicated by several recent studies that revealed abnormalities of RB expression, cellular disposition, or function, which are based on the interactive properties with SV40 large T antigen, DNA binding, and other factors discussed above.[267] Breast cancers, in particular, frequently possess RB gene deletions leading to truncation or loss of RB mRNA.[268,269] Even cases with seemingly normal RB gene structure show a proportion of RB-negative cells when tested by immunohistochemistry with anti-RB antibody.[270]

Similar observations have been made in small cell carcinoma of lung,[271] bladder,[206] and prostate.[272] Other studies have suggested that abnormalities of RB might be limited to this subset of human tumors, not including common malignancies such as colon carcinoma, melanoma, and even breast carcinoma.[273] However, breast carcinoma has clearly been shown to frequently have RB abnormalities, as noted above, and even colon carcinoma has been shown to overexpress RB mRNA.[274] Thus, the limited involvement of the RB gene in human cancer, as previously suggested,[273] may be overly restrictive. In fact, there is substantial evidence that such limited involvement is not the case.

An important point in this regard is the original observation that the RB gene segment is abnormal in both RMS and sporadic osteosarcoma.[275] By implication, other sarcomas might be expected to be involved as well. Subsequent studies have borne this out. A wide variety of sporadic osteosarcomas and soft tissue sarcomas (including MFH, liposarcoma, undifferentiated sarcoma, and synoviosarcoma) have all been shown to possess frequent (as high as 43% in osteosarcoma) abnormalities of the RB gene or RB mRNA.[266,275-278]

C. ROLE OF THE RB GENE IN RMS

Of greatest importance in this chapter, however, is the potential role of the RB gene in RMS. To date, there is little direct evidence, but sporadic reports serve to demonstrate that the malignant behavior of RMS is also potentially mediated, at least in part, by the RB gene. In particular, RMS, like osteosarcoma, has also been observed to occur as a second malignancy in patients with familial retinoblastoma. More importantly, analysis of 69 cases of a variety of soft tissue sarcomas, including leiomyosarcoma, malignant peripheral nerve sheath tumor, and particularly a RMS, showed heterozygous deletion of the RB gene.[279] However, widespread lack of RB protein in sarcomas of bone and soft tissues in children, particularly RMS, has not been observed.[280] Further studies have shown normal expression of the 4.7S RB mRNA in all of a group of embryonal and alveolar RMS cell lines[281] as well as some level of expression of phosphorylated, 115-kDa RB protein in all cases.[281a] These findings indicate that a common defect of the RB gene in RMS is likely to be considerably more subtle than that observed in osteosarcoma and adult sarcomas, as noted above.

D. OTHER SUPPRESSOR GENES

A discussion of tumor suppressor genes would be incomplete without consideration of one other important, well-characterized gene, p53. This gene is usually located on chromosome 17p, which is a frequent site for deletions and other cytogenetic abnormalities in human cancer. Unlike both the putative Wilms' tumor gene and the RB gene, p53 was originally identified as an oncogene, because of its ability to transform early passage normal cells.[282,283] However, subsequent studies showed that this determination was inadvertently performed using a mutant, not wild type, p53, and that the wild type did not complement *ras* in tumor formation.[284] Quite the contrary, the wild type of p53 was clearly shown to have tumor-suppressive effects.[285-287]

Eventually, it was determined that the wild type differed from the mutated form of p53, in this case at a single site, aa 135, where a normal valine was replaced by a mutant alanine.[288] Subsequent studies of mutated p53 in a variety of tumors have demonstrated that all known mutations are contained within four of five domains that show striking sequence conservation across species lines.[287,288] It thus appears that mutation functionally inactivates the gene. Also, gross deletions are less common, although they are not excluded, in view of the high incidence of deletions of chromosome 17p.

The mode of action of p53 has been explored, and it bears reasonable similarity to the RB gene. Like RB protein, the p53 protein (of 53 kDa mass, as indicated by its name) is a SV40 large T antigen-binding nuclear phosphoprotein. p53 is phosphorylated by the same cdc2 kinase which is suspected of phosphorylating RB protein, and is known to phosphorylate SV40 large T antigen.[283,284,289] Usually, expression of p53 falls to low levels with advancing embryonic development, and is quite low in normal adult tissues.[290]

The p53 protein from amino acid residues 312 to 323 (SSSPQPKKKP) contains a serine phosphorylation site (aa315). This region is also implicated in nuclear localization, as it is in SV40 large T. Thus, both phosphorylation and nuclear targeting of p53 appear to be affected by mutations that render the protein nonfunctional. Unlike RB protein, however, p53 is not a DNA binding protein.[291]

It was noted that p53 protein is bound to SV40 large T in untransformed but not in transformed cells, which is reminiscent of the SV40 large T-mediated inactivation of RB protein.[284] Furthermore, SV40 large T forms oligomeric complexes with both p53 and RB protein, thereby presumably inactivating both of them.[292] However, p53 and RB protein do not form oligomeric complexes between themselves. This scheme thus suggests that SV40 large T and other proteins like it inactivate at least two tumor suppressor genes, p53 and RB, by complexing with either or both of them. The fact that mutated p53 protein functions as an oncogene only strengthens this argument. In that case, mutated p53 is presumed to complex with wild type p53, thereby diluting out its tumor-suppressive effect.[293]

The simple schema outlined above may well be true to a large extent. However, it fails to account for the observation that overexpression of even the normal, wild type human p53 in murine cells in culture renders the cells tumorigenic.[293] It would appear that the role of normal p53 in maintenance of the normal cell phenotype is dose-dependent, since too little or too much can both lead to tumorigenesis. The precise mechanisms responsible for this process are not yet known.

E. p53 IN CANCER

It is now well known that mutated p53 protein plays a role in malignant transformation of a variety of animal and human cells. Mutant alleles expressed at high levels have been found in tumors of lung, bone, and lymph nodes in transgenic mice transfected with a mutant gene,[294] as well as in spontaneously occurring human, chronic myelocytic leukemia.[295] Likewise, mutated p53 has also been detected in a diverse array of solid tumors including tumors of the brain, breast, lung, colon, and liver.[288,296-301] However, of greater importance in this discussion is the involvement of p53 in human RMS. Circumstantial evidence for this derived from studies of osteosarcoma, where p53 mutations and loss were found.[302,303] Point mutations of p53 have been identified in both RD and *RMS* rhabdomyosarcoma cell lines,[303a] and nearly half of RMS tumors studied have similarly shown one or more abnormalities of p53: loss of heterozygosity, lack of expression or point mutations.[303b]

F. GENERAL CONCLUSIONS

The role of suppressor genes in normal development and malignant progression is currently an area of intense interest among tumor cell biologists, molecular geneticists, and others who are studying the underlying genetic mechanisms of cancer. It is likely that childhood cancer will be a particularly fruitful area of investigation. It may shed light on the role of these and other suppressor genes in the etiology of cancers in adults as well. Tumors, like RMS, that present in both embryonal and "adult" (alveolar) forms, may prove to be of particular interest, since divergent mechanisms of transformation may be responsible for these clinically distinct neoplasms.

VI. OTHER RECENT DEVELOPMENTS IN TUMOR BIOLOGY

A. GROWTH FACTORS

Growth factors have been identified as members of the oncogene family, particularly as a result of studies on p28 of simian sarcoma virus *(sis)*, where a strong sequence homology between platelet-derived growth factor (PDGF) and v-*sis* was identified.[304-308] These observations ultimately led to the recognition of an entire family of closely related growth factor receptors to which both PDGF and a host of other growth factors bind.[309] These factors and their receptors represent the proximal portion of the signal transduction pathway, which mirrors the families of oncogenes described above and shown in Figure 3.

The availability of various purified growth factors and defined media led to the identification of two growth factors with inhibitory effects on myogenesis. These are fibroblast growth factor (FGF)[310-312] and TGF-β.[313-315]

FGF appears to play a role in normal myogenesis, since it has been detected immunocytochemically in striated muscle cells and their precursors.[316] A temporal correlation between levels of FGF and muscle cell differentiation suggested a role of this growth factor in the regulation of muscle cell development.[316] Human RMS cell lines RD and A204 were found to produce and express FGF *in vitro*.[317] This factor stimulates proliferation of RMS cells as well as bovine vascular endothelial cells. FGF and TGF-β were also isolated from another cell line, A673.[318-320] The A673 cell line is often referred to as RMS,[77,320] but it is actually a primitive neuroectodermal tumor of the chest wall (Askin tumor).[320a] Thus, the role of this growth factor and its receptor is by no means specific for or limited to myoblasts and RMS.

The mechanism by which FGF and TGF-β inhibit myogenesis is unknown, although it is clear that each one operates through signal transduction pathways.[171,321] TGF-β, in particular, was found to down-regulate MyoD1 expression in some muscle cell lines.[322] This down-regulation appears to be dose-dependent, since at lower doses TGF-β has no effect on MyoD1, but rather regulates pathways of slow calcium channels.[323]

Another pair of growth factors involved in normal muscle growth and maturation are insulin-like growth factor (IGF) I and II, which stimulate both growth and differentiation via a receptor-mediated mechanism.[324-326] High levels of IGF-II expression have been observed in RMS cell lines RD and A204, as well as in tumors. This finding was attributed to an autocrine growth factor mechanism.[327,328] Like FGF, IGF has also been identified in the non-RMS cell line A673[329] and in Wilms' tumor,[330-334] as well as fetal kidney, liver, adrenal, and striated muscle.[333,334] The gene for IGF-II was localized to the short arm of chromosome 11p, in the region of the Wilms' tumor and Beckwith-Wiedemann syndrome loci. This finding provoked speculation that IGF-II is somehow linked to this cluster of fetal or embryonal tumors. However, the finding of IGF-II expression and mitogenic stimulation in a variety of adult tumors, such as breast carcinoma,[335,336] small cell carcinoma of lung,[337,338] and leiomyosarcoma,[339] clearly indicated that IGF-II is not linked to any specific group of tumors.

B. GENETIC CONTROL OF MYOGENESIS

Genetic control of myogenesis is currently an extremely active field of investigation. This is not only because of its relevance to normal tissue differentiation, but also because it has become a paradigm of molecular genetic control of gene expression, in general, in higher eukaryotes. Probably no other system, except immunoglobulin gene rearrangement in hematopoietic ontogeny, has been so successfully dissected at the genetic level. This area of research originated from studies on the effect of the chemotherapeutic agent 5-azacytidine on DNA methylation and the subsequent alterations of gene expression and cell phenotype, which was analogous to the studies on differentiating agents and myogenesis described earlier. The cells first investigated were nonmyogenic mouse 3T3 and 10T-$\frac{1}{2}$ cells. After treatment, these cells were noted to develop a markedly myogenic, as well as adipocytic and chondrocytic, phenotype.[340-343] The genes responsible were not identified at the time, but the results clearly implicated three separate regulatory loci, one for each phenotype. The findings also suggested that as few as one to three hypomethylation events per cell were sufficient to activate the hypothesized muscle locus.[344]

Following confirmation of this prescient observation, cDNA from 5-azacytidine-treated 10T-$\frac{1}{2}$ cells was transfected into untreated 10T-$\frac{1}{2}$ cells. The myogenic conversion rate (1:15,000) indicated that 5-azacytidine-induced demethylation of a single locus was sufficient to account for the induced myogenesis.[345] Later, the specific cDNA was identified by screening a myocyte cDNA library with cDNA isolated from proliferating myoblasts of three isolates. One was shown to induce myogenesis on transfection into a number of cells, and was identified as MyoD1.[125,345] The specific cDNA was also noted to have a 22-amino acid sequence with striking sequence homology to c-*myc*. Thus, a suitable candidate gene for control of myogenesis had been identified.

Subsequent molecular genetic analysis of myogenous cells used probes with highly conserved sequences with extensive homology to *myc* oncogenes, which were hybridized to genomic DNA of various species under reduced stringency conditions to allow binding to genes with only partial sequence homology. These molecular genetic studies led to the discovery of an entire family of myogenic regulatory genes (muscle determination genes) that occur in human, mouse, rat, chicken, and, undoubtedly, in most other vertebrate cells. Several of these myogenic genes have been cloned. They include the original mouse MyoD1 gene,[125] the avian MyoD1[346] and the human MyoD1[124] (or Myf-3),[347] rat[348] or mouse[126] myogenin or the human homologue (Myf-4),[347] the avian CMD,[346] the presumed early myogenic determination gene (myd),[349] a later human myogenic gene (Myf-5),[347] as well as the recently described Myf-6, a late myogenesis gene,[350] and the MRF-4 gene.[351] All these genes encode nuclear binding proteins that share sequence similarities with other important regulatory molecules, including the *myc* oncoproteins.[352] They all possess a unique tertiary configuration, the HLH motif.[353] They are also related to the *achaete-scute* complex in *Drosophila,* which appears to be involved in neuronal determination and in development of the nervous system.[352]

Although muscle determination genes may serve as diagnostic markers for RMS,[123] caution is adivsed in the interpretation of such data. For example, although both MyoD1 and myogenin are skeletal muscle-specific,[125,348] myogenin has been detected earlier than MyoD1 in the developing mouse embryo. On the other hand, in mouse limb bud explants, MyoD1 and myogenin are both absent initially in cells capable of myogenous differentiation.[354] These experiments suggest the existence of regulatory genes that act earlier than myogenin and MyoD1 in myogenesis.[355] Furthermore, it appears that myogenin can substitute for MyoD1.[354] This concept is supported by the fact that both of these factors dimerize and can form heterodimers with one another, or they may form homodimers of one or the other, since both are members of the HLH family. Thus, either factor can potentially confer the myogenic phenotype on uncommitted cells. Analysis of only one factor could lead to the erroneous conclusion that the tumor in question is nonmyogenic or, in the case of childhood sarcomas, that it is something other than a RMS. Furthermore, a tumor not expressing either factor might still be a RMS, if an even earlier gene, such as Myd,[349] is expressed but MyoD1 and myogenin are not.

It is conceivable that primitive RMSs may exist which do not express any of the known muscle determination genes. Such an occurrence has been demonstrated in C2 myoblasts (derived from the original Yaffe myoblast line[356,357]), where inducible myoblasts express no MyoD1.[358] This has probably also been demonstrated in A204 cells, where the original tissue has been reviewed and various muscle-specific proteins detected in the original tumor tissue (that it, muscle-specific actin, desmin, creatin kinase-MM, and myoglobin).[358a] Despite this, the cell line is negative for MyoD1, while all other RMS cell lines examined were positive.[359] Thus, sole reliance on MyoD1 as a single determinant of RMS is suspect until more is known of MyoD1 and other myogenic determinant gene expression in this tumor system.

The mode of action of muscle determination genes is unknown. However, a hierarchy in their appearance and function has been proposed. For example, since myd is thought to activate MyoD1, it has been speculated that MyoD1 is more distal in the regulatory pathway and is, therefore, activated by myd, which may be initially activated by hypomethylation.[349] MyoD1 can then act as a positive transcriptional regulator by binding to sites of several muscle-specific genes,[360] or it may act as a positive autoregulator of its own promoter.[361] Reciprocal activation of MyoD1 and myogenin, on the other hand, has suggested the existence of a loop mechanism. This loop either stabilizes the myogenic process[126] or amplifies the expression of these genes to a critical level necessary for activation of the myogenic program.[361]

As mentioned above, transfection experiments with muscle determination genes result in increased levels of expression of the MyoD1 geneins, and negative modulators of myogenesis, such as the H-*ras* or *fos* oncogenes[362,363] and FGF, inhibit of MyoD1 expression.[322] Thus, it is reasonable to suggest that MyoD1 may act as a common effector of terminal differentiation in already determined muscle cells. This hypothesis is also supported by experiments in permissive and inducible myoblasts *in vitro*. MyoD1 is constitutive in the permissive cells, but it is absent from the myoblastic stage of the inducible cells, appearing only in their terminally differentiated stages.[358] As mentioned earlier, MyoD1 alone is insufficient to account for myogenesis in every case. MyoD1 apparently functions *in vivo* as a dimer.[365,366] It then binds to a specific DNA sequence that has been shown to be an enhancer for muscle creatine kinase (MCK), among other genes.[360,367]

It has also become apparent that heterodimerization of either myogenin or MyoD1 with members of another ubiquitous immunoglobulin enhancer protein family, either E12 or E47, results in a heterodimer complex with markedly greater affinity for the MCK enhancer.[368] This complex is thus capable of up-regulating expression of either MyoD1 or myogenin and MCK. It now appears that this positive regulation is offset by negative regulation mediated by a similar HLH protein, termed Id, that lacks the critical 10- to 20-amino acid base region required for DNA binding.[369] The role of nonmuscle immunoglobulin gene expression-related enhancer proteins, such as E12 and E47, and their implications for the muscle specificity of the system are currently an area of intense interest. It is clear that there is more to expression of skeletal muscle differentiation than MyoD1.

Differentiation experiments in RMS cell lines using 5-azacytidine as a differentiating agent have also shown elevated levels of MyoD1 expression in relation to morphologic differentiation.[370] This finding suggests the presence of a regulatory pathway similar to the one in normal muscle development. The above experiments also suggest that quantitative expression of MyoD1 may be used as a differentiation marker. On the other hand, transfection experiments in the RD line with MyoD1 have shown morphologic differentiation as a result of positive autoregulation, but there were no differences in tumorigenicity in the nude mouse.[359] This observation supports the notion that coordinate morphologic differentiation and increased MyoD1 expression are not necessarily associated with decreased tumorigenicity, which is in contrast to observations on degree of differentiation and prognosis in children with RMSs.[149] Additional differentiation experiments in human RMSs are in progress, however. These studies include a variety of known differentiating agents such as retinoic acid,[40,84] dimethylformamide,[73] TPE,[371] and dibutyryl-cyclic AMP, as well as antineoplastic drugs such as 5-azacytidine.[370]

C. NEURAL DIFFERENTIATION IN RMS

It has been thought that a common function of all muscle determination genes and their products is their ability to confer a myogenic phenotype on cells of all germ layers, including neuroectodermal cells.[346] However, recent studies cast doubt on this simple interpretation. It has been shown that introduction of a functional MyoD1 gene in liver cells is not sufficient to induce a myogenous phenotype, but if sufficient numbers of fibroblasts are present in a subsequent heterokaryon fusion, muscle gene expression will occur.[353] This study, as well as an earlier one,[372] clearly indicates that not all cell types are responsive to MyoD1 alone. In particular, human kidney and tumor cell lines were not able to express muscle specific proteins after forced expression of MyoD1. Likewise, several tissues, including nerve, continued to express their tissue specific genes simultaneously with muscle specific genes.

These observations are particularly interesting in view of the existence of tumors containing malignant myogenous and neuroectodermal elements, such as medullomyoblastoma intracranially[373] and malignant ectomesenchymoma in soft tissues[374,375] or bone.[375] Also, some RMSs have the potential to express a neural phenotype.[377] Furthermore, MyoD1 regulates expression of the acetylcholine receptor-α subunit, and the myogenic gene family is closely related to the neuronal family of regulatory genes in *Drosophila, achaete-scute*. Thus, MyoD1, and probably other regulatory factors like it, can induce a variety of phenotypes, either alone or in concert with one another. Moreover, the spontaneous appearance of mixed myogenic-neuroectodermal phenotypic tumors is not only explicable, but perhaps expected in these embryonal tumors. In fact, the propensity for such mixed phenotype is perhaps most evident in the neonatal period, since most such tumors so far reported occur in this age group. Recent studies suggest that such tumors are much more frequent among poorly differentiated sarcomas of infancy and early childhood than previously believed.[382]

VII. FINAL NOTE

It is apparent from the preceding review that RMS *in vitro* represents a rich repertoire of opportunities for experimental studies. In addition, recent work on allied fields of biological research appear to be converging on this tumor system. At the same time, a highly organized clinical cooperative study, the Intergroup Rhabdomyosarcoma Study (IRS), has made possible laboratory and clinical investigation of this relatively rare and enigmatic tumor. This situation offers a promising opportunity to meld state-of-the-art basic laboratory research with fruitful clinical investigation and, as such, is unique among human tumor systems, with the possible exception of neuroblastoma. The authors hope that reviews, such as this chapter and this book, will foster such studies.

VIII. SUMMARY

This chapter discussed experimental models of RMS, including tumors induced in experimental animals, cell lines derived from such tumors, cell lines developed from human tumors, and xenografts in athymic or nude mice of both human primary tumors and cell lines. There was a section on animal tumors and cell lines and a section on human tumors. Biological aspects reviewed include patterns of growth and metastasis, adhesion properties of tumor cells, cytogenetics, light and electron microscopy, and immunocytochemistry. Possible applications of these findings in chemotherapy, radiotherapy, and induction of tumor differentiation were reviewed. In addition, a separate section on recent developments discussed newer findings in the areas of cytogenetics, molecular cytogenetics, cytoskeletal differentiation, and oncogenes. Relevance of these developments to RMS was shown for tumor suppressor genes (anti-oncogenes), growth factors, genetic control of myogenesis in both skeletal muscle and RMS, and neural differentiation in RMS.

Several major conclusions arise from these discussions. RMS *in vitro*, whether in animal systems or as human cell lines, represents an important model for exploration of the basic biology of the tumor and also has provided information of possible use in therapy. The clinical applications of findings derived from experimental chemotherapy, radiotherapy, and even induction of differentiation in models of RMS *in vitro* or as xenografts continue to evolve.

In addition, major advances have been made in understanding the relation of the genesis of RMS to skeletal muscle differentiation, as well as in elucidating properties of invasion and metastasis, cytogenetics, and molecular genetics of this tumor. These advances were possible only through the studies of RMS preparations in long- or short-term culture. RMS *in vitro* emerges as an essential tool for the investigation and improved understanding of this important malignant tumor of infants, children, and adolescents.

REFERENCES

1. **Gilman, J. P. W. and Ruckerbauer, G. M.,** Metal carcinogenesis. I. Observations on the carcinogenicity of a refinery dust, cobalt oxide, and colloidal thorium dioxide, *Cancer Res.,* 22, 152, 1962.
2. **Heath, J. C. and Webb, M.,** Content and intracellular distribution of the inducing metal in the primary rhabdomyosarcomata induced in the rat by cobalt, nickel and cadmium, *Br. J. Cancer,* 21, 768, 1967.
3. **Webb, M., Heath, J. C., and Hopkins, T.,** Intranuclear distribution of the inducing metal in primary rhabdomyosarcomata induced in the rat by nickel, cobalt and cadmium, *Br. J. Cancer,* 26, 274, 1972.
4. **Sen, P. and Costa, M.,** Induction of chromosomal damage in Chinese hamster ovary cells by soluble and particulate nickel compounds: preferential fragmentation of the heterochromatic long arm of the X-chromosome by carcinogenic crystalline NiS particles, *Cancer Res.,* 45, 2320, 1985.
5. **Gilman, J. P. W.,** Metal carcinogenesis. II. A study on the carcinogenic activity of cobalt, copper, iron, and nickel compounds, *Cancer Res.,* 22, 158, 1962.
6. **Hermens, A. F. and Barendsen, G. W.,** Cellular proliferation patterns in an experimental rhabdomyosarcoma in the rat, *Eur. J. Cancer,* 3, 361, 1967.
7. **Sweeney, F. L., Pot-Deprun, J., Poupon, M.-F., and Chouroulinkov, I.,** Heterogeneity of the growth and metastatic behavior of cloned cell lines derived from a primary rhabdomyosarcoma, *Cancer Res.,* 42, 3776, 1982.

8. **Pot-Deprun, J., Poupon, M.-F., Sweeney, F. L., and Chouroulinkov, I.,** Growth, metastasis, immunogenicity, and chromosomal content of a nickel-induced rhabdomyosarcoma and subsequent cloned cell lines in rats, *J. Natl. Cancer Inst.,* 71, 1241, 1983.

9. **Antoine, E., Pauwels, C., Verrelle, P., Lascaux, V., and Poupon, M. F.,** In vivo emergence of a highly metastatic tumour cell line from a rat rhabdomyosarcoma after treatment with an alkylating agent, *Br. J. Cancer,* 57, 469, 1988.

10. **Poupon, M.-F., Judde, J. G., Pot-Deprun, J., Sweeney, F., and Lespinats, G.,** Variable susceptibility to NK activity of cloned cell lines derived from a primary rat rhabdomyosarcoma: relationship to metastatic potential, *Br. J. Cancer,* 48, 75, 1983.

11. **Gabbert, H. E., Gerharz, C. D., Engers, R., Müller, K. W., and Moll, R.,** Terminally differentiated postmitotic tumor cells in a rat rhabdomyosarcoma cell line, *Virchows Arch. B,* 55, 255, 1988.

12. **Korach, S., Poupon, M.-F., Du Villard, J.-A., and Becker, M.,** Differential adhesiveness of rhabdomyosarcoma-derived cloned metastatic cell lines to vascular endothelial monolayers, *Cancer Res.,* 46, 3624, 1986.

13. **Lissitzky, J. C., Bouzon, M., Loret, E., Poupon, M. F., and Martin, P. M.,** Laminin-mediated adhesion in metastatic rat rhabdomyosarcoma cell lines involves prominent interactions with the laminin E8 fragment, *Clin. Exp. Metastasis,* 7, 469, 1989.

14. **Bouzon, M., Lissitzky, J.-C., Kopp, F., and Martin, P.-M.,** Laminin-induced capping and receptor expression at cell surface in a rat rhabdomyosarcoma cell line: involvement in cell adhesion and migration on laminin substrates, *Exp. Cell Res.,* 185, 482, 1989.

15. **Liotta, L. A., Rao, C. N., and Wewer, U.,** Biochemical interactions of tumor cells with the basement membrane, *Annu. Rev. Biochem.,* 55, 1037, 1986.

16. **Liotta, L. A.,** Mechanisms of cancer invasion and metastasis, *Cancer Growth Prog.,* 3, 58, 1989.

17. **Moczar, E., Becker, M., and Poupon, M. F.,** Modulation of proteoglycan metabolism by hydrocortisone and by growth factors in rhabdomyosarcoma cell lines of different metastatic potentials, *Clin. Exp. Metastasis,* 3, 235, 1985.

18. **Redini, F., Moczar, E., and Poupon, M. F.,** Cell surface glycosaminoglycans of rat rhabdomyosarcoma lines with different metastatic potentials and of non-malignant rat myoblasts, *Biochim. Biophys. Acta,* 883, 98, 1986.

19. **Redini, F., Moczar, E., Antoine, E., and Poupon, M. F.,** Binding and internalization of exogenous glycosaminoglycans in weakly and highly metastatic rhabdomyosarcoma cells, *Biochim. Biophys. Acta,* 991, 359, 1989.

20. **Moczar, M., Poupon, M. F., and Moczar, E.,** Hyaluronate-binding proteins in weakly and highly metastatic variants of rat rhabdomyosarcoma cells, *Clin. Exp. Metastasis,* 8, 129, 1990.

21. **Uriel, J., Poupon, M. F., and Geuskens, M.,** Alphafoetoprotein uptake by cloned cell lines derived from a nickel-induced rat rhabdomyosarcoma, *Br. J. Cancer,* 48, 261, 1983.

22. **Geuskens, M., Naval, J., and Uriel, J.,** Ultrastructural studies of the intracellular translocation of endocytosed alpha-foetoprotein (AFP) by cytochemistry and of the uptake of ^{3}H-arachidonic acid bound to AFP by autoradiography in rat rhabdomyosarcoma cells, *J. Cell. Physiol.,* 128, 389, 1986.

23. **Nath, N., Basrur, P. K., and Limebeer, R.,** A new cell line derived from nickel sulfide-induced rat rhabdomyosarcoma, *In Vitro,* 7, 158, 1971.

24. **Yamashiro, S., Gilman, J. P. W., Basrur, P. K., and Abandowitz, H. M.,** Growth and cytogenetic characteristics of nickel sulphide-induced rhabdomyosarcomas in rats, *Acta Pathol. Jpn.,* 28, 435, 1978.

25. **Christie, N. T., Sen, P., and Costa, M.,** Chromosomal alterations in cell lines derived from mouse rhabdomyosarcomas induced by crystalline nickel sulfide, *Biol. Metals,* 1, 43, 1988.

26. **Christie, N. T., Tummolo, D. M., Biggart, N. W., and Murphy, E. C. J.,** Chromosomal changes in cell lines from mouse tumors induced by nickel sulfide and methyl-cholanthrene, *Cell Biol. Toxicol.,* 4, 427, 1988.

27. **Corbeil, L. B.,** Differentiation of rhabdomyosarcoma and neonatal muscle cells in vitro, *Cancer,* 20, 572, 1967.

28. **Altmannsberger, M., Weber, K., Droste, R., and Osborn, M.,** Desmin is a specific marker for rhabdomyosarcomas of human and rat origin, *Am. J. Pathol.,* 118, 85, 1985.

29. **Hildebrand, H. F. and Biserte, G.,** Ultrastructural investigation of Ni_3S_2-induced rhabdomyosarcoma in Wistar rat. Comparative study with emphasis on myofibrillar differentiation and ciliar formation, *Cancer,* 42, 528, 1978.

30. **Hildebrand, H. F. and Biserte, G.,** Cylindrical laminated bodies in nickel-subsulphide-induced rhabdomyosarcoma in rabbits, *Eur. J. Cell Biol.,* 19, 276, 1979.

31. **Babai, F., Skalli, O., Schurch, W., Seemayer, T. A., and Gabbiani, G.,** Chemically induced rhabdomyosarcomas in rats. Ultrastructural, immunohistochemical, biochemical features and expression of α-actin isoforms, *Virchows Arch. B,* 155, 263, 1988.

32. **Kosmehl, H., Langbein, L., and Katenkamp, D.,** Histological and immunohistochemical findings in experimental rhabdomyosarcomas. Comparisons between original tumors, tumor recurrences and allotransplants in nude mice, *Exp. Pathol.,* 36, 81, 1989.

33. **Langbein, L., Kosmehl, H., and Katenkamp, D.,** Lectin histochemistry of experimental murine rhabdomyosarcomas, *Acta Histochem.,* 86, 93, 1989.
34. **Langbein, L., Kosmehl, H., Kiss, F., Katenkamp, D., and Neupert, G.,** Cytokeratin expression in experimental murine rhabdomyosarcomas. Intermediate filament pattern in original tumors, allotransplants, cell culture and re-established tumors from cell culture, *Exp. Pathol.,* 36, 23, 1989.
35. **Kosmehl, H., Langbein, L., and Katenkamp, D.,** Experimental rhabdomyosarcoma with regions like malignant fibrous histiocytoma (MFH)-a true double phenotypic pattern?, *J. Pathol.,* 160, 135, 1990.
36. **Markov, D. V. and Hadjiolov, D. C.,** Fine structure of 7, 12-dimethylbenz(a)anthracene-induced rhabdomyoblastoma in Syrian hamster, *Arch. Geschwulstforsch.,* 37, 344, 1971.
37. **Markov, D. V. and Hadjiolov, D. C.,** The fine structure of a transplantable rhabdomyoblastoma in Syrian hamster, *Arch. Geschwulstforsch.,* 40, 122, 1972.
38. **Markov, D. V. and Hadjiolov, D. C.,** Differentiation of malignant myoblasts in 7, 12-dimethylbenz(a)anthracene-induced rhabdomyoblastomas. An electron microscopic study, *Arch. Geschwulstforsch.,* 48, 521, 1978.
39. **Gerharz, C. D., Gabbert, H., Moll, R., Mellin, W., Engers, R., and Gabbiani, G.,** The intraclonal and interclonal phenotypic heterogeneity in a rhabdomyosarcoma cell line with abortive imitation of embryonic myogenesis, *Virchows Arch. B,* 55, 193, 1988.
40. **Gabbert, H. E., Gerharz, C.-D., Biesalski, H. K., Engers, R., and Luley, C.,** Terminal differentiation and growth inhibition of a rat rhabdomyosarcoma cell line (BA-HAN-1C) in vitro after exposure to retinoic acid, *Cancer Res.,* 48, 5264, 1988.
41. **Gerharz, C. D., Gabbert, H., Engers, R., and Luley, C.,** Long-term differentiation induction in a rat rhabdomyosarcoma cell line with retinoic acid and FCS-depleted growth medium, *Verh. Dtsch. Ges. Pathol.,* 72, 218, 1988.
42. **Reinhold, H. S.,** Quantitative evaluation of the radiosensitivity of cells of a transplantable rhabdomyosarcoma in the rat, *Eur. J. Cancer,* 2, 33, 1966.
43. **Perk, K. and Moloney, J. B.,** Pathogenesis of a virus-induced rhabdomyosarcoma in mice, *J. Natl. Cancer Inst.,* 37, 581, 1966.
44. **Perk, K., Moloney, J. B., and Jenkins, E. G.,** Virus-induced rhabdomyosarcoma transplantation studies in weanling BALB/c mice, *J. Natl. Cancer Inst.,* 40, 337, 1968.
45. **Perk, K., Gazdar, A. F., and Russell, E. R.,** Studies on a transplantable murine rhabdomyosarcoma, *J. Natl. Cancer Inst.,* 54, 1207, 1975.
46. **Azzarello, G., Sartore, S., Saggin, L., Gorza, L., D'Andrea, E., Chieco-Bianchi, L., and Schiaffino, S.,** Myosin isoform expression in rat rhabdomyosarcoma induced by Moloney murine sarcoma virus, *J. Cancer Res. Clin. Oncol.,* 113, 417, 1987.
47. **Nameroff, M. A., Reznik, M., Anderson, P., and Hansen, J. L.,** Differentiation and control of mitosis in a skeletal muscle tumor, *Cancer Res.,* 30, 596, 1970.
48. **Friedmann, I. and Bird, E. S.,** Electron-microscope investigation of experimental rhabdomyosarcoma, *J. Pathol.,* 97, 375, 1969.
49. **Bruni, C. and Rust, J. N.,** Fine structure of dividing cells and of nondividing, differentiating cells of nickel sulfide-induced rhabdomyosarcomas, *J. Natl. Cancer Inst.,* 54, 687, 1975.
50. **Gerharz, C. D., Gabbert, H. E., Biesalski, H. K., Engers, R., and Luley, C.,** Fetal calf serum and retinoic acid affect proliferation and terminal differentiation of a rat rhabdomyosarcoma cell line (BA-HAN-1C), *Br. J. Cancer,* 59, 61, 1989.
51. **Gerharz, C. D., Gabbert, H. E., Engers, R., Ramp, U., Mayer, H., Biesalski, H. K., and Luley, C.,** Heterogeneous response to differentiation induction in different clonal subpopulations of a rat rhabdomyosarcoma cell line (BA-HAN-1), *Cancer Res.,* 49, 7132, 1989.
52. **Gabbert, H. E., Gerharz, C. D., Ramp, U., Hoffmann, J., Oster, O., Oesch, F., and Doehmer, J.,** Enhanced expression of the proto-oncogenes *fos* and *raf* in the rhabdomyosarcoma cell line *ba-han-1cf* after differentiation induction with retinoic acid and n-methylformamide, *Int. J. Cancer,* 45, 724, 1990.
53. **Freeman, A., and Johnson, W.,** A comparative study of childhood rhabdomyosarcoma and virus-induced rhabdomyosarcoma in mice, *Cancer,* 28, 1490, 1968.
54. **Pauwels, C., Rebischung, J.-L., Jasmin, C., and Poupon, M.-F.,** Enhanced cloning efficiency of murine rhabdomyosarcoma cells after chlorozotocin treatment: relationship with enhanced lung metastasis, *J. Natl. Cancer Inst.,* 74, 817, 1985.
55. **Pauwels-Vergely, C. and Poupon, M.-F.,** Immunogenic capacity of tum variants isolated from a rat rhabdomyosarcoma, *Br. J. Cancer,* 56, 7, 1987.
56. **Pauwels-Vergely, C. and Poupon, M.-F.,** Chlorozotocin-induced selection of autocrine and multidrug resistant variants from a rat rhabdomyosarcoma, *Anticancer Res.,* 8, 137, 1988.
57. **Reinhold, H. S.,** A cell dispersion technique for use in quantitative transplantation studies with solid tumours, *Eur. J. Cancer,* 1, 67, 1965.
58. **Barendsen, G. W. and Broerse, J. J.,** Experimental radiotherapy of a rat rhabdomyosarcoma with 15 MeV neutrons and 300 kV X-rays. I. Effects of single exposures, *Eur. J. Cancer,* 5, 373, 1969.

59. **Moulder, J. E. and Fischer, J. J.,** Determination of an optimal treatment plan for rat rhabdomyosarcomas, *Radiology,* 107, 439, 1973.

60. **Barendsen, G. W., Roelse, H., Hermens, A. F., Madhuizen, H. T., van Peperzeel, H. A., and Rutgers, D. H.,** Clonogenic capacity of proliferating and nonproliferating cells of a transplantable rat rhabdomyosarcoma in relation to its radiosensitivity, *J. Natl. Cancer Inst.,* 51, 1521, 1973.

61. **Curtis, S. B. and Tenforde, T. S.,** Assessment of tumour response in a rat rhabdomyosarcoma, *Br. J. Cancer,* 41(Suppl. 4), 266, 1980.

62. **Jung, H., Beck, H.-P., Brammer, I., and Zywietz, F.,** Depopulation and repopulation of the R1H rhabdomyosarcoma of the rat after X-irradiation, *Eur. J. Cancer,* 17, 375, 1981.

63. **Tenforde, T. S., Afzal, S. M. J., Parr, S. S., Howard, J., Lyman, J. T., and Curtis, S. B.,** Cell survival in rat rhabdomyosarcoma tumors irradiated in vivo with extended-peak silicon ions, *Radiat. Res.,* 92, 208, 1982.

64. **Afzal, S. M. J., Tenforde, T. S., Parr, S. S., and Curtis, S. B.,** PLD repair in rat rhabdomyosarcoma tumor cells irradiated in vivo and in vitro with high-LET and low-LET radiation, *Radiat. Res.,* 107, 354, 1986.

65. **Martin, D. F., Porter, E. A., Fischer, J. J., and Rockwell, S.,** Effect of a perfluorochemical emulsion on the radiation response of BA1112 rhabdomyosarcoma, *Radiat. Res.,* 112, 45, 1987.

66. **Tenforde, T. S., Montoya, V. J., Afzal, S. M. J., Parr, S. S., and Curtis, S. B.,** Response of rat rhabdomyosarcoma tumors to split doses of mixed high- and low-LET radiation, *Int. J. Radiat. Oncol. Biol. Phys.,* 16, 1529, 1989.

67. **Reynolds, C. P., Reynolds, D. A., Frenkel, E. P., and Smith, R. G.,** Selective toxicity of 6-hydroxydopamine and ascorbate for human neuroblastoma in vitro: a model for clearing marrow prior to autologous transplant, *Cancer Res.,* 42, 1331, 1982.

68. **Reynolds, C. P., Matthay, K. K., Crouse, V. L., Wilbur, J. R., Shurin, S. B., and Seeger, R. C.,** Response of neuroblastoma bone marrow metastases to 13-cis-retinoic acid, *Proc. ASCO,* 9, 54, 1990.

69. **Friend, C. and Freedman, H. A.,** Effects and possible mechanism of action of dimethylsulfoxide on Friend cell differentiation, *Biochem. Pharmacol.,* 27, 1309, 1978.

70. **Marks, P. A. and Rifkind, R. A.,** Erythroleukemic differentiation, *Annu. Rev. Biochem.,* 47, 419, 1978.

71. **Rabson, A. S., Stern, R., Tralka, T. S., Costa, J., and Wilczek, J.,** Hexamethylene bisacetamide induces morphologic changes and increased synthesis of procollagen in cell line from glioblastoma multiforme, *Proc. Natl. Acad. Sci. U.S.A.,* 74, 5060, 1977.

72. **Dexter, D. L., Barbosa, J. A., and Calabresi, P.,** N,N-dimethylformamide-induced alteration of cell culture characteristics and loss of tumorigenicity in cultured human colon carcinoma cells, *Cancer Res.,* 39, 1020, 1979.

73. **Dexter, D. L.,** N,N-dimethylformamide-induced morphological differentiation and reduction of tumorigenicity in cultured mouse rhabdomyosarcoma cells, *Cancer Res.,* 37, 3136, 1977.

741. **Dexter, D. L., Konieczny, S. F., Lawrence, J. B., Shaffer, M., Mitchell, P., and Coleman, J. R.,** Induction by butyrate of differentiated properties in cloned murine rhabdomyosarcoma cells, *Differentiation,* 18, 115, 1981.

75. **Lazarides, E. and Capetanaki, Y. G.,** The striated muscle cytoskeleton: expression and assembly in development, in *Molecular Biology of Muscle Development,* Emerson, C., Fischman, D. A., Nadal-Ginard, B., and Siddiqui, M. A. O., Eds., Alan R. Liss, New York, 1986, 749.

76. **McAllister, R. M., Melnyk, J., Finklestein, J. Z., Adams, E. C. J., and Gardner, M. B.,** Cultivation in vitro of cells derived from a human rhabdomyosarcoma, *Cancer,* 24, 520, 1969

77. **Giard, D. J., Aaronson, S. A., Todaro, G. J., Arnstein, P., Kersey, J. H., Dosik, H., and Parks, W. P.,** In vitro cultivation of human tumors: establishment of cell lines derived from a series of solid tumors, *J. Natl. Cancer Inst.,* 51, 1417, 1973.

78. **Dickman, P. S. and Lazarides, E.,** Cytoskeletal differentiation in cultured rhabdomyosarcoma, *Lab. Invest.,* 60(Abstr.), 24A, 1989.

79. **Nelson-Rees, W. A., McAllister, R. M., and Gardner, M. B.,** Clonal aspects of the c-type virus-releasing cells of a cultured human rhabdomyosarcoma line (RD114) in vitro, *Nature New Biol.,* 236, 147, 1972.

80. **Stephens, R., Traul, K., Lowry, G., Zelljadt, I., and Mayyasi, S.,** Differential morphology of the RD virus from the human rhabdomyosarcoma, RD-114B cell line demonstrated by negative staining electron microscopy, *Nature New Biol.,* 240, 212, 1972.

81. **Chapman, A. L., Bogner, P., and Behbehani, A. M.,** A study of a new human tumor cell line (rhabdomyosarcoma), *Proc. Soc. Exp. Biol. Med.,* 146, 1087, 1974.

82. **Sekiguchi, M., Shiroko, Y., Suzuki, T., Imada, M., Miyahara, M., and Fujii, G.,** Characterization of a human rhabdomyosarcoma cell strain in tissue culture, *Biomed. Pharmacother.,* 39, 372, 1985.

83. **Garvin, A. J., Drew, S. W., Hintz, D. S., and Sens, D. A.,** Tissue culture as a diagnostic technique for soft-tissue sarcoma of childhood, *Arch. Pathol. Lab. Med.,* 108, 308, 1984.

84. **Garvin, A. J., Stanley, W. S., Bennett, D. D., Sullivan, J. L., and Sens, D. A.,** The in vitro growth, heterotransplantation, and differentiation of a human rhabdomyosarcoma cell line, *Am. J. Pathol.,* 125, 208, 1986.

85. **Clayton, J., Pincott, J. R., van den Berghe, J., and Kemshead, J. T.,** Comparative studies between a new human rhabdomyosarcoma cell line, jr-1 and its tumour of origin, *Br. J. Cancer,* 54, 83, 1986.

86. **Motoyama, T., Watanabe, H., and Yamamoto, T.,** Embryonal rhabdomyosarcoma in nude mice and in vitro, *Acta Pathol. Jpn.,* 36, 1495, 1986.

87. **Nanni, P., De Giovanni, C., Nicoletti, G., Del Re. B., Scotlandi, K., and Lollini, P. L.,** Human rhabdomyosarcoma cells in nude mice as a model for metastasis and differentiation, *Invasion Metastasis,* 9, 231, 1989.

88. **De Giovanni, C., Nanni, P., Nicoletti, G., Ceccarelli, C., Scotlandi, K., Landuzzi, L., and Lollini, P. L.,** Metastatic ability and differentiative properties of a new line of human embryonal rhabdomyosarcoma (CCA), *Anticancer Res.,* 9, 1943, 1989.

89. **Nanni, P., Schiaffino, S., De Giovanni, C., Nicoletti, G., Prodi, G., Del Re, B., Eusebi, V., Ceccarelli, C., Saggin, L., and Lollini, P.-L.,** RMZ: a new cell line from a human alveolar rhabdomyosarcoma. In vitro expression of embryonic myosin, *Br. J. Cancer,* 54, 1009, 1986.

90. **Schiaffino, S., Gorza, L., Sartore, S., Saggin, L., and Carli, M.,** Embryonic myosin heavy chain as a differentiation marker of developing human skeletal muscle and rhabdomyosarcoma. A monoclonal antibody study, *Exp. Cell Res.,* 163, 211, 1986.

91. **Kelland, L. R., Bingle, L., Edwards, S., and Steel, G. G.,** High intrinsic radiosensitivity of a newly established and characterised human embryonal rhabdomyosarcoma cell line, *Br. J. Cancer,* 59, 160, 1989.

92. **Sugimoto, T., Swada, T., Arakawa, S., Matsumura, T., Sakamoto, I., Takeuchi, Y., Reynolds, C. P., Kemshead, J. T., and Helson, L.,** Possible differential diagnosis of neuroblastoma from rhabdomyosarcoma and Ewing's sarcoma by using a panel of monoclonal antibodies, *Jpn. J. Cancer Res.,* 76, 301, 1985.

93. **Alitalo, K., Myllylä, R., Sage, H., Pritzl, P., Vaheri, A., and Bornstein, P.,** Biosynthesis of type V procollagen by A204, a human rhabdomyosarcoma cell line, *J. Biol. Chem.,* 257, 9016, 1982.

94. **Scarpa, S., Modesti, A., and Triche, T. J.,** Extracellular matrix synthesis by undifferentiated childhood tumor cell lines, *Am. J. Pathol.,* 129, 74, 1987.

95. **Krieg, T., Timpl, R., Alitalo, K., Kurkinen, M., and Vaheri, A.,** Type III procollagen is the major collagenous component produced by a continuous rhabdomyosarcoma cell line, *FEBS Lett.,* 104, 405, 1979.

96. **Stracca-Pansa, V., Dickman, P. S., Zamboni, G., Bevilacqua, P. A., and Ninfo, V.,** Extracellular matrix of small round cell tumors of childhood: an immunohistochemical study of 67 cases, presented to the 17th Int. Congr. International Academy of Pathology, Dublin, Ireland, September 4 to 9, 1988 and in preparation.

97. **Lazarus, H., Tegeler, W., Mazzone, H. M., Leroy, J. G., Boone, B. A., and Foley, G. E.,** Determination of sensitivity of individual biopsy specimens to potential inhibitory agents: evaluation of some explant culture methods as assay systems, *Cancer Chemother. Rep.,* 50, 543, 1966.

98. **Masuda, S., Shinohara, N., and Chuman, H.,** Antitumor effects of CDDP on human rhabdomyosarcoma transplanted in nude mice, *Fukuoka Acta Med.,* 73, 541, 1982.

99. **Takizawa, T., Matsui, T., Maeda, Y., Okabe, S., Mochizuki, M., Tanaka, A., Kawaguchi, K., Fukayama, M., Funata, N., Koike, M., and Mastuda, T.,** X-radiation-induced differentiation of xenotransplanted human undifferentiated rhabdomyosarcoma, *Lab. Invest.,* 60, 22, 1989.

100. **Houghton, J. A., Houghton, P. J., and Webber, B. L.,** Growth and characterization of childhood rhabdomyosarcomas as xenografts, *J. Natl. Cancer Inst.,* 68, 437, 1982.

101. **Houghton, J. A., Houghton, P. J., and Green, A. A.,** Chemotherapy of childhood rhabdomyosarcomas growing as xenografts in immune-deprived mice, *Cancer Res.,* 42, 535, 1982.

102. **Houghton, J. A., Cook, R. L., Lutz, P. J., and Houghton, P. J.,** Melphalan: a potential new agent in the treatment of childhood rhabdomyosarcoma, *Cancer Treat. Rep.,* 69, 91, 1985.

103. **Hazelton, B. J., Houghton, J. A., Parham, D. M., Douglass, E. C., Torrance, P. M., Holt, H., and Houghton, P. J.,** Characterization of cell lines derived from xenografts of childhood rhabdomyosarcoma, *Cancer Res.,* 47, 4501, 1987.

104. **Houghton, P. J., Tharp, R., Houghton, J. A., Holland, J. F., and Bekesi, J. G.,** Evaluation of 3-(p-fluorophenyl)-L-alanyl-3-[m-bis-(2-chloroethyl)aminophenyl]-L-alanyl-L-methionine ethyl ester HCl(PTT.119) against xenografts of human rhabdomyosarcoma, *Cancer Chemother. Pharmacol.,* 22, 201, 1988.

105. **Horowitz, M. E., Etcubanas, E., Christensen, M. L., Houghton, J. A., George, S. L., Green, A. A., and Houghton, P. J.,** Phase II testing of melphalan in children with newly diagnosed rhabdomyosarcoma: a model for anticancer drug development, *J. Clin. Oncol.,* 6, 308, 1988.

106. **DeGregorio, M. W., Lui, G. M., Macher, B. A., and Wilbur, J. R.,** Uptake, metabolism, and cytotoxicity of doxorubicin in human Ewing's sarcoma and rhabdomyosarcoma cells, *Cancer Chemother. Pharmacol.,* 12, 59, 1984.

107. **Nyce, J.,** Drug-induced DNA hypermethylation and drug resistance in human tumors, *Cancer Res.,* 49, 5829, 1989.

108. **Sandor, R.,** Inhibition of human rhabdomyosarcoma-cell growth in agar by dibutyryl cyclic AMP, *J. Natl. Cancer Inst.,* 51, 257, 1973.
109. **Sandberg, A. A., Turc, C. C., and Gemmill, R. M.,** Chromosomes in solid tumors and beyond, *Cancer Res.,* 48, 1049, 1988.
110. **Molenaar, W. M., Dam, M. A., Kamps, W. A., and Cornelisse, C. J.,** DNA-aneuploidy in rhabdomyosarcomas as compared with other sarcomas of childhood and adolescence, *Hum. Pathol.,* 19, 573, 1988.
111. **Lai, J. L., Savary, J. B., Deminatti, M., Demaille, M. C., and Baranzelli, M. C.,** Translocation (2;13)(q37;q14) in rhabdomyosarcoma: a new case (letter), *Cancer Genet. Cytogenet.,* 25, 371, 1987.
112. **Lizard-Nacol, S., Mugneret, F., Volk, C., Turc-Carel, C., Favrot, M., and Philip, T.,** Translocation (2;13)(q37;q14) in alveolar rhabdomyosarcoma: a new case (letter), *Cancer Genet. Cytogenet.,* 25, 373, 1987.
113. **Rowe, D., Gerrard, M., Gibbons, B., and Malpas, J. S.,** Two further cases of t(2;13) in alveolar rhabdomyosarcoma indicating a review of the published chromosome breakpoints, *Br. J. Cancer,* 56, 379, 1987.
114. **Douglass, E. C., Valentine, M., Etcubanas, E., Parham, D., Webber, B. L., Houghton, P. J., Houghton, J. A., and Green, A. A.,** A specific chromosomal abnormality in rhabdomyosarcoma, *Cytogenet. Cell Genet.,* 45, 148, 1987.
115. **Engel, R., Ritterbach, J., Schwabe, D., and Lampert, F.,** Chromosome translocation (2;13)(q37;q14) in a disseminated alveolar rhabdomyosarcoma, *Eur. J. Pediatr.,* 148, 69, 1988.
116. **Wang-Wuu, S., Soukup, S., Ballard, E., Gotwals, B., and Lampkin, B.,** Chromosomal analysis of sixteen human rhabdomyosarcomas, *Cancer Res.,* 48, 983, 1988.
117. **Seidal, T., Mark, J., Hagmar, B., and Angervall, L.,** Alveolar rhabdomyosarcoma: a cytogenetic and correlated cytological and histological study, *Acta Pathol. Microbiol. Immunol. Scand. Sect. A,* 90, 345, 1982.
118. **Whang-Peng, J., Triche, T. J., Knutsen, T., Miser, J., Kao-Shan, S., Tsai, S., and Israel, M. A.,** Cytogenetic characterization of selected small round cell tumors of childhood, *Cancer Genet. Cytogenet.,* 21, 185, 1986.
119. **Hayashi, Y., Inaba, T., Hanada, R., and Yamamoto, K.,** Translocation 2;8 in a congenital rhabdomyosarcoma (letter), *Cancer Genet. Cytogenet.,* 30, 343, 1988.
120. **Moriyama, M., Shuin, T., Kubota, Y., Satomi, Y., Sugio, Y., and Kuroki, Y.,** A case of rhabdomyosarcoma of the bladder with a (2;5) chromosomal translocation in peripheral lymphocytes, *Cancer Genet. Cytogenet.,* 22, 177, 1986.
121. **Koufos, A., Hansen, M. F., Copeland, N. G., Jenkins, N. A., Lampkin, B. C., and Cavenee, W. K.,** Loss of heterozygosity in three embryonal tumours suggests a common pathogenetic mechanism, *Nature,* 316, 330, 1985.
122. **Scrable, H. J., Witte, D. P., Lampkin, B. C., and Cavenee, W. K.,** Chromosomal localization of the human rhabdomyosarcoma locus by mitotic recombination mapping, *Nature,* 329, 645, 1987.
123. **Scrable, H., Witte, D., Shimada, H., Seemayer, T., Wang-Wuu, S., Soukup, S., Koufos, A., Houghton, P., Lampkin, B., and Cavenee, W.,** Molecular differential pathology of rhabdomyosarcoma, *Genes Chromosomes Cancer,* 1, 23, 1989.
124. **Scrable, H. J., Johnson, D. K., Rinchik, E. M., and Cavenee, W. K.,** Rhabdomyosarcoma-associated locus and myod1 are syntenic separate loci on the short arm of human chromosome 11, *Proc. Natl. Acad. Sci. U.S.A.,* 87, 2182, 1990.
124a. **Cavenee, W.,** personal communication to the author, 1990.
125. **Davis, R. L., Weintraub, H., and Lassar, A. B.,** Expression of a single transfected cDNA converts fibroblasts to myoblasts, *Cell,* 51, 987, 1987.
126. **Edmondson, D. G. and Olson, E. N.,** A gene with homology to the myc similarity region of myod1 is expressed during myogenesis and is sufficient to activate the muscle differentiation program, *Genes Dev.,* 3, 628, 1989.
127. **Sapienza, C., Paquette, J., Tran, T. H., and Peterson, A.,** Epigenetic and genetic factors affect transgene methylation imprinting, *Development,* 107, 165, 1989.
128. **Sapienza, C.,** Genome imprinting and dominance modification, *Ann N.Y. Acad. Sci.,* 564, 24, 1989.
129. **Sapienza, C., Tran, T. H., Paquette, J., McGowan, R., and Peterson, A.,** A methylation mosaic model for mammalian genome imprinting, *Prog. Nucleic Acid Res. Mol. Biol.,* 36, 145, 1989.
130. **Hall, J. G.,** Genomic imprinting: review and relevance to human diseases, *Am. J. Hum. Genet.,* 46, 857, 1990.
131. **Scrable, H., Cavenee, W., Ghavimi, F., Lovell, M., Morgan, K., and Sapienza, C.,** A model for embryonal rhabdomyosarcoma tumorigenesis that involves genome imprinting, *Proc. Natl. Acad. Sci. U.S.A.,* 86, 7480, 1989.
132. **Brown, K. W., Williams, J. C., Maitland, N. J., and Mott, M. G.,** Genomic imprinting and the Beckwith-Wiedemann syndrome (letter), *Am. J. Hum. Genet.,* 46, 1000, 1990.

133. **Knudson, A. J.,** Mutation and cancer: statistical study of retinoblastoma, *Proc. Natl. Acad. Sci. U.S.A.,* 68, 820, 1971.

134. **Knudson, A. J. and Strong, L. C.,** Mutation and cancer: a model for Wilms' tumor of the kidney, *J. Natl. Cancer Inst.,* 48, 313, 1972.

135. **Knudson, A. G., Jr. and Meadows, A. T.,** Regression of neuroblastoma IV-S: a genetic hypothesis, *N. Engl. J. Med.,* 302, 1254, 1980.

136. **Li, F. P. and Fraumeni, J. J.,** Rhabdomyosarcoma in children: epidemiologic study and identification of a familial cancer syndrome, *J. Natl. Cancer Inst.,* 43, 1365, 1969.

137. **Li, F. P. and Fraumeni, J. J.,** Soft-tissue sarcomas, breast cancer, and other neoplasms. A familial syndrome?, *Ann. Intern. Med.,* 71, 747, 1969.

138. **Li, F. P., Fraumeni, J. J., Mulvihill, J. J., Blattner, W. A., Dreyfus, M. G., Tucker, M. A., and Miller, R. W.,** A cancer family syndrome in twenty-four kindreds, *Cancer Res.,* 48, 5358, 1988.

139. **Adelstein, R. S., Conti, M. A., Daniel, J. L., and Anderson, W., Jr.,** The interaction of platelet actin, myosin and myosin light chain kinase, in *Biochemistry and Pharmacology of Platelets,* CIBA Foundation Symp. 35 (New Series), Vol. 35, Elsevier/North-Holland, Amsterdam, 1975, 101.

140. **Whalen, R. G., Sell, S. M., Butler-Browne, G. S., Schwartz, K., Bouveret, P., and Pinset-Härström, I.,** Three myosin heavy-chain isozymes appear sequentially in rat muscle development, *Nature,* 292, 805, 1981.

141. **Biral, D., Damiani, E., Margreth, A., and Scarpini, E.,** Myosin subunit composition in human developing muscle, *Biochem. J.,* 224, 923, 1984.

142. **Sartore, S., Gorza, L., and Schiaffino, S.,** Fetal myosin heavy chains in regenerating muscle, *Nature,* 298, 294, 1982.

143. **Molenaar, W. M., Oosterhuis, J. W., Oosterhuis, A. M., and Ramaekers, F. C. S.,** Mesenchymal and muscle-specific intermediate filaments (vimentin and desmin) in relation to differentiation in childhood rhabdomyosarcomas, *Hum. Pathol.,* 16, 838, 1985.

144. **Capetanaki, Y. G., Ngai, J., and Lazarides, E.,** Regulation of the expression of the genes coding for the intermediate filament subunits vimentin, desmin and glial fibrillary acidic protein, in *Molecular Biology of the Cytoskeleton,* Borisy, G. G., Cleveland, D., and Murphy, D., Eds., Cold Spring Harbor Laboratory, Cold Spring Harbor, NY, 1984, 415.

145. **Gard, D. L. and Lazarides, E.,** The synthesis and distribution of desmin and vimentin during myogenesis in vitro, *Cell,* 19, 263, 1980.

146. **Tokuyasu, K. T., Maher, P. A., and Singer, S. J.,** Distributions of vimentin and desmin in developing chick myotubes in vivo. II. Immunoelectron microscopic study, *J. Cell Biol.,* 100, 1157, 1985.

147. **Nelson, W. J. and Lazarides, E.,** Assembly and establishment of membrane-cytoskeleton domains during differentiation. Spectrin as a model system, *Cell Membranes,* 2, 219, 1984.

148. **Newton, W. A., Jr., Soule, E. H., Hamoudi, A. B., Reiman, H. M., Shimada, H., Beltangady, M., and Maurer, H.,** Histopathology of childhood sarcomas, Intergroup Rhabdomyosarcoma Studies I and II: clinicopathologic correlation, *J. Clin. Oncol.,* 6, 67, 1988.

149. **Schmidt, D., Reimann, O., Treuner, J., and Harms, D.,** Cellular differentiation and prognosis in embryonal rhabdomyosarcoma, *Virchows Arch. A,* 409, 183, 1986.

150. **Dickman, P. S. and Triche, T. J.,** Immunocytochemistry and prognosis in pediatric soft tissue sarcomas: primitive rhabdomyosarcoma vs. primitive soft tissue sarcoma, in preparation.

151. **Bishop, J. M.,** Retroviruses and cancer genes, *Adv. Cancer Res.,* 37, 1, 1982.

152. **Bishop, J. M.,** Cellular oncogenes and retroviruses, *Annu. Rev. Biochem.,* 52, 301, 1983.

153. **Land, H., Parada, L. F., and Weinberg, R. A.,** Cellular oncogenes and multistep carcinogenesis, *Science,* 222, 771, 1983.

154. **Friend, S. H., Dryja, T. P., and Weinberg, R. A.,** Oncogenes and tumor-suppressing genes, *N. Engl. J. Med.,* 318, 618, 1988.

155. **Weinberg, R. A.,** Oncogenes, antioncogenes, and the molecular bases of carcinogenesis, *Cancer Res.,* 49, 3713, 1989.

156. **Thiele, C. J., McKeon, C., Triche, T. J., Ross, R. A., Reynolds, C. P., and Israel, M. A.,** Differential proto-oncogene expression characterizes histopathologically indistinguishable tumors of the peripheral nervous system, *J. Clin. Invest.,* 80, 804, 1987.

157. **McKeon, C., Thiele, C. J., Ross, R. A., Kwan, M., Triche, T. J., Miser, J. S., and Israel, M. A.,** Indistinguishable patterns of protooncogene expression in two distinct but closely related tumors: Ewing's sarcoma and neuroepithelioma, *Cancer Res.,* 48, 4307, 1988.

158. **McAllister, R. M.,** Search for oncogenes in human rhabdomyosarcoma cells, *Prog. Immunobiol. Stand.,* 5, 237, 1972.

159. **Cook, B., O'Sullivan, F., Leung, J., Morse, P., Graham, B., and Chapman, A. L.,** Transformation of human embryo cells with the use of cell-free extracts of a human rhabdomyosarcoma cell line (HUS-2): brief communication, *J. Natl. Cancer Inst.,* 60, 979, 1978.

160. **Karpas, A. and Tuckerman, E.,** Transformation of human fibroblasts with D.N.A. of cultured human rhabdomyosarcoma cells, *Lancet,* 1, 1138, 1974.

161. **Hall, A., Marshall, C. J., Spurr, N. K., and Weiss, R. A.,** Identification of transforming gene in two human sarcoma cell lines as a new member of the *ras* gene family located on chromosome 1, *Nature,* 303, 396, 1983.

162. **Marshall, C. J., Hall, A., and Weiss, R. A.,** A transforming gene present in human sarcoma cell lines, *Nature,* 299, 171, 1982.

163. **Pulciani, S., Santos, E., Lauver, A. V., Long, L. K., Aaronson, S. A., and Barbacid, M.,** Oncogenes in solid human tumours, *Nature,* 300, 539, 1982.

164. **Chardin, P., Yeramian, P., Madaule, P., and Tavitian, A.,** N-*ras* gene activation in the RD human rhabdomyosarcoma cell line, *Int. J. Cancer,* 35, 647, 1985.

165. **Suarez, H. G., Nardeux, P. C., Andeol, Y., and Sarasin, A.,** Multiple activated oncogenes in human tumors, *Oncogene Res.,* 1, 201, 1987.

166. **Leibovitch, M. P., Leibovitch, S. A., Hillion, J., Guillier, M., Schmitz, A., and Harel, J.,** Possible role of c-*fos*, c-n-*ras* and c-*mos* proto-oncogenes in muscular development, *Exp. Cell Res.,* 170, 80, 1987.

167. **Olson, E. N., Spizz, G., and Tainsky, M. A.,** The oncogenic forms of n-*ras* or h-*ras* prevent skeletal myoblast differentiation, *Mol. Cell. Biol.,* 7, 2104, 1987.

168. **Payne, P. A., Olson, E. N., Hsiau, P., Roberts, R., Perryman, M. B., and Schneider, M. D.,** An activated c-ha-ras allele blocks the induction of muscle-specific genes whose expression is contingent on mitogen withdrawal, *Proc. Natl. Acad. Sci. U.S.A.,* 84, 8956, 1987.

169. **Clegg, C. H. and Hauschka, S. D.,** Heterokaryon analysis of muscle differentiation: regulation of the postmitotic state, *J. Cell Biol.,* 105, 937, 1987.

170. **Schneider, M. D. and Olson, E. N.,** Control of myogenic differentiation by cellular oncogenes, *Mol. Neurobiol.,* 2, 1, 1988.

171. **Druker, B. J., Mamon, H. J., and Roberts, T. M.,** Oncogenes, growth, factors, and signal transduction, *N. Engl. J. Med.,* 321, 1383, 1989.

172. **Slamon, D. J., de Kernion, J. B., Verma, I. M., and Cline, M. J.,** Expression of cellular oncogenes in human malignancies, *Science,* 224, 256, 1984.

173. **Yokota, J., Tsunetsugu-Yokota, Y., Battifora, H., Le Fevre, C., and Cline, M. J.,** Alterations of *myc*, *myb*, and Ha-*ras* protooncogenes in cancers are frequent and show clinical correlation, *Science,* 231, 261, 1986.

174. **Tsuda, H., Shimosato, Y., Upton, M. P., Yokota, J., Terada, M., Ohira, M., Sugimura, T., and Hirohashi, S.,** Retrospective study on amplification on n-*myc* and c-*myc* genes in pediatric solid tumors and its association with prognosis and tumor differentiation, *Lab. Invest.,* 59, 321, 1988.

175. **Yamada, H., Sakamoto, H., Taira, M., Nishimura, S., Shimosato, Y., Terada, M., and Sugimura, T.,** Amplifications on both c-Ki-*ras* with a point mutation and c-*myc* in a primary pancreatic cancer and its metastatic tumors in lymph nodes, *Jpn. J. Cancer Res.,* 77, 370, 1986.

176. **Dias, P., Kumar, P., Marsden, H. B., Gattamaneni, H. R., and Kumar, S.,** N- and c-*myc* oncogenes in childhood rhabdomyosarcoma (letter), *J. Natl. Cancer Inst.,* 82, 151, 1990.

177. **Benz, C. C., Scott, G. K., Santos, G. F., and Smith, H. S.,** Expression of c-*myc*, c-Ha-*ras*1, and c-*erb*B-2 proto-oncogenes in normal and malignant human breast epithelial cells, *J. Natl. Cancer Inst.,* 81, 1704, 1990.

178. **Leder, A., Pattengale, P. K., Kuo, A., Stewart, T. A., and Leder, P.,** Consequences of widespread deregulation of the c-*myc* gene in transgenic mice: multiple neoplasms and normal development, *Cell,* 45, 485, 1986.

179. **Prochownik, E. V. and Kukowska, J.,** Deregulated expression of c-*myc* by murine erythroleukaemia cells prevents differentiation, *Nature,* 322, 848, 1986.

180. **Schneider, M. D., Payne, P. A., Ueno, H., Perryman, M. B., and Roberts, R.,** Dissociated expression of c-*myc* and a *fos*-related competence gene during cardiac myogenesis, *Mol. Cell. Biol.,* 6, 4140, 1986.

181. **Keath, E. J., Caimi, P. G., and Cole, M. D.,** Fibroblast lines expressing activated c-*myc* oncogenes are tumorigenic in nude mice and syngeneic animals, *Cell,* 39, 339, 1984.

182. **Coppola, J. A. and Cole, M. D.,** Constitutive c-*myc* oncogene expression blocks mouse erythroleukaemia cell differentiation but not commitment, *Nature,* 320, 760, 1986.

183. **Schwab, M., Varmus, H. E., Bishop, J. E., Grzeschik, K.-H., Naylor, S. L., Sakaguchi, A. Y., Brodeur, G., and Trent, J.,** Chromosome localization in normal human cells and neuroblastomas of a gene related to c-*myc*, *Nature,* 308, 288, 1984.

184. **Schwab, M., Ellison, J., Busch, M., Rosenau, W., Varmus, H. E., and Bishop, J. M.,** Enhanced expression of the human gene N-*myc* consequent to amplification of DNA may contribute to malignant progression of neuroblastoma, *Proc. Natl. Acad. Sci. U.S.A.,* 81, 4940, 1984.

185. **Brodeur, G. M., Seeger, R. C., Schwab, M., Varmus, H. E., and Bishop, J. M.,** Amplification of N-*myc* in untreated human neuroblastomas correlates with advanced disease stage, *Science,* 224, 1121, 1984.

186. **Brodeur, G. M., Seeger, R. C., Schwab, M., Varmus, H. E., and Bishop, J. M.,** Amplification of N-*myc* sequences in primary human neuroblastomas: correlation with advanced disease stage, *Prog. Clin. Biol. Res.,* 175, 105, 1985.

187. **Seeger, R. C., Brodeur, G. M., Sather, H., Calton, A., Siegel, S. E., Wong, K. Y., and Hammond, D.,** Association of multiple copies of the N-*myc* oncogene with rapid progression of neuroblastomas, *N. Engl. J. Med.,* 313, 1111, 1985.

188. **Brodeur, G. M., Fong, C. T., Morita, M., and Griffith, R.,** Molecular analysis and clinical significance of N-*myc* amplification and chromosome 1p monosomy in human neuroblastomas, *Prog. Clin. Biol. Res.,* 271, 3, 1988.

189. **Garson, J. A., Clayton, J., McIntyre, P., and Kemshead, J. T.,** N-*myc* oncogene amplification in rhabdomyosarcoma at relapse, *Lancet,* 1, 1496, 1986.

189a. **Kemshead, J. T.,** personal communication to the author, 1990.

190. **Mitani, K., Kurosawa, H., Suzuki, A., Hayashi, Y., Hanada, R., Yamamoto, K., Komatsu, A., Kobayashi, N., Nakagome, Y., and Yamada, M.,** Amplification of n-*myc* in a rhabdomyosarcoma, *Jpn. J. Cancer Res.,* 77, 1062, 1986.

191. **Hayashi, Y., Sugimoto, T., Horii, Y., Hosoi, H., Inazawa, J., Kemshead, J. T., Inaba, T., Hanada, R., Yamamoto, K., Gown, A. M., et al.,** Characterization of an embryonal rhabdomyosarcoma cell showing amplification and over-expression of the n-*myc*, *Int. J. Cancer,* 45, 705, 1990.

192. **Kouraklis, G., Triche, T. J., and Tsokos, M.,** Alveolar vs. embryonal rhabdomyosarcoma: growth in nude mice and *myc* oncogene expression, *Fed. Proc.,* 46 (Abstr.), 742, 1987.

193. **Sejersen, T., Sumegi, J., and Ringertz, N. R.,** Density-dependent arrest of DNA replication is accompanied by decreased levels of c-*myc* mRNA in myogenic but not in differentiation-defective myoblasts, *J. Cell. Physiol.,* 125, 465, 1985.

194. **Sejersen, T., Wahrmann, J. P., Sumegi, J., and Ringertz, N. R.,** Change in expression of oncogenes (*sis, ras, myc,* and *abl*) during in vitro differentiation of 16 rat myoblasts, *Prog. Cancer Res. Ther.,* 32, 243, 1985.

195. **Endo, T. and Nadal, G. B.,** Transcriptional and posttranscriptional control of c-*myc* during myogenesis: its mRNA remains inducible in differentiated cells and does not suppress the differentiated phenotype, *Mol. Cell. Biol.,* 6, 1412, 1986.

196. **Alemà, S., Casalbore, P., Agostini, E., and Tatò, F.,** Differentiation of PC12 phaeochromocytoma cells induced by v-*src* oncogene, *Nature,* 316, 557, 1985.

197. **Casalbore, P., Agostini, E., Alemà, S., Falcone, G., and Tatò, F.,** The v-*myc* oncogene is sufficient to induce growth transformation of chick neuroretina cells, *Nature,* 326, 188, 1987.

198. **Curran, T. and Morgan, J. I.,** Superinduction of c-*fos* by nerve growth factor in the presence of peripherally active benzodiazepines, *Science,* 229, 1265, 1985.

199. **Mulvagh, S. L., Michael, L. H., Perryman, M. B., Roberts, R., Schneider, M. D.,** A hemodynamic load in vivo induces cardiac expression of the cellular oncogene, c-*myc*, *Biochem. Biophys. Res. Commun.,* 147, 627, 1987.

200. **Starksen, N. F., Simpson, P. C., Bishopric, N., Coughlin, S. R., Less, W. M., Escobedo, J. A., and Williams, L. T.,** Cardiac myocyte hypertrophy is associated with c-*myc* protooncogene expression, *Proc. Natl. Acad. Sci. U.S.A.,* 83, 8348, 1986.

201. **Engström, W., Barrios, C., Willems, J. S., Möllermark, G., Kängström, L. E., Eliasson, I., and Larsson, O.,** Expression of the *myc* protooncogene in canine rhabdomyosarcoma, *Anticancer Res.,* 7, 1109, 1987.

202. **Knudson, A. G.,** Hereditary cancers of man, *Cancer Invest.,* 1, 187, 1983.

203. **Knudson, A. G.,** Model hereditary cancers of man, *Prog. Nucleic Acid Res. Mol. Biol.,* 29, 17, 1983.

204. **Kaneko, Y., Egues, M. C., and Rowley, J. D.,** Interstitial deletion of short arm of chromosome 11 limited to Wilms' tumor cells in a patient without aniridia, *Cancer Res.,* 41, 4577, 1981.

205. **Koufos, A., Hansen, M. F., Lampkin, B. C., Workman, M. L., Copeland, N. G., Jenkins, N. A., and Cavenee, W. K.,** Loss of alleles at loci on human chromosome 11 during genesis of Wilms' tumour, *Nature,* 309, 170, 1984.

206. **Knudson, A. G., Meadows, A. T., Nichols, W. W., and Hill, R.,** Chromosomal deletion and retinoblastoma, *N. Engl. J. Med.,* 295, 1120, 1976.

207. **Mikkelsen, T. and Cavenee, W. K.,** Suppressors of the malignant phenotype, *Cell Growth Differentiation,* 1, 201, 1990.

208. **Sager, R.,** Genetic suppression of tumor formation: a new frontier in cancer research, *Cancer Res.,* 46, 1573, 1986.

209. **Fearon, E. R., Cho, K. R., Nigro, J. M., Kern, S. E., Simons, J. W., Ruppert, J. M., Hamilton, S. R., Preisinger, A. C., Thomas, G., Kinzler, K. W., and Vogelstein, B.,** Identification of a chromosome 18q gene that is altered in colorectal cancers, *Science,* 247, 49, 1990.

210. **Solomon, E.,** A genetic model for colorectal tumorigenesis, *Cell,* 61, 759, 1990.

211. **Fearon, E. R. and Vogelstein, B.,** A genetic model for colorectal tumorigenesis, *Cell,* 61, 759, 1990.

212. **Baker, S. J., Fearon, E. R., Nigro, J. M., Hamilton, S. R., Preisinger, A. C., Jessup, J. M., van Tuinen, P., Ledbetter, D. H., Barker, D. F., Nakamura, Y., White, R., and Vogelstein, B.,** Chromosome 17 deletions and p53 gene mutations in colorectal carcinomas, *Science,* 244, 217, 1989.

213. **Francke, U.,** A gene for Wilms tumour?, *Nature,* 343, 692, 1990.

214. **Gessler, M., Poustka, A., Cavenee, W., Neve, R. L., Orkin, S. H., and Bruns, G. A.,** Homozygous deletion in Wilms tumours of a zinc-finger gene identified by chromosome jumping, *Nature,* 343, 774, 1990.

215. **Call, K. M., Glaser, T., Ito, C. Y., Buckler, A. J., Pelletier, J., Haber, D. A., Rose, E. A., Kral, A., Yeger, H., Lewis, W. H., Jones, C., and Housman, D. E.,** Isolation and characterization of a zinc finger polypeptide gene at the human chromosome 11 Wilms' tumor locus, *Cell,* 60, 509, 1990.

216. **Rose, E. A., Glaser, T., Jones, C., Smith, C. L., Lewis, W. H., Call, K. M., Minden, M., Champagne, E., Bonetta, L., Yeger, H., and Housman, D. E.,** Complete physical map of the WAGR region of 11p13 localizes a candidate Wilms' tumor gene, *Cell,* 60, 495, 1990.

217. **Wadey, R. B., Pal, N., Buckle, B., Yeomans, E., Pritchard, J., and Cowell, J. K.,** Loss of heterozygosity in Wilms' tumor involves two distinct regions of chromosome 11, *Oncogene,* 5, 901, 1990.

218. **Weissman, B. E., Saxon, P. J., Pasquale, S. R., Jones, G. R., Geiser, A. G., and Stanbridge, E. J.,** Introduction of a normal human chromosome 11 into a Wilms' tumor cell line controls its tumorigenic expression, *Science,* 236, 175, 1987.

219. **Balaban, G., Gilbert, F., Nichols, W., Meadows, A. T., and Shields, J.,** Abnormalities of chromosome #13 in retinoblastomas from individuals with normal constitutional karyotypes, *Cancer Genet. Cytogenet.,* 6, 213, 1982.

220. **Benedict, W. F., Banerjee, A., Mark, C., and Murphree, A. L.,** Nonrandom chromosomal changes in untreated retinoblastomas, *Cancer Genet. Cytogenet.,* 10, 311, 1983.

221. **Cavenee, W. K., Dryja, T. P., Phillips, R. A., Benedict, W. F., Godbout, R., Gallie, B. L., Murphree, A. L., Strong, L. C., and White, R. L.,** Expression of recessive alleles by chromosomal mechanisms in retinoblastoma, *Nature,* 305, 779, 1983.

222. **Godbout, R., Dryja, T. P., Squire, J., Gallie, B. L., and Phillips, R. A.,** Somatic inactivation of genes on chromosome 13 is a common event in retinoblastoma, *Nature,* 304, 451, 1983.

223. **Dryja, T. P., Cavenee, W., White, R., Rapaport, J. M., Petersen, R., Albert, D. M., and Bruns, G. A.,** Homozygosity of chromosome 13 in retinoblastoma, *N. Engl. J. Med.,* 310, 550, 1984.

224. **Dryja, T. P., Rapaport, J. M., Joyce, J. M., and Petersen, R. A.,** Molecular detection of deletions involving band q14 of chromosome 13 in retinoblastomas, *Proc. Natl. Acad. Sci. U.S.A.,* 83, 7391, 1986.

225. **Benedict, W. F., Srivatsan, E. S., Mark, C., Banerjee, A., Sparkes, R. S., and Murphree, A. L.,** Complete or partial homozygosity of chromosome 13 in primary retinoblastoma, *Cancer Res.,* 47, 4189, 1987.

226. **Friend, S. H., Bernards, R., Rogelj, S., Weinberg, R. A., Rapaport, J. M., Albert, D. M., and Dryja, T. P.,** A human DNA segment with properties of the gene that predisposes to retinoblastoma and osteosarcoma, *Nature,* 323, 643, 1986.

227. **Fung, Y. K., Murphree, A. L., T'Ang, A., Qian, J., Hinrichs, S. H., and Benedict, W. F.,** Structural evidence for the authenticity of the human retinoblastoma gene, *Science,* 236, 1657, 1987.

228. **Bookstein, R., Lee, E. Y., To, H., Young, L. J., Sery, T. W., Hayes, R. C., Friedmann, T., and Lee, W. H.,** Human retinoblastoma susceptibility gene: genomic organization and analysis of heterozygous intragenic deletion mutants, *Proc. Natl. Acad. Sci. U.S.A.,* 85, 2210, 1988.

229. **T'Ang, A., Wu, K. J., Hashimoto, T., Liu, W. Y., Takahashi, R., Shi, X. H., Mihara, K., Zhang, F. H., Chen, Y. Y., Du, C., et al.,** Genomic organization of the human retinoblastoma gene, *Oncogene,* 4, 401, 1989.

230. **Lee, W. H., Shew, J. Y., Hong, F. D., Sery, T. W., Donoso, L. A., Young, L. J., Bookstein, R., and Lee, E. Y.,** The retinoblastoma susceptibility gene encodes a nuclear phosphoprotein associated with DNA binding activity, *Nature,* 329, 642, 1987.

231. **Wang, N. P., Chen, P.-L., Huang, S., Donoso, L. A., Lee, W.-H., and Lee, E. Y.,** DNA-binding activity of retinoblastoma protein is intrinsic to its carboxyl-terminal region, *Cell Growth Differentiation,* 1, 233, 1990.

232. **Hong, F. D., Huang, H. J., To, H., Young, L. J., Oro, A., Bookstein, R., Lee, E. Y., and Lee, W. H.,** Structure of the human retinoblastoma gene, *Proc. Natl. Acad. Sci. U.S.A.,* 86, 5502, 1989.

233. **Xu, H. J., Hu, S. X., Hashimoto, T., Takahashi, R., and Benedict, W. F.,** The retinoblastoma susceptibility gene product: a characteristic pattern in normal cells and abnormal expression in malignant cells, *Oncogene,* 4, 807, 1989.

234. **Lee, E. Y., Bookstein, R., Young, L. J., Lin, C. J., Rosenfeld, M. G., and Lee, W. H.,** Molecular mechanism of retinoblastoma gene inactivation in retinoblastoma cell line Y79, *Proc. Natl. Acad. Sci. U.S.A.,* 85, 6017, 1988.

235. **Goddard, A. D., Balakier, H., Canton, M., Dunn, J., Squire, J., Reyes, E., Becker, A., Phillips, R. A., and Gallie, B. L.,** Infrequent genomic rearrangement and normal expression of the putative RB1 gene in retinoblastoma tumors, *Mol. Cell. Biol.,* 8, 2082, 1988.

236. **Dunn, J. M., Phillips, R. A., Becker, A. J., and Gallie, B. L.,** Identification of germline and somatic mutations affecting the retinoblastoma gene, *Science,* 241, 1797, 1988.

237. **Dunn, J. M., Phillips, R. A., Zhu, X., Becker, A., and Gallie, B. L.,** Mutations in the RB1 gene and their effects on transcription, *Mol. Cell. Biol.,* 9, 4596, 1989.

238. **Yandell, D. W., Campbell, T. A., Dayton, S. H., Petersen, R., Walton, D., Little, J. B., McConkie, R. A., Buckley, E. G., and Dryja, T. P.,** Oncogenic point mutations in the human retinoblastoma gene: their application to genetic counseling, *N. Engl. J. Med.,* 321, 1689, 1989.

239. **Reik, W. and Surani, M. A.,** Genomic imprinting and embryonal tumors, *Nature,* 338, 112, 1989.

240. **Zhu, X. P., Dunn, J. M., Phillips, R. A., Goddard, A. D., Paton, K. E., Becker, A., and Gallie, B. L.,** Preferential germline mutation of the paternal allele in retinoblastoma, *Nature,* 340, 312, 1989.

241. **Toguchida, J., Ishizaki, K., Sasaki, M. S., Nakamura, Y., Ikenaga, M., Kato, M., Sugimot, M., Kotoura, Y., and Yamamuro, T.,** Preferential mutation of paternally derived RB gene as the initial event in sporadic osteosarcoma, *Nature,* 338, 156, 1989.

242. **Shew, J.-Y., Lin, B. T.-Y., Chen, P.-L., Tseng, B. Y., Yang-Feng, T. L., and Lee, W.-H.,** C-terminal truncation of the retinoblastoma gene product leads to functional inactivation, *Proc. Natl. Acad. Sci. U.S.A.,* 87, 6, 1990.

243. **Lillie, J. W. and Green, M. R.,** Transcription activation by the adenovirus E1a protein, *Nature,* 338, 39, 1989.

244. **Green, M. R.,** When the products of oncogenes and anti-oncogenes meet, *Cell,* 56, 1, 1989.

245. **DeCaprio, J. A., Ludlow, J. W., Figge, J., Shew, J. Y., Huang, C. M., Lee, W. H., Marsilio, E., Paucha, E., and Livingston, D. M.,** SV40 large tumor antigen forms a specific complex with the product of the retinoblastoma susceptibility gene, *Cell,* 54, 275, 1988.

246. **Whyte, P., Buchkovich, K. J., Horowitz, J. M., Friend, S. H., Raybuck, M., Weinberg, R. A., and Harlow, E.,** Association between an oncogene and an anti-oncogene: the adenovirus E1A proteins bind to the retinoblastoma gene product, *Nature,* 334, 124, 1988.

247. **Dyson, N., Howley, P. M., Münger, K., and Harlow, E.,** The human papilloma virus-16 E7 oncoprotein is able to bind to the retinoblastoma gene product, *Science,* 243, 934, 1989.

248. **Münger, K., Werness, B. A., Dyson, N., Phelps, W. C., Harlow, E., and Howley, P. M.,** Complex formation of human papillomavirus E7 proteins with the retinoblastoma tumor suppressor gene product, *EMBO J.,* 8, 4099, 1989.

249. **Huang, S., Wang, N. P., Tseng, B. Y., Lee, W. H., and Lee, E. H.,** Two distinct and frequently mutated regions of retinoblastoma protein are required for binding to SV40 T antigen, *EMBO J.,* 9, 1815, 1990.

250. **Hu, Q. J., Dyson, N., and Harlow, E.,** The regions of the retinoblastoma protein needed for binding to adenovirus E1A or SV40 large T antigen are common sites for mutations, *EMBO J.,* 9, 1147, 1990.

251. **Egan, C., Bayley, S. T., and Branton, P. E.,** Binding of the Rb1 protein to E1A products is required for adenovirus transformation, *Oncogene,* 4, 383, 1989.

252. **Horowitz, J. M., Yandell, D. W., Park, S.-H., Canning, S., Whyte, P., Buchkovich, K., Harlow, E., Weinberg, R. A., and Dryja, T. P.,** Point mutational inactivation of the retinoblastoma antioncogene, *Science,* 243, 937, 1989.

253. **Ludlow, J. W., DeCaprio, J. A., Huang, C. M., Lee, W. H., Paucha, E., and Livingston, D. M.,** SV40 large T antigen binds preferentially to an underphosphorylated member of the retinoblastoma susceptibility gene product family, *Cell,* 56, 57, 1989.

254. **Chen, P. L., Scully, P., Shew, J. Y., Wang, J. Y., and Lee, W. H.,** Phosphorylation of the retinoblastoma gene product is modulated during the cell cycle and cellular differentiation, *Cell,* 58, 1193, 1989.

255. **Mihara, K., Cao, X. R., Yen, A., Chandler, S., Driscoll, B., Murphree, A. L., T'Ang, A., and Fung, Y. K.,** Cell cycle-dependent regulation of phosphorylation of the human retinoblastoma gene product, *Science,* 246, 1300, 1989.

256. **Buchkovich, K., Duffy, L. A., and Harlow, E.,** The retinoblastoma protein is phosphorylated during specific phases of the cell cycle, *Cell,* 58, 1097, 1989.

257. **DeCaprio, J. A., Ludlow, J. W., Lynch, D., Furukawa, Y., Griffin, J., Piwnica, W. H., Huang, C. M., and Livingston, D. M.,** The product of the retinoblastoma susceptibility gene has properties of a cell cycle regulatory element, *Cell,* 58, 1085, 1989.

258. **Furukawa, Y., DeCaprio, J. A., Freedman, A., Kanakura, Y., Nakamura, M., Ernst, T. J., Livingston, D. M., and Griffin, J. D.,** Expression and state of phosphorylation of the retinoblastoma susceptibility gene product in cycling and noncycling human hematopoietic cells, *Proc. Natl. Acad. Sci. U.S.A.,* 87, 2770, 1990.

259. **Akiyama, T. and Toyoshima, K.,** Marked alteration in phosphorylation of the RB protein during differentiation of human promyelocytic HL60 cells, *Oncogene,* 5, 179, 1990.

260. **Ludlow, J. W., Shon, J., Pipas, J. M., Livingston, D. M., and DeCaprio, J. A.,** The retinoblastoma susceptibility gene product undergoes cell cycle-dependent dephosphorylation and binding to and release from SV40 large T, *Cell,* 60, 387, 1990.

261. **Taya, Y., Yasuda, H., Kamijo, M., Nakaya, K., Nakamura, Y., Ohba, Y., and Nishimura, S.,** In vitro phosphorylation of the tumor suppressor gene RB protein by mitosis-specific histone H1 kinase, *Biochem. Biophys. Res. Commun.,* 164, 580, 1989.

262. **Cooper, J. A. and Whyte, P.,** RB and the cell cycle: entrance or exit?, *Cell,* 58, 1009, 1989.

263. **Laiho, M., DeCaprio, J. A., Ludlow, J. W., Livingston, D. M., and Massague, J.,** Growth inhibition by TGF-β linked to suppression of retinoblastoma protein phosphorylation, *Cell,* 62, 175, 1990.

264. **Pietenpol, J. A., Stein, R. W., Moran, E., Yaciuk, P., Schlegel, R., Lyons, R. M., Pittelkov, M. R., Münger, K., Howley, P. M., and Moses, H. L.,** TGF-beta 1 inhibition of c-*myc* transcription and growth in keratinocytes is abrogated by viral transforming proteins with pRB binding domains, *Cell,* 61, 777, 1990.

265. **Huang, H. J., Yee, J. K., Shew, J. Y., Chen, P. L., Bookstein, R., Friedmann, T., Lee, E. Y., and Lee, W. H.,** Suppression of the neoplastic phenotype by replacement of the RB gene in human cancer cells, *Science,* 242, 1563, 1988.

266. **Sumegi, J., Uzvolgyi, E., and Klein, G.,** Expression of the RB gene under the control of MuLV-LTR suppresses tumorigenicity of WERE-Rb-27 retinoblastoma cells in immunodefective mice, *Cell Growth Differentiation,* 1, 247, 1990.

267. **Marx, J.,** Eye cancer gene linked to new malignancies, *Nature,* 241, 293, 1988.

268. **Lee, E. Y., To, H., Shew, J. Y., Bookstein, R., Scully, P., and Lee, W. H.,** Inactivation of the retinoblastoma susceptibility gene in human breast cancers, *Science,* 241, 218, 1988.

269. **T'Ang, A., Varley, J. M., Chakraborty, S., Murphree, A. L., and Fung, Y. K.,** Structural rearrangement of the retinoblastoma gene in human breast carcinoma, *Science,* 242, 263, 1988.

270. **Varley, J. M., Armour, J., Swallow, J. E., Jeffreys, A. J., Ponder, B. A., T'Ang, A., Fung, Y. K., Brammar, W. J., and Walker, R. A.,** The retinoblastoma gene is frequqently altered leading to loss of expression in primary breast tumours, *Oncogene,* 4, 725, 1989; published erratum appears in *Oncogene,* 5(2), 245, 1990.

271. **Hensel, C. H., Hsieh, C.-L., Gazdar, A. F., Johnson, B. E., Sakaguchi, A. Y., Nalor, S. L., Lee, W.-H., and Lee, E. Y.-H. P.,** Altered structure and expression of the human retinoblastoma susceptibility gene in small cell lung cancer, *Cancer Res.,* 50, 3067, 1990.

272. **Bookstein, R., Shew, J.-Y., Chen, P.-L., Scully, P., and Lee, W.-H.,** Suppression of tumorigenicity of human prostate carcinoma cells by replacing a mutated RB gene, *Science,* 247, 712, 1990.

273. **Horowitz, J. M., Park, S.-H., Bogenman, E., Cheng, J.-C., Yandell, D. W., Kaye, F. J., Minna, J. D., Dryja, T. P., and Weinberg, R. A.,** Frequent inactivation of the retinoblastoma anti-oncogene is restricted to a subset of human tumor cells, *Proc. Natl. Acad. Sci. U.S.A.,* 87, 2775, 1990.

274. **Gope, R., Christensen, M. A., Thorson, A., Lynch, H. T., Smyrk, T., Hodgson, C., Wildrick, D. M., Gope, M. L., and Boman, B. M.,** Increased expression of the retinoblastoma gene in human colorectal carcinomas relative to normal colonic mucosa, *J. Natl. Cancer Inst.,* 82, 310, 1990.

275. **Weichselbaum, R. R., Beckett, M., and Diamond, A.,** Some retinoblastomas, osteosarcomas, and soft tissue sarcomas may share a common etiology, *Proc. Natl. Acad. Sci. U.S.A.,* 85, 2106, 1988.

276. **Toguchida, J., Ishizaki, K., Sasaki, M. S., Ikenaga, M., Sugimoto, M., Kotoura, Y., and Yamamuro, T.,** Chromosomal reorganization for the expression of recessive mutation of retinoblastoma susceptibility gene in the development of osteosarcoma, *Cancer Res.,* 48, 3939, 1988.

277. **Reissmann, P. T., Simon, M. A., Lee, W.-H., and Slamon, D. J.,** Studies of the retinoblastoma gene in human sarcomas, *Oncogene,* 4, 839, 1989.

278. **Mendoza, A. E., Shew, J. Y., Lee, E. Y., Bookstein, R., and Lee, W. H.,** A case of synovial sarcoma with abnormal expression of the human retinoblastoma susceptibility gene, *Hum. Pathol.,* 19, 487, 1988.

279. **Stratton, M. R., Williams, S., Fisher, C., Ball, A., Westbury, G., Gusterson, B. A., Fletcher, C. D., Knight, J. C., Fung, Y. K., Reeves, B. R., and Cooper, C. S.,** Structural alterations of the RB1 gene in human soft tissue tumours, *Br. J. Cancer,* 60, 202, 1989.

280. **Hachitanda, Y., Aoyama, C., Mihara, K., Shimada, H., Fung, Y., Murphree, A. L., and Triche, T. J.,** Expression of the Rb1 gene product in retinoblastoma and childhood sarcomas, *Lab. Invest.,* 62(Abstr.), 41A, 1990.

281. **DeChiara, A., Lopez-Terrada, D., Cohen, V., T'ang, A., Fung, T., and Triche, T.,** Expression of the retinoblastoma (RB) gene in childhood rhabdomyosarcomas, *Mod. Pathol.,* 4(Abstr.), 108A, 1991.

281a. **DeChiara, A.,** unpublished observations, 1990.

282. **Lane, D. P. and Benchimol, S.,** p53: oncogene or anti-oncogene?, *Genes Dev.,* 4, 1, 1990.

283. **Soussi, T., de Fromentel, C. C., and May, P.,** Structural aspects of the p53 protein in relation to gene evolution, *Oncogene,* 5, 945, 1990.

284. **Finlay, C. A., Hinds, P. W., Tan, T. H., Eliyahu, D., Oren, M., and Levine, A. J.,** Activating mutations for transformation by p53 produce a gene product that forms an hsc70-p53 complex with an altered half-life, *Mol. Cell. Biol.,* 8, 531, 1988.

285. **Levine, A. J.,** Tumor suppressor genes, *Bioessays,* 12, 60, 1990.

286. **Eliyahu, D., Michalovitz, D., Eliyahu, S., Pinhasi, K. O., and Oren, M.,** Wild-type p53 can inhibit oncogene-mediated focus formation, *Proc. Natl. Acad. Sci. U.S.A.,* 86, 8763, 1989.

287. **Finlay, C. A., Hinds, P. W., and Levine, A. J.,** The p53 proto-oncogene can act as a suppressor of transformation, *Cell,* 57, 1083, 1989.

288. **Nigro, J. M., Baker, S. J., Preisinger, A. C., Jessup, J. M., Hostetter, R., Cleary, K., Bigner, S. H., Davidson, N., Baylin, S., Devilee, P., Glover, T., Collins, F. S., Weston, A., Modali, R., Harris, C. C., and Vogelstein, B.,** Mutations in the p53 gene occur in diverse human tumour types, *Nature,* 342, 705, 1989.

289. **Addison, C., Jenkens, J. R., and Sturzbecher, H.-W.,** The p53 nuclear localisation signal is structurally linked to a p34cdc2 kinase motif, *Oncogene,* 5, 423, 1990.

290. **Louis, J. M., McFarland, V. W., May, P., and Mora, P. T.,** The phosphoprotein p53 is down-regulated post-transcriptionally during embryogenesis in vertebrates, *Biochim. Biophys. Acta,* 950, 395, 1988.

291. **Deppert, W., Steinmayer, T., and Richter, W.,** Cooperation of SV40 large T antigen and the cellular protein p53 in maintenance of cell transformation, *Oncogene,* 4, 1103, 1989.

292. **Ewen, M. E., Ludlow, J. W., Marsilio, E., DeCaprio, J. A., Millikan, R. C., Cheng, S. H., Paucha, E., and Livingston, D. M.,** An N-terminal transformation-governing sequence of SV40 large T antigen contributes to the binding of both p11ORb and a second cellular protein, p120, *Cell,* 58, 257, 1989.

293. **Tuck, S. P. and Crawford, L.,** Overexpression of normal human p53 in established fibroblasts leads to their tumorigenic conversion, *Oncogene Res.,* 4, 81, 1989.

294. **Lavigueur, A., Maltby, V., Mock, D., Rossant, J., Pawson, T., and Bernstein, A.,** High incidence of lung, bone, and lymphoid tumors in transgenic mice overexpressing mutant alleles of the p53 oncogene, *Mol. Cell. Biol.,* 9, 3982, 1989.

295. **Ahuja, H., Bar, E. M., Advani, S. H., Benchimol, S., and Cline, M.J.,** Alterations in the p53 gene and the clonal evolution of the blast crisis of chronic myelocytic leukemia, *Proc. Natl. Acad. Sci. U.S.A.,* 86, 6783, 1989.

296. **Cattoretti, G., Rilke, F., Andreola, S., D'Amato, L., and Delia, D.,** p53 expression in breast cancer, *Int. J. Cancer,* 41, 178, 1988.

297. **Iggo, R., Gatter, K., Bartek, J., Lane, D., and Harris, A. L.,** Increased expression of mutant forms of p53 oncogene in primary lung cancer, *Lancet,* 335, 675, 1990.

298. **Takahashi, T., Nau, M. M., Chiba, I., Birrer, M. J., Rosenberg, R. K., Vinocour, M., Levitt, M., Pass, H., Gazdar, A. F., and Minna, J. D.,** p53: a frequent target for genetic abnormalities in lung cancer, *Science,* 246, 491, 1989.

299. **Thompson, A. M., Steel, C. M., Chetty, U., Hawkins, R. A., Miller, W. R., Carter, D. C., Forrest, A. P., and Evans, H. J.,** p53 gene mRNA expression and chromosome 17p allele loss in breast cancer, *Br. J. Cancer,* 61, 74, 1990.

300. **Bartek, J., Iggo, R., Gannon, J., and Lane, D. P.,** Genetic and immunochemical analysis of mutant p53 in human breast cancer cell lines, *Oncogene,* 5, 893, 1990.

301. **Bressac, B., Galvin, K. M., Liang, T. J., Isselbacher, K. J., Wands, J. R., and Ozturk, M.,** Abnormal structure and expression of p53 gene in human hepatocellular carcinoma, *Proc. Natl. Acad. Sci. U.S.A.,* 87, 1973, 1990.

302. **Masuda, H., Miller, C., Koeffler, H. P., Battifora, H., and Cline, M. J.,** Rearrangement of the p53 gene in human osteogenic sarcomas, *Proc. Natl. Acad. Sci. U.S.A.,* 84, 7716, 1987.

303. **Romano, J. W., Ehrhart, J. C., Duthu, A., Kim, C. M., Appella, E., and May, P.,** Identification and characterization of a p53 gene mutation in a human osteosarcoma cell line, *Oncogene* 4, 1483, 1989.

303a. **Stratton, M. R., Moss, S., Warren, W., Patterson, H., Clark, J., Fisher, C., Fletcher, C. D. M., Ball, A., Thomas, M., Gusterson, B. A., and Cooper, C. S.,** Mutation of the p53 gene in human soft tissue sarcomas: association with abnormalities of the RB1 gene, *Oncogene,* 5, 1297, 1990.

303b. **Mulligan, L. M., Matlashewski, G. J., Scrable, H. J., and Cavenee, W. K.,** Mechanisms of p53 loss in human sarcomas, *Proc. Natl. Acad. Sci. U.S.A.,* 87, 5863, 1990.

304. **Deuel, T. F., Huang, J. S., Huang, S. S., Stroobant, P., and Waterfield, M. D.,** Expression of a platelet-derived growth factor-like protein in simian sarcoma virus transformed cells, *Science,* 221, 1348, 1983.

305. **Waterfield, M. D., Scrace, G. T., Whittle, N., Stroobant, P., Johnsson, A., Wasteson, A., Westermark, B., Heldin, C. H., Huang, J. S., and Deuel, T. F.,** Platelet-derived growth factor is structurally related to the putative transforming protein p28*sis* of simian sarcoma virus, *Nature,* 304, 35, 1983.

306. **Robbins, K. C., Antoniades, H. N., Devare, S. G., Hunkapiller, M. W., and Aaronson, S. A.,** Structural and immunological similarities between simian sarcoma virus gene product(s) and human platelet-derived growth factor, *Nature,* 305, 605,1983.

307. **Doolittle, R. F., Hunkapiller, M. W., Hood, L. E., Devare, S. G., Robbins, K. C., Aaronson, S. A., and Antoniades, H. N.,** Simian sarcoma virus onc gene, v-*sis*, is derived from the gene (or genes) encoding a platelet-derived growth factor, *Science,* 221, 275, 1983.

308. **Niman, H. L.,** Antisera to a synthetic peptide of the *sis* viral oncogene product recognize human platelet-derived growth factor, *Nature,* 307, 180, 1984.

309. **Yarden, Y., Escobedo, J. A., Kuang, W. J., Yang, F. T., Daniel, T. O., Tremble, P. M., Chen, E. Y., Ando, M. E., Harkins, R. N., Francke, U., Fried, V. A., Ullrich, A., and Williams, L. T.,** Structure of the receptor for platelet-derived growth factor helps define a family of closely related growth factor receptors, *Nature,* 323, 226, 1986.

310. **Clegg, C. H., Linkhart, T. A., Olwin, B. B., and Hauschka, S. D.,** Growth factor control of skeletal muscle differentiation: commitment to terminal differentiation occurs in G1 phase and is repressed by fibroblast growth factor, *J. Cell Biol.,* 105, 949, 1987.

311. **Lathrop, B., Olson, E., and Glaser, L.,** Control by fibroblast growth factor of differentiation in the BC3H1 muscle cell line, *J. Cell Biol.,* 100, 1540, 1985.

312. **Wice, B., Milbrandt, J., and Glaser, L.,** Control of muscle differentiation in BC3H1 cells by fibroblast growth factor and vanadate, *J. Biol. Chem.,* 262, 1810, 1987.

313. **Florini, J. R., Roberts, A. B., Ewton, D. Z., Falen, S. L., Flanders, K. C., and Sporn, M. B.,** Transforming growth factor-beta. A very potent inhibitor of myoblast differentiation, identical to the differentiation inhibitor secreted by Buffalo rat liver cells, *J. Biol. Chem.,* 261, 16509, 1986.

314. **Massagué, J., Cheifetz, S., Endo, T., and Nadal, G. B.,** Type beta transforming growth factor is an inhibitor of myogenic differentiation, *Proc. Natl. Acad. Sci. U.S.A.,* 83, 8206, 1986.

315. **Olson, E. N., Sternberg, E., Hu, J. S., Spizz, G., and Wilcox, C.,** Regulation of myogenic differentiation by type beta transforming growth factor, *J. Cell Biol.,* 103, 1799, 1986.

316. **Joseph-Silverstein, J., Consigli, S. A., Lyser, K. M., and Ver Pault, C.,** Basic fibroblast growth factor in the chick embryo: immunolocalization to striated muscle cells and their precursors, *J. Cell Biol.,* 108, 2459, 1989.

317. **Schweigerer, L., Neufeld, G., Mergia, A., Abraham, J. A., Fiddes, J. C., and Gospodarowicz, D.,** Basic fibroblast growth factor in human rhabdomyosarcoma cells: implications for the proliferation and neovascularization of myoblast-derived tumors, *Proc. Natl. Acad. Sci. U.S.A.,* 84, 842, 1987.

318. **Dart, L. L., Smith, D. M., Meyers, C. A., Sporn, M. B., and Frolik, C. A.,** Transforming growth factors from a human tumor cell: characterization of transforming growth factor beta and identification of high molecular weight transforming growth factor alpha, *Biochemistry,* 24, 5925, 1985.

319. **Fryling, C. M., Iwata, K. K., Johnson, P. A., Knott, W. B., and Todaro, G. J.,** Two distinct tumor cell growth-inhibiting factors from a human rhabdomyosarcoma cell line, *Cancer Res.,* 45, 2695, 1985.

320. **Iwata, K. K., Fryling, C. M., Knott, W. B., and Todaro, G. J.,** Isolation of tumor cell growth-inhibiting factors from a human rhabdomyosarcoma cell line, *Cancer Res.,* 45, 2689, 1985.

320a. **Litton, M., Triche, T. J., et al.,** unpublished data, 1990.

321. **Olwin, B. B. and Hauschka, S. D.,** Identification of the fibroblast growth factor receptor of Swiss 3T3 cells and mouse skeletal muscle myoblasts, *Biochemistry,* 25, 3487, 1986.

322. **Vaidya, T. B., Rhodes, S. J., Taparowsky, E. J., and Konieczny, S. F.,** Fibroblast growth factor and transforming growth factor beta repress transcription of the myogenic regulatory gene MyoD1, *Mol. Cell Biol.,* 9, 3576, 1989.

323. **Shih, H. T., Wathen, M. S., Marshall, H. B., Caffrey, J. M., and Schneider, M. D.,** Dihydropyridine receptor gene expression is regulated by inhibitors of myogenesis and is relatively insensitive to denervation, *J. Clin. Invest.,* 85, 781, 1990.

324. **Tollefsen, S. E., Lajara, R., McCusker, R. H., Clemmons, D. R., and Rotwein, P.,** Insulin-like growth factors (IGF) in muscle development. Expression of IGF-I, the IGF-I receptor, and an IGF binding protein during myoblast differentiation, *J. Biol. Chem.,* 264, 13810, 1989.

325. **Tollefsen, S. E., Sadow, J. L., and Rotwein, P.,** Coordinate expression of insulin-like growth factor II and its receptor during muscle differentiation, *Proc. Natl. Acad. Sci. U.S.A.,* 86, 1543, 1989.

326. **McCusker, R. H., Camacho, H. C., and Clemmons, D. R.,** Identification of the types of insulin-like growth factor-binding proteins that are secreted by muscle cells in vitro, *J. Biol. Chem.,* 264, 7795, 1989.

327. **Helman, L. T., Israel, M. A., and El-Badry, O. M.,** Growth inhibition of rhabdomyosarcoma cells by an antibody to the IGF type I receptor, *Proc. Am. Assoc. Cancer Res.,* 30(Abstr.), 62, 1990.

328. **El-Badry, O. M., Minniti, C., Kohn, E. C., Houghton, P. J., Daughaday, W. H., and Helman, L. J.,** Insulin-like growth factor II acts as an autocrine growth and motility factor in human rhabdomyosarcoma tumors, *Cell Growth Differentiation,* 1, 3215, 1990.

329. **Romanus, J. A., Tseng, L. Y., Yang, Y. W., and Rechler, M. M.,** The 34 kilodalton insulin-like growth factor binding proteins in human cerebrospinal fluid and the a673 rhabdomyosarcoma cell line are human homologues of the rat brl-3a binding protein, *Biochem. Biophys. Res. Commun.,* 163, 875, 1989.

330. **Reeve, A. E., Eccles, M. R., Wilkins, R. J., Bell, G. I., and Millow, L. J.,** Expression of insulin-like growth factor-II transcripts in Wilms' tumour, *Nature,* 317, 258, 1985.

331. **Gansler, T., Furlanetto, R., Gramling, T. S., Robinson, K. A., Blocker, N., Buse, M. G., Sens, D. A., and Garvin, A. J.,** Antibody to type I insulin-like growth factor receptor inhibits growth of Wilms' tumor in culture and in athymic mice, *Am. J. Pathol.,* 135, 961, 1989.

332. **Irminger, J. C., Schoenle, E. J., Briner, J., and Humbel, R. E.,** Structural alteration of the insulin-like growth factor II-gene in Wilms tumour, *Eur. J. Pediatr.,* 148, 620, 1989.
333. **Scott, J., Cowell, J., Robertson, M. E., Priestley, L. M., Wadey, R., Hopkins, B., Pritchard, J., Bell, G. I., Rall, L. B., Graham, C. F., and Knott, T. J.,** Insulin-like growth factor-II gene expression in Wilms' tumour and embryonic tissues, *Nature,* 317, 260, 1985.
334. **Paik, S., Rosen, N., Jung, W., You, J. M., Lippman, M. E., Perdue, J. F., and Yee, D.,** Expression of insulin-like growth factor-II mRNA in fetal kidney and Wilms' tumor. An in situ hybridization study, *Lab. Invest.,* 61, 522, 1989.
335. **Cullen, K. J., Yee, D., Sly, W. S., Perdue, J., Hampton, B., Lippman, M. E., and Rosen, N.,** Insulin-like growth factor receptor expression and function in human breast cancer, *Cancer Res.,* 50, 48, 1990.
336. **Osborne, C. K., Coronado, E. B., Kitten, L. J., Arteaga, C. I., Fuqua, S. A., Ramasharma, K., Marshall, M., and Li, C. H.,** Insulin-like growth factor-II (IGF-II): a potential autocrine/paracrine growth factor for human breast cancer acting via the IGF-I receptor, *Mol. Endocrinol.,* 3, 1701, 1989.
337. **Jaques, G., Kiefer, P., Rotsch, M., Hennig, C., Göke, R., Richter, G., and Havemann, K.,** Production of insulin-like growth factor binding proteins by small-cell lung cancer cell lines, *Exp. Cell Res.,* 184, 396, 1989.
338. **Macaulay, V. M., Everard, M. J., Teale, J. D., Trott, P. A., Van, W. J., Smith, I. E., and Millar, J. L.,** Autocrine function for insulin-like growth factor I in human small cell lung cancer cell lines and fresh tumor cells, *Cancer Res.,* 50, 2511, 1990.
339. **Daughaday, W. H., Emanuele, M. A., Brooks, M. H., Barbato, A. L., Kapadia, M., and Rotwein, P.,** Synthesis and secretion of insulin-like growth factor II by a leiomyosarcoma with associated hypoglycemia, *N. Engl. J. Med.,* 319, 1434, 1988.
340. **Constantinides, P. G., Jones, P. A., and Gevers, W.,** Functional striated muscle cells from non-myoblast precursors following 5-azacytidine treatment, *Nature,* 267, 364, 1977.
341. **Constantinides, P. G., Taylor, S. M., and Jones, P. A.,** Phenotypic conversion of cultured mouse embryo cells by aza pyrimidine nucleosides, *Dev. Biol.,* 66, 57, 1978.
342. **Taylor, S. M. and Jones, P. A.,** Multiple new phenotypes induced in 10T$^1/_2$ and 3^{-}3 cells treated with 5-azacytidine, *Cell,* 17, 771, 1979.
343. **Taylor, S. M. and Jones, P. A.,** Changes in phenotypic expression in embryonic and adult cells treated with 5-azacytidine, *J. Cell Physiol.,* 111, 187, 1982.
344. **Konieczny, S. F., and Emerson, C. J.,** 5-Azacytidine induction of stable mesodermal stem cell lineages from 10T$^1/_2$ cells: evidence for regulatory genes controlling determination, *Cell,* 38, 791, 1984.
345. **Lassar, A. B., Paterson, B. M., and Weintraub, H.,** Transfection of a DNA locus that mediates the conversation of 10T$^1/_2$ fibroblasts to myoblasts, *Cell,* 47, 649, 1986.
346. **Lin, Z. Y., Dechesne, C. A., Eldridge, J., and Paterson, B. M.,** An avian muscle factor related to myod1 activates muscle-specific promoters in nonmuscle cells of different germ-layer origin and in brdu-treated myoblasts, *Genes Dev.,* 3, 986, 1989.
347. **Braun, T., Bober, E., Buschhausen, D. G., Kohtz, S., Grzeschik, K. H., Arnold, H. H., and Kotz, St. K. S.,** Differential expression of myogenic determination genes in muscle cells: possible autoactivation by the Myf gene products, EMBO J., 8, 3617, 1989; published erratum appears in *EMBO J.,* 8(13), 4358, 1989.
348. **Wright, W. E., Sassoon, D. A., and Lin, V. K.,** Myogenin, a factor regulating myogenesis, has a domain homologous to MyoD, *Cell,* 56, 607, 1989.
349. **Pinney, D. F., Pearson, W. S., Konieczny, S. F., Latham, K. E., and Emerson, C. J.,** Myogenic lineage determination and differentiation: evidence for a regulatory gene pathway, *Cell,* 53, 781, 1988.
350. **Braun, T., Bober, E., Winter, B., Rosenthal, N., and Arnold, H. H.,** Myf-6, a new member of the human gene family of myogenic determination factors: evidence for a gene cluster on chromosome 12, *EMBO J.,* 9, 821, 1990.
351. **Rhodes, S. J. and Konieczny, S. F.,** Identification of MRF4: a new member of the muscle regulatory factor gene family, *Genes Dev.,* 3, 2050, 1989.
352. **Candy, M., Vässin, H., Brand, M., Tuma, R., Jan, L. Y., and Jan, Y. N.,** *daughterless,* a *Drosophila* gene essential for both neurogenesis and sex determination has sequence similarities to *myc* and the *achaete-scute* complex, *Cell,* 55, 1061, 1988.
353. **Schäfer, B. W., Blakely, B. T., Darlington, G. J., and Balu, H. M.,** Effect of cell history on response to helix-loop-helix family of myogenic regulators, *Nature,* 344, 454, 1990.
354. **Sassoon, D., Lyons, G., Wright, W. E., Lin, V., Lassar, A., Weintraub, H., and Buckingham, M.,** Expression of two myogenic regulatory factors myogenin and MyoD1 during mouse embryogenesis, *Nature,* 341, 303, 1989.
355. **Blau, H. M.,** Hierarchies of regulatory genes may specify mammalian development, *Cell,* 53, 673, 1988.
356. **Yaffe, D. and Saxel, O.,** Serial passaging and differentiation of myogenic cells isolated from dystrophic mouse muscle, *Nature,* 270, 725, 1977.

357. **Yaffe, D. and Saxel, O.,** A myogenic cell line with altered serum requirements for differentiation, *Differentiation,* 7, 159, 1977.

358. **Montarras, D., Pinset, C., Chelly, J., Kahn, A., and Gros, F.,** Expression of MyoD1 coincides with terminal differentiation in determined but inducible muscle cells, *EMBO J.,* 8, 2203, 1989.

358a. **Triche, T. J.,** unpublished data, 1990.

359. **Hiti, A. L., Bogenmann, E., Gonzales, F., and Jones, P. A.,** Expression of the MyoD1 muscle determination gene defines differentiation capability but not tumorigenicity of human rhabdomyosarcomas, *Mol. Cell Biol.,* 9, 4722, 1989.

360. **Lassar, A. B., Buskin, J. N., Lockshon, D., Davis, R. L., Apone, S., Hauschka, S. D., and Weintraub, H.,** Myod is a sequence-specific dna binding protein requiring a region of myc homology to bind to the muscle creatine kinase enhancer, *Cell,* 58, 823, 1989.

361. **Thayer, M. J., Tapscott, S. J., Davis, R. L., Wright, W. E., Lassar, A. B., and Weintraub, H.,** Positive autoregulation of the myogenic determination gene MyoD1, *Cell,* 58, 241, 1989.

362. **Konieczny, S. F., Drobes, B. L., Menke, S. L., and Taparowsky, E. J.,** Inhibition of myogenic differentiation by the h-*ras* oncogene is associated with the down regulation of the myod1 gene, *Oncogene,* 4, 473, 1989.

363. **Lassar, A. B., Thayer, M. J., Overell, R. W., and Weintraub, H.,** Transformation by activated *ras* or *fos* prevents myogenesis by inhibiting expression of myod1, *Cell,* 58, 659, 1989.

365. **Murre, C., McCaw, P. S., and Baltimore, D.,** A new DNA binding and dimerization motif in immunoglobulin enhancer binding, daughterless, MyoD, and *myc* proteins, *Cell,* 56, 777, 1989.

366. **Murre, C., McCaw, P. S., Vaessin, H., Caudy, M., Jan, L., Jan, Y. N., Cabrera, C. V., Buskin, J. N., Hauschka, S. D., Lassar, A. B., Weintraub, H., and Baltimore, D.,** Interactions between heterologous helix-loop-helix proteins generate complexes that bind specifically to a common DNA sequence, *Cell,* 58, 537, 1989.

367. **Davis, R. L., Cheng, P. F., Lassar, A. B., and Weintraub, H.,** The MyoD DNA binding domain contains a recognition code for muscle-specific gene activation, *Cell,* 60, 733, 1990.

368. **Brennan, T. J. and Olson, E. N.,** Myogenin resides in the nucleus and acquires high affinity for a conserved enhancer element on heterodimerization, *Genes Dev.,* 4, 582, 1990.

369. **Benezra, R., Davis, R. L., Lockshon, D., Turner, D. L., and Weintraub, H.,** The protein Id: a negative regulator of helix-loop-helix DNA binding proteins, *Cell,* 61, 49, 1990.

370. **Noguera, R., Navarro, S., Mims, S., and Tsokos, M.,** Action of 5-azacytidine and transforming growth factor-β on human rhabdomyosarcoma cell lines, *Lab. Invest.,* 62(Abstr.), 74A, 1990.

371. **Aguanno, S., Bouchè, M., Adamo, S., and Molinaro, M.,** 12-O-tetradecanoylphorbol-13-acetate-induced differentiation of a human rhabdomyosarcoma cell line, *Cancer Res.,* 50, 3377, 1990.

372. **Weintraub, H., Tapscott, S. J., Davis, R. L., Thayer, M. J., Adam, M. A. Lassar, A. B., and Miller, A. D.,** Activation of muscle-specific genes in pigment, nerve, fat, liver, and fibroblast cell lines by forced expression of myod, *Proc. Natl. Acad. Sci. U.S.A.,* 86, 5434, 1989.

373. **Smith, T. W. and Davidson, R. I.,** Medullomyoblastoma: a histologic, immunohistochemical, and ultrastructural study, *Cancer,* 54, 323, 1984.

374. **Schmidt, D., Mackay, B., Osborne, B. M., and Jaffe, N.,** Recurring congenital lesion of the cheek, *Ultrastruct. Pathol.,* 3, 85, 1982.

375. **Kawamato, E. H., Weidner, N., Agostini, R. M., Jr., and Jaffe, R.,** Malignant ectomesenchymoma of soft tissue. Report of two cases and review of the literature, *Cancer,* 59, 1791, 1987.

376. **Scheele, P. J., Von Kuster, L. C., and Krivchenia, G., II,** Primary malignant mesenchymoma of bone, *Arch. Pathol. Lab. Med.,* 114, 614, 1990.

377. **Miettinen, M. and Rapola, J.,** Immunohistochemical spectrum of rhabdomyosarcoma and rhabdomyosarcoma-like tumors. Expression of cytokeratin and the 68-kd neurofilament protein, *Am. J. Surg. Pathol.,* 13, 120, 1989.

378. **Shvemberger, I. N.,** Conversion of malignant cells into normal ones, *Int. Rev. Cytol.,* 103, 341, 1986.

379. **Johnson, W., Jurand, J., and Hiramoto, R.,** Immunohistologic studies of tumors containing myosin, *Am. J. Pathol.,* 47, 1139, 1965.

380. **Schoenberger, O. L. and Beikirch, S.,** Cell cycle phases of two human lung tumor cell lines derived from squamous cell carcinoma and pulmonary metastasis of a rhabdomyosarcoma (HS 24 and HS 57) and N-acetylalanine aminopeptidase activity, *Cancer Biochem. Biophys.,* 10, 337, 1989.

381. **White, L. and Cox, D.,** Chromosome changes in a rhabdmoyosarcoma during recurrence and in cell culture, *Br. J. Cancer,* 21, 684, 1967.

382. **Hachitanda, Y., Aoyama, C., Triche, T., and Shimada, H.,** The most primitive form of ectomesenchymoma: an immunohistochemically and untrastructurally identified entity, *Lab. Invest.,* 64(Abstr.), 5, 1991.

Section II
Clinical Manifestations and Diagnosis of Rhabdomyosarcoma

Chapter 4

RHABDOMYOSARCOMA IN CHILDREN: CLINICAL SYMPTOMS, DIAGNOSIS, AND STAGING

Francoise Flamant, Bernard Luboinski, Dominique Couanet, and Heither McDowell

TABLE OF CONTENTS

I. INTRODUCTION

Rhabdomyosarcoma (RMS) is a tumor of the young child, although it can be present at any age from birth up until adulthood. The median age at diagnosis in the series of the International Society of Pediatric Oncology (SIOP) was 5 years, as opposed to a median age of 7 years in the Intergroup Rhabdomyosarcoma Study (IRS). This difference may be attributed to the older age limit of 21 years permitted for registration of patients in the IRS study.

In both series there is a male predominance, the male/female ratio being 1.7:1.0 in the SIOP study.

II. GENERAL PRINCIPLES OF DIAGNOSIS

The histological diagnosis of this tumor is made by microscopic examination of a biopsy of the suspect tissue. The biopsy must be large and not too superficial, particularly in the head and neck tumors, where the tumor can be surrounded by inflammatory tissue. In these cases it is useful to obtain a pathological examination (frozen section) during the operative procedure to ensure that a representative specimen of tumor tissue has been removed. In some cases of small localized tumors, the biopsy constitutes total excision. In such cases, it must be a large excision with tumor-free margins. Also, a good description and accurate details concerning the orientation of the tumor must be given to the pathologist so that examination of the margins confirms the occurrence of total excision. Such a biopsy procedure is therapeutic and can be the most efficacious part of treatment if the tumor is totally removed with microscopically free margins.

If primary surgical excision is impossible and if the localization of the tumor allows it, the specimen may be obtained by a percutaneous fine needle biopsy under guidance by CT scan or ultrasonography. Use of needle biopsy avoids laparotomy or thoracotomy for abdominal or thoracic tumors. The advantage of this technique is that it is a nonsurgical procedure, causing little pain to the child, and can be performed quickly. The disadvantages are the difficulty of interpretation of a small specimen, especially for a general histopathologist, and the inability to do cytogenetic or molecular biological studies on such a small specimen.

The diagnosis can also be made from cytological examination of the bone marrow, or from ascitic or pleural fluid in situations where growth of the tumor is producing life-threatening complications, such as asphyxia in a thoracic or cervical tumor, and a prompt diagnosis is necessary. Myoblastic cells are readily recognizable in these cytological samples.

Delineation of the total extent of the tumor is necessary before initiating treatment. RMSs tend to involve the contiguous tissues and to destroy the adjacent bone marrow structures very rapidly. Regional spread is defined by use of a CT scan, by magnetic resonance imaging (MRI), or both. Bone destruction is more accurately defined on CT scan than on MRI, whereas soft tissue and intracranial involvement (in head and neck tumors) is more clearly seen on MRI. If bone lesions are mainly osteolytic, without osteoblastic reaction, these metastases will be detected only by conventional radiographs.

Thus, in some cases CT and MRI are complementary, but in the majority of patients it is only necessary to perform a CT scan to define regional extension. In addition, ultrasonography can be useful in pelvic tumors.

RMSs frequently involve adjacent lymph nodes, and the rate of lymph node spread is different according to the site of the tumor. It is often difficult to appreciate lymph node involvement, but this must be evaluated accurately. In the past, lymphangiography was performed in patients with limb tumors to investigate the presence of lymph node involvement by the tumor. Lymphangiography has now been superseded by CT scan of the abdomen

TABLE 1
Various Sites of Head and Neck
Rhabdomyosarcomas

Parameningeal sites, 63%
  Nasopharynx
  Nasal cavity
  Paranasal sinus
  Middle ear, mastoid
  Pterygoid fossa
  Orbit with intracranial tumor or with bone destruction

Nonparameningeal sites, 37%
  Parotid gland
  Oropharynx
  Orocavity
  Larynx
  Soft tissues of head and neck

and pelvis, which is now preferred by most pediatric radiologists. For the other sites, CT scan adequately reveals lymph node spread. If a lymph node is clinically palpable and is located in the course of drainage of a RMS, then cytological examination or even biopsy of this node must be performed to ascertain whether involvement is present.

In the head and neck, RMSs situated in sites adjacent to the meninges can involve this membrane by contiguity; these sites of tumor origin are called "parameningeal" sites and are listed in Table 1. In such patients, an examination of the cerebrospinal fluid (CSF) is necessary to ascertain the presence of myoblastic cells.

Distant metastases of RMSs are principally found in the lungs, but they are also found in bone, subcutaneous tissue, and bone marrow. More rarely metastases can occur in the liver, abdomen, or brain. Brain metastases are very rarely present at the time of primary presentation of the tumor, but seem to be more commonly associated with primary tumors of the limbs.

Thus, pretreatment assessment begins with a physical examination, including measurement of height, weight, and blood pressure, as well as noting the site and size of the tumor, presence of enlarged lymph nodes, and presence of any congenital anomalies. Biopsy of any suspicious lymph nodes should be carried out.

Laboratory studies should consist of serum creatinine and electrolytes (including calcium and magnesium), urine analysis, hemoglobin level, hematocrit, total leukocyte count and differential, and platelet count. CSF cytology should be examined in the presence of parameningeal tumors of the head and neck. Bone marrow aspiration should be done in all patients, but for stage IV tumors a trephine biopsy should also be obtained.

Radiological examinations include chest X-ray, CT scan of the primary site, and MRI for head and neck, pelvic, and limb tumor. Ultrasound examination should be done for abdominal and pelvic RMSs, with three-dimensional measurement of the tumors. Abdominal/pelvic CT scans are needed for limb tumors. Technetium bone scan, with plain X-ray of any abnormal sites, and brain CT scan are needed for extremity tumors. Finally, local examination under general anesthesia is needed for assessment of vaginal RMSs in little girls.

III. CLINICAL MANIFESTATIONS AND DIAGNOSIS OF TUMORS IN EACH SITE

The initial symptoms depend on the location and extent of the tumor. RMSs can be located anywhere in the body where mesenchymal tissue is found. No region is excluded,

TABLE 2
Classification of 289 Cases of
Rhabdomyosarcoma According to Anatomic
Sites of the Original Tumor

Site of primary	Number of cases	%
Orbit	26	9
Head and neck nonparamenin-geal	30	10
Head and neck parameningeal	53	18
Genitourinary	73	25
Bladder-prostate	29	
Vagina-paratesticular uterus	44	
Limbs	42	15
Other	65	23

From SIOP 1984—1988.

not even the brain where a few cases of this primitive tumor have been observed.[1] The first objective was to establish a classification system that precisely defines the location of a tumor. However, there are times when it is difficult to determine sites of origin of certain tumors, particularly expansive tumors which are classified differently by different clinicians. For example, a RMS involving both the thoracic and abdominal sides of the diaphragm and the retroperitoneum would be considered by some as an intrathoracic tumor, while others would call it an abdominal tumor.

Because of this discrepancy, it is often not possible to compare results using location of the tumor alone. As a result, an international effort was made through SIOP to unify classification of limited and regional localization of RMSs, and an international definition of anatomical sites was adopted in 1986. These sites are listed as follows: (1) orbit (without bone or intracranial involvement); (2) head and neck (excluding parameningeal sites); (3) head and neck (parameningeal sites; see Table 1); (4) genitourinary (including, first, bladder and prostate and second, vagina, vulva, uterus, and paratesticular); (5) extremities; (6) others (consisting of the wall of the trunk, as well as intrathoracic, intra-abdominal, pelvic, perineal, and paravertebral regions).

The relative frequency of the various localizations is given in Table 2, which summarizes results from the SIOP study 1984—1988 on these tumors. About half were situated in the head and neck, if the orbit is included. The next most frequent site was in tissues derived from the urogenital sinus (vagina, bladder, and prostate), which was followed by tumors originating in the extremities. A detailed code of localization has been published[2] which allows physicians to define precisely the site and extension of tumors for each anatomical site and to indicate possible secondary invasion.

A. ORBITAL RMS

RMSs of the orbit are characterized by their symptomatology, evolution, and the specific problems that they pose in diagnosis and therapy. They can evolve at any age. They develop in the motor muscles of the eye and rapidly give rise to ocular symptoms, such as ex-ophthalmus and strabismus. However, occasionally the tumor is visible at the side of the eye. The diagnosis is suspected on CT scan which reveals an intraorbital mass. The mass is extraconical and appears hyperdense on CT after injection with contrast. It may compress the ocular globe and optic nerve, distorting or breaking the orbital walls.

It is necessary to determine whether there is any internal extension of the tumor toward the ethmoid. One should look for evidence of posterior extension of the tumor to the sphenoidal cleft which would impose the risk of meningeal invasion, but such involvement is rare in tumors in this localization (being present in only 10% of cases in the 1975 SIOP series, not published). Toward the base, destruction of the orbital floor is accompanied by lysis of the suborbital canal and invasion of the maxillary sinus (Figure 1). In these cases, the tumor is classified as being parameningeal and is treated as such.

It is usually easy to exclude the diagnosis of an angioma, although diagnosis by clinical examination alone can be difficult. RMS is the most frequent malignant tumor of this region. The differential diagnosis includes a lymphosarcoma or, rarely, a germ cell tumor. Orbital bone tumors (such as Ewing's sarcoma, bone metastases of neuroblastoma, or Langerhans' cell histiocytosis) can closely simulate an intraorbital tumor when the tumor involves intraorbital soft tissue. A biopsy is indispensable when presence of biological markers cannot be detected. The surgeon should use a lateral approach if the tumor has arisen from that area. In the majority of cases a neurosurgical approach is needed.

Extension of orbital RMSs to lymph nodes is rare in the absence of bone or intracranial extension.

RMSs of the orbit also include tumors of the eyelids (Figure 2), which may consist of an apparently benign small nodule in the eyelid. If the nodule does not disappear within a few days, then one is obliged to carry out a total excision and complete histopathological examination.

B. RMS OF THE HEAD AND NECK

Great importance is laid in specifically defining the site of origin of tumors in this region. Site of origin is important because future prognosis depends on the structures involved, the possible extension, and whether the base of the skull or the meninges are invaded.

For example, a RMS localized to the maxillary sinus has a better prognosis than one that has already involved the orbit. It is often difficult to precisely define the origin of some of these tumors which rapidly destroy surrounding anatomical structures. In some cases the exact origin of the tumor is uncertain. Therefore, it is appropriate to describe the tumor according to its assumed origin and its extension as laid out in the published code, such as maxillary sinus, orbit, nasal fossa.

A plain skull X-ray is not helpful. Only a CT scan or MRI will allow precise determination of the site and extension of the tumor. These two imaging studies, CT and MRI, are indispensable for assessment of RMSs of the head and neck. The CT scan clearly defines bone destruction.

MRI is very useful to examine the soft tissues, for distinguishing between inflammation and tumor, and for detection of intracranial extension. However, a precise technique is needed which includes premedication in children younger than 4 years. Intravenous contrast, as used in CT scan, is used for the MRI and must be included in the examination to give the most information. Both axial and coronal cuts should be made. One advantage of the MRI is that it is not necessary to move the child to obtain coronal or oblique views.

The imaging studies must include not only the tumor, but all regions of possible extension, as well as satellite cervical lymphadenopathy. In any RMS of the ear, nose, and throat region, it is also imperative to examine by CT scan or MRI all intracranial structures, the base of the skull, and the upper cervical region.

Accurate assessment of cervical lymphadenopathy should include cytological (needle biopsy) or surgical biopsy examination of both enlarged lymph nodes and also the smallest node clinically palpable to assess their histology. The site of lymphadenopathy relates to locations of primary tumors. Thus, enlargement of submaxillary or digastric lymph nodes occurs in buccal tumors, and posterior cervical lymphadenopathy is present in nasopharyngeal or middle ear tumors.

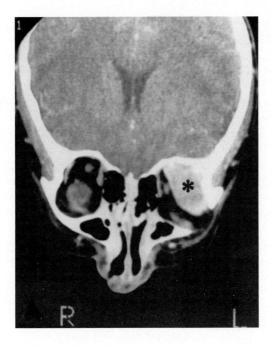

A

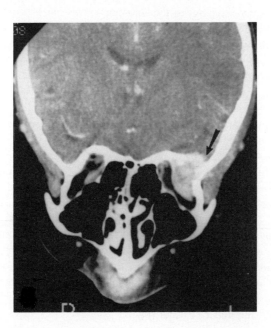

B

FIGURE 1.   A 14-year-old boy with orbital RMS. (A) CT scan with iodine contrast, coronal section shows extraconical, dense, solid mass displacing the musculoaponeurotic aspect of the left orbit (*); (B) CT scan, a more posterior section, shows osteolysis of the large wing of the sphenoid with intracranial extension (arrow).

97

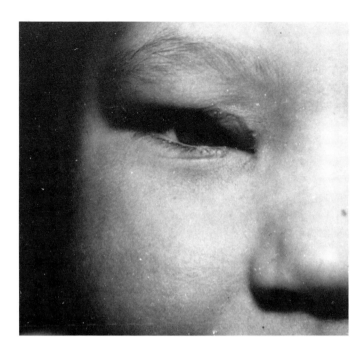

FIGURE 2.   A 2-year-old girl with a RMS of the lower eyelid after biopsy.

C. RMS OF THE NASOPHARYNX
1. Symptoms

Symptoms are often insidious. The history may be benign. There may be clear rhinorrhea which persists despite symptomatic treatment, accompanied by the voice changing to a nasal quality; or, serous otitis media may be the first symptom resulting from tumoral obstruction of the eustachian tube without evidence of tumor invasion. An inflammatory otitis media may also be a primary presentation, which is persistent despite antibiotic treatment, and remains unilateral. Examination of the throat may show protrusion of the soft palate or the tonsils.

The most alarming symptoms, and also ones that present late, include repeated epistaxis, neurological signs affecting the sixth (abducens) and the third (oculomotor) cranial nerves, and persistent headache. Finally, there may be the appearance of the tumor as a piece of tissue protruding from the nostrils by involvement of the nasal cavity or protrusion from the ear canal from a tumor of the middle ear. Sudden blindness can occur as a result of intracranial extension involving the optic chiasm.

2. Imaging Studies

Negative standard examinations are of little use. CT scan is the first line-effective examination. It reveals the tumor in the nasopharynx, gives guidance for the surgical biopsy, and contributes to determining the extent of the tumor. After injection with an iodine contrast, the tumor appears as isodense or hyperdense on CT. Heterogeneity in appearance is related to size of the tumor. The more voluminous the tumor is, the more tissue necrosis is usually present. Necrotic areas appear hypodense (sometimes the density of liquid) and are located at the center of the mass (Figure 3). The tumor promotes swelling or protrusion of the muscular structures in the pterygomaxillary and parapharyngeal regions.

The tumor can also destroy the neighboring bones. By anterior extension, the tumor erodes the posterior basin of the maxilla and pterygoid apophysis. By growth laterally, it invades the ascending branch of the inferior maxilla. With growth superiorly, it invades the

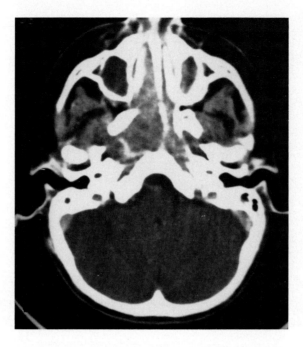

A

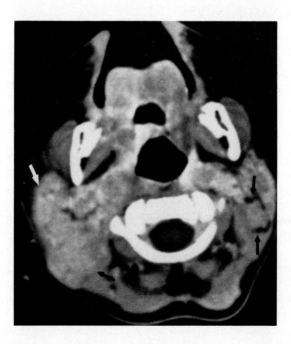

B

FIGURE 3.   A 3-year-old boy with nasopharyngeal RMS. CT scan, axial
section with contrast shows: (A) a mass occupying the nasopharyngeal
space with an anterior spread to the nasal fossae, plus an inflammatory
reaction in the paranasal sinuses; (B) enlargement of retromandibular lymph
nodes on both sides (arrows).

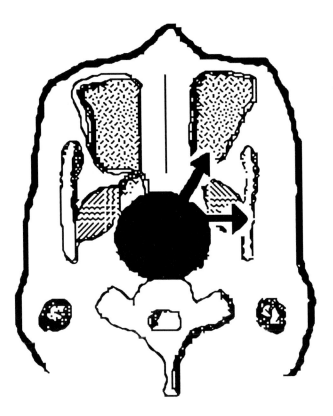

FIGURE 4. Schema showing anterior and lateral extension in a naso-pharyngeal RMS.

body of the sphenoid and the internal part of the sphenoidal wing. This may cause widening of the holes of the foramen of the sphenoid bone oval and anterior tearing with possible intracranial extension toward the cavernus sinus, the sella turcica, or temporal fossa (Figures 4 and 5). This intracranial invasion appears hyperdense after intravenous injection of contrast media.

The MRI is complementary to the CT scan, but provides better visualization of the composition of the tumor and its relation to the jugular and carotid vessels. Using a spin echo sequence at short repetition time (TR) (T1 weighted), the tumor gives a dull signal. With a spin echo sequence at long TR and long echo time (TE) in a T2 weighted sequence, a moderately bright signal is given. In these scans there is clear distinction of sinus inflammation which produces a high signal. The tumor increases its signal after intravenous injection of gadolinium-DPTA, which allows a more precise examination of intracranial spread.

3. Differential Diagnosis

In an early stage tumor, the condition most difficult to exclude is a simple adenoidal hypertrophy. This diagnosis is quickly eliminated as the tumor increases in size. These authors believe that histopathological examination of all hypertrophied adenoidal structures is indispensable. RMS must be distinguished from undifferentiated carcinoma of the naso-pharynx, which is more frequent in Mediterranean populations, and has a rapid rate of growth and extension associated with the presence of bilateral cervical lymphadenopathy. This tumor is also associated with previous Epstein-Barr virus infection. In addition, the presence of lymphosarcoma must also be excluded, as well as presence of a benign myxoid fibroma, although this tumor is extremely rare.

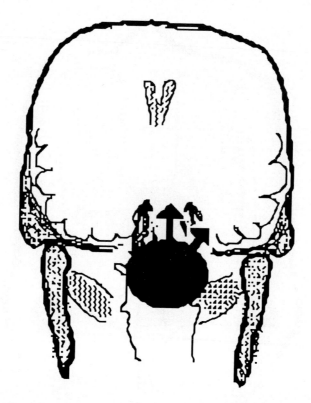

FIGURE 5. Schema showing superior extension through the sphenoid bone of a nasopharyngeal RMS.

The diagnosis of RMS is substantiated by a biopsy carried out under general anesthesia, ensuring that a deep segment of tissue is taken. Superficial specimens often only show benign inflammatory tissue, expecially when the tumor is deeply situated. In addition, biopsy of any suspicious lymph nodes should be carried out.

D. RMS OF THE SINUSES AND NASAL FOSSAE

Because of the rapidity with which the symptoms develop with a RMS in this region, one can determine their location and origin precisely.

Tumors arising in the nasal passages cause noisy breathing or complete nasal obstruction, which is unilateral at first but may progress to involve both sides. These symptoms may be accompanied by serous rhinorrhea which may lead to serosanguinous rhinorrhea, epistaxis, and finally visible evidence of the tumor in the nasal vestibule. When the tumor is visible, biopsy is easy and can be done without general anesthesia. However, if the biopsy is too superficial, then only necrotic and inflammatory tissue will be obtained.

RMS may also arise in the sinuses of the face and pterygomaxillary space. These cavities are anatomically deep and, therefore, clinical symptoms present late in the course of the disease, especially in pterygomaxillary tumors. These tumors cause rapid bony destruction and the symptoms are a result of this bone invasion. Superior extension of tumors of the maxillary sinus involves the orbital floor, while lateral extension into the nasal spaces and the ethmoid space results in neurological symptoms. Extension of tumor into the orbit results in strabismus, exophthalmus (Figure 6), or a swelling around the edge of the orbit. Anterior extension of tumors of the maxillary sinus produces a swollen cheek and causes loss of sensation in the lips due to suborbital invasion of the fifth (trigeminal) cranial nerve. Inferior extension of the tumor appears as a submucous swelling in the vault of the palate or in the

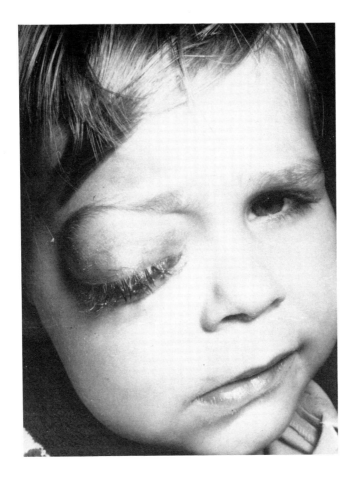

FIGURE 6. A 3-year-old boy with a paranasal RMS involving the orbit.

vestibule of the posterior-superior gingival space. This leads to gingival ulceration and then bony destruction, with increased mobility and dislocation of the teeth.

Medial extension gives destruction of the intersinonasal bone, with the same symptoms as those of a tumor arising from the nasal fossae.

Posterior extension of tumor toward the pterygomaxillary space results in the destruction of the posterior wall of the maxillary sinus and can remain asymptomatic for a long time. Invasion of the pterygomaxillary space finally becomes evident with the development of trismus, by invasion of the pterygoid muscles of mastication, and the occurrence of pain and altered sensation of the fifth cranial nerve. An even larger extension of tumor produces neurological signs relating to the ninth, tenth, eleventh, and twelfth cranial nerves and should alert the physician that a tumor may be their cause. It is this symptomatology that one finds, without signs relating to the nose, in RMSs originating from the pterygomaxillary space. That is to say that for this site the appearance of clinical signs is extremely late.

The ethmoid sinuses are never a primary site for this tumor, but a place of extension for RMSs originating from the maxillary sinus or nasal fossae. Extension of tumors into the ethmoid sinuses is extremely dangerous since it can allow the tumor to come into direct contact with the cribiform plate, which offers little resistance to intercranial spread.

Similarly, the sphenoidal and frontal sinuses are never a site of origin for RMSs, mainly because the frontal sinuses are not developed before the age of 10 years.

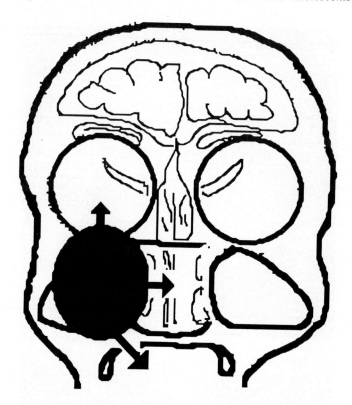

FIGURE 7.   Schema showing superior, lateral, and inferior extension of a paranasal RMS.

1. Diagnosis

The problem of biopsy depends of the site of origin. The biopsy is easy to perform if the tumor is present in the nasal space. However, a surgical operation is required if the tumor is located in the maxillary sinus. To biopsy a tumor of the maxillary sinus, the tumor is approached by route of Caldwell Luc: through a transbuccal opening of the anterior wall of the maxillary sinus. For tumors limited in the pterygomaxillary space, the problem is more difficult. The biopsy necessitates a surgical approach with opening of the anterior maxillary wall and passing the sinus, leaving by the posteroexternal wall. Since this procedure is very difficult, one must be guided by the use of histological examinations at the time of surgery (frozen section) to ensure that representative tumor tissue, and not peritumoral fibrosis, is obtained. A preoperative CT scan is indispensable in helping to define the site of the tumor, and the operation is aided by the use of an operating microscope.

2. Imaging Studies

Radiological examination allows the presumed site of origin and extension of the tumor to be defined.

CT scan is very useful for locating bone destruction. In RMSs of the maxillary sinus (Figure 7), there is lysis of bones of the sinus, posterior destruction of the pterygoid apophysis, upward invasion of the orbital floor, invasion of the nasal fossae, and downward extension into the infrastructure of the hard palate (Figure 8). For tumors of the pterygomaxillary space (Figure 9) there is forward invasion of the pterygoid apophysis and the posterior basin of the maxillary sinus, as well as lysis or subluxation of the rising branch of the inferior maxilla from the outside. In tumors arising in the greater wing of the sphenoid, the CT scan may show upward extension to the floor of the temporal fossa (Figure 10). For

RMSs of the nasal fossae (Figure 11) there may be upward extension of tumors of the ethmoid, extension to the nasopharynx and posteriorly by the choanae, and destruction of the nasal septum from the outside.

MRI gives the most information concerning the base of the skull and any intracranial extensions. In particular, at the level of the anterior shelf, frontal invasion occurs via the cribiform plate. By the sphenoidomaxillary cleft, invasion of the orbit and the anterior part of the floor of the temporal fossa is possible. At the level of the middle shelf, sphenoidal extension can cross to the oval foramena. These small holes can be broken anteriorly by tumor extension toward the cavernous sinus or the internal part of the temporal fossa, resulting in destruction of the greater sphenoidal wing and invasion of the temporal fossa. Finally, with posterior destruction of these holes, extension into the posterior fossa is possible. In all these situations, MRI can identify the alteration of all meningeal and cranial structures, including the adjacent perilesional cerebral edema.

3. Differential Diagnosis

In tumors arising in the facial sinuses, it is necessary to distinguish between a maxillary sinus inflammatory lesion without bony involvement and an inflammatory lesion in which a RMS has evolved. MRI, using a setting of T2 (T2 weighted), allows distinction between the increased signal of inflammatory lesions (identical to CSF) vs. an actual tumor mass. This characteristic increased signal can be used to examine the sinus cavities, and with the absence of a clearly definable mass, a malignant process can be excluded. A malignant tumor which can be localized in a facial sinus is perhaps more likely to be a RMS than a lymphoma. Burkitt's lymphoma is the most frequent type of lymphoma in this location, with its characteristic history and signs and its predilection for children of African origin.

One must also consider the possibility of benign tumors, such as adenomas and fibro-myxomas of the nasal fossae, in cases where there is no osseous involvement.

Osteodystrophic lesions can give a pseudosarcomatous appearance. Therefore, the imaging examination of choice in tumors having this histopathologic composition is the CT scan because of its ability to identify various bony lesions. A pseudotumorous or "frosted glass" appearance of bones at the base of the skull precedes massive facial deformation and the occurrence of multiple nerve compression.

E. RMS OF THE MIDDLE EAR

Early signs of a RMS in the middle ear are ordinary. In the beginning there is a picture of otitis media, consisting of a serous or serosanguinous discharge, auricular pain which may be a little more intense than expected, and a diminution in hearing. Suspicion is aroused by the lack of evidence for infection, the absence of anterior nasopharyngeal symptoms (rhinorrhea and coryza), and its unilaterality.

These apparently benign clinical symptoms should not deter a thorough examination of the ears, nose, and throat from being carried out. Such an examination is needed in view of the rapidity with which the tumor can destroy the tympanic membrane and rapidly oblate the external auditory canal by external extension. All tissue that is found within the auditory canal must be biopsied and examined histologically. This also applies to any polyps found in the area; they too should be biopsied to establish their benign histology.

At an advanced stage, the tumor can have the appearance of mastoiditis, with pain, retroauricular subcutaneous swelling, and appearance of an infectious process. Again, a systematic biopsy and histopathological examination should be done, and surgical exploration of the mastoid is needed even if it seems to contain only infection. The symptomatology may be mild, but a paralysis of the seventh (facial) cranial nerve soon leads one to suspect a serious pathology.

Presentation of a massive tumor in this region shows total paralysis of the seventh cranial

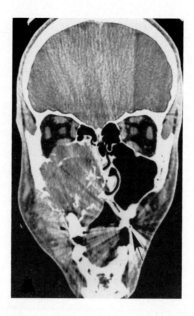

A

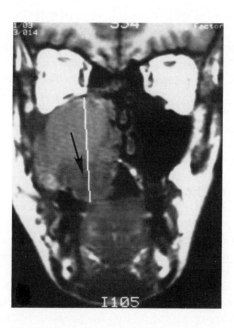

B

FIGURE 8.   A 15-year-old boy with a paranasal RMS. (A) CT scan with contrast, coronal section shows a solid mass destroying the right paranasal sinus, involving the inferior orbital wall, the nasal fossae, and the palatine roof (arrow). Note the dental artifacts due to metallic prosthesis. Coronal (B) and axial (C) T1-weighted MRI without contrast. There is better visualization of the soft tissue tumor spread without appearance of metallic dental artifacts. Note the heterogeneous appearance of the mass, being cystic, necrotic, and solid (black arrow). However, bone structures are less visible on MRI than on CT.

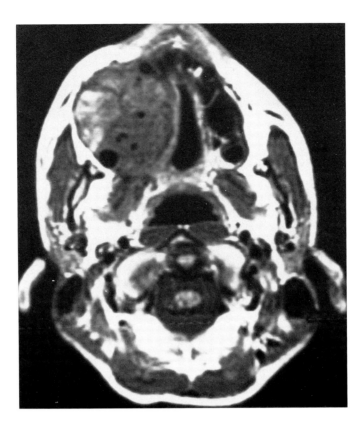

FIGURE 8C (continued)

nerve, extension into the nasopharynx by the eustachian tube, destruction of the petrous bone, and intracranial extension into the temporal lobe. Invasion can also occur inferiorly and behind the maxillary sinus, involving the parotid gland.

1. Imaging Studies

Radiologically, determining the size and extent and, particularly, tracing the spread of a RMS of the ear require many fine cuts using the CT scanner (1 mm thickness). These fine cuts are needed in order to methodically analyze the different compartments of the ear, not only the external auditory canal, but also the tympanic membrane and the internal ear. Destruction of the ossicles, intrusion into the eustachian tube with extension toward the nasopharynx, and mastoid invasion with lysis of walls of the mastoid cells can all occur (Figure 12).

The internal ear is protected for a considerable time. Intracranial extension appears after the destruction of the petrous pyramids. Tumor growth may be continuous toward the posterior part of the temporal fossa, and later may even involve the posterior fossa. Unfortunately, MRI does not give cuts less than 3 mm in thickness and this is a limiting factor for the use of MRI for analyzing pathology in this location.

2. Diagnosis

Procuring a piece of tissue for biopsy of a lesion in the external auditory canal is easy. Conversely, a full surgical exploration is needed in the presence of signs of mastoiditis, or extension of tumor to this area. Lesions in this location are the most difficult for the histopathologist to diagnose, particularly when details of the clinical history are not provided. A misdiagnosis of inflammation can easily be reached.

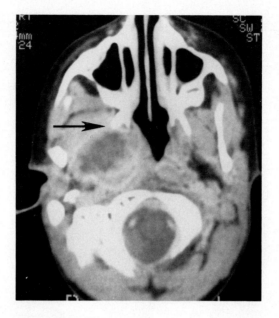

A

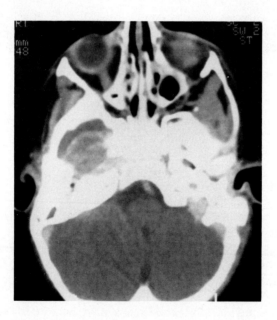

B

FIGURE 9.   A 6-year-old girl with a pterygomaxillary RMS. Axial CT
scan with contrast infusion shows: (A) a space-occupying heterogeneous
mass in the right pterygomaxillary fossa causing erosion of the external
wing of the pterygoid (black arrow) and lateral displacement of the right
nasopharyngeal wall; (B) scan at the level of the temporal fossa shows
hyperdense intracranial extension through the oval foramen.

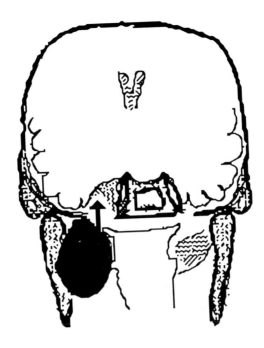

FIGURE 10. Schema showing superior extension to the internal aspect of the temporal fossa and to the cavernous sinus of a pterygomaxillary RMS.

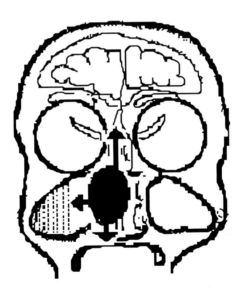

FIGURE 11. Schema showing extension of a RMS of the nasal fossae.

All forms of chronic otitis media are included in the differential diagnosis, which may include a polyp. However, when polyps are present there is a long history of otitis in the past and the otitis is bilateral.

F. RMS OF THE PAROTID GLAND

Tumors in this site cause swelling of the parotid, being located retromandibular and sublobular. Benign parotid tumors are rare in children, and if the swelling is accompanied

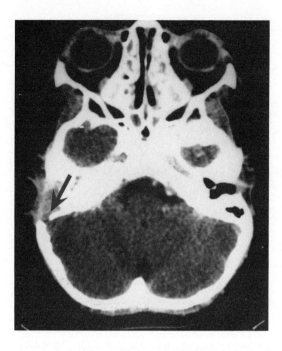

FIGURE 12.   A 5-year-old boy with RMS of the right ear. Axial CT scan with iodine contrast shows space-occupying mass involving the right middle ear with a lysis of the mastoid (arrow).

by paralysis of the seventh cranial nerve, then the malignant nature of the mass is assured. If the tumor arises from the deep lobe of the parotid gland, the first sign may be a swelling at the level of the soft palate, or the occurrence of pharyngeal discomfort on swallowing.

In the presence of any parotid swelling, meticulous examination of the oropharynx is necessary in order to estimate the size and extent of the tumor. The tumor also may extend to the external auditory canal, resulting in the appearance of tissue externally, or it may extend to the pterygomaxillary space giving the symptoms already described for tumors of this site.

1. Imaging Studies

As used for tumors in the other locations, radiological examinations are mainly CT scan and MRI. These techniques give precise information on extension of tumor to the pterygomaxillary space, base of the skull, and parapharyngeal space. However, extension of tumor to the parapharyngeal space is often clinically silent. Sialography can be useful. Also, ultrasound shows the volume of the tumor, but not the precise structures involved. CT scan, or preferably MRI, precisely defines the relation of the tumor to the surrounding bony structures. However, above all CT or MRI show the relation of the blood vessels and seventh cranial nerve along with enlargement of tumor in the deep spaces under the parotid and toward the posterior parapharyngeal space (Figure 13).

2. Diagnosis

Differential diagnosis includes all lymphomas, both Hodgkin's disease and non-Hodgkin's lymphomas, and also all other nonrhabdomyosarcomatous mesenchymal malignant tumors, adenocarcinoma, or mucoepithelial tumor. Also, intraparotid adenopathy due to metastases from another tumor may be seen. Infections due to viruses and other infectious microorganisms are easy to exclude because of their chronicity (such as in recurring chronic parotitis of childhood), their pain, and accompanying fever.

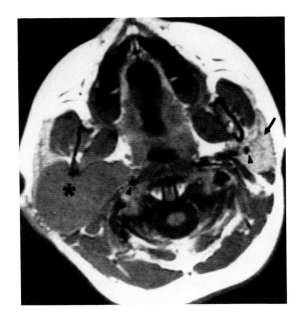

FIGURE 13. An 11-year-old girl with RMS of the parotid gland. Axial
T1-weighted MRI shows a parotid mass occupying the superficial and deep
part of the salivary gland (*). Normal contralateral parotid gland (black
arrow) is normal in appearance. The external carotid arteries (arrow heads)
are evident.

Surgical biopsy is needed so that the gland can be totally examined. In performing the
biopsy, care should be taken to avoid causing seventh nerve damage, which is a significant
risk.

Histological examination of tissue (frozen section) during surgery should be employed
to ensure that tumor tissue is obtained so that a definitive diagnosis can be made by the
pathologist. Whether the tumor is benign (adenoma) or malignant (adenocarcinoma) or
mucoepithelial (dermoid), a complete surgical resection should be carried out, allowing
examination of both deep and superficial lobes.

G. RMS OF ORAL CAVITY AND OROPHARYNX

The sites of origin are mainly the mobile part of the tongue, the gingival region and
intermaxillary cleft, the cheek, soft palate, and the tonsils (Figure 14). Very rarely, the
mouth floor may be involved. The tumor may cause interference with chewing or swallowing.
The lesion may be visible to the naked eye and perhaps infected or ulcerated. The diagnosis
may be established by clinical findings, and a biopsy is easy to perform. A careful examination of the ears, nose, and throat is the most reliable way to define any extension, since
radiological examinations are difficult in children due to the mobility of the structures.

A CT scan can determine the presence of bone and gingival invasion. However, coronal
cuts can be obtained more easily by MRI, which reveal any extension of tumor into the
pterygomaxillary space from primary tumors arising in the intermaxillary space. From this
finding, presence of a malignant tumor may be suspected before the appearance of trismus.
CT scan can easily detect spread to the parapharyngeal spaces and nasopharynx from a tumor
originating in the lateral walls of the oropharynx and the tonsillar region. However, CT
cannot, with equal accuracy, assess a primary tumor of the maxillary sinus or the extension
of a jaw RMS to the maxillary sinus or pterygomaxillary space. Furthermore, this tumor
may appear as a cheek swelling, imitating an extension of a RMS of the maxillary sinus.

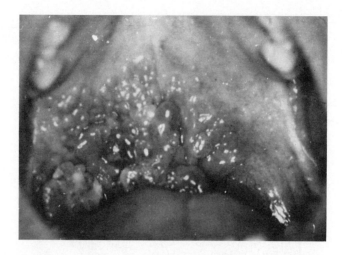

FIGURE 14.   An 11-year-old boy with a RMS of the soft palate. Anterosuperior view (with opened mouth) of the soft palate with the tumor.

At the beginning, symptoms of RMSs of this region are often wrongly considered as being due to dental problems and therefore the tumor is diagnosed late. A RMS of the tongue can sometimes be difficult to differentiate from a benign lesion (such as an Abrikosoff tumor), fibromatosis, or a schwannoma. Other diagnoses include a malignant fibrohistiocytoma or a fibrosarcoma. Concerning the cheek, benign infectious lesions are most common and can be diagnosed, while in the tonsils the main differential diagnosis is that of an abscess, but there are signs of infection or findings suggesting a non-Hodgkin's lymphoma.

1. RMS of the Larynx

This localization for RMS is extremely rare. Up until 1976, only 14 cases worldwide and 6 cases at the Institut Gustave-Roussy[6] were observed. The first symptom is dysphonia, sometimes accompanied by dysphagia, together with gradual progression to pharyngolaryngeal obstruction. Difficulty in swallowing indicates extension of tumor around the larynx. Direct laryngoscopy should be carried out under general anesthesia in order to visualize the tumor and to obtain a biopsy. The tumor has a subglottic and submucous location. Because of motion artifacts, CT scan is not helpful in these cases for detecting paralaryngeal extension.

A RMS must be differentiated from laryngeal cysts, laryngoceles, lymphangiomas, or an epithelial tumor, which are all very rare in children.

2. RMS of the Soft Tissues of Head and Neck

These are swellings of the neck, face, or scalp (Figure 15). They can be accompanied by regional lymphadenopathy. A particular site for RMS is the nasolabial fold (Figure 16). A biopsy must be performed; or complete surgical excision may be carried out if it can be done as a primary procedure and without any damage to surrounding structures. A CT scan is essential to detect tumor extension not only into the deep soft tissues, but also into the maxilla. One must take care not to confuse a RMS in this region with an angioma, a lipoma, chronic lymphadenopathy, congenital cysts, or a fibromatosis.

Although showing similar histology, RMS of the soft tissues of the head and neck are diverse clinical entities with very different prognoses depending on their location. These tumors are subdivided into two groups: nonparameningeal and parameningeal. Parameningeal tumors carry the significant risk of spread to the meninges through the foramen at the base of the skull or by destruction of contiguous bony structures. The international definition of parameningeal localization accepted in 1986 (by the SIOP workshop) is based on anatomical

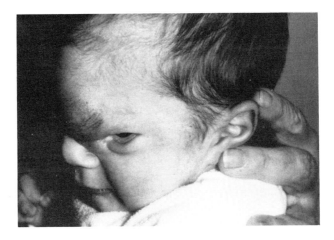

FIGURE 15.   A 1-month-old girl with RMS of soft tissue of the forehead.

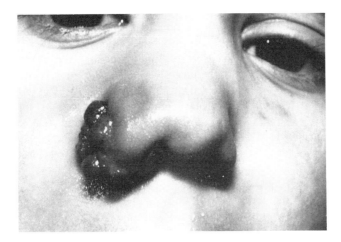

FIGURE 16.   A 2-year-old boy with a RMS of the nasal fold.

sites. These sites are the facial sinuses and nasal fossae, the middle ear and mastoid, the pterygomaxillary space, and the nasopharynx.

All nonparameningeal tumors spreading to parameningeal sites are considered to have the same risk as a parameningeal tumor. Therefore, they receive the same treatment. An example of this is an orbital RMS with intracranial extension. However, parameningeal tumors at different sites carry different risks and they are subdivided again into three categories: (1) sites that do not include bony invasion of the base of the skull (such as a localized maxillary sinus tumor); (2) sites likely to have basal skull erosion; and (3) tumors that have intracranial extension on CT scan or clinical signs of intracranial extension.

These three groups have a different prognosis, and the latter two have the worst. In fact, before 1986 SIOP considered only the last two categories as ''parameningeal''; but SIOP has now adopted the above definition in deference to recommendations of the IRS for the purpose of consistency and for ease in comparing results of clinical studies by IRS and SIOP.

H. RMS OF THE GENITOURINARY SYSTEM

These tumors are divided into two categories on account of their very different prognoses being either RMS of the bladder and prostate or tumors of the vulvovagina, uterus, and paratesticle.

1. RMS of the Bladder and Prostate

In most boys, the RMS arises in the neck of the bladder and then invades the prostate. Often the distinction between a primary prostatic and a primary bladder RMS is difficult to define by clinical findings. It was easier to determine the site of the primary tumor when the initial treatment was surgical.

Clinically, the first signs are urinary abnormalities, including dysuria, polyuria, and particularly episodes of retention, either complete or partial. In the absence of a palpable pelvic tumor, rectal examination may reveal the tumor when one finds a hard mass situated in front of the neck of the bladder. In the imaging investigation of these tumors of the bladder and surrounding structures, ultrasound has increasingly replaced intravenous urography. Ultrasound shows the tumor mass, identifies its local extension, and reveals any involvement of the urogenital system superiorly up to the kidneys.

Biopsy must be carried out to confirm the diagnosis and is possible using an endoscope. If the tumor is too superficial to allow histological diagnosis at first attempt, the biopsy must be repeated. If biopsy by cystoscopy is unsuccessful, then, despite the risk of tumor dispersion at the site, a cystotomy should be done. The transrectal route is dangerous because of the risk of dissemination of gut organisms, which could easily provoke a life-threatening sepsis in a child who will soon be made neutropenic by chemotherapy. Differential diagnosis consists of bladder polyps (rare in children), certain benign tumors of the bladder, and occasionally a septic granulomatosis. Also, appendicular abscesses in the form of pseudo-tumors encased in the pouch of Douglas can simulate a retrobladder or bladder tumor.

Urinary retention can also occur in a tumor confined to the urethra. Such a tumor may be detected by cytoscopy, CT scan, or better by MRI using coronal and sagittal cuts to distinguish any spread to prostate or surrounding tissues. Very rarely, a RMS of the dome of the bladder may be found which presents with hematuria. Biopsy is needed for the diagnosis. Usually a cystotomy is done, but if the tumor is very large, a needle biopsy is adequate. If the tumor is small, a partial cystectomy is the procedure of choice. It is in these tumors of the bladder dome that invasion of the peritoneum and abdominal structures occurs. This occurs when the tumor does not extend interiorly into the bladder, but instead the tumor arises from the muscularis muscle and spreads exteriorly. Therefore, it is important in these cases to do a surgical biopsy by laparotomy in order to detect any peritoneal spread and intra-abdominal involvement.

When the ureters are involved or compressed by the tumor, children with a vesicoprostatic tumor present with pain bilateral hydronephrosis, and renal insufficiency. This is a situation where diagnosis is urgent. A needle biopsy is the quickest and easiest way to identify the tumor, followed by bilateral pyelostomy before beginning treatment. Bladder tumors are less frequent in girls (there being only 18 girls and 91 boys in the international SIOP RMS workshop on nonmetastatic bladder or prostate tumors).[12] Signs include hematuria or appearance of tumor tissue at the vulva. There may be secondary spread, and in some cases the primary site is difficult to determine, between a vaginal tumor invading the bladder or a tumor from the bladder invading the vagina.

Imaging studies allow these distinctions to be made. If the tumor is of moderate size, ultrasonography is useful. However, CT scan visualizes various pelvic structures more precisely, and can determine the site of origin by anatomical landmarks not effaced by the tumor mass. Anatomical structures visualized on CT include the wall and lumen of the bladder, the bladder neck, the uterus, the vagina, the obturator muscle, the ischiorectal space, the superior pelvorectal space, and the iliac vascular axis. When the tumor mass fills the entire pelvis, it is difficult to localize the site of origin of the tumor. Reduction in size

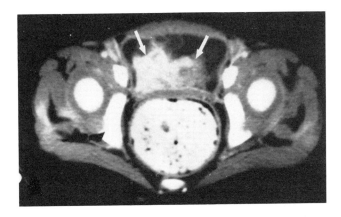

A

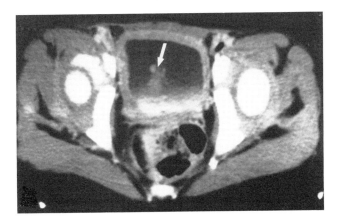

B

FIGURE 17. A 5-year-old boy with a vesicoprostatic RMS. CT scan with axial section after bolus iodine injection shows: (A) lobulated hyperdense mass occupying the lumen of the bladder (white arrows). After chemotherapy (B), there is regression of the tumor (white arrows).

of the tumor after chemotherapy can help in precisely defining the extent of the tumor as more anatomical landmarks become visible (Figure 17).

On ultrasonography, the tumor is echodense and the tumor on CT scan is either isodense or discretely hypodense compared to muscle before injection of intravenous contrast. Following contrast injection, the tumor becomes hyperdense and heterogeneous, which allows good examination of its contours. A dull signal is produced by the tumor on MRI using the settings weighted at T1 and a bright signal is produced in T2-weighted images after injection with gadolinium (Figure 18).

The route of lymph node spread is to the hypogastric or external iliac nodes, or only the lumboaortic nodes may be involved. The frequency of nodal involvement for RMSs of the bladder and vesicoprostate is difficult to determine precisely now when definitive surgery is often delayed until after chemotherapy. Lymph node invasion is assessed using CT scan to visualize the iliac axes and the lumboaortic nodes (Figure 19). Initially, gross lymphadenopathy allows easy detection of involved nodes, but when the tumor is very large and

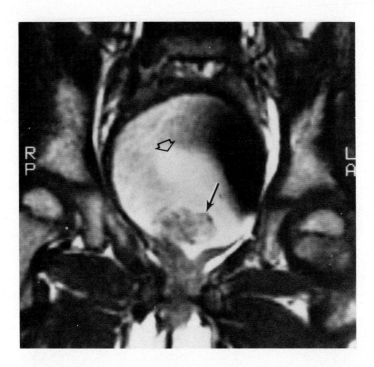

FIGURE 18.   A 3-year-old boy with RMS of the bladder. T1-weighted coronal MRI after gadolinium contrast injection shows a mass inside the bladder (arrow) overlying the bladder neck. There is opacification due to gadolinium contrast in the bladder (open arrow).

lymphadenopathy is limited to adjacent nodes, it may be difficult to distinguish the enlarged lymph nodes from the tumor. It is usually possible to identify involved lymph nodes at some distance from the tumor in the bladder or prostate, such as the lumboaortic nodes, for example; or, involved nodes may become recognizable after reduction chemotherapy, when they are more clearly separated from the tumor. The nodes appear polylobular, solid, and in contact with the opaque vascular axes, which they displace.

Tumors of this location, the bladder and prostate, do not include those arising from the pelvic walls.

2. Paratesticular RMS

These are discovered early by the appearance of a nontransilluminant mass, although a hydrocele can be associated.

Surgical intervention by the scrotal route incurs a risk of intrascrotal dissemination. Therefore, orchidectomy is carried out using the inguinal route, with the spermatic cord being cut as high as possible in the inguinal canal. Histological examination of both the cord and the tumor mass should be carried out to define the stage.

Differential diagnosis includes a testicular germ cell tumor which very often secretes α-feto protein (AFP), and whose diagnosis can be confirmed before orchidectomy. The surgical approach is the same.

Studies to determine possible spread of the tumor are done using ultrasonography, and CT scan of the lumboaortic region is done to detect lymphatic invasion. The authors believe that systematic surgical lymphadenectomy is unnecessary in cases in whom there is complete excision of the tumor along with a section of tumor-free cord and the chest X-ray is normal.[8,9] This recommendation is not in accordance with the IRS.[10] The difference in attitude is based

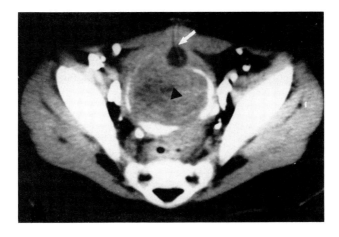

A

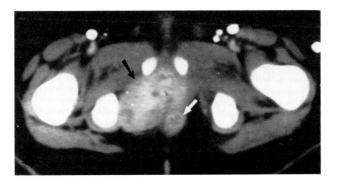

B

FIGURE 19. A 3-year-old boy with RMS of the bladder. Axial CT scan with iodine contrast. (A) Scan at the level of the bladder shows a mass in the bladder (arrow heads). Percutaneous cystotomy tube is seen (white arrow); (B) scan at the level of the perineum shows hyperdense lymphadenopathy (black arrow) displacing the perineal structures. The anal canal (white arrow) is seen.

on the fact that the IRS studies showed presence of tumor-involved nodes in 40% of patients after systematic lymphadenectomy performed as part of initial surgery in paratesticular RMSs, but without taking into account the local spread. In the SIOP protocol, nodal involvement is assessed radiologically for those who have localized tumor, that is, those whose tumor is completely excised and has no evidence of cord involvement at the upper margin. In effect, it is proposed that microscopic nodal involvement will be eradicated by the systemic chemotherapy these patients receive. If, however, the tumor is stage II, with local or regional invasion (particularly with invasion of the cord), lymphadenectomy is imperative and should be done either initially or following chemotherapy.

3. RMS of Vagina, Vulva, and Uterus

RMS of the vagina or vulva is most frequent in the first few years of life.[3] They are manifested by vulval inflammation because the tumor tissue appears exteriorly, there may genital bleeding, or both signs may be present. If the tumor arises from the vulva, it consists of a firm nodule imbedded in the labial folds or it may be periclitoric in location.

TABLE 3
Classification of 42 Cases of
Rhabdomyosarcoma of the
Extremities According to Anatomic
Sites of Origin

Upper extremities

Hand	5
Forearm	8
Arm	3
Axilla	1
Total	17

Lower extremities

Foot	7
Leg	8
Thigh	6
Groin	2
Buttock	2
Total	25

From SIOP 1984—1988

For all suspicious tissue and swellings, a vaginal examination under general anesthesia allows biopsy and reveals the full extent of the tumor, particularly for vaginal tumors. Such examination also shows vulval extension, location of tumor in the vagina, and spread of tumor to the neck of the uterus. Also, any apparently abnormal lymph nodes should be biopsied, which may be carried out during the same period of general anesthesia. Pelvic CT scan completes the workup for determining possible intrapelvic or intravesical extension of the tumor.

Vulva nodules should have primary surgical excision including a wide margin of normal tissue. However, in the experience at the Institut Gustave-Roussy, total excision is never complete microscopically.

Intrauterine RMSs are quite rare and tend to occur in adolescent girls around the time of puberty.[5] They present by vaginal extrusion of tumor tissue followed by hemorrhage, or they may be first detected as a pelvic mass. Biopsy is done vaginally, either by sampling of visible tumor tissue or by uterine curretage. When the size and maturity of the child allow, a hysteroscopy is the best route of access for biopsy of a completely intrauterine RMS.

I. RMS OF THE EXTREMITIES

RMSs of the legs are more frequent than those of the arms. For the SIOP study, the classification of tumors of the extremities according to anatomic sites is given in Table 3.

The presenting complaint often results from a traumatic event, with swelling more or less confined to a muscle, or giving the appearance of being subcutaneous in origin (Figure 20). The swelling can appear as a bruise, suggesting a hematoma. All new swellings of limbs need a biopsy in order to make a definitive diagnosis of their etiology. One must also be aware that often only upon further questioning is a history of local trauma revealed. It may be that this event, the accidental trauma, merely rendered the tumor detectable. Also, it is possible that trauma is such a common event in children that one would always find a traumatic event preceding the appearance of a tumor.

The best imaging study for local definition of tumors of the limbs is MRI. For this purpose, the MRI should use many different cuts in different plains to allow precise visualization of extension of the tumor into the anatomical compartments of the limb, to show

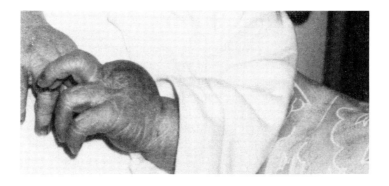

FIGURE 20. RMS of the dorsum of the hand in a newborn.

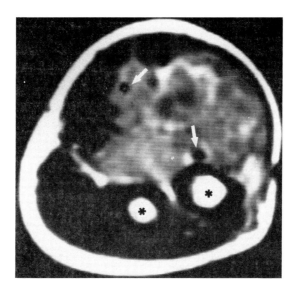

FIGURE 21. A 6-year-old boy with RMS of the forearm. Axial MRI with gadolinium contrast shows a hyperintense mass occupying the anterior aspect of the forearm, including the arteries (white arrows), as compared to the hypointense surrounding msucles (radius and cubitus) (*).

the tumor's relationship to muscles, aponeurotic tissue, blood vessels, nerves, and joints (Figure 21).

Studies to detect lymph node involvement must be carefully carried out. Close examination of the local nodal region often gives the impression of being uninvolved, but the first nodal involvement is found in the inguinal and axillary regions. All clinically suspicious nodes should be examined cytologically, and if at all possible such nodes should be biopsied before beginning therapy. Examination of pelvic lymphadenopathy for RMSs of the lower extremities is carried out with a CT scan. The lymph node spread of this tumor is by involvement of contiguous nodes.

The differential diagnosis includes a benign lipoma or a hematoma, which can be easily distinguished from a RMS using MRI and CT. On ultrasonography the fatty composition of a lipoma is very echogenic, but with the CT scan and MRI it is possible to distinguish fatty tissue of a lipoma from that of a tumor composed of other tissues. A lipoma gives a dull signal (d $= -100$ to -150 units), which is very characteristic on CT scan, and a bright signal identical to fatty subcutaneous tissue on MRI. A hematoma is hyperintense in both T1 and T2 sequences on MRI.

Either a biopsy or total excision of the lesion is required, since another type of aggressive nonrhabdomyosarcomatous mesenchymal malignant tumor may be present, such as synovial sarcoma, fibrosarcoma, malignant fibrohistiocytoma, neuroepithelioma, or clear cell tumor of the tendons and aponeuroses. The tumor may also be benign fibroma. The only definitive way of distinguishing these tumors is by histopathological examination. Of note, however, malignant nonrhabdomyosarcomatous mesenchymal tumors usually tend to appear in older age groups and are more localized. Last, non-Hodgkin's lymphoma must be excluded, and the metastases of another tumor, such as cutaneous metastasis of a lymphoma or a neuroblastoma, should be considered.

J. RMS OF OTHER SITES

RMS from all other sites, for which precise individual sites of origin are at times difficult to establish, are grouped together.

1. RMS of the Thorax

RMSs of the thoracic wall with spread to the lung are difficult to distinguish from primaries of the lung or mediastinum which have extended to the surrounding walls.

Clinical signs may be dyspnea or thoracic pain of variable intensity according to position, with the development of pleuritic pain, sometimes accompanied by a fever or general malaise. A swelling of the thoracic wall may be visible, being located intercostally or intraclavicularly, or the swelling may be situated in a location that is difficult to palpate, such as over the scapula. In all these situations, a CT scan detects the exact extent of the tumor. Examination of the mediastinum and thoracic wall by CT using many cuts in different plains not only detects pleural effusions, but can separate an inflammatory lesion from a reaction of neighboring tissues, or a lesion directly contiguous with the tumor. In the case of a small pleural effusion that is not clinically detectable, it is important to analyze a sample of the fluid in order to determine whether the effusion is reactive, or if the fluid contains malignant cells.

If the tumor is posteriorly situated, particular note should be made of any intraspinal involvement. Such a tumor can give rapid rise to a life-threatening situation, producing signs of spinal cord compression which would require urgent treatment. These neurological signs can be the presenting complaint and the etiology must be determined quickly before a paraplegia ensues. An emergency mediastinal MRI is indicated. It is necessary to detect any significant subarachnoid or extradural extension of tumor and any degree of compression on the dura, and to determine the level of the compression with relationship to the spinal cord (the filum terminale is at the level of L1).

Pericardial or paracardiac extension of a RMS requires an echocardiograph in order to confirm any direct pericardial or cardiac involvement. A primary RMS arising within the heart is extremely rare, there being only one such patient in the SIOP-84 study. Intrabronchial tumors are also extremely rare. At the thoracic site, the differential diagnosis is that of a nonmalignant tumor such as a lipoma (which is distinguishable by a CT scan), bronchial malformations, and cysts. Thus, often the diagnosis of RMS is late, the tumor having been thought to be a breast opacity or a pleural effusion as a result of an infection. In the presence of any radiological abnormality which does not respond to antibiotic treatment, one must always consider carrying out a CT scan, which will quickly show any tumor.

Other differential diagnoses include malignant tumors which are not evident on clinical or X-ray examination. A Ewing's sarcoma of a rib extending into soft tissues can be confused with RMS of the chest wall which has spread to adjacent structures. Some radiological findings can indicate spread of the tumor, but there are no definite radiological criteria to define the origin of a malignant tumor invading into soft tissue. This is important since the histological diagnosis can be inconclusive between Ewing's sarcoma and a poorly differentiated RMS. In such a case, an appropriate specimen of fresh tissue for cytogenetic examination is needed to show the characteristic chromosomal abnormalities of Ewing's sarcoma. In these patients, another biopsy should be attempted and if impossible, a decision should be reached based on clinical findings as well as the results of laboratory studies.

A thoracic neuroblastoma may also present in the same way as a Ewing's sarcoma or a RMS. A CT scan shows the position of a posterior mediastinal tumor and will indicate whether the tumor is involving the thoracic wall. CT scan of a neuroblastoma will reveal any characteristic intratumoral calcifications and, eventually, these scans will show extension of tumor into the arachnoid space, which frequently occurs. However, confirmation of the presence of a neuroblastoma is supported by presence of elevated levels of urinary VMA, HVA, and dopamine, as well as MIBG-positive scintigraphy. Last, the diagnosis of other nonrhabdomyosarcomatous mesenchymal tumors requires careful histopathological examination. These tumors include neuroepitheliomas, Askin's tumor, extraosseus Ewing's tumor, fibrosarcoma, schwannoma, synovial sarcoma (which is rare at this site), and clear cell tumor of tendons and aponeuroses.

2. RMS of the Diaphragm

RMS arising from the diaphragm gives a picture of a thoracoabdominal tumor with extension superiorly or inferiorly (Figure 22). It can be situated medially and spread paracardially where it is difficult to distinguish tumor from enlarged lymph nodes. MRI using saggital cuts gives the best visual definition of this area and the diaphragm. A pleural effusion always accompanies such a tumor.

3. RMS of the Abdominal or Pelvic Wall

The patient may complain of pain due to nerve root compression (such as in the paravertebral region) or there may be a visible swelling imbedded in the abdominal wall. A CT scan, or better an MRI, will show the size, situation, and extent of the tumor. This site poses the same problems relating to extension of the tumor as tumors in the thorax. In particular, there may be intraspinal invasion by paravertebral tumors or by extension of an intra-abdominal tumor. Involvement of axillary and cervical nodes is assessed clinically as well as radiographically by a CT scan. Diagnostic possibilities are the same as those for tumors of the thoracic wall, excluding Askin's tumor which by definition is situated in the thorax, but synovial sarcomas are more frequent in the abdominal wall.

4. Intra-Abdominal or Intra-Abdominopelvic RMS

These tumors can be large on presentation, filling the abdomen or pelvis. They may present as a distinct mass or maybe more diffuse and accompanied by ascites. The tumor may be confined to a particular part of the abdomen or pelvis, or it may have already spread to involve other structures. Intraperitoneal tumors occur, but more frequently they are retroperitoneal in location.

As in the assessment of RMSs in other sites, a CT scan is indispensable in defining the characteristics of the tumor and its extension, including evidence of lymphatic spread. CT detects not only the site and size of the tumor, but also delineates its relationship with other structures, such as the kidneys, uterus, and bladder. For intraperitoneal tumors, CT reveals the presence of ascites. Ultrasonography allows anatomical guidance in performing paracentesis to obtain ascitic fluid, and there is need to confirm the presence of dissemination of tumor cells.

The differential diagnosis includes other abdominal tumors, especially extrarenal tumors. Benign tumors are rare in this location. Neuroblastoma, the main other tumor to be considered, may show raised urinary catecholamines and, if it is nonsecretory, there may be

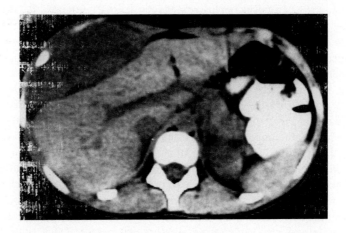

A

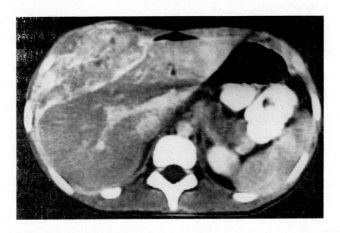

B

FIGURE 22.   A 14-year-old girl with a diaphragmatic RMS. (A) CT scan
without contrast shows heterogeneous hypodense mass notching the surface
of the right lobe of the liver; (B) CT scan with iodine contrast shows
heterogeneous hyperdense mass with a surrounding shell.

neuroblasts in the bone marrow or there may be positive findings on MIBG scintigraphy.
Malignant germ cell tumors are distinguished by their secretion of AFP, and presence of a
mature teratoma is suggested by its calcification. Other malignant mesenchymal tumors are
very rare in the region. A preferential site is paravesical, with the tumor pressing down on
the bladder without actually invading the bladder. The site of origin of the tumor is sometimes
difficult to determine at first examination. A second CT scan performed after the first course
of chemotherapy hopefully confirms that the tumor is smaller; and this follow-up scan may
define the anatomical paravesical origin of the tumor more clearly.

The diagnosis is made by a biopsy carried out by ''mini'' surgical laparotomy. In cases
of great urgency, such as when there is internal obstruction or severe hydronephrosis, a
needle biopsy suffices if a large enough piece of tissue is obtained. Peritoneal dissemination
of the tumor is not visualized by either CT scan or ultrasonography, which only establishes
the presence or absence of ascites. A tumor with peritoneal dissemination, with nodules on

the peritoneum, is classified as stage IV. In this case, a paracentesis should be done to confirm whether malignant cells are present in the ascites.

In principle, primary RMSs of the intestines do not occur, since in this organ a sarcomatous tumor would be a leiomyosarcoma or rarely an adenocarcinoma, or an extension of a contiguous RMS.

A particular site of interest for a RMS in this area are tumors of the biliary ducts, either intra- or extrahepatic in location, or even tumors originating in intrahepatic tissue. The clinical picture is that, or acute or subacute biliary obstruction with cholestasis, or presence of an intrahepatic mass if the tumor lies far from the porta hepatis. Often the symptoms alone suggest a diagnosis of acute cholecystitis.

An excellent examination for the liver is ultrasonography, perhaps complemented by a CT scan. However, it is still difficult to differentiate the tumor from normal intrahepatic or biliary tissue. A well-defined examination, including assessment for possible lymph node involvement, should also be carried out, since this information will strongly influence future management. Diagnosis is done by needle biopsy, or by open surgical biopsy, when the surgeon may be able to divert biliary flow and relieve the obstruction. In a localized tumor, full surgical excision with hepatectomy should be an option, particularly if histologic examination (frozen section) during surgery confirms the diagnosis of RMS, and total resection of the tumor is possible.

Intrahepatic RMS has a differential diagnosis which includes benign tumors, such as hamartomas and lymphangiomas, whose presence may be suspected by findings on radiological examination. An important criterion for identifying a malignant intrahepatic tumor is invasion of the biliary tree either proximally or distally. Such a tumor may be detected by ultrasound examination when the lesion is small; otherwise it may be visualized by CT scan and MRI. These scans do not identify particular histological types, but give information on spread, especially to the bile ducts and porta hepatis. CT and MRI also show the relationship of the tumor to hepatic vessels and to the inferior vena cava, in addition to revealing retrohepatic extension.

Other benign hepatic tumors displace the blood vessels. If it is an angioma, the characteristic features observed in CT scan and MRI are centripetal contrast enhancement appearing a minute after iodine injection on CT scan, plus a brilliant signal on MRI using a T2 setting. Adenomas are rare in children and have a specific arterial hypervascular phase. Malignant tumors include hepatoblastomas, which generally tend to secrete AFP. More rare in occurrence are tumors of the surrounding structures of the liver, such as a malignant germ cell tumor and an adrenocortical tumor. Possible presence of a neuroblastoma and Wilms' tumor is more easily excluded.

5. RMS of the Perineum

Perineal RMSs are situated deeply and give rise to compression of the rectum and difficulty in defecation. The tumor can appear as a swelling or nodule perianally, sometimes affecting the function of the anal sphincter. Its precise position and size are documented by a CT scan. If the tumor is small in size, then total surgical excision should be an option, but if the tumor involves the sphincter muscle, then biopsy alone should be done. Invasion of the perineum can come from a genitourinary, pelvic, or buttock primary.

K. SPECIAL CLINICAL PRESENTATIONS

Involvement of the bone marrow often gives misleading clinical symptoms which cause a delay in diagnosis. It occurs most often in older children who present with general symptoms, such as fever, arthralgia, nonspecific pain, and anemia. The first impression may be that of rheumatoid arthritis or acute leukemia. The primary tumor can be very small and pass unnoticed during a detailed examination. Diagnosis is reached on examination of the

TABLE 4
IRS Clinical Grouping Classification

Group	Description
I	Localized disease, completely resected
	Confined to organ or muscle of origin
	Infiltration outside organ or muscle of origin; regional nodes not involved
II	Comprised or regional resection of three types including
	Grossly resected tumors with microscopic residual, no evidence of regional node involvement
	Regional disease, completely resected, in which nodes may be involved, and/or extension of tumor into an adjacent organ present; no microscopic residual
	Regional disease with involved nodes, grossly resected, but with evidence of microscopic residual
III	Incomplete resection or biopsy with gross residual disease
IV	Distant metastases, present at onset

bone marrow, when the finding of abnormal nonhematopoietic cells prompts one to search for the primary tumor. In these cases, the most frequent type is alveolar RMS, but other types may also occur. Hypercalcemia following bone destruction may be present, and the condition resembles a paraneoplastic syndrome found in certain tumors in adults. Prompt treatment with chemotherapy is needed, in view of the rampant nature of this complication.[7] Disseminated intravascular coagulation (DIC) also occurs and recedes with treatment. Therefore, prompt diagnosis is needed.

IV. STAGING CLASSIFICATION

As for other tumors, a staging classification is necessary for RMS for two reasons. First, it is necessary to classify the tumor and its gravity in order to make the best choice from the different modalities of treatment. The second reason is to be able to compare the results of treatment in different countries. Two systems of staging have been used throughout the world.

First, a postsurgical staging system known as the IRS Grouping System (Table 4) was adopted with some modifications in many cancer centers throughout the world. Second, there is the presurgical staging system known as the TNM-UICC staging system (Table 5) which is used by SIOP and, with minor modifications, also by the cancer center at Stanford.[4]

Comparison between the two systems, presurgical (TNM) and postsurgical (IRS), is difficult because they are based on different criteria. Thus, the IRS grouping system is based on a treatment modality, namely, surgery. Accurate staging depends on information provided by the surgeon, as well as on certain currently prevailing concepts regarding treatment.

The TNM system offers the best description of the tumor and its degree of initial extension before any treatment is given. This staging system was adopted by both European and American members who participated in an international workshop, which was organized by SIOP in 1986 for reconciling some criteria concerning assessment of RMSs.[11]

The main reason for adopting this TNM presurgical staging system is that this staging method retains its value to compare patients, even if other prognostic factors are added to it afterward in order to define treatment groups. Therefore, other prognostic factors can change with time (such as the presence of favorable and unfavorable histology), or a new prognostic factor can appear (such as DNA ploidy), but the TNM description of the tumor never changes.

The TNM staging system could be the basis of comparison of the results of therapy between clinical studies carried out in several countries, or for studies carried out in the same country over a period of time.

In addition to the TNM pretreatment staging system there is a postsurgical pathologic

TABLE 5
SIOP UICC Soft Tissue Sarcoma Clinical Staging System: A TNM Classification for Malignant Tumors

Stage		Description
I	T1	Tumor confined to the organ or tissue of origin
	N0	No evidence of regional lymph node involvement
	M0	No evidence of distant metastasis
II	T2	Tumor involving one or more contiguous organs or tissues or with adjacent malignant effusion
	N0	
	M0	
III	Any T	
	N1	Evidence of regional lymph node involvement
	M0	
IV	Any T	
	Any N	
	M1	Evidence of distant metastasis

TABLE 6
Postsurgical TNM (pTNM) Histopathological Classification of Malignant Tumors

pT	Primary tumor
pT0	No evidence of tumor found on histological examination of specimen
pT1	Tumor limited to organ or tissue of origin; excision complete and margins histologically free
pT2	Tumor with invasion beyond the organ or tissue of origin; excision complete and margin histologically free
pT3	Tumor with or without invasion beyond the organ or tissue of origin; excision incomplete

> pT3a: evidence of microscopic residual tumor
> pT3b: evidence of macroscopic residual tumor
> pT3c: adjacent malignant effusion regardless of the size
> pT3x: the extent of invasion cannot be assessed

TNM classification (pTNM). This postsurgical TNM classification takes into account the quality of the resection after the primary surgery has been done and thus serves as a complement to the therapeutic guidelines (Table 6).

V. SUMMARY

RMSs can be located anywhere where mesenchymal tissue exists, that is to say, anywhere in the body. As a result, clinical symptoms are variable and often misleading.

This chapter discusses the principle symptoms caused by tumors in various locations, together with the differential diagnosis and the frequency of tumors in various sites.

The internationally recognized staging system now employed is based on the TNM system.

REFERENCES

1. **Bradford, R., Crockard, H. A., and Isaacson, P. G.,** Primary rhabdomyosarcoma of the central nervous system case report, *Cancer,* 54, 2132, 1984.
2. **Donaldson, S. S., Draper, G. S., Flamant, F., et al.,** Topography of childhood tumors. Pediatric coding system, *Pediatr. Hematol. Oncol.,* 3, 249, 1986.

3. **Flamant, F., Gerbaulet, A., Nihoul-Fekete, C., et al.,** Long-term sequelae of conservative treatment by surgery, brachytherapy and chemotherapy for vulvar and vaginal rhabdomyosarcoma in children, *J. Clin. Oncol.,* 8, 1867, 1990.

4. **Harmer, M. H.,** TNM classification of paediatric tumors, in *International Union Against Cancer,* Geneva, Switzerland, 1982.

5. **Hays, D. M., Shimada, H., Raney, R. B., et al.,** Sarcomas of the vagina and uterus: the Intergroup Rhabdomyosarcoma study, *J. Pediatr. Surg.,* 20, 721, 1985.

6. **Kato, M., Flamant, F., Terrier-Lacombe, M. J., et al.,** Rhabdomyosarcoma of the larynx in children; a series of 5 patients treated in the Institut Gustave-Roussy Villejuif, France, *Med. Pediatr. Oncol.,* 19, 2, 110, 1991.

7. **Leblanc, A., Caillaud, J. M., Hartmann, O., et al.,** Hypercalcemia preferentially occurs in unusual forms of childhood non-Hodgkin lymphomas, rhabdomyosarcomas, and Wilms' tumors; a study of 11 cases, *Cancer,* 54, 2132, 1984.

8. **Olive, D., Flamant, F., Zucker, J. M., et al.,** Para-aortic lymphadenectomy is not necessary in the treatment of localized paratesticular rhabdomyosarcoma, *Cancer,* 54, 1283, 1984.

9. **Olive-Sommelet, D.,** For the International Society of Pediatric Oncology: paratesticular rhabdomyosarcoma, in *Dialogues in Pediatric Urology,* Vol. 12 (No. 11), William J. Miller Associates, New York, 1989.

10. **Raney, A. B., Hays, D. M., Lawrence, W., et al.,** Paratesticular rhabdomyosarcoma in children, *Cancer,* 42, 729, 1978.

11. **Rodary, C., Flamant, F., Donaldson, S. S., et al.,** An attempt to use a common staging system in rhabdomyosarcoma; a report of an international workshop initiated by the International Society of Pediatric Oncology (SIOP), *Med. Pediatr. Oncol.,* 17, 210, 1989.

12. **Rodary, C., Flamant, F., Treuner, J., et al.,** Bladder salvage in 109 non-metastatic bladder and/or prostate rhabdomyosarcoma; a report of the International SIOP Workshop on RMS, *Med. Pediatr. Oncol.,* 18(Abstr.), 405, 1990.

Chapter 5

DIAGNOSTIC IMAGING OF RHABDOMYOSARCOMA

Lakshmana Das Narla and James W. Walsh

TABLE OF CONTENTS

I. INTRODUCTION

Rhabdomyosarcoma (RMS), the most common pediatric soft tissue sarcoma, is unique among childhood tumors because it can occur in virtually any primary site, except the brain and kidney. The most common sites of origin of RMS, in order of frequency, are as follows: head and neck, genitourinary tract, extremities, trunk, retroperitoneum, thorax, hepatobiliary tract, perineum, and anal region. RMSs extend locally and infiltrate along fascial planes into surrounding tissues. Metastases typically result from hematogenous spread to lungs, bone, bone marrow, liver, breast, and brain, although lymphatic spread to regional lymph nodes can also occur (Figure 1). Definitive diagnosis is established by histopathologic examination of the tumor.

The purposes of diagnostic imaging are both to define the extent of the disease for staging and treatment and to provide a baseline for measuring response to therapy. In the past, radiologic evaluation of RMSs had consisted of plain films, voiding cystourethography, excretory urography, barium enema, and lymphangiography. Now both computed tomography (CT) and magnetic resonance imaging (MRI) are making significant contributions to the current diagnostic workup of these tumors.[1,2]

II. DIAGNOSTIC IMAGING

Diagnostic workup begins with a plain film to demonstrate a soft tissue mass, with displacement of normal viscera, and obliteration and distortion of normal fat planes (Figure 2). Calcification is occasionally seen within the mass and is the result of hemorrhage into the tumor. Also, bone destruction due to adjacent tumor invasion can be delineated on conventional plain films.

III. RADIONUCLIDE EVALUATION

Bone scanning with Technetium 99^m-labeled phosphate is used for evaluation of skeletal metastases. Metastases from neural crest tumors usually show increased radionuclide activity. Occasionally, the tumor itself may take up the isotope and appear as a focal area of increased activity (Figure 3). Some of the factors that may be responsible for uptake of isotope by soft tissue tumors are tumor neovascularity with altered permeability, binding of phosphate compounds by mitochondria, and binding of the radiopharmaceutical to soluble proteins resulting from denatured macromolecules.

Great variations in sensitivity and specificity were observed when bone scans and plain films were used for detection of skeletal metastases.[3,4] Nevertheless, the metastatic workup of the child with RMS should include both a skeletal survey and a bone scan. Gallium scanning has the greatest sensitivity in assessment of RMSs of the extremities and the poorest in delineation of this tumor in the head and neck. Both the liver-spleen scan and the brain scan have been replaced by CT.

IV. CT AND MRI

Further diagnostic workup of children with RMS depends on the site of tumor origin. CT is preferred for evaluation of tumors of the middle ear, orbit, hepatobiliary system, and retroperitoneum. Magnetic resonance imaging is the procedure of choice for evaluation of nasopharyngeal, genitourinary, and extremity RMSs. CT is used when MRI is not available.

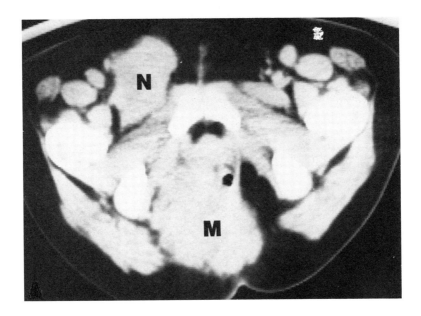

A

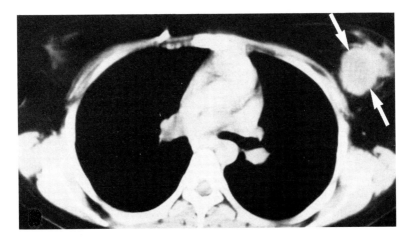

B

FIGURE 1. Pelvic RMS in a 15-year-old girl. (A) CT scan through the symphysis pubis shows a large mass (M) in the right ischiorectal fossa and right inguinal lymph node (N) metastases; (B) 2 years after pelvic irradiation, follow-up chest CT for lung metastases shows a mass in the left breast (arrows). Excisional biopsy confirmed the presence of a metastasis.

V. HEAD AND NECK

RMSs involving the head and neck are divided into three categories: (1) orbital; (2) parameningeal (middle ear, paranasal sinuses, and nasopharynx); and (3) all other head and neck sites.

A. ORBITS
Orbital RMSs arise either from extraocular muscles or from other pluripotential mesenchymal elements. The role of MRI in orbital tumors is still being evaluated. However,

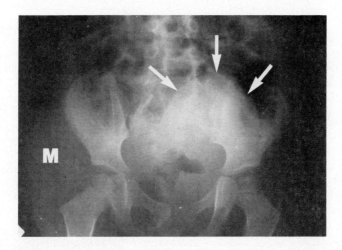

FIGURE 2.   Pelvic RMS. A 15-month-old girl with a palpable mass in the right gluteal region. Plain X-ray film shows a soft tissue mass (M) in the right gluteal muscles distorting normal fat planes. The mass extends into the central and left pelvis with superior displacement of bowel loops (arrows).

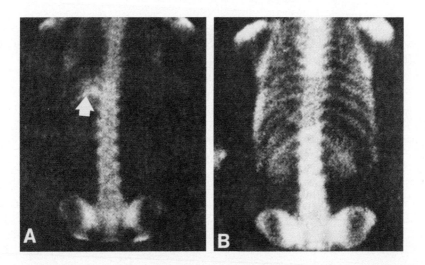

FIGURE 3.   Thoracic RMS. (A) Posterior bone scan image shows increased uptake of isotope in the left paravertebral mass (arrow); (B) repeat bone scan shows resolution of the mass 6 months after treatment.

CT, because of its excellent spatial resolution of bony orbital components and its axial as well as coronal scan planes, is the current imaging modality of choice. CT accurately defines the anatomic location of the orbital mass, reveals involvement of various intraorbital structures, and defines tumor extension into such periorbital regions as the sinuses, nasal cavity, and intracranial compartment. Coronal CT scans are useful for evaluation of lesions in the orbital roof or floor, and for showing their relationship to adjacent structures such as paranasal sinuses, anterior cranial fossae, and the nasal cavity.

On CT, most orbital RMSs appear as poorly defined, inhomogeneous soft tissue masses which distort soft tissue planes and destroy bone locally. Use of intravenous contrast enhances these tumors to the same degree as adjacent muscle.[5] Bone destruction associated with RMSs is easily seen on CT scans with the use of appropriate window and level settings. The differential diagnosis of orbital bone destruction associated with a soft tissue mass includes neuroblastoma, leukemia, and histiocytosis. Neuroblastoma is differentiated from orbital RMS by its relatively high CT attenuation values and the rarity of preseptal extension, which is more common with RMSs. A hemangioma may mimic an orbital RMS on CT, but it is differentiated both by its varying attenuation values and its significant enhancement after injection of intravenous contrast.

In difficult diagnostic cases, thin needle aspiration biopsies can be done under CT guidance without significant complications. CT is also valuable for following tumor regression after chemotherapy and radiation therapy, as well as for showing bone healing after radiation therapy. Follow-up CT scans at 3 months after therapy is the appropriate time to assess treatment response and to determine the patient's prognosis. CT and, to a greater extent, MRI are also useful to delineate leukoencephalopathy secondary to chemotherapy or irradiation.

B. PARAMENINGEAL

The worst prognostic indicator in head and neck RMSs is meningeal involvement, which has an incidence of 35%. Either CT or MRI can be used to confirm and define the extent of meningeal involvement.

RMSs of the orbit spread to the meninges by eroding the superior orbital fissure. Middle ear tumors may extend through the tegmen tympani to involve the middle cranial fossa meninges, or they may extend through the posterior mastoid to reach the posterior cranial fossa. Because of its superior resolution for bone detail and its ability to do thin sections in both axial and coronal planes, CT is also the preferred modality for evaluation of RMSs of the middle ear and temporal bone (Figure 4).

RMSs of the nasal cavity, paranasal sinus, and nasopharynx reach the meninges by extending through the basal foramina, by destroying the roofs of the paranasal sinuses and breaking through the orbital floor, and by eventual intracranial extension through the superior orbital fissue (Figure 5). Invasion of the base of the skull is seen in 35% of patients with nasopharyngeal RMSs. It usually involves the cavernous sinus and is associated with cranial nerve palsies (Figure 6). Lymph node involvement occurs in 50% of patients.

MRI, because of its superior resolution of soft tissue contrast, lack of ionizing radiation, absence of beam-hardening artifacts, and inherent multiplanar imaging capability, is the modality of choice for evaluating nasopharyngeal RMSs. On MRI, the signal intensity of tumor is intermediate between muscle and fat on T1-weighted images.[6] While small areas of bony destruction are difficult to perceive on MRI compared to findings on CT, visualization of tumor extension into the cranial vault is more easily appreciated on coronal MRI.

VI. GENITOURINARY SYSTEM

In girls, RMSs can arise from the bladder, cervix, vagina, and vulva. When it originates from the vagina, the tumor can protrude as a polypoid, grape-like mass, the so-called sarcoma botyroides (Figure 7). In boys, RMSs arise in the prostate gland and bladder (Figures 8 and 9). When the tumor arises posteriorly at the trigone or near the bladder neck, urinary retention may occur as a presenting symptom. If a mural tumor erodes into the mucosa, patients can also present with hematuria.

The traditional workup of genitourinary RMSs consisted of a voiding cystourethrogram, which showed multiple bladder-filling defects (Figure 9A). The causes of multiple filling defects in the bladder are listed in Table 1.[7] More recently, ultrasonography (US), because of its nonionizing radiation, easy availability, and multiple scan planes, is often the initial study to confirm the presence of genitourinary RMSs. On ultrasound examination, RMS of

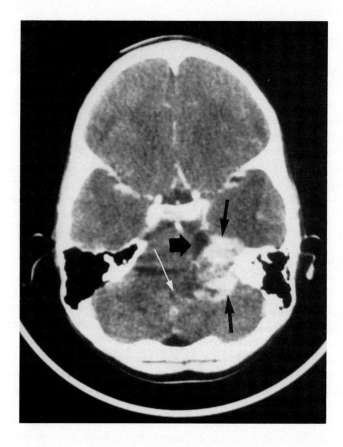

FIGURE 4.   RMS of the temporal bone. Contrast-enhanced axial CT image shows an irregularly enhancing mass (black arrows) destroying the petrous apex, with cystic component medially (black arrowhead) and associated deformity of the brain stem (white arrow). (Courtesy of Dr. Daniel Eggleston.)

the bladder appears as a polypoid solid echogenic mass with a heterogeneous echo texture (Figure 9B). Small sonolucent foci in the mass usually represent necrosis or hemorrhage within the tumor.

The tumor often extends to either pelvic sidewall and invades the posterior bladder wall, causing focal bladder wall thickening. CT or MRI is often used for further assessment of local extent of the tumors and for detection of regional lymph node metastases. CT directly depicts soft tissue masses in relation to surrounding pelvic organs. Also, decubitus or prone scans may be useful in separating normal pelvic structures from an adjacent mass or in determining tumor fixation and invasion of nearby organs.[8] In older girls, a vaginal tampon, by distending the vagina, may be helpful in delineating the tumor.

As in nasopharyngeal RMSs, MRI is gradually replacing CT as the imaging modality of choice for evaluation of RMSs in the pelvis (Figure 9C). Standard axial images are used to delineate the bladder floor, prostate gland, seminal vesicles, uterine corpus, cervix, and vagina. Sagittal images are important to detect bladder-rectal invasion and tumors of the bladder dome or base. Coronal images outline cephalocaudad tumor extent, the lateral bladder walls, and the relationships between the vagina and uterus or between the prostate and seminal vesicles.

Coronal images also confirm enlargement of the common iliac nodes and the external and internal iliac nodes, as well as revealing inguinal adenopathy typically detected on axial

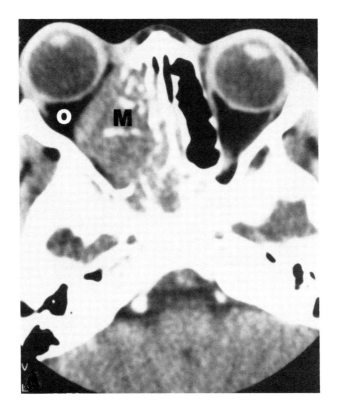

A

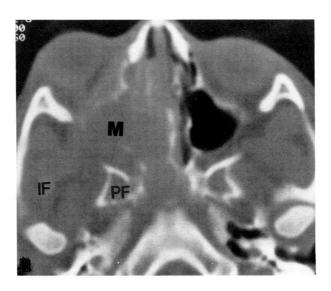

B

FIGURE 5. (A) RMS of the paranasal sinus. Axial CT shows a mass (M) in the right ethmoid and sphenoid sinuses with bony destruction and mass extension into the orbit (O); (B) axial CT with bone window settings shows extension of mass (M) into pterygopalatine fossa (PF) and infra-temporal fossa (IF) with associated bone destruction.

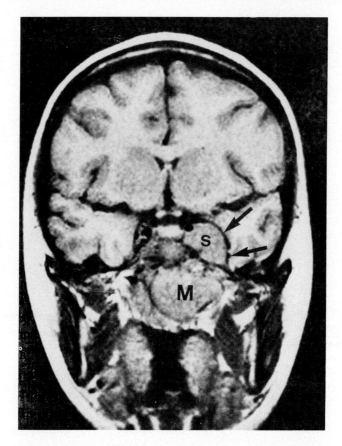

FIGURE 6.   Nasopharyngeal RMS in a 12-year-old child. Coronal T1-weighted MR image shows a nasopharyngeal mass (M) with tumor extension through the skull base into the left cavernous sinus (S). The dura forming the lateral boundary of cavernous sinus is displaced laterally (arrows). (Courtesy of Dr. Ira F. Braun.)

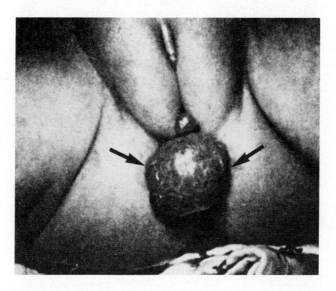

FIGURE 7.   RMS (arrows) arising from the vagina, having the typical appearance of a sarcoma botryoides.

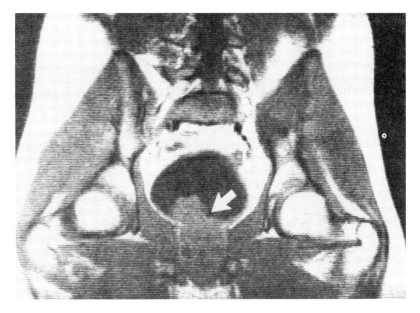

FIGURE 8. RMS of the prostate. T1-weighted coronal MRI shows a mass arising from prostate gland with direct extension into the bladder (arrow). (Courtesy of Dr. J. P. Kuhn.)

images. T1-weighted sequences are used to achieve high spatial resolution and to detect local tumor invasion of the peripelvic fat and pelvic adenopathy. T2-weighted sequences are useful for demonstrating the total extent of the neoplasm and to detect invasion of surrounding organs, such as the bladder wall, seminal vesicles, prostate gland, uterus, or vagina.

VII. PATHWAYS OF RHABDOMYOSARCOMA SPREAD IN THE PELVIS

The fascial investments of the illiopsoas, obturator internus, and pyriformis muscles, and the natural openings of the pelvis, such as the sciatic notch and obturator foramen, provide pathways for tumor spread in the pelvis.[9] The sciatic notch serves as a pathway between the true pelvis and the gluteal region or posterior thigh, whereas the obturator foramen serves as a natural opening between the inguinal region and the perineum (Figure 10).

A. LYMPH NODES

Although sarcomas characteristically spread by hematogenous dissemination, they can also metastasize to regional lymph nodes (Table 2). The incidence of lymph node involvement in RMS varies according to the site of the primary tumors: for paratesticular tumors 50%; for tumors of the extremity 20%; for tumors of the trunk 17%; for genitourinary tumors 10%; and for head and neck tumors 3%. Orbital RMSs do not metastasize to lymph nodes. On CT, enlargement of the lymph nodes is the major criterion for diagnosing metastatic involvement, and retroperitoneal and pelvic nodes 1.5 cm or greater in diameter are considered to be abnormal (Figures 1A and 10B). In the neck, lymph nodes greater than 1.0 cm are considered to be abnormal. However, minimal lymph node enlargement is not always due to tumor; this enlargement may be seen in chronic lymphadenitis or in reactive hyperplasia. In equivocal cases, examination of CT-guided aspiration cytology can be used to document presence of lymph node metastases.

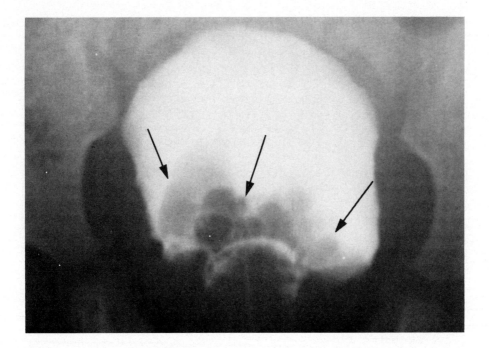

A

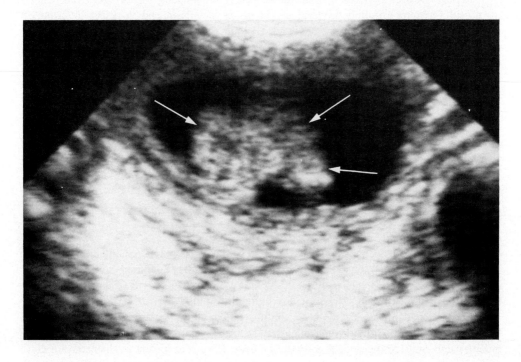

B

FIGURE 9.   RMS of the bladder in 2-year-old boy who presented with hematuria after a fall. (A) Voiding cystourethrogram shows multiple filling defects (arrows) in the bladder which proved to be RMS on cytoscopic biopsy; (B) transverse ultrasonogram shows a polypoid echogenic mass (arrows) in the bladder; (C) T2-weighted coronal MRI shows high-intensity tumor (T) confined to the bladder with intact bladder wall muscle (arrows).

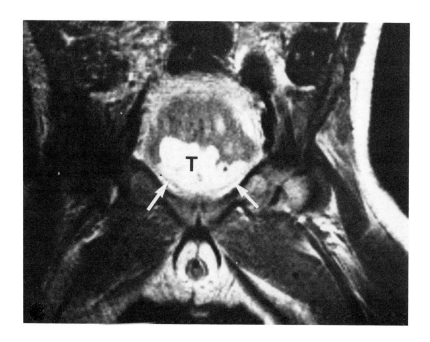

FIGURE 9C (continued)

TABLE 1
Differential Diagnosis of
Bladder-Filling Defects

Congenital anomalies
    Bilateral ectopic ureteroceles
    Multiple hemangiomas
Inflammatory lesions
    Cystitis glandularis
    Cystitis cystica
    Cytoxan-induced cystitis
Benign tumors
    Neurofibroma
    Fibroma
Malignant tumors
    RMS of the bladder and prostate
    Leukemia
    Neuroblastoma
Miscellaneous conditions
    Lucent foreign bodies
    Radiolucent stones
    Blood clots

Since CT cannot detect tumor in normal size nodes, some centers have used lymphangiography to demonstrate the internal architecture of lymph nodes and to delineate the defects associated with metastatic disease. Abnormal lymphangiographic findings include: peripheral filling defects or node replacement; foamy lace-like nodes; interruption of opacified lymphoic channels with formation of collateral vessels; displacement of lymphatic channels; and stasis and persistent opacification of channels. However, in the pelvis, internal iliac and obturator lymph nodes are not usually opacified at lymphangiography, and this is the major disadvantage.[10] Hence, lymphangiography is not commonly used in the workup of pelvic RMSs.

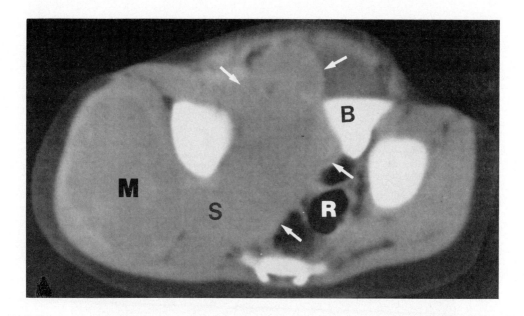

A

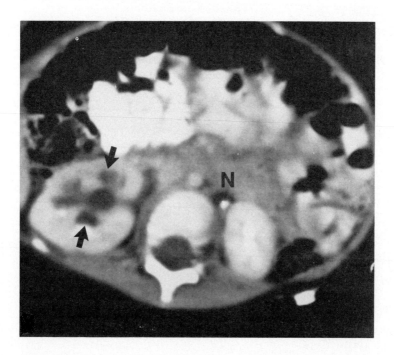

B

FIGURE 10.   Pelvic RMS in a 15-month-old girl. (A) CT scan through the true pelvis shows a large soft tissue mass (M) in the right gluteal region extending through the sciatic notch (S) into the pelvis (arrows). Bladder (B) and rectum (R) are markedly displaced to the left. (B) CT scan at the level of the kidneys shows hydronephrosis of the right kidney (arrows) due to the pelvic mass, together with an enlarged left para-aortic node (N).

TABLE 2
Sarcomas that Frequently Metastasize to Lymph Nodes

RMS
Synovial sarcoma
Clear cell sarcoma
Epithelioid sarcoma
Hemangiopericytoma
Malignant fibrous histiocytoma

VIII. SUMMARY

In summary, cross-sectional imaging techniques such as US, CT, and MRI have replaced conventional excretory urography, barium enema, and voiding cystourethography in the diagnostic workup of RMS. The bone scan and skeletal survey maintain their roles in the evaluation of bone metastases. The new imaging modalities are better able to define the extent, as well as local and regional spread of these tumors. MRI, because of its multiplanar imaging capability, soft tissue contrast resolution, and lack of ionizing radiation, has become the primary imaging modality of choice for most types of RMSs.

ACKNOWLEDGMENT

The authors gratefully acknowledge the help of Ms. Louise Logan for secretarial services.

REFERENCES

1. **Baker, M. E., Silverman, P. M., and Korobkin, M.,** Computed tomography of prostatic and bladder rhabdomyosarcoma, *J. Comput. Assist. Tomogr.,* 94, 780, 1985.
2. **Dietrich, R. B. and Kangarloo, H.,** Pelvic abnormalities in children; assessment with MR imaging, *Radiology,* 163, 367, 1987.
3. **Weinblatt, M. E. and Miller, J. H.,** Radionuclide scanning in children with rhabdomyosarcoma, *Med. Pediatr. Oncol.,* 9, 293, 1981.
4. **Quddus, F. E., Espinola, D., and Kramer, S. S.,** Comparison between X-ray and bone scan detection of bone metastases in patients with rhabdomyosarcoma, *Med. Pediatr. Oncol.,* 11, 125, 1983.
5. **Latack, J. T., Hutchinson, R. J., and Heyn, R. M.,** Imaging of rhabdomyosarcoma of the head and neck, *A.J.N.R.,* 8, 353, 1987.
6. **Braun, I. F.,** MRI of the nasopharynx, *Radiol. Clin. N. Am.,* 27, 315, 1989.
7. **Grunebaum, M. and Varsano, I.,** Multiple bladder filling defects in children with cystitis, *Pediatr. Radiol.,* 4, 93, 1975.
8. **Siegel, M. J., Glasier, C. M., and Sagel, S. S.,** CT of pelvic disorders in children, *Am. J. Roentgenol.,* 137, 1139, 1989.
9. **Ammann, A. M. and Walsh, J. W.,** Normal anatomy and technique of pelvic examination, in *Computed Tomography of the Pelvis,* Walsh, J., Ed., Churchill Livingstone, New York, 1985, 1.
10. **Bergiron, C., Markovitis, P., and Benjaafar, M.,** Lymphography in childhood rhabdomyosarcoma, *Radiology,* 133, 627, 1979.

Chapter 6

PROGNOSTIC FACTORS IN RHABDOMYOSARCOMA

Lisa A. Garnsey and Edmund A. Gehan

TABLE OF CONTENTS

I. INTRODUCTION

Knowledge of the prognostic factors of rhabdomyosarcoma (RMS) patients is important for the planning and analysis of clinical studies.[1] In the planning of clinical trials, knowing the patient characteristics related to prognosis is useful in selecting therapy for specific subgroups of patients. This information also provides a rational basis for stratifying patients as to prognosis. In analyzing clinical studies, there are three reasons why prognostic factors might be utilized: (1) they provide a basis for comparing treatments in subgroups of patients that have a similar prognosis; (2) heterogeneity among patients can be explained by prognostic characteristics, so that an analysis adjusting for these characteristics can reduce the residual random variation and make comparisons between treatments more precise; and (3) interactions between treatments and prognostic variables may be detected, so that subgroups of patients may be found in which various therapies differ in efficacy.

RMS is a common solid tumor of childhood, accounting for 4 to 8% of malignant diseases in children under the age of 15 years.[2] Since the advent in 1972 of the multimodality clinical trials of the Intergroup Rhabdomyosarcoma Committee, there have been dramatic improvements in survival for patients with this tumor. In a study (Intergroup Rhabdomyosarcoma Study-II, IRS-II) completed in 1984, the percentage of patients surviving 5 years was 70% for those with nonmetastatic disease and 27% for those who had metastases.[3]

An early study identified extent of disease, localized vs. metastatic, and primary site as being prognostic features of major importance.[4] These findings were confirmed in subsequent studies.[5-12] The prognostic importance of local invasiveness of the primary neoplasm and tumor size was also established.[5]

In this chapter, a comprehensive review of the prognostic factors derived and assessed in the various RMS studies will be given. Second, a detailed univariate and multivariate analysis of patient characteristics will be carried out for the two completed studies (IRS-I and -II) of the Intergroup Rhabdomyosarcoma Committee.[3,13] The overall objective is to summarize the current state of knowledge concerning prognostic factors of RMS patients. This review should provide a rational basis for more efficient planning, analysis, and interpretation of clinical studies in childhood RMS.

II. REVIEW OF LITERATURE

Table 1 summarizes the patient characteristics related to survival in various large series or clinical trials of patients who were diagnosed with RMS when less than 21 years of age. The characteristics are organized into three groups according to the strength of their relationship to prognosis. These groups are (1) characteristics strongly related to survival ($p < 0.01$ or implied), (2) characteristics related to survival ($p < 0.10$ or significance stated but not specified), and (3) characteristics not related to prognosis. The attributes examined in assessing prognostic factors and the statistical methods used differed among the studies. However, an overall perspective of patient characteristics was accomplished that was the basis for the analysis of prognostic factors in IRS-I and -II.

A. PATIENT CHARACTERISTICS STRONGLY RELATED TO SURVIVAL

Characteristics included here are extent of disease, primary site, tumor invasiveness, and tumor size.

A comparison of patients by disease extent is not possible because different staging systems were used for the various reported studies. Nonetheless, it is clear that classification of disease extent, regardless of the staging system, was the most consistent factor related to survival. Whether defined as "extent of disease", "stage", or "clinical group", prognosis was generally most favorable in patients with localized disease. Prognosis was least favorable in patients who had metastases at the time of diagnosis. Patients with regional involvement had an intermediate prognosis.

The location of the primary tumor was strongly associated with prognosis in nearly all studies. The relationship between site and survival is summarized in Table 2. Tumors of the orbit were most consistently associated with a favorable prognosis, followed by tumors arising in genitourinary sites. Patients with tumors in head and neck sites generally had an intermediate prognosis. With the exception of one study,[6] patients with tumors of the trunk or extremities consistently had poor survival outcomes.

Tumor invasiveness (TNM stage T1 or T2) was examined and reported separately in only one study which involved an early subset of IRS-II patients.[5] In this subset, the survival experience of children with tumors confined to the organ or tissue of origin was much more favorable than it was in patients in which contiguous organs or structures were involved ($p = 0.004$). Local invasiveness of the tumor is considered in the UICC staging system which was used by other studies examined.[7-9] The survival experience of stage I patients (i.e., those with noninvasive tumors) reported in these studies was also significantly better than that for patients with more invasive tumors.

In two successive studies (IRS-I and -II), patients with larger tumors had an increased risk of death.[10] This finding supported the importance of tumor size demonstrated in the analysis of an early subset of IRS-I patients.[5]

B. PATIENT CHARACTERISTICS RELATED TO SURVIVAL

These characteristics include histology, sex, and lymphocyte count.

The histologic type of the tumor was shown to be related to survival in many studies. This finding was confirmed and expanded upon in a study of pathologic subtype in 1626 patients from studies of the IRS. It was shown that patients with botryoid RMSs had the most favorable prognosis, those with the embryonal type or extraosseous Ewing's sarcoma had an intermediate prognosis, and patients with the alveolar subtype had the worst prognosis.[14]

An association between poorer survival and female sex was noted by certain studies,[8-10] although others who examined this characteristic[6,11] found no relationship between gender and outcome.

For patients enrolled on the first IRS study,[10] lymphocyte count over 2000/mm^3 was associated with a more favorable outcome.

C. PATIENT CHARACTERISTICS GENERALLY NOT RELATED TO SURVIVAL

These characteristics include age, lymph node involvement, and race.

The age of the patient was related to survival in two of the ten studies reviewed. In a relatively small study (less than 100 patients), it was observed that children under 7 years of age had better survival experience than those older than 7 years. Others[10] reported that older children had poorer survival than younger children in certain subgroups (clinical groups I, II, and IV) of IRS-II. Hence, among children, a consistent relationship of age to survival has not been found.

Involvement of the lymph nodes is an important characteristic in staging patients according to the UICC system, and stage has a strong relationship to survival in the studies utilizing UICC staging.[7-9] However, in other studies[5,8,12] that examined the direct relationship of lymph node involvement to survival, there was no evident association between this characteristic and outcome. In one study,[5] only 7% of the patients (28 out of 402) had clinically positive regional lymph nodes. Thus, it is possible that a relationship would have been found if more patients had been examined for histologic evidence of lymph node involvement. Future studies should permit a more precise characterization of the prognostic importance of this feature.

TABLE 1
Relationship of Patient Characteristics to Prognosis Based on a Review of the Literature

No. of patients	Time period	Patient characteristics and their relationship to survival			Ref.
		Strongly related	Related	Not related	
78	1946—1966	Extent of disease	Primary site Histology Age		4
61	1947—1969	Extent of disease	Primary site Histology	Age	11
385	1971		Extent of disease Primary site	Histology Age Sex Race	6
345	1955—1981	Stage[a] Primary site[b]		Histology Sex Age	7
73	1974—1981	Stage[a] Histology	Primary site[b] Sex	Age	9
281	1975—1983	Clinical stage[a] Primary site	Sex	Pathology Age Lymph node involvement Cytology	8 (multivariate results)
686	1972—1978	Size (group I) Primary site (group III) Clinical group	Size (groups II and IV) Primary site (group IV) Histology (groups I and II) Sex (group II) Lymphocyte count (group II) Clinical subgroup (group II)	Age	10 (IRS-I) (multivariate results)
554	1972—1978	Primary site (groups III and IV) Lymphocyte count (group I) Clinical group	Primary site (group I) Lymphocyte count (group II) Clinical subgroup (group II) Sex (groups II and IV)	Age Lymph node involvement	12
1002	1978—1984	Histology (group I) Age (group IV) Primary site (groups III and IV)	Histology (group III) Age (groups I and II)	Sex Lymphocyte count Clinical subgroup	10 (IRS-I) (multivariate results)

505	1978–1982	Size (group III) Clinical group Clinical group Primary site Tumor invasiveness	Size	Histology Lymph node involvement	5 (Strat. Log rank tests except for primary site)

a   UICC-TNM staging classification;[7-9] St. Jude staging system;[9] Barts/Marsden staging system.[9]
b   Not independent of stage.

TABLE 2

Ordering of Primary Sites[a] by Their Relationship to Prognosis Based on the Literature Review

Authors

Ordering of sites	Sutow[4]	Jaffe[11]	Neifeld[6]	Kingston[9]	Rodary[8]	Crist[10] IRS-I	Crist[10] IRS-II
Favorable	Orbit	Orbit	Extremities	Orbit	Vagina/paratestis	Orbit	Orbit
	GU/vagina	Body wall	HN/GU	Paratestis	Orbit	GU	HN (non-PM)
	Extremities	HN/GU	Trunk	Vagina	HN (non-PM)	HN (non-PM)	GU
	Head	Extremities		HN	Bladder/prostate	Extremities	HN (PM)
				Limb/trunk	Body walls	HN (PM)	Extremities
				Pelvic/perineal	Limbs	Other	Other
					Pelvis		
Unfavorable					HN (PM)		

Note: The article by Flamant and Hill[7] stated that site (not adjusting for stage) was significant (*p* <0.001), but did not specifically state which sites were favorable and which were unfavorable.

a   GU = genitourinary, PM = parameningeal, HN = head and neck.

TABLE 3
Clinical Grouping Classification

Extent of disease	Clinical group	Classification
	I	Localized disease, completely resected (regional nodes not involved)
		Confined to organ or muscle of origin
		Infiltration outside the muscle or organ of origin
	II	Compromised or regional resection
		Grossly resected tumors with "microscopic" residual, no evidence of regional node involvement
Nonmetastatic		Regional disease with involved nodes, grossly resected but with evidence of "microscopic" residual
		Regional disease, completely resected with no "microscopic" residual tumor (regional nodes involved and/or extension of tumor into an adjacent organ)
	III	Incomplete resection or biopsy with gross residual disease
Metastatic	IV	Distant metastatic disease present at onset

In the only study reporting on the relationship of race to outcome, no association between this characteristic and survival was noted.[6]

III. PATIENTS AND METHODS

Patient characteristics have been investigated for their relationship to prognosis in children entered into one of two successive IRSs, IRS-I (1972—1978) and IRS-II (1978—1984). Eligibility criteria for the two studies were identical. These criteria required that each patient have a confirmed diagnosis of RMS, extraosseous Ewing's sarcoma, or undifferentiated sarcoma. The patients had to be younger than 21 years of age, and had to have received no prior chemotherapy or radiation therapy. In IRS-I, 833 patients were registered of whom 686 (82%) were eligible for analysis; and in IRS-II 1002 out of 1115 patients (90%) were eligible.

For both studies, patients were assigned to clinical groups based on extent of disease and type of surgery performed (Table 3). Treatment regimens were then randomly assigned to each patient according to the clinical grouping. The schema and treatment schedules for the two studies are shown in Figures 1 and 2.

Survival time was measured from the start of treatment to death or from start of treatment to last date of contact for surviving patients. For patients in clinical groups III or IV, disease-free status was defined as the complete disappearance of all clinical evidence of tumor for a minimum of 4 weeks based upon clinical examinations and imaging studies. Patients in clinical groups I or II were classified as disease-free at the start of treatment based on their surgical results. For those patients who achieved complete remission (CR), disease-free survival (DFS) time was calculated as the length of time from the start of treatment to the recurrence of local disease, the appearance of metastases, or the occurrence of death. Otherwise, DFS was set equal to zero since the patient never achieved disease-free status. Hence, the curves for DFS begin at the CR rate at time zero and characterize the proportion of patients alive and disease-free at various time points after the start of treatment. However, it should be noted that since clinical group III and IV patients do not achieve complete remission at time zero, interpretation of the DFS curve is meaningful only after that point in time when all patients have been on study long enough to achieve CR, a maximum of about 2 years.

Curves for survival and DFS were calculated using the method of Kaplan and Meier,[15] and tests of the statistical significance of the differences between curves were accomplished

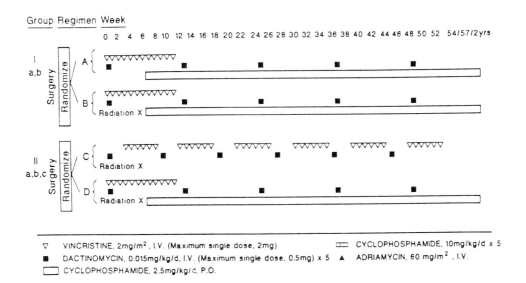

FIGURE 1.   Schema of treatment schedule, drugs and doses, and length of therapy by clinical groups for IRS-I (1972 to 1978).

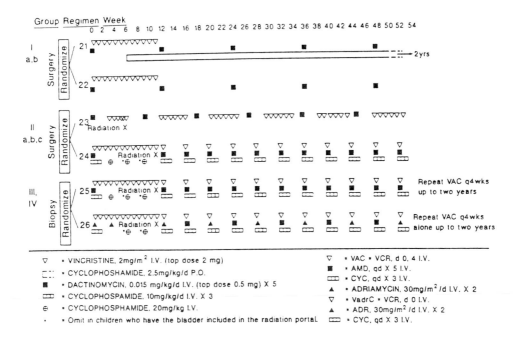

FIGURE 2.   Schema of treatment schedule, drugs and doses, and length of therapy by clinical groups for IRS-II (1978 to 1984).

using log-rank[16] and generalized Wilcoxon tests.[17] Chi-square tests[18] and Mantel-Haenszel chi-square statistics for linear trend[19] were used to compare the frequency distributions of characteristics between groups of patients.

The relationship between various patient attributes and outcome was initially investigated separately within each study in a univariate analysis according to extent of disease, classified as either nonmetastatic or metastatic. Those characteristics consistently associated with prognosis were then entered into a stepwise multivariate regression model developed by

Cox.[20] The purpose of this calculation was to determine the combination of variables that when taken together, best fit the combined data of IRS-I and IRS-II. Since the multivariate model was fit in a stepwise fashion, the order in which the patient characteristics entered the equation generally indicates the relative importance of each characteristic in predicting outcome, while adjusting for those variables already entered. However, "statistically significant prognostic variables do not necessarily add much to the predictive power of the model".[21] Hence, the proportion of variation explained (PVE) by the set of covariates was computed for each successive model using the "V_1" method proposed by Schemper.[22] Those variables entered in the successive stepwise multivariate regression model which improved the PVE by more than 20% were kept in the final model.

The general form of Cox's proportional hazards regression model can be written as follows:

$$\ln \frac{\lambda_i(t)}{\lambda_0(t)} = b_1 (x_1 - \bar{x}_1) + \ldots + b_k (x_k - \bar{x}_k)$$

In this equation, the b's are regression coefficients estimated in the model. The x_i's are the values of the relevant patient characteristics, with $\bar{x}_i$'s denoting average values of these variables. The quantity $\lambda_i(t)/\lambda_0(t)$ may be termed a "relative risk" or the ratio of chance of death or relapse per unit of time for a patient with a specific set of characteristic(s), relative to a patient having average values of the characteristics. A high value of this quantity indicates that the prognosis is poor. Hence, values of patient characteristics that tend to increase the relative risk are associated with decreased duration of survival or DFS. An indication of the magnitude of the importance of each characteristic can be obtained by determining the ratio of the relative risk when the characteristic is at its least favorable value to that when the characteristic is at its most favorable level. The higher this ratio is above 1.0, the greater the differences in prognoses for patients having unfavorable vs. favorable values of this attribute.

All computations were performed using Statistical Analysis System (SAS) software on a mainframe IBM 4281 computer, and two-sided statistical tests have been used throughout. There are articles containing good discussions of additional technical details concerning the identification of prognostic factors and the use of regression models in clinical oncology.[1,23] Others discuss the PVE in survival data models.[21,22]

IV. RESULTS

This analysis of prognostic factors differs from others[5,10,12] of the Intergroup Rhabdomyosarcoma Committee. The difference is that results are presented for patients grouped according to the general extent of disease (metastatic or nonmetastatic) at the time of start of treatment rather than by clinical group. Nonmetastatic patients are those in clinical groups I to III, while metastatic patients are in clinical group IV (Table 3). Prognosis is considered first by study (IRS-I and II) and disease extent; then prognosis is considered according to individual patient characteristics within each study and disease-extent grouping. Finally, a multivariate analysis was performed by combining the studies (IRS-I and -II), with a separate analysis of a subgroup of IRS-II patients from an earlier study.[5]

A. RELATIONSHIP OF STUDY AND EXTENT OF DISEASE TO PROGNOSIS

The survival (Figure 3) and DFS (Figure 4) experience for patients treated in IRS-II was consistently better than that observed for IRS-I. However, the improvement in outcome was statistically significant only for the survival comparison of the nonmetastatic patients ($p = 0.03$).

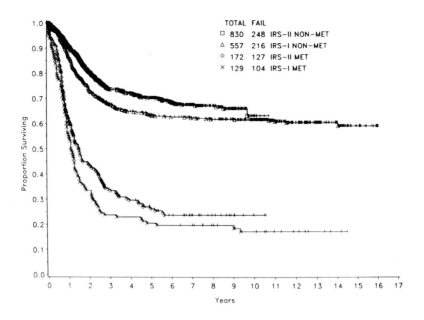

FIGURE 3. Kaplan-Meier estimates of survival by study and disease extent.

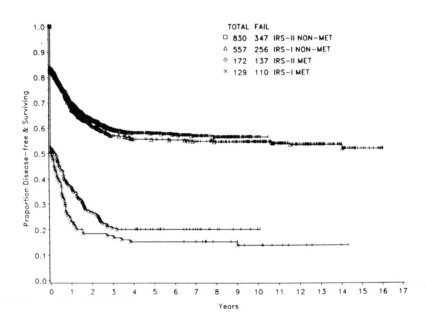

FIGURE 4. Kaplan-Meier estimates of DFS by study and disease extent.

1. Nonmetastatic Patients

For nonmetastatic patients, the CR rates were 84% (468 out of 557) in IRS-I and 83% (685 out of 830) in IRS-II. The percentages of patients that were disease-free and DFS at 5 years were 55% for IRS-I and 58% for IRS-II (Figure 4). The percentages of patients surviving 5 years or more were 63% for IRS-I and 70% for IRS-II (Figure 3), the latter representing a significant improvement ($p = 0.03$).

2. Metastatic Patients

The prognosis for metastatic patients was much poorer than that for nonmetastatic

TABLE 4

Variable Codes Used for the Univariate and Multivariate Regression Analyses

	Code for analysis	
Characteristic	**Univariate**	**Multivariate**
Extent of disease	1 = clinical group I	1 = clinical group I
	2 = clinical group II	2 = clinical group II
	3 = clinical group III	3 = clinical group III
Primary site[a]	For each of the following categories,	0 = more favorable sites
	0 = no and 1 = yes	(orbit, HN [non-PM], GU [non-BP])
	Orbit and eye	1 = less-favorable sites (GU [BP],
	HN (non-PM)	extremity, HN [PM], other)
	Gu (non-BP)	
	GU (BP)	
	Extremity	
	HN (PM)	
	Other	
Tumor size, cm	For each of the following categories,	0 = ≤5
	0 = no and 1 = yes	1 = >5
	<3	
	3—5	
	>5	
Histology[b]	For each of the following categories,	0 = botryoid/embryonal
	0 = no and 1 = yes	1 = alveolar, embryonal, or other
	Alveolar	
	Botryoid/embryonal	
	Embryonal	
	Other	
Age, years[b]	0 = <1	For each of the following categories,
	1 = 1—<5	0 = no and 1 = yes
	2 = 5—<10	<1
	3 = 10—<15	1—10 (reference group)
	4 = ≥15	≥10
Sex	1 = male, 2 = female	Not entered
Lymphocyte Count	1 = <2000/mm³, 2 = ≥2000/mm³	Not entered
Race		Not entered
Caucasian	0 = no, 1 = yes	
Negro	0 = no, 1 = yes	
Other	0 = no, 1 = yes	
Nodal involvement[c]		0 = no, 1 = yes
Tumor invasiveness[c]		1 = T1, 2 = T2

[a] HN = head and neck, GU = genitourinary, BP = bladder/prostate, PM = parameningeal.

[b] Due to low frequencies, the following groups were combined: metastatic patients — botryoid/embryonal and embryonal groups; IRS-I metastatic patients: age <1 year and age 1—10 years.

[c] IRS-II[5] subgroup analysis.

patients. The CR rates were 50% (65 out of 129) in IRS-I and 52% (90 out of 172) in IRS-II. The percentages of DFS patients at 5 years were 15% for IRS-I and 20% for IRS-II (Figure 4), with the percentages of patients surviving 5 years or more being 21% in IRS-I and 26% in IRS-II (Figure 3).

B. RELATIONSHIP OF INDIVIDUAL PATIENT CHARACTERISTICS TO PROGNOSIS

Table 4 gives a list of the patient characteristics investigated in the univariate analysis. Table 5 indicates which of the patient characteristics were significantly related to prognosis in IRS-I and IRS-II, respectively.

TABLE 5
Results of the Univariate Analysis

	IRS-I Survival (favorable subgroups)	IRS-I DFS (favorable subgroups)	IRS-II Survival (favorable subgroups)	IRS-II DFS (favorable subgroups)
Nonmetastatic Patients				
Very strongly related (p <0.001)	Clinical group (I) Primary site (orbit, GU/non-BP) Tumor size (3—5 cm)	Clinical group (I) Primary site (orbit, GU/non-BP) Tumor size (3—5 cm)	Clinical group (I) Primary site (orbit, HN, GU/non-BP) Tumor size (<5 cm) Age (1—10 years) Histology (botryoid/embryonal)	Clinical group (I) Primary site (orb, HN, GU/non-BP) Tumor size (<5 cm) Age (1—10 years)
Strongly related (p <0.01)	Histology (botryoid/embryonal)	Histology (botryoid/embryonal)	Race (Caucasian or other)	Histology (botryoid/embryonal or embryonal) Race (Caucasian)
Related (p <0.05)	Age (>1 year)		Sex Lymphocyte count	Sex Lymphocyte count
Not related (p >0.05)	Race Sex Lymphocyte count	Age Race Sex Lymphocyte count		
Metastatic Patients				
Strongly related (p <0.01)	Primary site (orbit, GU/non-BP)		Primary site (HN, GU/non-BP, GU/BP, Age (<10 years)	Primary site (HN, GU/non-BP, GU/BP)
Related (p <0.05)	Tumor size (>5 cm)			
Not related (p >0.05)	Histology Age Race Sex Lymphocyte count	Primary site Tumor size Histology Age Race Sex Lymphocyte count	Tumor size Histology Race Sex Lymphocyte count	Tumor size Histology Age Race Sex Lymphocyte count

1. Nonmetastatic Patients

For nonmetastatic patients, clinical group, primary site, and tumor size were all very strongly related ($p < 0.001$) to survival as well as to DFS in both IRS-I and IRS-II. The percentage of surviving and DFS patients at 5 years decreased with increasing clinical group number. Thus, patients in clinical group I had the most favorable outcome while those in clinical group III experienced the least favorable prognosis. The most favorable patients by primary site were those with tumors arising in the orbit, head and neck (nonparameningeal), and genitourinary organs (nonbladder/prostate). Patients with tumors less than 5 cm in diameter had a better prognosis than those with tumors that were 5 cm in diameter or larger.

2. Metastatic Patients

For metastatic patients in IRS-I and IRS-II (Table 5), primary site of the tumor was the only patient characteristic significantly related to survival in both studies. While the numbers of patients with tumors in some primary sites were small, genitourinary patients generally had favorable survival, while patients with disease in the extremities exhibited the worst survival.

C. RELATIONSHIP OF MULTIPLE PATIENT CHARACTERISTICS TO PROGNOSIS

The data from IRS-I and IRS-II were combined for the purpose of investigating the relationship of multiple patient characteristics to outcome (both for survival and DFS). Only those patient characteristics demonstrating a consistent relationship to outcome in both studies were included in the multivariate analyses. For nonmetastatic patients, the variables considered included clinical group, primary site, histology, age, and tumor size. For metastatic patients, the same variables were considered for entry into the multivariate regression models. Interaction terms involving two patient characteristics were also considered for the multivariate models after selecting the important individual variables.

1. Nonmetastatic Patients

There were known values of all the patient characteristics (Table 4) for 1225 of the 1387 nonmetastatic IRS-I and II patients. Within this subgroup, the frequency distributions of patient characteristics, as well as the pattern of events (relapses and deaths) were similar to those for the patients that had some unknown patient characteristics. For the survival model, there was a total of 409 deaths (33%), and for the DFS model, there were 516 failures in the form of relapses, metastases, or deaths (42%).

Table 6 gives the listing of order of entry of patient characteristics in the Cox regression models for survival and DFS. For both survival and DFS, primary site and clinical group were the first two variables to be selected, which indicated the major importance of these two characteristics. The other statistically significant variables entered in the survival model, in order of prognostic significance, were: tumor size, age under 1 year, tumor histology, study number (IRS-I or IRS-II), age 10 years or older, and interaction of site and age under 1 year. Only tumor size substantially increased the predictive ability of the model and was included in the final model along with primary site and clinical group. In the DFS model, age 10 years or older, age less than 1 year, tumor histology, study number, and tumor size were significant in the Cox regression model. However, none of these patient characteristics resulted in an important increase in the PVE.

The Cox multivariate regression model for survival in nonmetastatic patients is as follows:

$$\ln \frac{\lambda_i(t)}{\lambda_0(t)} = 1.1440 \text{ (primary site} - 0.6751) + 0.5108 \text{ (clinical group}$$

$$- 2.3739) + 0.4379 \text{ (tumor size} - 0.3429)$$

TABLE 6
Results of the Cox Multivariate Regression Models in IRS-I and IRS-II Combined

Prognosis	Characteristic	Regression coefficient	p	Relative risks[a] Unfavorable	Favorable	Ratio
		Nonmetastatic patients				
Survival	Site	1.1440	<0.001	1.60	0.38	4.22
	Clinical group	0.5108	<0.001	1.38	0.50	2.78
	Tumor size	0.4379	0.001	1.33	0.86	1.55
DFS	Clinical group	0.5340	<0.001	1.40	0.48	2.91
	Site	0.6579	<0.001	1.28	0.64	1.93
	Age ≥10	0.3039	0.002	1.24	0.91	1.36
		Metastatic Patients				
Survival	Primary site	0.8235	0.001	1.12	0.49	2.28
	Age ≥10	0.3356	0.023	1.19	0.85	1.40
DFS	No variables entered					

[a]   Nonmetastatic — Unfavorable: GU (BP), extremities, HN (PM), and other primary sites; clinical group III; tumor size >5 cm. Favorable: orbit, HN (non-PM), and GU (non-BP) primary sites; clinical group I; tumor size ≤5 cm.
Metastatic — Unfavorable: GU/BP, extremities, parameningeal, and other primary sites; age ≥10 years. Favorable: orbit, HN, and GU/non-BP primary sites; age <10 years.

From the regression coefficients and the codes for each patient characteristic (Table 4), the variables with an important favorable relationship to survival are as follows: primary site (orbit, head and neck [nonparameningeal], and genitourinary [nonbladder/prostate]), clinical group I, and tumor size under 5 cm. For DFS, the variables with a favorable relationship to survival are clinical group I and the same sites as for survival.

2. Metastatic Patients

Among the 301 patients with metastatic disease, 254 had known values for all of the patient characteristics considered for entry into the model. Among these 254 patients, there were 191 deaths (75%) for the survival analysis and 204 relapses, metastases, or deaths (80%) for the analysis of DFS.

When Cox's regression model was fit to these patients, there were two variables associated with improved survival: primary site (orbit, head and neck [nonparameningeal], and genitourinary [nonbladder/prostate]) and age (less than 10 years) and no interaction terms. There were no patient characteristics significantly related to DFS.

3. Lawrence Subset of IRS-II Patients[5]

In the 505 patients, data were recorded concerning patient characteristics not generally available in large series of RMS patients. These characteristics included tumor invasiveness, tumor size, lymph node involvement, and histologic type.[5] There was a significant relationship to survival for all of these features, except for lymph node involvement.

A Cox regression model was fit to the data for the 393 nonmetastatic RMS patients, of which 123 (31%) died. The patient characteristics entered the regression model in the following order: primary site (orbit, head and neck [nonparameningeal], and genitourinary [nonbladder/prostate], favorable), tumor size (less than 5 cm, favorable), age group (10 years or older, unfavorable), and clinical group (increasing number, unfavorable). However, only primary site of the tumor contributed substantially to the predictive power of the model.

V. DISCUSSION

There is no universally accepted staging system for RMS.[9] However, classification of the extent of disease was the most consistent factor related to survival in the studies reviewed, and this finding was confirmed in the current analysis. For nonmetastatic patients, the risk of relapse or death was nearly three times higher for patients with incomplete resections or biopsies with gross residual disease (clinical group III) than it was for patients with completely resected localized disease (clinical group I).

The strong association between primary site and prognosis noted in several of the previous studies was also borne out in this analysis. Based on the univariate results, orbit, head and neck (nonparameningeal), and genitourinary (nonbladder/prostate) sites were grouped together in the multivariate analysis. In both the nonmetastatic and the metastatic patient groups, this combination of sites was consistently associated with more favorable outcomes than genitourinary (bladder/prostate), extremity, head and neck (parameningeal), and other sites. In some previous studies,[4,6,9,11] head and neck sites were associated with generally less favorable outcomes than were other primary sites. However, a distinction is made between parameningeal and nonparameningeal head and neck sites within the IRS studies, since patients with nonparameningeal head and neck sites generally have more favorable outcomes than patients with parameningeal head and neck sites.

In two analyses of the IRS data,[5,10] a strong association between tumor size and survival was established, demonstrating that patients with larger tumors were generally at an increased risk of death. Tumor size also had a strong relationship to prognosis in the current univariate analysis of the IRS-I and IRS-II data. This characteristic contributed substantially to the predictive ability of the multivariate model of survival, but not to the model for DFS.

Other patient characteristics have been associated with outcome in previous studies, including histology,[4,9-11] sex,[8-10,12] lymphocyte count,[10,12] and age.[4,10] In the current analysis, neither sex nor lymphocyte count was related to outcome in the univariate models, and these patient characteristics were not included in the final multivariate models. Histology and age were related to prognosis in the univariate model. Both of these patient characteristics entered the Cox multivariate regression model for the nonmetastatic patients, while age entered for the metastatic patients.

However, as one author warned, "It is easy to be misled by highly significant p-values of covariates in the adequately fitting model" which may "discourage the search for better prognostic variables" or "encourage the use of new costly assessments and procedures that add little to the predictive ability of a model based on simpler clinical variables."[21] Hence, since neither histology nor age significantly increased the predictive ability of the non-metastatic model with clinical group, primary site, and tumor size (survival model), these prognostic factors were not included in the final multivariate models. Age did add to the predictive ability of the metastatic survival model and is included in the list of important prognostic factors for this group of patients.

Currently, a report is being prepared of 951 newly diagnosed nonmetastatic RMS patients under 21 years of age from four different cooperative study groups (IRS, SIOP, Italy, and FRG [Germany]) in order to identify the most important pretreatment characteristics for use in predicting survival. In a Cox regression analysis, tumor invasiveness (T status) and primary site were the only significant predictive factors. Tumor size was not included since data for this variable were not available from all centers. Tumor invasiveness was not a significant prognostic factor in the multivariate analysis of the subset of IRS-II patients.[5] However, this is undoubtedly because of its high correlation with tumor size which did enter the model.

VI. CONCLUSIONS

In light of the findings from this analysis, we recommend that disease extent and location of the primary tumor be included as prognostic factors to be considered when planning, analyzing, or interpreting clinical studies of childhood RMS. Tumor size was determined to be important in the analysis of survival of nonmetastatic patients, and age was influential in the metastatic model of survival. Hence, these patient characteristics should probably also be included in this list. While this analysis did not establish the separate importance of tumor invasiveness as a predictor of outcome, this may be due to an analysis based on limited data. Thus, further investigation of this parameter would be useful.

Finally, it should be emphasized that the above list of significant prognostic factors is not meant to be final. Rather, further investigation of new and, perhaps, better prognostic factors may lead to increased insight into the biology of this disease. This new information may lead to improved treatment for subsets of patients categorized by different sets of prognostic factors.

REFERENCES

1. **Armitage, P. and Gehan, E. A.,** Statistical methods for the identification and use of prognostic factors, *Int. J. Cancer,* 13, 16, 1974
2. **Maurer, H. M. and Ragab, A. H.,** Rhabdomyosarcoma, in *Clinical Pediatric Oncology,* Sutow, W. W., Fernbach, D. J., and Vietti, T. J., Eds., C. V. Mosby, St. Louis, 1984, 622.
3. **Maurer, H. M., Gehan, E. A., Beltangady, M., et al.,** The Intergroup Rhabdomyosarcoma Study II, *Cancer,* in press.
4. **Sutow, W. W., Sullivan, M. P., Reid, H. L., et al.,** Prognosis in childhood rhabdomyosarcoma, *Cancer,* 25, 1384, 1970.
5. **Lawrence, W., Gehan, E. A., Hays, D. M., et al.,** Prognostic significance of staging factors of the UICC staging system in childhood rhabdomyosarcoma; a report from the Intergroup Rhabdomyosarcoma Study (IRS-II), *J. Clin. Oncol.,* 5, 46, 1987.
6. **Neifeld, J. P., Maurer, H. M., Godwin, D., et al.,** Prognostic variables in pediatric rhabdomyosarcoma before and after multi-modal therapy, *J. Pediatr. Surg.,* 14, 699, 1979.
7. **Flamant, F. and Hill, C.,** The improvement in survival associated with combined chemotherapy in childhood rhabdomyosarcoma, *Cancer,* 53, 2417, 1984.
8. **Rodary, C., Rey, A., Olive, D., et al.,** Prognostic factors in 281 children with nonmetastatic rhabdomyosarcoma (RMS) at diagnosis, *Med. Pediatr. Oncol.,* 16, 71, 1988.
9. **Kingston, J. E., McElwain, T. J., and Malpas, J. S.,** Childhood rhabdomyosarcoma: experience of the Children's Solid Tumor Group, *Br. J. Cancer,* 48, 195, 1983.
10. **Crist, W. M., Garnsey, L., Beltangady, M. S., et al.,** Prognosis in children with rhabdomyosarcoma; a report of the Intergroup Rhabdomyosarcoma Studies I and II, *J. Clin. Oncol.,* 8, 443, 1990.
11. **Jaffe, N., Filler, R. M., Farber, S., et al.,** Rhabdomyosarcoma in children; improved outlook with a multidisciplinary approach, *Am. J. Surg.,* 125, 482, 1973.
12. **Gehan, E. A., Glover, F. N., Maurer, H. M., et al.,** Prognostic factors in children with rhabdomyosarcoma, *Natl. Cancer Inst. Monogr.,* 56, 83, 1981.
13. **Maurer, H. M., Beltangady, M., Gehan, E., et al.,** The Intergroup Rhabdomyosarcoma Study I, *Cancer,* 61, 209, 1988.
14. **Newton, W. A., Soule, E. H., Hamoudi, A. B., et al.,** Histopathology of childhood sarcomas, Intergroup Rhabdomyosarcoma Studies I and II; clinical pathologic correlation, *J. Clin. Oncol.,* 6, 67, 1988.
15. **Kaplan, E. L. and Meier, P.,** Non-parametric estimation from incomplete observations, *J. Am. Stat. Assoc,* 53, 457, 1958.
16. **Mantel, N.,** Evaluation of survival data and two new rank order statistics arising in its consideration, *Cancer Chemother. Rep.,* 50, 163, 1966.
17. **Gehan, E. A.,** A generalized Wilcoxon test for comparing arbitrarily singly-censored samples, *Biometrika,* 52, 203, 1965.
18. **Fleiss, J. L.,** *Statistical Methods for Rates and Proportions,* 2nd ed., John Wiley & Sons, New York, 1981, 14.
19. **Mantel, N. and Haenszel, W.,** Statistical aspects of the analysis of data from retrospective studies of disease, *J. Natl. Cancer Inst.,* 22, 719, 1959.
20. **Cox, D. R.,** Regression models and life tables, *J. R. Stat. Soc. (Br.),* 34, 187, 1972.

21. **Korn, E. L. and Simon, R.,** Measures of explained variation for survival data, *Stat. Med.,* 9, 487, 1990.
22. **Schemper, M.,** The explained variation in proportional hazards regression, *Biometrika,* 77, 216, 1990.
23. **Simon, R.,** Use of regression models; statistical aspects, in *Cancer Clinical Trials; Methods and Practice,* Buyse, M., Sylvester, R., and Staguet, M., Eds., Oxford University Press, New York, 1984, 444.

Section III
Treatment

Chapter 7

PHARMACOLOGIC CONSIDERATIONS AND NEW AGENT THERAPY

Robert L. Saylors, III and Teresa J. Vietti

TABLE OF CONTENTS

I. INTRODUCTION

Despite the impressive gains made in the use of combined modality therapy for childhood rhabdomyosarcoma (RMS) in the cooperative group (IRS) studies, approximately 35% of patients remain uncured.[1] It is hoped that this number can be reduced through further advances in radiation therapy and improved surgical techniques. However, the primary focus of current clinical investigations is the development of new chemotherapeutic agents active against RMS and the administration of previously proven agents in innovative ways. Preliminary findings indicate that this approach may result in further improvement in survival, particularly for high risk patients.[2] In this chapter, the authors will first review the available data from experimental and theoretical studies concerning action of chemotherapeutic drugs and their interaction in treatment of RMS. Then they will review the available data on new agents that are effective in treatment of this tumor.

II. PHARMACOLOGIC CONSIDERATIONS IN THERAPY

Prior to the administration of any agent, the interrelationship of patient, tumor, and chemotherapeutic agent to be administered must be considered (Figure 1). For example, if the patient is to receive a myelosuppressive drug, the blood counts must be adequate. If a drug to be given is primarily excreted by the kidneys, renal function must be adequate and appropriate hydration should be given (Figure 1).

Among tumor factors that must be considered, the first is histology, if effective agents are to be selected or if antitumor efficacy is to be established (as in the case of phase II agents). A second group of tumor factors to be considered are the growth fractions of the tumor cells (Figure 2). The proliferative compartment of the cell cycle is the most susceptible to the effects of chemotherapy and radiation therapy. Those cells in the G_0 phase of the cell cycle most closely resemble the normal host cells and are the most resistant to chemotherapy. Although cells in G_0 phase may remain quiescent for a long period of time, they will eventually move back into the proliferative compartment (Figure 2).

Cells in the nonproliferative compartment are fully differentiated. These cells are unimportant because they cannot resume proliferation. The necrotic fraction consists of cells that are dead or dying. The necrotic core is surrounded by a zone of poorly vascularized and poorly oxygenated cells which are arrested in G_1 phase of the cell cycle. They are thus resistant to chemotherapy. It is this zone that can become revascularized, converting it to a proliferative compartment which will then be sensitive to chemotherapy.

After tumor sensitivity, the most critical characteristic of the chemotherapeutic drugs to be tried is related to pharmacokinetics. Following administration, the distribution of the drug throughout body tissues, binding of the drug to tissue proteins, peak level achieved and decay of this level over time, and other pharmacokinetic parameters must be considered. A useful calculation can be performed by plotting the peak drug level and the decay to nontoxic levels as related to time. The result of this calculation is the area under the decay curve for the drug, known as the AUC. If the AUC required to exert a lethal effect in animals is known, then presumably a similar AUC would be required in humans to exert an antitumor effect.

After administration of a chemotherapeutic agent and attainment of a peak level, there is an exponential decay in plasma concentration of the agent. This decay can generally be fitted to a biphasic or triphasic curve. In a triphasic curve, the initial decay to one half of the peak level is known as the $\alpha T^{1}/_{2}$, the intermediate decrease is known as the $\beta T^{1}/_{2}$, and the final exponential drop is the $\gamma T^{1}/_{2}$. Because the AUC for the $\gamma T^{1}/_{2}$ has a much longer time course for most drugs, this final period of excretion becomes the most important level both in terms of antitumor effect and host toxicity.

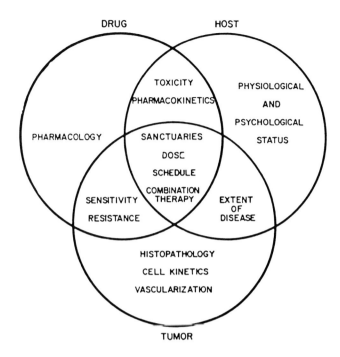

FIGURE 1.   Drug, tumor, and host factors and their interactions that
influence effectiveness of chemotherapy. (From Fernbach, D. J. and Vietti,
T. J., *Clinical Pediatrics Oncology,* 3rd ed., Mosby, St. Louis, MO,
1991. With permission.)

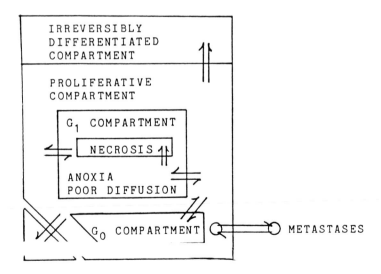

EXFOLIATION

FIGURE 2.   Diagrammatic visualization of various compartments of a tumor. (From Fernbach, D. J. and Vietti, T. J., *Clinical Pediatrics Oncology,* 3rd ed., Mosby, St. Louis, MO,
1991. With permission.)

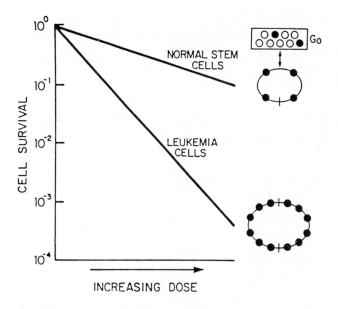

FIGURE 3. Dose-response relationship for a cycle specific agent demonstrating the differential sensitivity for nonproliferating cells as compared to proliferating cells. Solid circles indicate cells killed by the agent. (From Fernbach, D. J. and Vietti, T. J., *Clinical Pediatrics Oncology,* 3rd ed., Mosby, St. Louis, MO, 1991. With permission.)

It is also important to consider the kinetics of cell kill when selecting a chemotherapeutic regimen. Alkylating agents kill cells in any phase of the cell cycle, resulting in an exponential cell kill with increasing dose. There is a preferential cell kill for rapidly dividing cells. Thus, the exponential curve for the tumor cells is much steeper than the curve for the cells in a stem cell compartment which are not proliferating (Figure 3). If tolerated, these agents should be given as a single dose and the dose should not be repeated until there is host recovery. The antimetabolites, on the other hand, are phase specific agents which kill cells only during the phase of DNA synthesis (Figure 4). These agents should be given either by multiple doses over a specified time interval or by continuous infusion. There are drugs, such as actinomycin D and the anthracyclines, which are phase specific in action in tissue culture but cause exponential cell kill *in vivo*. This occurs because these agents have extraordinarily long $\gamma T^{1}/_{2}$ intervals, with lethal levels of drug persisting in the host for several days (Figures 3 and 4).

When two or more agents are used together, the clinician should consider whether the toxic effect on the patient or the lethal effect on the tumor will be enhanced (synergistic), additive, less than additive, or even antagonistic. Generally, when giving combination chemotherapy, the clinician uses drugs which do not have similar toxicities. In this way, one hopes to produce an acceptable degree of toxicity in the patient, together with enhanced destruction of the tumor. For example, synergistic cell kill occurs when vincristine and prednisone are used to induce remission in children with acute lymphoblastic leukemia. Less than additive cell kill occurs when two phase specific agents are used together, such as hydroxyurea and cytosine arabinoside (Ara C), both of which kill cells only during the phase of DNA synthesis. However, by proper sequencing of these agents, giving hydroxyurea first followed by cytosine arabinoside 6 h later, enhanced cell kill will occur. This is because hydroxyurea initially blocks the cells at the G_1S junction, thus synchronizing the cells in a single phase of growth. When hydroxyurea is stopped, all cells then start through DNA synthesis and are killed by the subsequent addition of cytosine arabinoside.

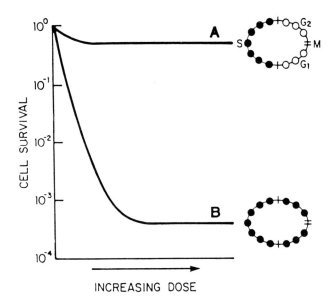

FIGURE 4.   Survival of proliferating cells following (A) a single exposure
to an S-phase specific agent and (B) repeated exposure over a period of
time greater than the median cell cycle time. Solid circles indicate cells
killed by the agent. (From Fernbach, D. J. and Vietti, T. J., *Clinical
Pediatrics Oncology*, 3rd ed., Mosby, St. Louis, MO, 1991. With permission.)

Another example of the enhancement of cell kill by giving two drugs is the use of
cisplatin and etoposide in combination. Cisplatin, an alkylating agent, causes breaks in the
DNA chain, while etoposide, an inhibitor of DNA topoisomerase II, prevents repair of the
DNA damage. Yet another example of drug interaction resulting in synergistic cell kill can
be found in the combination of methotrexate and cytosine arabinoside, which is currently
used to treat acute lymphoblastic leukemia. When methotrexate is given to cells and followed
by cytosine arabinoside, the conversion of cytosine arabinoside to cytosine arabinoside
triphosphate (Ara-CTP) is augmented, thus enhancing the lethal effect of the drug. An
antagonistic drug interaction results when methotrexate is given prior to or along with L-
asparaginase. This is due to the effect asparaginase has on arresting DNA synthesis, which
is the phase of the cell cycle during which methotrexate exerts its lethal effect.

At the time of diagnosis, most of the malignant neoplasms in children are relatively
sensitive to chemotherapy. Unfortunately, in a significant number of children mutant clones
resistant to chemotherapeutic agents later emerge and the child eventually dies of uncontrolled
growth of the neoplasm. It is not clear whether these drug-resistant clones are present at the
time of diagnosis or if they develop during therapy. It is known, however, that at the time
of diagnosis the tumor cell burden is generally between 10^{10} and 10^{12} malignant cells. It is
theorized, with some experimental support, that one drug-resistant clone is formed for every
10^5 to 10^7 malignant cells. It is also possible that mutant clones are induced by chemotherapy,
particularly by regimens employing mutagens such as alkylating agents. Utilizing these data,
a mathematical rationale was constructed for the scheduling of intensive multiagent chemotherapy early in the treatment course.[3]

A. DRUG RESISTANCE

It is of interest to consider the mechanisms by which tumor cells may become drug-
resistant. One may theorize that at any step along the pathway, from binding of a chemotherapeutic agent to its receptor at the cell surface to its terminal effect, mutations may occur

which will render the target cell resistant to the drug's action. Indeed, examples of many of these possible mutations are known. For instance, patients with acute lymphoblastic leukemia who become resistant to corticosteroids do so as a result of the loss of the cytoplasmic steroid receptor. Another example of a site of drug resistance is the increase of dihydrofolate reductase levels in cells exposed to methotrexate. The elevated levels of dihydrofolate reductase circumvent the block in folate metabolism induced by methotrexate in these cells and lessen the therapeutic effect of regimens employing the drug.[4]

The most intriguing mechanism of drug resistance concerns the phenomenon of the multiple drug resistance (MDR) phenotype. It was known that cells resistant to certain drugs, such as methotrexate, are generally sensitive to other chemically unrelated chemotherapeutic agents. Selection of cells resistant to certain other agents, such as actinomycin D, vincristine, or adriamycin, on the other hand, results in isolation of cells which are resistant to a whole spectrum of other compounds.

Recent work from several laboratories has confirmed that this type of multiple drug resistance is due to increased levels on the cell surface of a transport protein known as the P-glycoprotein. It has further been learned that the increased levels of the P-glycoprotein result from amplification of the gene encoding this protein, which is known as the mdr1 gene.[5] This receptor has been identified and characterized as an energy-dependent multidrug efflux pump, which can be inhibited by a variety of agents, such as verapamil, quinidine, and reserpine. This finding has generated enthusiasm for the clinical trial of these agents in an effort to reverse the MDR phenotype.[6,7] Other uses of this information include attempts to predict which patients will fail chemotherapy based on the patient's expression of the P-glycoprotein or amplification of the mdr1 gene.[8]

III. NEW AGENTS

Selection of agents for phase I and II trials begins when the agent has been shown to have antitumor activity in animals, with use of a reliably reproducible regimen and associated with an acceptable degree of toxicity. Almost all trials of new phase I agents designed to establish the optimal dose for phase II trials are initially performed in adults. The regimen (that is, the timing and method of drug administration) chosen is usually that which is most effective in treating tumors in animals. The usual starting dose in phase I trials is one tenth the lethal dose in animals, or the LD10. In subsequent patients the dose is doubled until some biologic effect is seen, or until the dose level that was observed to show some toxic effect in animals is reached. Subsequent dose increments are decreased to 20 to 30%. These increases are continued until the maximum dose is reached at which there is an acceptable degree of toxicity and at which the toxicity is reversible. This dose is known as the maximum tolerated dose (MTD).

Phase I trials in children are delayed until a known dose level shows a biologic effect in adults or a MTD is established for adults. The starting dose level in children is 80% of the MTD in adults, with subsequent dose escalations in 20 to 30% increments until the MTD for children is reached. Children are usually able to tolerate a per square meter dose level 20% higher than adults. Unless this dosage is translated to a per kilogram dosing regimen, a significantly higher (more toxic) total dose will result. This is a particular danger for the young children, due to their much higher ratio of surface area to weight. In fact, to prevent undue drug toxicity for children under 1 year of age, the dose should be translated to a per kilogram basis prior to administration.

A. NEW DRUGS

The clinical testing of agents found to be active *in vitro* and in xenograft models has identified a small group of new agents which show promise in the treatment of RMSs.

Among these drugs, the platinum compounds, either alone or in combination with etoposide, have been extensively tested. Sixteen patients with recurrent and progressive RMS resistant to the usual chemotherapeutic agents were given 3 mg/kg cisplatin every 3 weeks. Of these 16 patients, there was one complete response which lasted 2 months and two partial responses which lasted 2 months each.[9] Others then studied cisplatin plus etoposide in a group of 21 relapsed patients with RMS and obtained three durable complete responses (lasting 8, 9, and 11 months) and four shoft-lived partial responses.[10] These results were encouraging enough to allow the Intergroup Rhabdomyosarcoma Study (IRS) to pilot a regimen containing cisplatin plus etoposide, in addition to the standard regimen of VAC-Adria plus radiation, in a group of previously untreated patients. Of the 29 patients with RMS enrolled in this study, 21 of whom had the embryonal type and 8 the alveolar type, a total of 22 complete responses and 4 partial remissions were obtained.[11] This regimen is undergoing further trial in the current IRS study.

Other platinum compounds currently undergoing clinical trial include CHIP and carboplatinum. CHIP (*cis*-dichloro-*trans*-dihydroxy-bis-[isopropylamide] platinum IV, NSC 256927) is a second-generation cisplatin derivative which differs from the parent compound in that it has an octahedral platinum IV structure. The dose-limiting toxicity is myelosuppression, with a maximum tolerated dose of 350 mg/m^2 causing a median leukocyte depression to 2500/mm^3 and a median platelet nadir of 32,000/mm^3.[12] No appreciable renal or audiologic toxicity has been noted in studies reported thus far.

Carboplatinum (*cis*-diamino-1,1-cyclobutane dicarboxylate platinum II, NSC 241240, CBDCA) is another second-generation platinum analogue which has undergone extensive testing in adult solid tumors. This drug is currently used in many clinical situations in place of cisplatin. Carboplatinum has a similar spectrum of activity as the parent compound and its dose-limiting toxicity is myelosuppression. However, it causes no appreciable auditory, neurologic, or renal toxicity.[13] Both of these compounds, CHIP and carboplatinum, have been tested in phase II trials in RMS and may soon be incorporated into the next generation of phase III studies.

Another drug which has received a great deal of attention in the treatment of RMS is DTIC (dimethyl triazeno imidazole carboxamide, NSC-45388). DTIC is a synthetic purine analog. Its mechanism of action is unclear, though it appears to act principally as an alkylating agent.[14] The first clinical trial of DTIC in childhood RMS utilized a schedule of five consecutive daily doses of DTIC repeated every 3 weeks. Of the two patients in the study who had RMS, one had a response to the therapy.[14] The next study in which DTIC was used as a single agent in the treatment of RMS resistant to conventional therapy was reported in 1975.[15] Of the 11 patients treated in this study, only 1 achieved a partial response. As a result of the data generated by these two studies, it was concluded that DTIC had definite but minimal activity as a single agent against RMSs resistant to conventional chemotherapeutic agents. This finding warranted further evaluation of DTIC as a component of combination chemotherapy.

Studies in adult patients with all types of sarcomas indicated that the combination of DTIC plus adriamycin gave objective response rates of up to 41% without causing additional toxicity. Thus, this combination of drugs was chosen for further study in treating childhood RMS. The first studies using DTIC and adriamycin in children with resistant RMS obtained a total of 8 responses out of 18 children treated.[16,17] These results encouraged a trial of DTIC and adriamycin as initial therapy in a group of 26 patients with previously untreated RMS.[18] In this study, DTIC and adriamycin were given as the initial induction regimen, followed by alternation of these drugs with vincristine, actinomycin D, and cyclophosphamide (VAC) as maintenance therapy. Seventeen of the 26 patients had partial responses to this regimen, but there were no complete responses. Thus, this combination is inferior to other regimens which utilize combinations of VAC, with or without adriamycin. Testing of

DTIC is continuing in the current IRS study, which utilizes DTIC in addition to vigorous conventional therapy in a randomized arm for patients classified in groups 3 and 4.

Etoposide (VP-16-213) is another agent which has been extensively evaluated, given both alone and in combination with other agents, for activity against childhood RMS. Etoposide, a semisynthetic analog of podophyllin, shows activity against a wide variety of tumors. It appears to have two mechanisms of antineoplastic activity in growing cells. First, it delays transit of cells through the S-phase and arrests them in the late S or early G_2 phase of the growth cycle. Second, this drug induces concentration-dependent scission of DNA and prevents topoisomerase II-mediated repair of these breaks, leading to growth inhibition and cell death.[19-21]

The first studies in which etoposide was used in treatment of children with RMSs resistant to conventional therapy showed three complete or partial responses out of 16 patients.[22,23] These results, in addition to *in vitro* data suggesting synergy when given with other agents such as cisplatinum, led to trials using etoposide in combination with other agents for treating adults with refractory tumors. In addition to combination therapy utilizing conventional intravenous dosing regimens, it was recently shown that etoposide could be effectively given by daily oral administration.[24] In this study, 5 out of 16 patients with measurable tumors which were refractory to conventional chemotherapy had partial responses lasting 3 to 4 months in duration when given a regimen of etoposide administered orally for 21 consecutive days. When given in this manner, the maximum tolerated dose of etoposide was 50 mg/m²/ day and the dose-limiting toxicity was myelosuppression which occurred between days 21 and 28. Notably, four of the five responders had types of tumors which are usually considered unresponsive to etoposide when the drug is administered by conventional schedules.

Ifosfamide is another agent which has been through phase II trials and is currently being utilized in pilot studies for high risk RMS patients. Ifosfamide is an oxazaphosphorine in which one chloroethyl group is present on each nitrogen atom. Although it has a mechanism of action similar to its structural isomer, cyclophosphamide, it appears to be more active in several animal tumors.[25,26] The initial studies of ifosfamide indicated that hemorrhagic cystitis was the dose-limiting toxicity.[27] At first, this was a major problem which limited clinical use of ifosfamide, particularly in the patient who was to also receive bladder or pelvic radiation therapy. It was only with the development of effective protection from the urotoxic oxazaphosphorine metabolites, particularly acrolein and the 4-hydroxy metabolites, that clinically useful evaluation of ifosfamide could begin. The uroprotection currently utilized is MESNA (2-mercaptoethane sulfonate), which is a thiol compound which can be given orally or intraveneously. In the plasma, MESNA is rapidly converted to dimesna, which is again reduced to MESNA in the renal tubular epithelium. The MESNA is secreted into the urine where it reacts with the urotoxic ozazaphosphorine metabolites, preventing the hemorrhagic cystitis and allowing these drugs to be given in maximally myelosuppressive doses.[28,29]

Initial phase II studies of ifosfamide in patients with RMS resistant to standard chemotherapeutic agents showed moderate single agent activity. There were five partial responses out of 17 patients treated in a group of children who had been heavily pretreated with alkylating agents.[30-33] With its efficacy as a single agent thus established, ifosfamide was given in combination with other agents. In the most impressive trials, there were responses in six out of six patients (four partial responses and two complete responses) treated with vincristine and ifosfamide for RMSs resistant to conventional therapy.[34] These results led to further use of vincristine and ifosfamide, with the addition of actinomycin D in Europe for newly diagnosed patients.[35]

Ifosfamide has also been combined with etoposide to successfully treat a number of recurrent pediatric solid tumors. The rationale for this combination includes nonoverlapping nonhematopoietic toxicities, moderate myelosuppression of each drug used alone, and differing mechanisms of action. Whereas etoposide has specific cell cycle interaction, as described above, ifosfamide is a cell cycle nonspecific alkylating agent. In addition, it is theorized that etoposide may prevent the repair of DNA damage induced by ifosfamide through its interference with DNA topoisomerase II activity, as outlined above. The results of the first series of patients with RMS resistant to conventional therapy who were treated with this combination of drugs are very encouraging: 9 out of 13 patients responded, 3 with complete responses and 6 with partial responses.[36] When compared to a previous trial using ifosfamide alone, which had only 2 partial responses out of 9 patients treated, a statistically significant benefit for the combination is shown ($p = 0.04$).[36] The IRS is currently evaluating ifosfamide given in the drug pairs ifosfamide-Adriamycin and ifosfamide-etoposide as induction therapy for high risk RMS patients in an up-front phase II window (interval of treatment).

Melphalan, a bifunctional phenylalanine mustard alkylating agent with a broad spectrum of activity, has been tested for activity against childhood RMS in both laboratory models as well as in clinical trials. Studies in the mouse xenograft model indicated that melphalan should be a very active agent against RMS in a wide variety of dose ranges.[37] Not only did melphalan induce complete tumor regression in five out of six xenografts tested, one of which was taken from a heavily pretreated patient, it also showed more activity against RMS than any of the commonly used chemotherapeutic agents. This favorable experimental data, combined with the failure to demonstrate appreciable responses in 12 out of 13 heavily pretreated patients with recurrent tumors, led to a phase II study of melphalan in newly diagnosed, poor risk patients with RMS. Of the 13 children who received melphalan for 6 weeks (two courses), there were ten partial responses. This demonstration of significant single agent activity of a drug which would have been discarded in traditional phase II trials has led to a proposed modification in the scheme of new cancer chemotherapeutic drug development.[38] Another interesting report is that of a patient with RMS who was treated with high-dose melphalan followed by autologous bone marrow transplant and achieved a complete response.[39]

Use of methotrexate for RMS resistant to conventional drugs has also been reported. Two patients with pulmonary metastases of RMS showed partial response to methotrexate given in the dose range 50 to 500 mg/m^2 as a 6-h infusion.[40] This study was later expanded with nine additional patients, none of whom responded.[41] In Germany, four patients achieved dramatic responses when very high doses of methotrexate were given in combination with VAC with or without adriamycin, after the patients had progressed on regimens not containing methotrexate.[42] These studies indicating activity of methotrexate against RMS were added to older clinical and laboratory data showing that duration of exposure to methotrexate, rather than peak concentration, is the most important determinant of cell kill with this drug. Based on these findings, a study was begun utilizing low-dose methotrexate in patients with RMSs that are resistant to conventional chemotherapy.[43,44]

High-dose cytosine arabinoside (HiDAC) is another chemotherapeutic agent which has been evaluated in phase I trials, and is beginning phase II trials in pediatric solid tumors, including RMSs which are resistant to conventional chemotherapy. Though cytosine arabinoside has been used since 1963 to treat lymphoreticular malignancies, it has been only sporadically tested for activity against other solid tumors. There are several reasons to believe that this agent may be active when given in high doses in children with solid tumors. First, the pharmacokinetics of cytosine arabinoside given in high doses may act to circumvent the usual mechanisms of resistance, such as decreased cellular uptake, reduced phosphorylation of cytosine arabinoside to form the active agent, cytosine arabinoside triphosphate, decreased binding affinity of ara-CTP for DNA polymerase, and increased inactivation of the drug by deamination.[45,46]

A second factor is the reported activity in mouse neuroblastoma models in which cytosine arabinoside causes a dose-dependent inhibition of DNA synthesis when given in doses of

15 to 90 mg/kg/dose.[47] Last, there are phase I and II data in adult patients with refractory solid tumors indicating that high-dose cytosine arabinoside may have some efficacy in this clinical situation.[48,49] A phase II trial of HiDAC in advanced solid tumors, including RMSs, which are resistant to conventional therapy, is now being performed.

B. BIOLOGIC RESPONSE MODIFIERS

The newest class of agents for the treatment of all tumors, including RMS, is the biologic response modifiers. Among the agents available, interleukin-2 (IL-2) has been the most extensively studied in the treatment of solid tumors in adults. IL-2, previously known as T cell growth factor, is a 15.5-kD glycoprotein released by activated T cells in response to antigenic stimulus.[50] Initial enthusiasm for its clinical use was derived from the ability of IL-2 to correct the immunodeficiency in athymic nude mice and from initial studies indicating antitumor activity in the mouse.[51,52] The first report of a group of 25 patients treated with IL-2 showed that the dose-limiting toxicity was reached at a dose of 10^6 units/kg given by intravenous bolus or a dose of 3000 units/kg given as a continuous intravenous infusion over 24 h. This toxicity consisted of marked malaise and a capillary leak syndrome resulting in weight gain of 10 to 20% above pretreatment weight. There was minimal renal or hepatic toxicity. Hematologic toxicity was limited to mild anemia and thrombocytopenia with presence of a marked, though temporary, eosinophila. It is notable that two partial responses were seen in two patients with malignant melanoma metastatic to the lung.[53]

To improve upon these results obtained with interleukin-2 given alone, clinical trials were undertaken which further explored the observation that lymphocytes incubated with IL-2 (lymphokine activated killer cells, or LAK cells) develop the ability to lyse tumor cells.[54] In one study, 157 patients with metastatic cancer were given IL-2 either alone or in combination with LAK cells.[55] Of the 106 patients receiving the combination of LAK cells and interleukin-2, there were 33 responders, with a median duration of 10 months in the 8 patients with a complete response and a duration of 6 months in the patients who had lesser responses. Of the 46 patients who received IL-2 alone, there were seven responses. The toxicity resulting from IL-2 and LAK cell therapy was considerable, requiring critical care in the Intensive Care Unit in the majority of patients. These studies have established the clinical efficacy of IL-2 given alone or with LAK cells in the treatment of metastatic cancer resistant to conventional chemotherapy. These studies must now be extended to a wider variety of histologic types of tumors and to cancer patients at an earlier stage of therapy for their disease.

An exciting development in the treatment of all solid tumors, including RMS, is the utilization of hematopoietic growth factors (Figure 5). These agents are used to enhance the tolerance to chemotherapeutic agents which have myelosuppression as their major dose-limiting toxicity. The most intensively studied of these agents is GM-CSF, which stimulates proliferation and differentiation *in vitro* of neutrophil, eosinophil, and monocyte precursors. GM-CSF has also been shown to act as a neutrophil activator *in vitro*, inducing phagocytosis of bacteria,[56] as well as stimulating tumoricidal activity of macrophages.[57]

In a clinical trial, GM-CSF was administered following a course of myelosuppressive chemotherapy, followed by an identical course of chemotherapy without giving GM-CSF. This trial demonstrated a statistically significant shortening of the duration of the post-chemotherapy neutropenia and thrombocytopenia in patients given GM-CSF.[58] In another study, GM-CSF was given in conjunction with high-dose chemotherapy followed by autologous bone marrow transplantation. This study showed a dose-dependent increase in leukocyte count 14 days after autologous marrow infusion, in comparison with a historical control group of similarly treated patients who did not receive GM-CSF. No consistent effect on platelet counts was demonstrated.[59] GM-CSF is currently being given as daily subcutaneous injections, in a regimen designed to maintain constant low levels of circulating hor-

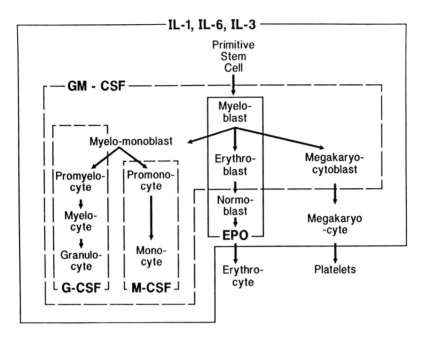

FIGURE 5. Interaction of the interleukines (IL-1, IL-3, and IL-6) with the colony-stimulating factors (CSFs). The abbreviations are G-CSF — granulocyte-CSF, GM-CSF — granulocyte-macrophage CSF, and EPO — erythropoietin. (From Fernbach, D. J. and Vietti, T. J., *Clinical Pediatrics Oncology*, 3rd ed., Mosby, St. Louis, MO, 1991. With permission.)

mone. In addition, a phase I dose-escalation study has been completed. This study demonstrated the significant effect of GM-CSF on the neutrophil, eosinophil, and lymphocyte populations, while failing to demonstrate a significant effect on numbers of monocytes or platelets, or on the hemoglobin level. It is hoped that this dosing regimen will allow more intensive chemotherapy to be safely administered to outpatients.

G-CSF has also been studied for its effect on accelerating postchemotherapy recovery of leukocyte counts. G-CSF has a theoretical advantage in that it is more lineage specific than GM-CSF, preventing the clonal expansion of the eosinophil and mast cell compartments which contributes to many of the undesired side effects of GM-CSF.[60] G-CSF also acts at a later stage of granulocyte differentiation than GM-CSF, evoking less anxiety regarding a drug-induced clonal expansion of a neoplastic granulocyte population resulting in myeloid leukemia (Figure 5). G-CSF has been studied in a group of 22 adult patients who were being given chemotherapy for treatment of transitional cell carcinoma of the urothelium. In these patients, G-CSF significantly reduced the number of days on which the absolute neutrophil count was less than $1000/mm^3$, it reduced the number of days patients were given antibiotics as treatment for fever and neutropenia, and it significantly increased the percentage of patients qualified to receive their planned chemotherapy on day 14 of the treatment cycle. An unexpected but encouraging finding was that the incidence of mucositis was significantly reduced in the G-CSF-treated group of patients who received methotrexate and anthracyclines.[61]

IV. SUMMARY

Current multimodality therapy for childhood RMS has resulted in cure of up to 65% of patients. Further improvements in outcome must come from utilization of new drugs and from incorporation of biologic response modifiers into therapeutic regimens, both as therapeutic agents and as protectants against the dose-limiting hematopoietic toxicities of many of the effective chemotherapeutic drugs. Among the chemotherapeutic agents we have reviewed, the most promising appear to be melphalan used alone or in combination and ifosfamide given in combination with etoposide. Though the therapeutic experience with biologic response modifiers has been limited, further study of IL-2 with or without LAK cells and other biologic therapies is proceeding on other solid tumors and may soon be utilized in the treatment of children with high risk RMS. The hematopoietic colony-stimulating factors may allow us to use much higher doses, and thus increase both the response and survival rates.

REFERENCES

1. **Maurer, H., Gehan, E., et al.,** Intergroup rhabdomyosarcoma study (IRS)-II. A final report, *Proc. Am. Soc. Clin. Oncol.,* 7, 255, 1988.
2. **Maurer, H., Gehan, E., et al.,** Intergroup rhabdomyosarcoma study (IRS)-III. A preliminary report of overall outcome, *Proc. Am. Soc. Clin. Oncol.,* 8, 296, 1989.
3. **Goldie, J. H., Coleman, A. J., and Gadauskas, G. A.,** Rationale for the use of alternating non-cross-resistant chemotherapy, *Cancer Treat. Rep.,* 66, 439, 1982.
4. **Bertino, J. R., Donohue, D. R., et al.,** Increased levels of dihydrofolic reductase in leucocytes of patients treated with amethopterin, *Nature,* 193, 140, 1962.
5. **Gottesman, M. M. and Pastan, I.,** The multidrug transporter, a double-edged sword, *J.Biol. Chem.,* 263, 12163, 1988.
6. **Gottesman, M. M. and Pastan, I.,** Clinical trials of agents that reverse multidrug-resistance, *J. Clin. Oncol.,* 7, 409, 1989.
7. **Dalton, W. S., Grogan, T. M., et al.,** Drug resistance in multiple myeloma and non-Hodgkin's lymphoma: detection of P-glycoprotein and potential circumvention by addition of verapamil to chemotherapy, *J. Clin. Oncol.,* 7, 415, 1989.
8. **Salmon, S. E., Grogan, T. M., et al.,** Prediction of doxorubicin resistance in vitro in myeloma, lymphoma, and breast cancer by P-glycoprotein staining, *J. Natl. Cancer Inst.,* 81, 696, 1989.
9. **Baum, E. S., Gaynon, P., Greenberg, L., Krivit, W., and Hammond, D.,** Phase II trial of cisplatin in refractory childhood cancer. Children's Cancer Study Group Report, *Cancer Treat. Rep.,* 65, 815, 1981.
10. **Carli, M., Perilongo, G., et al.,** Phase II trial of cisplatin and etoposide in children with advanced soft tissue sarcoma; a report from the Italian Cooperative Rhabdomyosarcoma Group, *Cancer Treat. Rep.,* 71, 525, 1987.
11. **Crist, W. M., Raney, R. B., et al.,** Intensive chemotherapy including cisplatin with or without etoposide for children with soft tissue sarcomas, *Med. Pediatr. Oncol.,* 15, 51, 1987.
12. **Creaven, P. J., Madajewicz, S., et al.,** Phase I clinical trial of cis-dichloro-transdihydroxy-bis-isopropylamine platinum (IV) (CHIP), *Cancer Treat. Rep.,* 67, 795, 1983.
13. **Muggia, F. M.,** Overview of carboplatin; replacing, complementing, and extending the therapeutic horizons of cisplatin, *Semin. Oncol.,* 16(Suppl. 5), 7, 1989.
14. **Luce, J. K., Thurman, W. G., Isaacs, B. L., and Talley, R. W.,** Clinical trials with the antitumor agent 5-(3,3-dimethyl-1-triazeno)imidazole-4-carboxamine (NSC-45388), *Cancer Treat. Rep.,* 54, 119, 1970.
15. **Finklestein, J. Z., Albo, V., Ertel, L., and Hammond, D.,** 5-(3,3-Dimethyl-1-triazeno)imidazole-4-carboxamine (NSC-45388) in the treatment of solid tumors in children, *Cancer Chemother. Rep.,* 59, 351, 1975.
16. **Gottlieb, J. A., Baker, L. H., et al.,** Chemotherapy with a combination of adriamycin and dimethyl triazeno imidazole carboxamide (DTIC), *Cancer,* 30, 1632, 1972.
17. **Cangir, A., Morgan, S. K., et al.,** Combination chemotherapy with adriamycin (NSC-123127) and dimethyl triazeno imidazole carboxamide (DTIC) (NSC-45388) in children with metastatic solid tumors, *Med. Pediatr. Oncol.,* 2, 183, 1976.
18. **Etcubanas, E., Horowitz, M., and Vogel, R.,** Combination of dacarbazine and doxorubicin in the treatment of childhood rhabdomyosarcoma, *Cancer Treat. Rep.,* 69, 999, 1985.
19. **Kalwinsky, D. K., Look, A. T., Ducore, J., and Fridland, A.,** Effects of epipodophyllotoxin VP-16-213 on cell cycle traverse, DNA synthesis, and DNA strand size in cultures of human leukemic lymphoblasts, *Cancer Res.,* 43, 1592, 1983.

20. **Chen, G. L., Yang, L., et al.,** Nonintercalative antitumor drugs interfere with the breakage-reunion reaction of mammalian DNA topoisomerase II, *J. Biol. Chem.,* 259, 13560, 1984.

21. **Ross, W., Rowe, T., et al.,** Role of topoisomerase II in mediating epidophyllotoxin-induced DNA cleavage, *Cancer Res.,* 44, 5857, 1984.

22. **Chard, R. L., Krivit, W., Bleyer, W. A., and Hammond, D.,** Phase II study of VP-16-213 in childhood malignant disease; a Children's Cancer Study Group Report, *Cancer Treat. Rep.,* 63, 1755, 1979.

23. **Nissen, N. L., Pajak, T. F., et al.,** Clinical trial of VP-16-213 (NSC 141540) intravenously twice weekly in advanced neoplastic disease, *Cancer,* 45, 232, 1980.

24. **Hainsworth, J. D., Johnson, D. H., Frazier, S. R., and Greco, F. A.,** Chronic daily administration of oral etoposide; a phase I trial, *J. Clin. Oncol.,* 7, 396, 1989.

25. **Goldin, A.,** Ifosfamide in experimental tumor systems, *Semin. Oncol.,* 9(Suppl. 1), 14, 1982.

26. **Colvin, M.,** The comparative pharmacology of cyclophosphamide and ifosfamide, *Semin. Oncol.,* 9(Suppl. 1), 2, 1982.

27. **Brock, N.,** The oxazaphosphorines, *Cancer Treat. Rev.,* 10(Suppl. A), 3, 1983.

28. **Ormstad, K., Orrenius, S., et al.,** Pharmacokinetics and metabolism of sodium 2-mercaptoethanesulfonate in the rat, *Cancer Res.,* 43, 333, 1983.

29. **Shaw, I. C. and Graham, M. I.,** Mesna; a short review, *Cancer Treat. Rev.,* 14, 67, 1987.

30. **Pinkerton, C. R., Rodgers, H., et al.,** A phase II study of ifosfamide in children with recurrent solid tumors, *Cancer Chemother. Pharmacol.,* 15, 258, 1985.

31. **Antman, H. K., Montella, D., Rosenbaum, C., and Schwen, M.,** Phase II trial of ifosfamide with mesna in previously treated metastatic sarcoma, *Cancer Treat. Rep.,* 69, 499, 1985.

32. **Pratt, C. B., Horowitz, M. E., et al.,** Phase II trial of ifosfamide in children with malignant solid tumors, *Cancer Treat. Rep.,* 71, 131, 1987.

33. **Magrath, I. T., Sandlund, J. T., et al.,** Treatment of recurrent sarcomas with ifosfamide, *Proc. Am. Soc. Clin. Oncol.,* 4, 136, 1985.

34. **deKraker, J. and Voute, P. A.,** Ifosfamide, mesna, and vincristine in paediatric oncology, *Cancer Treat. Rev.,* 10(Suppl. A), 165, 1983.

35. **Otten, J., Flament, F., et al.,** Treatment of malignant mesenchymal tumors of childhood with ifosfamide, vincristine, and dactinomycin (IVA) as front-line therapy; a preliminary report of the International Society of Pediatric Oncology (SIOP), *Proc. Am. Soc. Clin. Oncol.,* 6, 233, 1987.

36. **Miser, J. S., Kinsella, T. J., et al.,** Ifosfamide with mesna uroprotection and etoposide; an effective regimen in the treatment of recurrent sarcomas and other tumors of children and young adults, *J. Clin. Oncol.,* 5, 1191, 1987.

37. **Houghton, J. A., Cook, R. L., Lutz, P. J., and Houghton, P. J.,** Melphalan; a potential new agent in the treatment of childhood rhabdomyosarcoma, *Cancer Treat. Rep.,* 69, 91, 1985.

38. **Horowitz, M. E., Etcubans, E., et al.,** Phase II testing of melphalan in children with newly diagnosed rhabdomyosarcoma; a model for anticancer drug development, *J. Clin. Oncol.,* 6, 308, 1988.

39. **Lasarus, H. M., Herzig, R. H., et al.,** Intensive melphalan chemotherapy and cryopreserved autologous bone marrow transplantation for the treatment of refractory cancer, *J. Clin. Oncol.,* 1, 359, 1983.

40. **Pratt, C. B., Roberts, D., Shanks, E. C., and Warmath, E. L.,** Clinical trials and pharmacokinetics of intermittent high-dose methotrexate-"leucovorin rescue" for children with malignant tumors, *Cancer Res.,* 34, 3326, 1974.

41. **Pratt, C. B., Roberts, D., Shanks, E., and Warmath, E. L.,** Response, toxicity, and pharmacokinetics of high-dose methotrexate (NSC-740) with citrovorum factor (NSC-3590) rescue for children with osteosarcoma and other malignant tumors, *Cancer Chemother. Rep.,* 6, 13, 1975.

42. **Bode, U.,** Methotrexate as relapse therapy for rhabdomyosarcoma, *Am. J. Pediatr. Hematol. Oncol.,* 8, 70, 1986.

43. **Djerassi, I., Farber, S. Abir, E., and Neikirk, W.,** Continuous infusion of methotrexate in children with acute leukemia, *Cancer,* 20, 233, 1967.

44. **Keefe, D. A., Capizzi, R. L., and Rudnick, S. A.,** Methotrexate cytotoxicity for L5178Y/Asn-lymphoblasts: relationship of dose and duration of exposure to tumor cell viability, *Cancer Res.,* 42, 1641, 1982.

45. **Rustum, Y. M., Slocum, H. K., and Li, Z. R.,** Determinants of Ara-C action; biochemical considerations, *Prog. Clin. Biol. Res.,* 132, 107, 1983.

46. **Capizzi, R. L. and Cheng, Y. C.,** Sequential high-dose cytosine arabinoside and asparaginase in refractory acute leukemia, *Med. Pediatr. Oncol.,* Suppl. 1, 221, 1982.

47. **Sufrin, G. and Murphy, G. P.,** Pharmacokinetic studies in the chemotherapy of neuroblastoma using the C-1300 murine system, *Oncology,* 33, 173, 1976.

48. **Atkins, J., Muss, H., et al.,** A phase I study of high-dose Ara-C in patients with solid tumors, *Proc. Am. Soc. Clin. Oncol.,* 3, 42, 1984.

49. **Kirshner, J., Delosantos, R., et al.,** Phase I/II study of high dose Ara-C in solid tumors, *Proc. Am. Soc. Clin. Oncol.,* 3, 44, 1984.

50. **Smith, K. A.,** Interleukin-2: inception, impact, and implications, *Science,* 240, 1169, 1988.
51. **Wagner, H., et al.,** T cell derived helper factor allows *in vivo* induction of cytotoxic T-cells in nu/nu mice, *Nature,* 284, 278, 1980.
52. **Rosenberg, S. A., Mule, J. J., et al.,** Systemic administration of interleukin-2 leads to the regression of established tumor in mice, *J. Exp. Med.,* 61, 1169, 1985.
53. **Lotze, M. T., Yvedt, L. M., et al.,** Clinical effects and toxicity of interleukin-2 in patients with cancer, *Cancer,* 58, 2764, 1986.
54. **Lotze, M. T., Grimm, E. A., et al.,** Lysis of fresh and cultured autologous tumor by human lymphocytes cultured in T-cell growth factor, *Cancer Res.,* 41, 4420, 1981.
55. **Rosenberg, S. A., Lotze, M. T., et al.,** A progress report on the treatment of 157 patients with advanced cancer using lymphokine-activated killer cells and interleukin-2 or high-dose interleukin-2 alone, *N. Engl. J. Med.,* 316, 889, 1987.
56. **Fleischman, J., Golde, D. W., Weisbart, R. H., and Gasson, J. C.,** Granulocyte-macrophage colony-stimulating factor enhances phagocytosis of bacteria by human neutrophils, *Blood,* 68, 708, 1986.
57. **Grabstein, K. H., Urdal, D. L., et al.,** Induction of granulocyte tumorocidal activity by granulocyte-macrophage colony-stimulating factor, *Science,* 232, 506, 1986.
58. **Antman, K. S., Griffin, J. D., et al.,** Effect of recombinant human granulocyte-macrophage colony-stimulating factor on chemotherapy-induced myelosuppression, *N. Engl. J. Med.,* 319, 593, 1988.
59. **Brandt, S. J., Peters, W. P., et al.,** Effect of recombinant granulocyte-macrophage colony-stimulating factor on hematopoietic reconstitution after high-dose chemotherapy and autologous bone marrow transplantation, *N. Engl. J. Med.,* 318, 869, 1988.
60. **Clark, S. C. and Kamen, R.,** The human hematopoietic colony-stimulating factors, *Science,* 236, 1229, 1987.
61. **Gabrilove, J. L., Jakubowski, A., et al.,** Effect of granulocyte colony-stimulating factor on neutropenia and associated morbidity due to chemotherapy for transitional-cell carcinoma of the urothelium, *N. Engl. J. Med.,* 318, 1414, 1988.

Chapter 8

SURGICAL PRINCIPLES IN THE MANAGEMENT OF SARCOMAS IN CHILDREN

Walter Lawrence, Jr.

TABLE OF CONTENTS

I. INTRODUCTION

The principles of surgical management of sarcomas in children generally follow those that have been outlined for soft part sarcomas in the older age group, but these principles are modified somewhat by two important factors. The first differing clinical feature of childhood sarcomas that significantly affects their overall management, particularly in rhabdomyosarcoma (RMS), is the striking responsiveness of these tumors to chemotherapy. This observation contrasts with experience using chemotherapy for adult sarcomas. Soft part sarcomas in children, other than RMSs, may respond in only a more limited fashion. However, the marked responsiveness of childhood RMS to chemotherapy, given either alone or in combination with surgery and radiotherapy, clearly modifies our surgical approach to these lesions.

A second feature of these tumors that affects surgical management is the unusual anatomic distribution of sarcomas in children. Only one fifth of childhood RMSs arise in the extremities, which is by far the most frequent anatomic site for adult sarcomas. Also, the head and neck and the genitourinary tract are common primary sites for children. These latter anatomic locations for sarcomas in children raise special surgical problems in this age group.

II. BIOPSY

The first important surgical principle related to soft tissue masses is that of performing a biopsy to establish the exact diagnosis. Simple as a biopsy may seem, an improper biopsy procedure might give either incomplete information or compromise performance of the subsequent definitive resection. Thus, in tumors of the soft tissues of the head and neck, trunk, or extremities, one generally favors an *incisional* biopsy, as opposed to either needle biopsy or excisional biopsy. With incisional biopsy, adequate material for careful pathologic studies is obtained without extensive contamination of the surrounding soft tissues with tumor cells. Fine needle aspiration of these same anatomic sites may or may not be helpful in making a diagnosis. However, needle aspiration and core needle biopsy are less precise procedures than an incisional biopsy for determining histologic categorization of the tumor.

Excisional biopsy, or "enucleation", of any soft tissue tumor, other than very small lesions, is not advisable. This approach runs the risk of reducing the likelihood of success in obtaining a clear (tumor-free) histologic margin on all surfaces of the resected tissue at the time of a subsequent definitive resection. There is no palpable mass after excisional biopsy to use as a guide for determining operative margins at the time of definitive resection. Also, microscopic residual tumor is virtually always present, particularly if the tumor and its "pseudocapsule" have been enucleated. For these simple physical reasons, later adequate resection of the entire tumor may be extremely difficult to accomplish after "excisional" biopsy.

There are a number of exceptions to the preferential use of incisional biopsy for childhood sarcomas as related to certain unusual anatomic primary sites. These exceptions include the use of nasopharyngeal forceps biopsy, cystoscopic biopsy, forceps biopsy of the polypoid lesions of "sarcoma botryoides" of the vagina, and even use of needle biopsy of the prostate. The anatomic situation usually dictates the optimal approach to obtaining biopsy material. For example, excisional biopsy of the primary lesion by orchiectomy, combined with excision of the spermatic cord, is quite appropriate for the diagnosis and initial operative management of a paratesticular mass in a child, just as it is for a testis mass in an adult. However, excisional biopsy should be avoided in most other anatomic sites unless the primary lesion in question is quite small.

Frozen section diagnosis followed by immediate definitive resection should be avoided. Adequate pathologic study and evaluation should precede the definitive operation in most instances. These studies may include electron microscopy, immunohistochemistry, and other studies in addition to the standard paraffin-embedded histologic sections. Some of these newer histopathologic techniques are now being evaluated for improved classification of sarcomas; eventually, these techniques may become standard practice, as well as possibly leading to modifications of our treatment approach. However, an appropriate treatment plan must be based on an accurate and confident diagnosis, and frozen section diagnosis is not really adequate for this purpose.

III. PREOPERATIVE EVALUATION

Preoperative assessment of a patient with a biopsy-proven sarcoma requires a series of additional studies to establish the stage of the disease. Some studies may actually lead to a decision to eliminate surgery from the treatment plan due to the detection of distant metastases. Among the various soft tissue sarcomas, the frequency of distant spread is best documented for RMS; metastases were detected in about one fifth of patients entering the national clinical trial, the Intergroup Rhabdomyosarcoma Study (IRS). Complete preoperative assessment to detect such metastatic spread requires numerous diagnostic studies. These include bone marrow aspiration or biopsy, computerized tomographic (CT) examination of the lungs, CT of the liver, radionuclide bone scan, skeletal survey and (when appropriate) MRI of the head and spinal cord, plus examination of the cerebrospinal fluid. The local extent of the primary lesion, its size, and the clinical status of the regional lymph nodes are best evaluated for TNM (tumors, nodes, metastases) staging by adding CT of the appropriate region to a complete and thorough physical examination.

It has become apparent that pretreatment staging is necessary for optimal operative planning, as well as being essential to the conduct of the ongoing clinical trials that are designed to further improve treatment of these tumors. The use of prognostic factors, that have been identified both in the IRS and in the European studies, has led to more precise staging of childhood RMS (see Chapters 4 and 6).

IV. GENERAL PRINCIPLES OF OPERATIVE RESECTION

As will be noted later, the specific anatomic primary site usually affects details of the operation recommended, but there are some general principles of operative management that deserve emphasis. For tumors in most sites, the basic principle of wide resection of the primary tumor with an ''envelope'' of normal tissue should be followed at the initial operation whenever possible. Exceptions to this rule are the orbit and those anatomic sites where chemotherapy is now being given prior to actual definitive resection, such as with lesions arising in the bladder and the prostate. This approach of developing a generous anatomic margin of excision is more applicable generally to sites on the extremities and for some sections of the trunk, than it is for the more difficult head and neck, retroperitoneal, or pelvic areas. Adequate margins of normal tissue are required, however, to achieve good local control rates; resections that provide narrow margins are associated with more frequent local treatment failure when surgery is the only local therapy.

The actual determination of the margins to be achieved at the time of operation is dictated somewhat by the anatomic relationships of the sarcoma to vital structures of the region. Also, patients who have undergone total, but limited, biopsy excision of a soft tissue mass, which is found ultimately to be a sarcoma on pathologic study, should probably undergo a formal reoperation. The likelihood of gross or microscopic residual neoplasm, when simple resection of an undiagnosed soft tissue tumor has been carried out, is so high that such reoperation is recommended as the initial definitive approach to management.[1] Surgical findings from the IRS confirm this need to carry out a formal, planned reexcision of the operative site, if this is feasible. The goal is to achieve truly adequate margins of excision, whether the margins of resection from the original unplanned excision by microscopic study were reported to be free of tumor or not.[2] The problem, of course, is that the pathologic study of the operative margins is often quite incomplete when the initial operative procedure is not a definitive one for cancer. The report of a "negative" margin in this situation may be very misleading.

At the time of definitive resection of a neoplastic mass known to be a RMS, the type of resection will vary somewhat depending on the anatomic site. Wherever possible, however, this resection will include some overlapping skin, subcutaneous tissue, adjacent muscle and fibrous tissue, and the entire biopsy wound itself. Although this approach is an ideal one for either the initial resection or for reoperation after limited excisional biopsy, wide gross margins at all points around the sarcoma cannot be achieved anatomically in all patients. Only a narrow gross margin of excision may be possible in an anatomic area near a neurovascular bundle, or when the sarcoma arises in close proximity to bone or to vital organs. At the same time, the other resection margins may seem quite adequate in gross terms. This is the type of clinical situation where use of adjuvant radiation therapy has proved to be of benefit.

V. MANAGEMENT OF REGIONAL LYMPH NODES

The regional lymph nodes may be a site of metastasis for RMS, but clinicopathologic reviews of children with these tumors have yielded conflicting information regarding the frequency of this route of spread. A review of 1415 patients with nonmetastatic RMSs entered in IRS-I and IRS-II revealed that frequency of lymph node metastases from tumors in the extremities (12%) and genitourinary tract (24%) was somewhat higher than expected, while RMSs arising in the orbit (0%), head and neck region (7%), and trunk (3%) had a very low incidence of lymph node metastasis.[3] A subset of tumors in genitourinary sites, the paratesticular region, had a 26% incidence of lymphatic spread. All of these rates are minimum figures for the frequency of lymphatic spread, since many patients with nonpalpable regional nodes did not have a biopsy, particularly those included in the early phases of this study.

These findings demonstrate, however, that regional lymph node biopsy is especially indicated for tumors occurring in some anatomic sites, even when nodes are not palpable, such as with tumors of extremities and genitourinary sites. Likewise, operative management by dissection of the regional lymph nodes is considered appropriate for those patients who have either clinically involved regional lymph nodes or a positive regional lymph node biopsy without evidence of more distant spread. Paratesticular RMSs are a particular exception to this general approach. With paratesticular tumors, the regional lymph nodes are not accessible for adequate examination, and the frequency of lymphatic spread is high enough to justify lymph node sampling or dissection for all patients.

VI. OPERATION FOR SPECIFIC ANATOMIC SITES

A study of prognostic factors revealed that the anatomic site of the primary tumor is an important consideration.[4] There appear to be both "favorable" and "unfavorable" sites (Figure 1). The favorable sites, from the standpoint of survival rates, are nonparameningeal head and neck sites, the orbit, and genitourinary sites other than bladder and prostate (paratesticular, vaginal, uterine, and vulvae). Survival rates for patients in this favorable group of sites have been excellent for all stages, other than those with distant metastasis at the time of initial diagnosis. This was true even when surgery was omitted (as with orbital primaries), or when the operation was a conservative one. Other factors, such as tumor size, tumor invasiveness, or nodal status, had little impact on prognosis of this group.

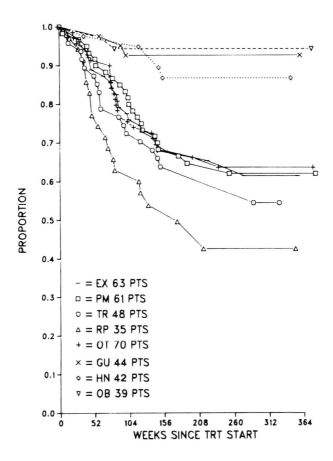

FIGURE 1. Survival curves by anatomic site of patients without metastases in IRS-II. The upper three curves represent genitourinary, orbital, and nonparameningeal head and neck sites. (From Lawrence, W., Jr., Gehan, E. A., Hays, D., et al., *J. Clin. Oncol.*, 5, 46, 1987. With permission.)

Patients with lesions in all other sites, including those in the extremities, parameningeal head and neck sites, bladder, prostate, trunk, and retroperitoneum, had a less favorable prognosis. Furthermore, other factors in the clinical staging process, such as tumor invasiveness, tumor size, and regional lymph node status, proved to be important prognostic variables. Because of variations in prognosis for the different anatomic sites, and the special surgical problems associated with variations in anatomic involvement in these sites, distinct differences in the operative approach are used for each of these anatomic locations.

A. ORBIT

This primary site has been effectively managed in the IRS by irradiation and chemotherapy after limited biopsy for diagnosis. Although there are some late effects from radiation, there appear to be no indications for orbital exenteration for RMS arising in this site. Long-term, disease-free survival results after radiation and chemotherapy are superb.

B. HEAD AND NECK

It has proven to be convenient to categorize RMSs arising in the head and neck region as parameningeal and nonparameningeal. Parameningeal tumors are those arising in the nasopharynx, paranasal sinuses, middle ear-mastoid, and pterygopalatine and infratemporal fossae; nonparameningeal tumors are those originating in the scalp, cheek, oral cavity, larynx, pharynx, and neck. Tumors in all head and neck sites are "difficult" from the standpoint of applying the general principles of resection that have been outlined, but, for some specific sites, these principles are either impractical or impossible. This is particularly true for the parameningeal sites. With tumors in these sites, complete resection with clear margins may not be anatomically feasible, as in tumors of the nasopharynx. Likewise, complete excision may not be practical due to the massive destruction of tissue that is required to achieve good margins by a craniofacial resection, as in tumors of the middle ear-mastoid, infratemporal fossae, etc.

Such procedures are often considered appropriate for adults with epithelial cancers, but they are less appealing, generally, for children's sarcomas, due partly to the responsiveness of these tumors to radiotherapy and chemotherapy. In these sites, the operation employed is usually either a biopsy or incomplete resection, the surgeon relying on nonoperative therapy for local control of the tumor. This conservative operative approach is frequently employed for sarcomas in nonparameningeal sites as well, with reliance on irradiation and chemotherapy. However, wide *en bloc* resection of the tumor with clear margins is preferred if this is anatomically feasible and the expected morbidity and cosmetic deformity are not too severe. RMSs arising in the neck region are often suitable for complete resection, with the hope of achieving clear microscopic margins. This is the preferred approach to tumors in this site when it is anatomically feasible.

C. EXTREMITIES

The general operative principles outlined earlier, including regional lymph node biopsy and/or dissection, apply to RMS arising in the extremity. However, total gross resection with clear margins cannot be accomplished in some situations without considerable loss of extremity function, or even the need for amputation. A limb-sparing operation is an important goal. This can be accomplished in most instances by utilizing radiation therapy for close margins of resection. However, total gross resection of the sarcoma is important if the patient is free of distant metastases.

A retrospective analysis was done on such patients with extremity sarcomas in whom gross disease was not resected, despite feasibility of resection by "radical" operation or amputation of some type. This study demonstrated a lower survival rate than that experienced by patients undergoing total gross resection.[5] This finding should encourage total gross resection of extremity RMSs, even if a radical operation with physical disability would be required. Close microscopically involved margins can be effectively treated by radiation therapy. It should be stressed, however, that it is preferable, when feasible, to consider reexcision of the primary site if pathologic study of the initial operative specimen reveals microscopic involvement of the margin. Drs. Hays and Weiner discuss the operative problems of extremity RMS in more detail in Chapter 21.

D. GENITOURINARY SITES

These include sites having an extremely favorable prognosis, such as the vagina, uterus, and paratesticular tissues, as well as the bladder-prostate RMSs, which have a slightly less favorable prognosis. An operative approach to these lesions is specific for each site; the approach is certainly different from those employed for RMSs arising in soft tissues elsewhere in the body.

A paratesticular mass should be resected by inguinal orchiectomy, with complete resection of the spermatic cord structures to the level of the internal ring. Resection of the scrotal skin is usually not necessary, except for a rare patient with neoplastic fixation to the scrotal skin, or a patient in whom a prior transcrotal approach has been employed for biopsy. This operative approach to paratesticular RMS is the same as that used for primary epithelial tumors of the testis in adults. Unilateral retroperitoneal lymph node sampling or dissection is indicated for all patients with paratesticular sarcomas. This is needed because of the frequency of regional lymphatic spread from this primary site and the clinical difficulty of determining the presence or absence of lymphatic spread without such a dissection. There is no general agreement on this point, and some investigators rely on lymphangiography and CT as means for selecting patients for node operations.[6]

The actual technique for node evaluation in this group of patients consists of a transabdominal unilateral resection of the spermatic vessels and the associated node-bearing tissue adjacent to the iliac and spermatic vessels. There is also resection of nodes along the aorta or vena cava from the level of the internal ring to the ipsilateral renal vein. Some surgeons favor complete bilateral retroperitoneal lymph node dissection because of possible "cross metastasis", but this dissection has the disadvantage of the significant sequelae of bilateral sympathetic nerve resection, including ejaculatory impotence. Both renal hilar areas can be included in a modification of unilateral dissection that deals with the concern of cross-metastasis, but this extension should not proceed any more caudad than the origin of the inferior mesenteric artery. It should be especially noted that ipsilateral inguinal lymph nodes are not a site of regional spread in patients with paratesticular RMS, unless there is actually scrotal involvement. Thus, inguinal node biopsy or dissection is not indicated except under unusual circumstances.

The optimal initial treatment of paratesticular RMS is surgical, as described above, with irradiation and chemotherapy to be carried out subsequently.

There are some special surgical problems that are worthy of further comment. The first problem is the operative management of the patient who has had an inappropriate transcrotal biopsy of a paratesticular mass, which ultimately proved to be RMS. In this situation, reoperation, including excision of the prior operative site, the hemiscrotum, and the spermatic cord structures to the inguinal ring, is an appropriate approach. In patients in whom it has been determined that postoperative regional radiation to the scrotal area is indicated (as in this case), the contralateral testis can be transposed surgically into a subcutaneous pocket in the adjacent thigh prior to this radiaton. The testis is then replaced in the scrotum after radiation therapy has been completed.

RMS of the vagina and uterus often presents as the "sarcoma botryoides", previously referred to in the discussion of biopsy techniques. Tumors originating in this extremely favorable site, from the standpoint of survival, and tumors with bladder-prostate primary sites are associated with significant disability if the principle of total gross resection is adhered to. In the early IRSs, this was the operative approach employed, and it frequently required either partial or total pelvic exenteration to achieve total gross removal of the primary lesion. A trial of preoperative chemotherapy then led to general acceptance of this approach, with the hope of reducing the extent of the subsequent operation and the subsequent disability resulting from loss of the bladder. Although the long-term benefits of scheduling irradiation and chemotherapy prior to the operation are still not fully established, it is the currently employed approach, and it does affect some of our surgical "ground rules".

At the time of clinical presentation of RMS in these "special" pelvic sites, some form of biopsy diagnosis must be established prior to initiating nonoperative therapy. For primary sites in the bladder or vagina, this can be accomplished by either endoscopic or forceps biopsies. For patients with primary prostatic RMS, core needle biopsy can be employed, but it is usually wise to obtain several cores in order to obtain sufficient pathologic material for accurate histologic study. If urinary tract obstruction is present at the time of the initial clinical presentation, catheters should be employed in the bladder and/or ureters to allow control of this problem prior to initiation of the presurgical chemotherapy program. Rapid resolution of this urinary obstruction frequently occurs soon after primary chemotherapy is initiated. This tends to encourage the use of simple intubation approaches rather than any formal operative urinary diversion.

The surgeon plays another important role in the overall management of patients with tumors in these special pelvic sites. This role involves the evaluation laparotomy that is performed at some time, usually about 16 to 20 weeks, following initiation of therapy with chemotherapy, either alone or combined with radiotherapy. The initial purpose of this laparotomy is to determine the actual response that has occurred, since physical examination and radiologic procedures have been shown to be inaccurate for assessing status of the tumor. This caveat has been demonstrated in a recent pilot trial of so-called "second look" surgery in the IRS.[7] Endoscopic procedures to evaluate tumor response may be performed under the same anesthetic as the laparotomy.

At a minimum, the operative procedure of second look should include examination of all intra-abdominal structures for evidence of metastases, evaluation of nodal spread by biopsy of the pelvic and para-aortic nodes, and biopsy of the previously involved primary site (using cystotomy for bladder or prostate lesions). If the site of origin of the prior tumor mass can be totally excised without performing pelvic exenteration, such an excision should be carried out at this time. Even if regression of the sarcoma has been grossly incomplete, showing only a partial response or "PR", any indicated surgical resection less radical than pelvic exenteration should be performed at this time. This procedure might include partial cystectomy in some patients, and for vaginal-uterine lesions the operation might include hysterectomy, partial or total vaginectomy, or both. For distal vaginal lesions, it might even be possible to resect the residual tumor and retain the uterus. Oophorectomy is not indicated unless there is gross ovarian involvement. The purpose of this resection, if it can be accomplished at the second look procedure, is total removal of remaining tumor tissue without disabling resection of normal structures.

When the procedures described above are successful in removing the remaining gross tumor mass, but "microscopic residual" remains on pathologic study, a secondary operative procedure should be seriously considered for removing the residual tumor. In many patients with pelvic primary lesions, this is not feasible. In patients with either microscopic involvement of the surgical margin that cannot be resolved by reoperation, or histologically positive regional nodes, local irradiation should follow this operation on patients who have primary esions of the vagina, uterus, prostate, or bladder.

In patients found to have a tumor that is too extensive at second look operation for any of the above operative procedures, postoperative radiation therapy should be employed rather than embarking upon anterior or total pelvic exenteration. Exenteration may be indicated at a later date, or at a later evaluation laparotomy, if radiation therapy does not control the tumor. In this setting, pelvic exenteration is a "salvage procedure", but it is probably more efficacious than a second line chemotherapy program if both the initial chemotherapy and the program of radiation therapy fail to control the local neoplastic disease.

E. OTHER SITES

The general principles of the operative approach to RMSs on the trunk are similar to that described under the section on general concepts of resection. Total gross resection and reexcision for better (tumor free) microscopic margins, when necessary and feasible, are the general standards for treatment of tumors at this site, also. This approach is similar to that employed for patients with RMSs of the extremities except that the radical approach of amputation is not available as an option for patients with trunk lesions (see Chapter 21). The surgical approach to RMSs of the perineum is similar, but tumors in this site are both uncommon and difficult to deal with surgically due to proximity of vital structures. Nevertheless, an attempt should be made to achieve total gross resection; the optimal operation is one that accomplishes clear (tumor-free) microscopic margins.

A few RMSs arise in unusual sites, such as the biliary tree, the gastrointestinal tract, or the retroperitoneal space. Surgical treatment of these sites is often quite difficult, due to anatomic considerations, but an attempt should be made to adhere to the general principles outlined above.

There are some uncommon clinical situations in which surgical resection of metastatic disease is appropriate. The lung is the most frequent metastatic site for which surgery is feasible. Thoracotomy for this purpose is indicated if there are no concurrent nonpulmonary metastases, and if thorough evaluation suggests that total excision of gross metastatic disease is possible. In patients with persistent pulmonary metastases after irradiation and/or chemotherapy, total gross excision of all metastases (unilateral or bilateral) by lung-conserving resection or resections is the principle to follow.

VII. SUMMARY

The general principles of surgical management of RMS in infants and children are similar to the operative approaches used for adult soft tissue sarcomas. However, the unusual features of some anatomic sites of origin of this tumor in children introduce special problems. Also, the overall results of multimodal therapy have been so encouraging, from the standpoint of survival data, that classic surgical principles utilized heretofore are often tempered by the observed responsiveness to chemotherapy and irradiation. The surgical ''ground rules'' that have been reviewed are subject to change as results from the cooperative clinical trials of therapeutic management of RMS mature.

REFERENCES

1. **Giuliano, A. E. and Eilber, F. R.,** The rationale for planned reoperation after unplanned total soft tissue excision of soft tissue sarcoma, *J. Clin. Oncol.,* 3, 1344, 1985.
2. **Hays, D. M., Lawrence, W., Jr., Wharam, M., et al.,** Primary re-excision for patients with ''microscopic residual'' tumor following initial excision of sarcomas of trunk and extremity sites, *J. Pediatr. Surg.,* 24, 5, 1989.
3. **Lawrence, W., Jr., Hays, D. M., Heyn, R., et al.,** Lymphatic metastases with childhood rhabdomyosarcoma; a report from the Intergroup Rhabdomyosarcoma Study, *Cancer,* 60, 910, 1987.
4. **Lawrence, W., Jr., Gehan, E. A., Hays, D., et al.,** Prognostic significance of staging factors of the UICC staging system in childhood rhabdomyosarcoma (a report from the IRS), *J. Clin. Oncol.,* 5, 46, 1987.
5. **Lawrence, W., Jr., Hays, D. M., Heyn, R., et al.,** Surgical lesions from the Intergroup Rhabdomyosarcoma Study (IRS) pertaining to extremity tumors, *World J. Surg.,* 12, 676, 1988.
6. **Olive, D., Flamont, F., Zucker, J. M., et al.,** Para-aortic lymphadenopathy is not necessary in the treatment of localized paratesticular rhabdomyosarcoma, *Cancer,* 54, 1283, 1984.
7. **Weiner, E. S., Hays, D., Lawrence, W., Jr., et al.,** Second look operations in children in groups III and IV rhabdomyosarcoma, *Proc. Am. Soc. Clin. Oncol.,* 8 (Abstr. 183), 304, 1989.

Chapter 9

RADIATION THERAPY GUIDELINES IN RHABDOMYOSARCOMA: RESULTS OF THE INTERGROUP RHABDOMYOSARCOMA STUDIES

Melvin Tefft

TABLE OF CONTENTS

I. REVIEW OF EARLY AND RECENT STUDIES

Past experience had indicated that radiation therapy achieved local control in approximately 90% of children with rhabdomyosarcoma (RMS) when treated with doses between 5000 and 6000 cGy.[1-5] However, certain chemotherapeutic agents have seemed to increase the injury of radiation to normal supporting tissues. Moreover, use of such concomitant chemotherapy and radiation therapy may allow for reduction of total radiation dose so that (1), the high rate of local tumor control is maintained and (2) there is less injury to normal tissues.

The Intergroup Rhabdomyosarcoma Study (IRS) has reviewed the experiences relative to local tumor control with combined chemotherapy and radiation, and have reported these data for one of the earlier studies.

When doses of 5000 to 6000 cGy were delivered initially to tissues encompassing entire muscle bundle compartments and organs of origin, it was observed that lower doses of radiation, on the order of 4000 cGy, might suffice for treatment of subclinical disease in patients with completely resected tumors. In patients with gross residual disease, successful treatment of the local sight of origin might be achieved with doses between 4500 to 5500 cGy. Also, volumes of irradiated tissues restricted to the site of tumor origin plus 3- to 5-cm margins seemed to be sufficient to achieve satisfactory local control of tumor for both subclinical and gross residual disease.[6]

A total of 291 patients were evaluated for dose efficacy and 317 were assessed for volume irradiated. It was reported that local control of subclinical disease could be achieved in 90% of patients with a dose of approximately 4000 cGy and with volumes which included the "tumor bed" plus a sufficient margin, but not including the entire muscle bundle compartment or organ of origin. Similarly, patients with gross residual disease were found to have local tumor control of 84% when given doses of radiation of less than 6000 cGy and with similarly reduced volumes of tissues irradiated. This experience allowed the author to evaluate prospectively and in a nonrandom manner the use of reduced doses of irradiation and volumes irradiated for patients with both subclinical and gross disease status in subsequent IRS studies.

Patients in later IRS studies received a radiation dose of 4000 cGy to restricted volumes, including the tumor bed with 3- to 5-cm margins. Patients with gross residual disease were given 4500 to 5500 cGy, depending on age and tumor size. Older patients and those with larger tumors received the higher doses in this range. A recent review of 496 patients from these later IRS studies showed similar excellent results for local control in patients with subclinical disease.[19] Thus, in future studies the author will continue to use these reduced doses of radiation and treatment volumes for these patients.

However, patients with gross residual disease appear to have somewhat higher rates of local failure when one accounts for all such patients, including those who never achieved a complete local response. This comparison included earlier patients who received doses as high as 6000 cGy to the entire muscle bundle compartment or organ of origin. In all IRS studies to date, patients who were given radiation treatment received fractions of 150 to 200 cGy (average 180 cGy) at a rate of one fraction per day, 5 days/week.

II. PILOT STUDIES

This most recent analysis has resulted in a prospective randomized pilot study, now ongoing, which attempts to improve the local control rate for patients with gross residual disease. Patients are randomized between the "lower doses" used in more recent IRS experience (that is, 4500 to 5500 cGy, at one fraction per day) vs. a hyperfractionation approach of 110 cGy per fraction, two fractions per day. The total dose to be delivered is

5490 cGy; fractions are given 6 to 8 h apart. This approach is meant to improve local tumor control, without adding increased injury to normal tissues.

Preliminary review has shown the occurrence of only a moderate and acceptable degree of acute toxicity from use of hyperfractionation. If these findings are verified in the ongoing pilot study, the latest formal IRS study will incorporate randomization of patients to receive hyperfractionated radiation. In addition, more intensive chemotherapy will be tried on a randomized basis in these patients.

Findings in 110 patients with gross residual disease were reviewed to evaluate the efficacy and safety of delaying radiation therapy during the first 6 weeks of chemotherapy.[7] Of these patients, 81% showed a complete or partial response to chemotherapy prior to starting radiation; 56% of these patients maintained the response. Because of these favorable results, in further IRS studies administration of radiation is delayed in most such patients.

Unpublished preliminary data indicate that patients with the embryonal type of RMS may have an improved local control rate, as compared to those with less favorable histopathologic types, such as alveolar RMS.[8] Preliminary and unpublished data indicate a less favorable local control rate in patients with completely excised tumors (group I) which have unfavorable histopathology and receive no radiation. Such patients now all receive radiation therapy to the local site at a dose of 4000 cGy. Reports of previous IRS studies have indicated that radiation may be omitted to patients in group I who have tumors with favorable histopathology.[9]

Certain subgroups of patients with RMS have been evaluated from the previous IRS studies. These include patients with tumors in parameningeal sites and tumors arising in the genitourinary tract.

III. PARAMENINGEAL TUMORS

Patients with parameningeal primary tumors, defined as those tumors arising in sites in the nasopharynx and accessory sinuses, middle ear, and temporal fossa, were found to have a 35% incidence of direct extension to adjacent meninges at the base of the brain.[10] The lethal nature of this disease was shown by a 90% mortality rate at a median of 9 months. Patients died with diffuse meningeal extension, including spinal subarachnoid spread. Attempts to retrieve these patients with craniospinal irradiation, either alone or combined with intrathecal chemotherapy (such as methotrexate), were not successful. However, it was also realized that approximately one third of these patients had less than an adequate dose of irradiation to the primary site, or less than adequate coverage by radiation of the meninges at the base of the brain.

Nearly all of these patients had either gross residual disease or metastatic disease. As part of the study design, radiation therapy was delayed during the more intensive 6 weeks of initial chemotherapy for these patients with extensive disease.

Modification of IRS guidelines then included starting radiation to the primary site and to the whole brain simultaneously, and concomitant with initial systemic chemotherapy. Chemotherapy included simultaneous intrathecal triple-drug chemotherapy. A dose of radiation of 3000 cGy in 4 weeks was to be delivered to the whole brain; a dose of 2400 cGy in 3 weeks was to be given to children less than 5 years of age. This course of radiation was followed by irradiation of a reduced volume of tissue, to include the primary site and 4 cm of adjacent meninges to a total dose of 4500 cGy. An additional boost to the primary site with a 1-cm margin of adjacent meninges raised the total dose to the primary tumor to 5500 cGy. Fractions of 180 cGy/day were to be delivered.

Spinal radiation was to commence on the sixth week, when systemic chemotherapy was less intensive. A dose of 3000 cGy in 4 weeks was recommended for treatment of the spinal subarachnoid.

Halfway through this amended study, evaluation of these patients indicated that approximately one half did not receive spinal radiation because of severe bone marrow suppression. None of the patients who failed to receive spinal radiation exhibited spinal relapse. At this point, the modified study was further amended to exclude routine spinal radiation, but to continue to give intrathecal chemotherapy. However, patients with established tumor seeding to the spinal cord were to receive radiation to the spinal axis. Few such patients were found to be present in this study.

Review of this experience showed a much improved overall survival rate for these patients. This experience was assessed in relation to prognostic risk factors.[11] As many as 76% of 68 patients with parameningeal tumors had complete remission and 68% were tumor free or alive at 3 years. However, meningeal involvement at diagnosis was an unfavorable sign. In patients without meningeal involvement, 81% were tumor free at 3 years as compared to tumor-free status in only 51% of patients who had established meningeal disease at diagnosis.

This evaluation allowed further IRS protocols to evaluate omitting spinal radiation in all patients with parameningeal RMSs except for the occasional patient who had abnormal cytological findings on spinal fluid examination. However, intrathecal chemotherapy was continued in those patients with significant risk factors for meningeal extension.

Radiotherapy of the cranial meninges was limited to radiating the cranial cavity in patients only when there was demonstrable evidence of intracranial extension. Radiation continued to be initiated on the first day of the protocol, being given concomitantly with systemic chemotherapy, except for those patients who had no evidence of extension of tumor to the base of the brain. Later, these patients with no extension to the base of the brain received radiation to the primary site, plus a margin including the adjacent 2 cm of brain meninges at the base of the brain. Treatment was given in a manner comparable to the radiotherapy given other patients with gross residual disease. Such radiation was delayed until the sixth week from the date the patient was placed on study. Preliminary data suggest that this approach is equally efficacious.

We believe that the most important factor which has improved the prognosis of these patients is better quality of radiation therapy. In the improved protocol, the radiation field includes the base-of-brain meninges, and radiation is started earlier in those patients who are at any significant risk for having intracranial extension.

Except for those with tumors in parameningeal sites, patients with tumors arising in the head and neck, most of whom have gross residual disease, have an excellent prognosis when treated with radiation combined with intensive chemotherapy. Approximately 88% of the 63 patients who were reviewed attained complete remission and were surviving at 5 years. Of these patients, 78% retained a complete remission at 5 years when treated with the doses of radiation mentioned previously, even without being given specific radiation coverage of adjacent regional lymph nodes. However, patients who present with lesions in the neck do less well, with only 46% of such cases surviving at 5 years.[12]

These findings led to trials using less intensive chemotherapy, such as regimens more consistent with those used in patients who have subclinical disease, in patients with head and neck primaries (exclusive of parameningeal sites), and in those with tumors presenting in the neck. Preliminary data indicate that an equal rate of local control and survival can be achieved with the use of this less intensive chemotherapy.

Patients with RMSs of the orbit have an excellent prognosis. A total of 127 such patients were reviewed and 93% were alive at 3 years: 94% of these children retained local control.[13] On the other hand, only 47% of children with RMS of the middle or external ear were free of disease at a median of 3.6 years at the time of the report.[14] However, these results were influenced to some extent by use of the earlier approach to radiation for patients with parameningeal tumors. Later results indicate improved survival, which was consistent with improvements noted following use of the new radiotherapy regimen for treatment of tumors in other parameningeal sites.

IV. GENITOURINARY TUMORS

Tumors arising in paratesticular sites have an excellent prognosis. Most patients have subclinical disease. Microscopic involvement of regional lymph nodes occurs in about 40% of cases. Patients with gross residual disease are mainly those who present with regional node involvement.

The 89% survival rate of these patients is based on the use of systemic chemotherapy and is related to whether local or regional lymph nodes were involved. Radiation therapy was given to most of these patients. Regional node involvement, including para-aortic nodes, has indicated that doses of radiation of 3000 cGy given over 4 weeks to the "hockey stick" portal should be delivered. Any residual gross tumor that was encompassable by a portal of approximately 6 × 6 cm was boosted by an additional radiation dose of 1500 cGy given in ten treatments.[15]

In anecdotal cases there were no regional failures in patients who showed involvement of surgically removed lymph nodes, when radiation was not given to seemingly uninvolved adjacent nodes. This has led us to ask whether regional nodal radiation may be omitted in patients who have no gross residual nodal involvement, in spite of having subclinical disease or gross tumors that were surgically removed.[16]

Patients who have transscrotal resection of paratesticular RMS are at risk for recurrence of the tumor in the scrotum. Such patients should have either (1) a hemiscrotectomy or (2) radiation therapy to the ipsilateral scrotum. Use of radiotherapy implies the need to transplant the contralateral testicle to the soft tissues of the thigh during radiation, with subsequent return of the testicle to the scrotum following radiation. The efficacy of preserving testicular function by this technique in these patients has not been determined.

In the past, patients with RMS of "special pelvic sites", such as vagina, uterus, bladder, and prostate, had been subjected to radical surgical procedures including exenteration. IRS studies have evaluated the usefulness of a combination of radiation and chemotherapy in such patients. It was found that preservation of normal structures such as the bladder may be possible with use of an intensive program of combined chemotherapy and radiation.[17,18]

However, patients with lesions of the bladder trigone and prostate may have false-negative biopsies at week 16 when routine surgical evaluation was to be done. IRS recommendations include routine radiation to such patients at week 6 irrespective of the finding of a negative biopsy. Beginning on week 16, these patients should receive radiation doses of 4500 cGy given over 5 weeks, similar to the doses of radiation delivered at week 16 to all patients who have tumors of special pelvic sites.

Thus, patients with RMS have been observed to benefit from use of a more conservative overall radiation dose and volume. Certain categories of patients seem to require a somewhat more intensive approach, with use of a radiation dose such as that given to patients with gross residual disease. Patients with tumors of the bladder, trigone, and prostate seem to require routine radiation therapy begun at week 6 from "on study".

Further IRS studies and detailed evaluation and review will be required to refine the delicate balance between optimum local control and minimum injury to normal tissues.

V. SUMMARY

Review of the results of past and ongoing IRS trials has indicated that radiation dose and volume may be reduced safely in certain categories of patients with RMS. Other patients seem to require a more intensive regimen of radiation. Factors which determine the choice of degree of radiation "intensity" include patient age, clinical group, site and/or size of primary tumor, and histopathology. Present pilot studies and planned prospective randomized studies will further address efficacy of newer radiation techniques, as well as evaluating long-term effects on normal tissue beyond those observations made in past IRS studies.

REFERENCES

1. **Conte, P. J. and Sagerman, R. H.,** Embryonal rhabdomyosarcoma of the middle ear with long-term survival, *N. Engl. J. Med.,* 284, 92, 1971.
2. **Donaldson, S. S., Castro, J. R., Wilbur, J. R., et al.,** Rhabdomyosarcoma of the head and neck in children, *Cancer,* 31, 26, 1973.
3. **Edland, R. W.,** Embryonal rhabdomyosarcoma, *Am. J. Roentgenol. Radium Ther. Nucl. Med.,* 93, 671, 1965.
4. **Edland, R. W.,** Embryonal rhabdomyosarcoma; 5 year survival of a patient treated by radiation and chemotherapy, *Am. J. Roentgenol. Radium Ther. Nucl. Med.,* 99, 400, 1967.
5. **Nelson, A. J., III,** Embryonal rhabdomyosarcoma; report of 24 cases and study of the effectiveness of radiation therapy on the primary tumor, *Cancer,* 22, 64, 1968.
6. **Tefft, M., Lindberg, R. D., and Gehan, E. A.,** Radiation therapy combined with systemic chemotherapy of rhabdomyosarcoma in children; local control in patients enrolled in the Intergroup Rhabdomyosarcoma Study, *Natl. Cancer Inst. Monogr.,* 56, 75, 1981.
7. **Tefft, M., Fernandez, C. H., and Moon, T. E.,** Rhabdomyosarcoma; response with chemotherapy prior to radiation in patients with gross residual disease, *Cancer,* 39, 665, 1977.
8. **Shimada, H.,** personal communication to the author, 1990.
9. **Maurer, H. M., Donaldson, M., Gehan, E. A., et al.,** (For the IRS Committee): the Intergroup Rhabdomyosarcoma Study: update — November, 1978, *Natl. Cancer Inst. Monogr.,* 56, 61, 1981.
10. **Tefft, M., Fernandez, C., Donaldson, M., et al.,** Incidence of meningeal involvement by rhabdomyosarcoma of the head and neck in children; a report of the Intergroup Rhabdomyosarcoma Study (IRS), *Cancer,* 42, 253, 1978.
11. **Raney, R. B., Jr., Tefft, M., Newton, W. A., et al.,** Improved prognosis with intensive treatment of children with cranial sarcoma arising in non-orbital parameningeal sites; a report from the Intergroup Rhabdomyosarcoma Study, *Cancer,* 59, 147, 1987.
12. **Wharam, M. D., Foulkes, M. A., Lawrence, W., Jr., et al.,** Soft tissue sarcoma of the head and neck in childhood; nonorbital and non-parameningeal sites. A report of the Intergroup Rhabdomyosarcoma Study (IRS)-1, *Cancer,* 53, 1016, 1984.
13. **Wharam, M., Beltangady, M., Hays, D., et al.,** Localized orbital rhabdomyosarcoma. An interim report of the Intergroup Rhabdomyosarcoma Study Committee, *Ophthalmology,* 94, 251, 1987.
14. **Raney, R. B., Jr., Lawrence, W., Jr., Maurer, H. M., et al.,** Rhabdomyosarcoma of the ear in childhood, A report from the Intergroup Rhabdomyosarcoma Study-I, *Cancer,* 51, 2356, 1983.
15. **Raney, R. B., Jr., Tefft, M., Lawrence, W., Jr., et al.,** (For the IRS Committee): paratesticular sarcoma in childhood and adolescence. A report from the Intergroup Rhabdomyosarcoma Studies I and II, 1973—1983, *Cancer,* 60, 2337, 1987.
16. **Tefft, M., Hayes, D., Raney, R. B., Jr., et al.,** Radiation to regional nodes for rhabdomyosarcoma of the genitoruinary tract in children: is it necessary? A report from the Intergroup Rhabdomyosarcoma Study I (IRS-1), *Cancer,* 45, 3065, 1980.
17. **Hays, D., Shimada, H., Raney, R. B., et al.,** (For the IRS Committee): clinical staging and treatment results in rhabdomyosarcoma of the female genital tract among children and adolescents, *Cancer,* 61, 1893, 1988.
18. **Raney, R. B., Hays, D., Tefft, M., et al.,** (For the IRS Committee): primary chemotherapy with or without radiation therapy, surgery or both for children with localized, residual sarcomas of the bladder, prostate, or vagina. Results of the Intergroup Rhabdomyosarcoma Study (IRS-II), *Cancer,* in press.
19. **Tefft, M.,** unpublished results.

Chapter 10

DRUG SENSITIVITY AND RESISTANCE IN THE XENOGRAFT MODEL

Peter J. Houghton, Julie K. Horton, and Janet A. Houghton

TABLE OF CONTENTS

I. INTRODUCTION

Because rhabdomyosarcoma (RMS), like many other solid tumors of childhood, is a relatively rare malignancy, certain restrictions arise in developing new therapies that are not encountered with the more frequently occurring tumors of adults. Clearly, it is not possible to evaluate large numbers of new chemical or biological entities as potential therapeutic agents in a systematic manner. Furthermore, evaluation by traditional phase II trials may be suboptimal for identifying potentially useful new drugs.[1,2] The focus then becomes one of utilizing the limited patient resources in a manner which will most likely lead to success in identifying new modalities.

Exactly how one approaches this problem is still controversial. In this chapter, the authors will review some of their studies. These studies demonstrate the feasibilty of developing histiotype specific preclinical models, their validation, their potential for identifying new therapeutic agents, and the strategy they adopted for assessing these leads in the clinic.

When model systems are considered that may have application for evaluation of new agents, or for developing multiple drug therapies using agents with known clinical utilities, certain demands can be made. These demands include: (1) that selectivity of drug action can be assessed; (2) that metabolic characteristics of the model parallel those of a particular cancer type; and (3) that the model reflects at least some of the intertumor variability observed in patients with the same tumor. As a minimum requirement, the model should identify those agents known to be clinically effective, and should retain the chemosensitivity/resistance profile of the tumor as seen in clinical studies.

II. A PRECLINICAL MODEL OF RMS

The approach the authors have taken is to heterograft surgical specimens into mice which have been immune-deprived to prevent graft rejection. Over the last 10 years, approximately 50 specimens of RMS have been transplanted, with about 40% giving rise to permanently transplantable tumor lines. In general, tumors have retained their original histology, degree of differentiation, chromosomal ploidy, and cytogenetic characteristics.[3-5] However, it is important that early transplant material is used, since with increasing serial transplantation in the mouse, characteristics of xenografts have a greater possibility of changing. Pertinent to their potential as therapeutically useful models is whether or not they retain their sensitivity to therapeutic agents. Although this appears to be a rather simple correlation to make, such studies have proven difficult due, in part, to the complexity of chemotherapy regimens used in the treatment of RMS. Such correlations have been made for several types of cancer, where responses to single agent therapy could be compared in the individual patient and in the respective xenograft.[6-9] For studies with RMSs, it has been necessary to compare the sensitivity of individual tumor lines to the drug with the expected response rate reported in clinical studies.

To parallel the heterogeneity of chemosensitivity observed clinically, the models necessarily become quite complex. Clearly, a tumor line derived from a single patient is unlikely to simulate the chemosensitivity profile of the same tumors as seen in clinical studies, although the National Cancer Institute has for some years used a single xenograft of colon, lung, and breast to do exactly that.[10] The number of tumor lines required to accurately simulate a clinical spectrum of any cancer may depend upon the histologic type in question. Routinely, the authors have used six lines of tumor established from untreated patients, and six lines derived at the time of relapse, or after phase I/II therapy. Thus, two models of RMS have been developed: the relapse model which should represent the phase II population and the "diagnosis" model representing untreated tumor.

TABLE 1
Responsiveness of Human Rhabdomyosarcoma Xenografts to Four Agents Used as Primary Therapy in the Clinical Disease

Agent/tumor[a]	Tumor line					
	HxRh12	HxRh18	HxRh28	HxRh30	HxRh35	HxRh39
Vincristine	+ + + + + +	+ + +	+ + + + + +	+ + + + + +	+ + + + +	+ +
Cyclophosphamide	+ +	+ + +	+ + + +	+ +	+	+ + + +
Actinomycin D	—	+ +	+ +	—	±	—
Doxorubicin	+ +	±	+ + +	—	—	+ +

Tumor response	Representation
No growth inhibition	—
Transient response, inhibition $<Td_2$[b]	±
Growth inhibition $\geq Td_2$	+
Growth inhibition $\geq 2 \times Td_2$	+ +
Growth inhibition $\geq 3 \times Td_2$	+ + +
Growth inhibition $\geq 3\ Td_2$ + volume regression $\geq 50\%$	+ + + +
Complete regression with subsequent regrowth	+ + + + +
Complete regression with no regrowth of any tumors during the period of observation (≥ 84 days)	+ + + + + +

Note: All tumor lines were established from previously untreated patients.

[a] All agents were given by the i.p. route at equitoxic doses.
[b] Td_2 = mean time for tumor volume to double.

From Houghton, J. A., Cook, R. L., Lutz, P. J., and Houghton, P. J., *Eur. J. Cancer Clin Oncol.,* 20, 955, 1984. With permission.

III. SENSITIVITY TO CONVENTIONAL CYTOTOXIC AGENTS

The chemosensitivity of tumors which comprise the diagnosis model are presented in Table 1. The model identifies, as active, those agents known to cause regressions of tumor in patients. Qualitatively, this group of tumors ranks vincristine as the most active agent and actinomycin D as the least active, which is in agreement with the clinical experience.[11] In these studies, mice bearing advanced tumors (larger than 1 cm³ in size) received a single dose of cytotoxic agent. Hence, the outcome did not represent results based on optimal therapy, but rather demonstrated the relative sensitivity of a given tumor to a series of agents administered at their maximally tolerated dose levels in the mouse. Thus, whereas actinomycin D demonstrated rather less activity in these experiments, administration on a weekly or a once-every-3-week schedule would probably have caused regression in some of these tumors.

Obviously, conditions for tumor growth in the mouse must differ from that of the original host. However, the contribution from the mouse in determining chemosensitivity of these RMS xenografts is of importance. That is, under conditions of growth in the mouse, do all tumor types respond in a similar manner? This can be addressed in two ways: first, the tumors established from specimens taken at relapse should maintain relative resistance to the diagnosis tumors as xenografts. Second, tumors intrinsically resistant to those agents known to be effective against RMS should, in the mouse, also be intrinsically resistant.

Responses of tumors heterografted at relapse to the same agents used in conventional therapy are shown in Table 2. These tumors are significantly less sensitive to treatment, and hence appear to retain their clinical characteristics with respect to chemosensitivity. These data indicate that the response of xenografted tumors is not merely a consequence of

TABLE 2

**Responsiveness[a] of Xenografts Established from
Previously Treated Patients**

Agent	Tumor line				
	Rh10	RD	LL	CB	Rh14
Vincristine	+	+ +	+	±	+ + + + +
Cyclophosphamide	—	+	+	+	+
Actinomycin D	—	—	—	—	—
Doxorubicin	—	—	±	±	—

[a]   Tumor response: see Table 1.

From Houghton, J. A. and Houghton, P. J., in *Rodent Tumor Models in Experimental Chemotherapy*, Kallman, R. F., Ed., Pergamon Press, Elmsford, NY, 1987, 199. With permission.

TABLE 3

**Responsiveness[a] of Human Colon Adenocarcinoma Xenografts to
Agents Used in Primary Treatment of Rhabdomyosarcoma**

Agent	Tumor line						
	AC$_4$	HC$_1$	GC$_3$	SJC$_3$A	SJC$_3$B	VRC$_5$	ELC$_2$
Vincristine	ND	ND	+	±	—	+	±
Actinomycin D	—	—	—	ND	ND	ND	—
Cyclophosphamide	—	—	—	ND	ND	ND	+ +
Doxorubicin	—	—	—	—	—	—	—

Note: ND = not determined.

[a]   Tumor response: see Table 1.

From Reference 12 with additional unpublished data.

their host environment. This conclusion is further supported when the responsiveness of xenografts derived from intrinsically resistant colon adenocarcinomas is examined (Table 3).[12] Each of the colon adenocarcinomas is quite unresponsive to both vincristine and doxorubicin (adriamycin), and thus retain the anticipated phenotype of the human disease.

IV. USING MODELS TO IDENTIFY NEW AGENTS

The data presented above suggest that RMSs growing as heterografts do indeed retain the chemosensitivity characteristics of the original tumor. Similar results have been reported with several other tumor types derived from adult malignancies.[9,13,14] It should, therefore, be feasible to use these as a preclinical phase II system to identify potentially useful agents for therapy of RMS. However, it would be wise to first consider the potential pitfalls of such an approach; in particular, the authors will consider the criteria that should be applied in determining the level of activity necessary to advance a compound into clinical trial.

As with any model, the xenograft system may predict false-positive or false-negative results. A false-positive result may be a consequence of host tolerance, such that far greater drug concentrations may be achieved in mice compared to humans. A false negative, on the other hand, could be generated for exactly the opposite reasons. The authors have used the colon adenocarcinoma model as an internal "negative control". That is, a drug should demonstrate far greater activity against RMS xenografts than against the colon tumors for it to be considered as a significant entity.

The authors have also applied similar criteria with respect to quantitating responses in the model in comparison to those responses used in the clinic. Thus, tumors are relatively advanced at the time therapy as initiated, and objective regressions are determined. To generate sufficient enthusiasm for extensive testing and a full pharmacokinetic study, a new compound would have to cause partial or complete regression in four out of six tumor lines used in the diagnosis (previously untreated) tumor panel.

An additional criterion that the authors recently adopted is that optimally a new compound is equally active against cell lines that demonstrate a classical multidrug-resistant phenotype.[15] The reason for this requirement is that RMS is routinely treated with three agents (vincristine, adriamycin, and actinomycin D) that are associated with this pleiotropic type of drug resistance. Consequently, it is of importance to identify new active agents where there is no cross-resistance with drugs used in conventional therapy. The use of an *in vitro* prescreen to select agents equally active against parent and multidrug-resistant cells provides a simple assay system for selecting agents for *in vivo* testing.

V. PROSPECTIVE IDENTIFICATION OF NEW AGENTS

Responsiveness of a panel of xenografts to several "new" agents is summarized in Table 4 and Figure 1. When these were examined, several had not received clinical evaluation against RMS, although some have subsequently entered clinical trial and have been found to cause regression of this tumor. These findings are of interest in that they demonstrate the potential capacity and the problems in identifying drugs for subsequent clinical evaluation. Melphalan, given at its maximum tolerated dose (42 mg/m^2), caused complete regression in five out of six tumor lines, whereas both DTIC and mitomycin C caused complete regression in only two out of six lines.[16] Both DTIC and mitomycin C demonstrate activity in the diagnosis model, although for DTIC, *N*-demethylation required for activation of DTIC may proceed more rapidly in the mouse as compared to man. Hence, for this agent, the model may overpredict antitumor activity in patients. In limited dose-ranging studies, it was found that the activity of DTIC was observed only at the maximally tolerated dose level. Unfortunately, there are no single agent trials of either mitomycin C or DTIC in previously untreated RMSs with which results in the xenograft model can be compared.

In contrast, a comprehensive dose-ranging study[17] showed the melphalan had significant activity over a fairly wide range of dose levels, although the dose-response relationship was again quite steep (Figure 2). Against tumors in the "relapse" model, only one line demonstrated significant tumor regression. Clinical evaluation of melphalan, given at conventional dose levels to children in relapse and against advanced disease at the time of diagnosis, have recently been reported.[1] At relapse, only 1 out of 13 patients demonstrated an objective response, whereas 16 out of 20 patients responded when treatment was given at the time of diagnosis.[1,1a] These results suggest that xenograft models may have value in identifying drugs which may fail to demonstrate activity against RMS at relapse, but which may have significant activity against disease at the time of diagnosis.

The activity of a novel agent currently under phase I evaluation in adults, *N*-(5-indanylsulfonyl)-*N*′-(4-chlorophenyl)-urea (ISCU), is included in Table 5. This diarylsulfonylurea has been shown to have significant activity against rodent solid tumors, and also against early and late stage xenografts of human colon adenocarcinomas.[18,18a] This drug is equally active against multidrug-resistant human cell lines resistant to anthracyclines and vinca alkaloids.[15] Although ISCU has less antitumor potency than either vincristine or melphalan, giving ISCU in optimal schedules of administration caused complete regression in all six RMS xenografts examined, with relatively mild toxicity. The efficacy of different schedules

TABLE 4
Responsiveness[a] of Xenografts of Childhood Rhabdomyosarcoma to "New" Agents

Agent/tumor	HxRh12	HxRh18	HxRh28	HxRh30	HxRh35	HxRh39	IRS49	IRS68
L-PAM	+++++	+++	+++++++	++++++	+++++++	+++++++	ND	ND
cis-DDP	+	++	++	+	+	++	ND	ND
Mitomycin C	—	+	++++	+	+++++	+++++	ND	ND
DTIC	+	+++	+++++	++++	+++++	+++	ND	ND
VP-16	+	+++	+++++	+	ND	ND	+++++	—

Note: Responses were determined as for Table 1. ND = not determined.

a   Agents administered as a single i.p. injection at equitoxic doses, except VP-16 which was administered daily for 5 days.

From Reference 16 with additional data.

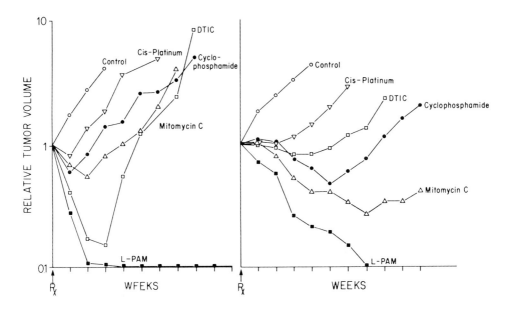

FIGURE 1. Responses of advanced xenografts of childhood RMS to "new" agents. Mice bearing advanced subcutaneous tumors received a single administration of each agent given at the maximum tolerated dose level. Tumor volumes were determined at intervals of 7 days. Left panel: Rh28 xenografts. Right panel: Rh39 xenografts. Each curve represents the mean growth of 10 to 14 tumors per treatment group and demonstrates tumor volume relative to that at the time of treatment. (From Houghton, J. A., Cook, R. L., Lutz, P. J., and Houghton, P. J., *Eur. J. Cancer Clin. Oncol.*, 20, 955, 1984. With permission.)

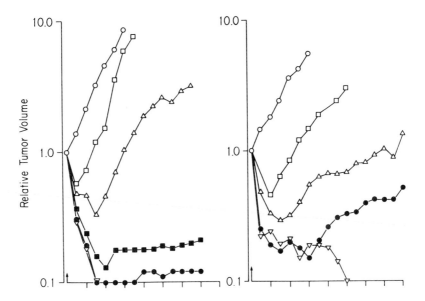

FIGURE 2. Response of Rh12 (left) and Rh30 (right) xenografts to various dose levels of melphalan. (▽) 16; (●) 13; (■) 10; (△) 7; (□) 4 mg/kg; (○) control. Each curve represents the mean growth of 12 to 14 tumors and shows tumor volume relative to the time of treatment. Abscissa: intervals of 14 days. (From Houghton, J. A., Cook, R. L., Lutz, P. J., and Houghton, P. J., *Cancer Treat. Rep.*, 69, 91, 1985. With permission.)

TABLE 5
**Responsiveness[a] of Xenografts of Childhood
Rhabdomyosarcoma to the Diarylsulfonylurea ISCU**

Tumor	mg/kg/dose		
	300	200	100

Schedule: BID × 10 days

Tumor	300	200	100
Rh12		+ + + +[a]	+ + +
Rh12/VCR-3[c]		+ + + +	ND[b]
Rh12/ifos		+ + + +	ND
Rh18		+ + + +	ND
Rh18/VCR-3		+ + + + + +	ND
Rh18/L-PAM		+ + +	ND
Rh28		+ + + + + +	+ + + + +
Rh28/L-PAM		+ + + + +	+ + +
IRS68		+ + + +	ND

Schedule: (BID × 5 days)₂

Tumor	300	200	100
Rh12		+ + + +	+ + +
Rh30	+ + + + + +	+ + + + + +	ND
IRS49		+ + + + + +	+ + + + + +
Rh18/VCR-3		+ + + + + +	+ + + + + +
IRS68	+ + + + +	+ + + + +	ND

Schedule: (BID × 5 days)₃[d]

Tumor	300	200	100
Rh18		+ + + + + +	+ + + + + +
Rh12		+ + + + +	+ + + +

[a] Tumor response criteria: see Table 1.
[b] ND = not determined.
[c] Suffix indicates subline resistant to vincristine (/VCR), ifosfamide (/ifos), or melphalane (/L-PAM).
[d] Subscript denotes number of courses.

From Houghton, P. J., Houghton, J. A., Myers, L., Cheshire, P. J., Howbert, J. J., and Grindley, G. B., *Cancer Chemother. Pharmacol.*, 25, 84, 1989. With permission.

is presented in Table 5. Toxicity in mouse (and in man) is limited to anemia and methemoglobinemia, without myelosuppression of gastrointestinal toxicity.

Thus, this agent, with novel activity and toxicity profiles, has potential in the treatment of childhood RMS. At this time, the mechanism of action of antitumor diarylsulfonylureas is poorly understood. However, preliminary findings suggest that these agents may be sequestered into mitochondria and accumulate in these organelles to high concentrations. A novel characteristic of this compound is that it appears to be equally cytotoxic to both proliferating and nonproliferating cells, thus demonstrating cytotoxicity independent of proliferation.[18a]

VI. DEVELOPMENT OF DRUG-RESISTANT XENOGRAFTS

Although the "relapse" model appears to be representative of resistance encountered in treating patients with RMSs, such experimental tumors are of limited value in determining which biochemical changes may lead to drug resistance. An alternative approach is to select sublines resistant to single agents by treating xenograft tumors in mice. Specifically, the authors have been interested in understanding intrinsic and acquired resistance to vinca alkaloids, the alkylating agent melphalan, and the chloroethylnitrosoureas. Two procedures for selecting resistant tumors have been used: (1) acute exposure where the poorest responding tumor is subsequently transplanted; and (2) chronic exposure to drug, which more readily simulates the clinical situation.[19-21] Drug-resistant sublines are approximately fourfold resistant and represent low level resistance which may have clinical significance.

VII. BIOCHEMICAL BASIS FOR TUMOR SENSITIVITY AND RESISTANCE TO VINCA ALKALOIDS

Resistance to vincristine is frequently associated with a decrease in uptake or decrease in retention of the drug in tumor cells mediated by an energy-dependent efflux pump.[22-24] Through gene transfection experiments, it has been shown that a single cDNA confers this multidrug resistance phenotype and encodes a transmembrane protein of 170 to 180 kDa (P-glycoprotein).[25] It is considered that this efflux glycoprotein has wide substrate specificity and thus accepts structurally diverse cytotoxic agents. These agents include vinca alkaloids, anthracyclines, many plant and bacterial alkaloids, and possibly certain lipid-soluble antifols.[26,27] Resistance due to increased synthesis of P-glycoprotein thus leads to a pleiotropic drug resistance phenotype known as multidrug resistance (MDR).

In the xenograft model, it is clear that for vincristine, tumor sensitivity is dependent upon drug retention.[28] The basis for vincristine sensitivity and resistance is depicted in Figure 3. The parameters that appear important are (1) that the level of drug in tumor cells exceeds some critical level required to inhibit mitosis, and (2) that this level is maintained until the cell enters mitosis.[29] For RMS xenografts (and some tumor cell lines) that the authors have examined, the cell cycle time is between 50 and 55 h.[14] Hence, for drugs such as vinca alkaloids, which after bolus administration are rapidly eliminated from plasma,[28,30] the drug must be bound tenaciously within tumor cells during transit through the cell cycle.

It is of interest that whereas RMS xenografts are very sensitive to vincristine, they are far less sensitive to vinblastine, a structurally similar antimitotic agent.[28] The basis for this differential is decreased retention of vinblastine compared to retention of vincristine in these tumors. The uptake and retention of vinblastine in vincristine-sensitive xenografts is similar to that of vincristine in the vincristine-resistant xenografts (Figure 3).[28] The biochemical basis for this difference in drug uptake and retention appears to relate, at least in part, to the binding affinity of these alkaloids to their intracellular target tubulin.[31] Thus, vinblastine binds with lesser affinity than vincristine and, accordingly, dissociates from this protein more readily. The unbound drug then equilibrates with the extracellular compartment which results in a loss of drug from the tumor.

VIII. MULTIDRUG RESISTANCE

The "classical" MDR phenotype demonstrates cross-resistance between vinca alkaloids, anthracyclines, and actinomycins, and may also include epipodophyllotoxins. The MDR phenotype is associated with overexpression of P-glycoprotein. There is increasing evidence that this phenotype exists as a significant clinical entity.[32-34] It was recently demonstrated that immunohistochemical detection of P-glycoprotein-positive rhabdomyoblasts is associated with a poor prognosis.[35]

As shown in Table 6, vincristine-resistant sublines developed *in vivo* are cross-resistant to adriamycin, suggesting the presence of a MDR phenotype. At this time, however, the authors have been unable to detect P-glycoprotein, or overexpression of the gene, *mdr1*, which encodes this protein.[25] It is quite possible that methods for detection of P-glycoprotein are insufficiently sensitive to detect this low level of resistance. In each tumor, however,

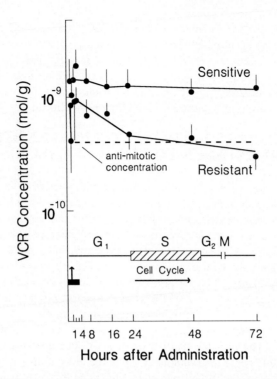

FIGURE 3. Proposed model for vincristine sensitivity of RMS xenografts. Bolus administration of vincristine (arrow) results in rapid clearance
of drug from plasma allowing only a transient exposure (depicted as heavy
bar) for tumor cells which are distributed throughout the cell cycle. Uptake
and retention of vincristine in sensitive and resistant tumors are shown
relative to the cell cycle (50 to 60 h). The broken line indicates the drug
concentration required to arrest cells in mitosis. Uptake and retention of
vinblastine in tumors responsive to vincristine are similar to that shown
for vincristine in the resistant tumor. (From Horton, J. K., Houghton, P.
J., and Houghton, J. A., *Biochem. Pharmacol.*, 37, 3995, 1988. With
permission.)

TABLE 6
Cross-Resistance Patterns in
Xenografts with Acquired Resistance
to Vincristine or Melphalan

	Response	
Tumor/agent[a]	Vincristine	Doxorubicin
Rh12	+ + + + + +	+ +
Rh12/VCR-3	+	—
Rh18	+ + +	+ +
Rh18/VCR-3	±	—
Rh18/L-PAM	—	—
Rh28	+ + + + +	+ + +[b]
Rh28/L-PAM	—	±[b]

Note: For response criteria see Table 1.
[a] Agents given as a single administration at a
maximum tolerated dose level.
[b] Doxorubicin administered twice with a 7-day
interval between doses.

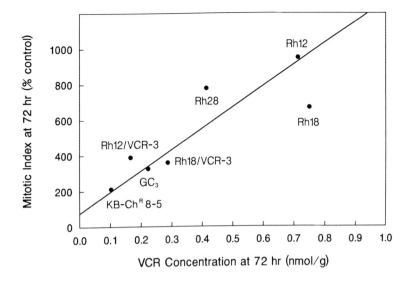

FIGURE 4. Relationship between vincristine concentration in tumor tissue and the mitotic index (expressed as a percentage of the control value) 72 h after a single administration of vincristine. Tumors with Rh prefix are RMSs, KB-Ch[R] 8-5 is a multidrug-resistant human cell line. (From Horton, J. K., Houghton, P. J., and Houghton, J. A., *Biochem. Pharmacol.*, 37, 3995, 1988. With permission.)

the retention of vincristine is decreased in the resistant subline. In resistant tumors, cells initially arrest in mitosis after vincristine treatment, although this accumulation is relatively short in duration. In contrast, in vincristine-sensitive xenografts, the mitotic index increases for at least 72 h after a single administration of the drug.[29] Indeed, the increase in mitotic index appears to correlate well with retention of vincristine and tumor sensitivity, as shown in Figure 4.

The authors have also demonstrated a MDR phenotype in RMSs which have an acquired resistance to melphalan.[20,36] As shown in Figure 5, the Rh28 RMS is sensitive to melphalan, vincristine, adriamycin, and VP-16 (etoposide). The melphalan-resistant subline of Rh28 (Rh28/LPAM) is cross-resistant to each of these agents, and thus demonstrates a pleiotropic resistance profile typical of P-glycoprotein-mediated resistance. Melphalan, a bifunctional alkylating agent, is not frequently associated with the P-glycoprotein associated MDR.[37] However, it has been reported that a subline of murine L1210 leukemia, selected for resistance to melphalan, is also cross-resistant to vincristine.[38] The mechanism causing resistance is not known at present, although there is no indication that the expression of *mdr1* is increased from analysis of mRNA levels. Also, there is no evidence that P-glycoprotein is increased from immunohistochemical studies using antibodies directed against internal or external epitopes or P-glycoprotein.

To examine this further, permanent cell lines were established from Rh28 and Rh28/LPAM xenografts. These cell lines were compared to a series of clones of KB cells which demonstrate different levels of MDR.[36] It is of note that *in vitro* both Rh28 lines demonstrate similar sensitivity to vincristine and to melphalan, thus these cell lines do not retain the differences seen *in vivo*. In addition, both cell lines are more sensitive than the parent "sensitive" KB cell line, which was used as an internal control representing a sensitive line. Interestingly, when inoculated into mice, Rh28/LPAM produces tumors that are completely resistant to both melphalan and vincristine. Thus, for this line, conditions of growth appear to influence drug sensitivity.

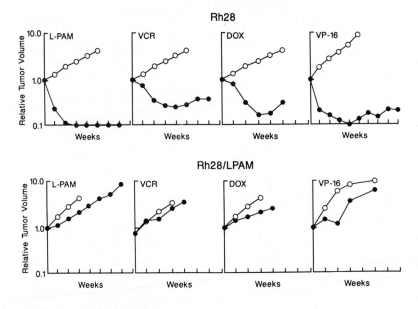

FIGURE 5.   Responses of Rh28 xenografts (top panel) and the melphalan-resistant derivative Rh28/LPAM (bottom panel). Mice bearing advanced tumors received a single administration of melphalan (LPAM) or vincristine (VCR). Doxorubicin was administered twice separated by 7 days, and etoposide (VP-16) was given daily for 5 days. Each treatment represents the maximum tolerated. Open symbols show growth of untreated tumors and drug-treated groups are shown as filled symbols. Each curve represents the mean of 10 to 14 tumors per group.

IX. RESISTANCE TO CHLOROETHYLNITROSOUREAS

Although chloroethylnitrosourea drugs are not generally considered as being useful in treatment of RMSs, a subset of tumors may indeed be quite sensitive to this class of agent.[39] As shown in Figure 6, several RMS xenografts demonstrated significant regression after treatment with 1-(2-chloroethyl)-3-(*trans*-4-methylcyclohexyl)-1-nitrosourea (methyl-CCNU). Of note was the complete regression of Rh28 xenografts following a single administration of the drug.

The chloroethylnitrosoureas exert their cytotoxic effects mainly through the production of DNA interstrand cross-links which are formed in a multistep reaction in which O^6-chloroethylguanine is thought to be the initial monoadduct. Recent evidence indicates that O^6-chloroethylguanine-DNA alkyltransferase (GATase) can repair this lesion, thus blocking the formation of cross-links.[40] Analysis of GATase in these xenografts revealed a distinct association between tumor response and levels of this repair enzyme (Figure 7). In this analysis, the estimated proportion of cells surviving treatment has been plotted against GATase activity. It was demonstrated that tumors with lower enzyme levels were progressively more sensitive to methylCCNU. The Rh28 tumor and the cell line derived *in vitro* appear deficient in this repair enzyme,[41] and they have been useful as tools in the identification of monoclonal antibodies that recognize GATase.[42] Several monoclonal antibodies that appear to recognize GATase are currently being characterized. These monoclonal antibodies offer the potential to select patients with RMS and other malignant tumors that may have tumors that are very sensitive to treatment with this class of alkylating agent.

X. TRANSLATING PRECLINICAL FINDINGS TO THE CLINIC

Xenograft models of RMS and other malignant tumors represent with considerable fidelity the tumors from which they were derived. With respect to chemosensitivity, xenograft

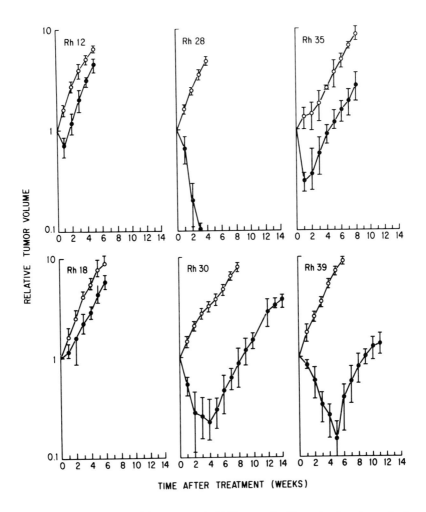

FIGURE 6. Time-course of drug response in RMS xenografts. Tumor-bearing mice received
a single administration of methylCCNU (●) or drug vehicle (○). Each curve represents the
mean response of 12 to 14 tumors. (From Brent, T. P., Houghton, P. J., and Houghton, J.
A., *Proc. Natl. Acad. Sci. U.S.A.*, 82, 2985, 1985. With permission.)

RMSs appear to be useful for identifying drugs which may have significant activity in
treating RMSs in patients, for understanding underlying mechanisms of tumor sensitivity
and resistance, and for examining alternative schedules for determining more effective drug
administration.

However, as with all preclinical experiments, it is a quantum leap to the clinic. Applying
xenograft-derived data to a chemosensitive and potentially curable tumor presents greater
problems than testing concepts against tumor types that are refractory to available therapy,
such as colorectal adenocarcinoma. The approach that the authors have adopted has recently
been reviewed[2] and is illustrated by the study with melphalan.

Melphalan was selected as a potentially interesting agent, based upon its significant
activity causing tumor regression in five out of six lines of diagnosis RMSs, and because
it had activity over a wide range of dose levels. In initial testing, melphalan showed little
activity as a phase II agent in relapsed RMSs.[1] However, studies in mice and children
demonstrated very similar pharmacokinetics (Figure 8), suggesting that the failure to demonstrate a significant activity was not due to species differences in metabolizing this drug.
An alternative explanation was that the patients included in the phase II study were resistant

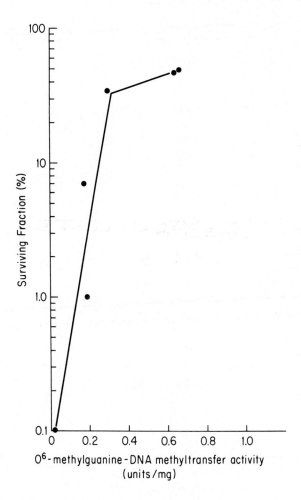

FIGURE 7. Relationship between the estimated surviving fraction of cells after methylCCNU treatment and GATase activity in tumor extracts. The surviving repopulation fraction was calculated from the volume-doubling times of untreated tumors and the growth delay of treated tumors. (From Brent, T. P., Houghton, P. J., and Houghton, J. A., *Proc. Nat. Acad. Sci. U.S.A.*, 82, 2985, 1985. With permission.)

to melphalan as a consequence of their prior therapy. All patients had been treated with vincristine, actinomycin D, and cyclophosphamide and 12 patients had also received adriamycin.[1] Thus, cross-resistance to melphalan was quite probable in these patients.

In patients considered to be at advanced stage and poor risk at the time of diagnosis, melphalan (45 mg/m²) showed very significant activity, producing objective responses in 16 out of 20 patients. These results indicated the value of developing preclinical models that may accurately represent specific types of cancer. A critical step in using these models was the pharmacokinetic comparison between species, which was determined during a phase I evaluation. For most new agents being developed in the U.S., pharmacokinetic data are available from phase I studies done in adults, which traditionally precede evaluation of new drugs in children. In cases where the pharmacokinetics and pharmacodynamics are similar in children and in mice, it may be appropriate to evaluate an agent in poor risk patients at diagnosis, even when the agent has shown poor activity in a traditional phase II setting.

In conclusion, the xenograft models of RMS appear to be representative of their clinical counterpart. They consitute a useful preclinical system for identification of new chemical

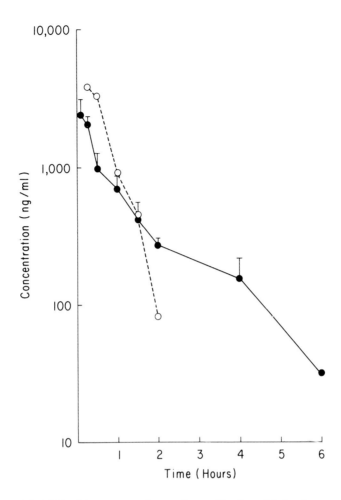

FIGURE 8. Mean concentration vs. time profiles for melphalan plasma dispostion in patients (solid line) and mice (broken line). Bars indicate standard deviations from the means. The area under curve (AUC) for patients was 175,000 μg/l/min, and the total systemic clearance was 232 ml/min/m². For mice the corresponding values were 170,000 μg/l/min and 235 ml/min/m². (From Horowitz, M. E., Etcubanas, E., Christensen, M., Houghton, J. A., George, S. L., Green, A. A., and Houghton, P. J., *J. Clin. Oncol.*, 6, 308, 1988. With permission.)

or biological agents that may have tissue-type selective activity. For rare tumors such as RMS, xenograft models may have particular value in allowing priority testing of new agents, and in determining therapeutically useful strategies for circumventing drug resistance.

XI. SUMMARY

RMSs heterotransplanted into mice have been evaluated as a preclinical model of childhood malignant disease. As xenografts, these tumors retain biological and biochemical characteristics of the donor tumor. Sensitivity to chemotherapeutic agents is representative of the known clinical responsiveness, and tumors transplanted at diagnosis are clearly more sensitive to conventional agents than are those heterografted from relapse specimens. These models have been useful for identifying new therapeutic agents for treating this tumor in children and for understanding the basis for chemosensitivity and resistance associated with several classes of antitumor agents.

ACKNOWLEDGMENTS

Studies referred to in this chapter were supported in part by American Cancer Society Award CH-423, and PHS Grants CA 23099 and CA 21765 from the National Cancer Institute, Bethesda, MD, and by the American Lebanese Syrian Associated Charities (ALSAC), Memphis, TN.

REFERENCES

1. **Horowitz, M. E., Etcubanas, E., Christensen, M., Houghton, J. A., George, S. L., Green, A. A., and Houghton, P. J.,** Predictability of pediatric rhabdomyosarcoma xenografts for melphalan activity in previously untreated patients: a model for development of cancer therapy, *J. Clin. Oncol.,* 6, 308, 1988.
1a. **Horiwitz, M. E.,** unpublished observations, 1989.
2. **Meyer, W. H., Houghton, P. J., Horowitz, M. E., Etcubanas, E., Pratt, C. B., Hayes, F. A., Thompson, E. I., Green, A. A., Houghton, J. A., Sandlund, J. T., and Crist, W. M.,** Use of investigational drugs as initial therapy for childhood solid tumors, in *Modern Trends in Human Leukemia,* Vol. 8, Neth, R., Ed., Springer-Verlag, Berlin, in press.
3. **Houghton, J. A., Houghton, P. J., and Webber, B. L.,** Growth and characterization of childhood rhabdomyosarcoma as xenografts, *J. Natl. Cancer Inst.,* 68, 437, 1982.
4. **Douglass, E. C., Valentine, M., Etcubanas, E., Parham, D. M., Webber, B. L., Houghton, P. J., Houghton, J. A., and Green, A. A.,** A specific chromosomal abnormality in rhabdomyosarcoma, *Cytogenet. Cell Genet.,* 45, 148, 1987.
5. **Hazelton, B. J., Houghton, J. A., Parham, D. M., Douglass, E. C., Torrance, P. M., Holt, H., and Houghton, P. J.,** Characterization of cell lines derived from xenografts of childhood rhabdomyosarcoma, *Cancer Res.,* 47, 4501, 1987.
6. **Giovanella, B. C., Stehlin, J. S., and Shepard, R. C.,** Experimental chemotherapy of human breast carcinomas heterotransplanted in nude mide, in *Proc. 2nd Int. Workshop on Nude Mice,* University of Tokyo Press, Tokyo, 1977, 475.
7. **Fodstad, O., Aass, N., and Pihl, A.,** Response to chemotherapy of human, malignant melanoma xenografts in athymic, nude mice, *Int. J. Cancer,* 25, 453, 1980.
8. **Shorthouse, A. J., Pekcham, M. J., Smyth, J. F., and Steel, G. G.,** The therapeutic response of bronchial carcinoma xenografts: a direct patient-xenograft comparison, *Br. J. Cancer,* 4(Suppl. 4), 142, 1980.
9. **Steel, G. G.,** How well do xenografts maintain the therapeutic response characteristics of the source tumor in the donor patient?, in *Rodent Tumor Models in Experimental Cancer Therapy,* Kallman, R. F., Ed., Pergamon Press, Elmsford, NY, 1987, 205.
10. **Goldin, A., Venditti, J. M., MacDonald, J. S., Muggia, F. M., Henney, J. E., and DeVita, V. T.,** Current results of the screening program at the Division of Cancer Treatment, National Cancer Institute, *Eur. J. Cancer,* 17, 129, 1981.
11. **Green, D. M. and Jaffe, N.,** Progress and controversy in the treatment of childhood rhabdomyosarcoma, *Cancer Treat. Rev.,* 5, 7, 1978.
12. **Houghton, J. A. and Houghton, P. J.,** The suitability and use of human tumor xenografts, in *Rodent Tumor Models in Experimental Chemotherapy,* Kallman, R. F., Ed., Pergamon Press, Elmsford, NY, 1987, 199.
13. **Nowak, K., Peckham, M. J., and Steel, G. G.,** Variation in response of xenografts of colo-rectal carcinoma to chemotherapy, *Br. J. Cancer,* 37, 576, 1978.
14. **Houghton, J. A. and Houghton, P. J.,** The xenograft as an intermediary model system: methods and advantages, in *Human Tumor Drug Sensitivity Testing in Vitro — Techniques and Clinical Applications,* Hill, B. T. and Dendy, P. P., Eds., Academic Press, New York, 1983, 179.
15. **Houghton, P. J., Houghton, J. A., Myers, L., Cheshire, P. J., Howbert, J. J., and Grindey, G. B.,** Evaluation of 5-(indanylsulfonyl)-N'-(4-chlorophenyl)-urea against xenografts of pediatric rhabdomyosarcoma, *Cancer Chemother. Pharmacol.,* 25, 84, 1989.
16. **Houghton, J. A., Cook, R. L., Lutz, P. J., and Houghton, P. J.,** Childhood rhabdomyosarcoma xenografts: response to DNA interacting agents and agents used in current therapy, *Eur. J. Cancer Clin. Oncol.,* 20, 955, 1984.
17. **Houghton, J. A., Cook, R. L., Lutz, P. J., and Houghton, P. J.,** L-Phenylalanine mustard (NSC 8806): a potential new agent in the treatment of childhood rhabdomyosarcoma, *Cancer Treat. Rep.,* 69, 91, 1985.

18. **Grindey, G. B.,** Identification of diarylsulfonylureas as novel anticancer drugs, *Proc. Am. Assoc. Cancer Res.,* 29, 535, 1988.

18a. **Houghton, P. J.,** unpublished observations, 1989.

19. **Houghton, J. A., Houghton, P. J., Hazelton, B. J., and Douglass, E. C.,** In situ selection of a human rhabdomyosarcoma resistant to vincristine with altered β-tubulins, *Cancer Res.,* 45, 2706, 1985.

20. **Horton, J. K., Houghton, P. J., and Houghton, J. A.,** Reciprocal cross-resistance in human rhabdomyosarcomas selected in vivo for primary resistance to vincristine and L-phenylalanine mustard, *Cancer Res.,* 47, 6288, 1987.

21. **Houghton, J. A., Houghton, P. J., Brodeur, G. M., and Green, A. A.,** Development of resistance to vincristine in a childhood rhabdomyosarcoma growing in immune-deprived mice, *Int. J. Cancer,* 28, 409, 1981.

22. **Fojo, A., Akiyama, S.-I., Gottesman, M. M., and Pastan, I.,** Reduced drug accumulation in multiply drug-resistant human KB carcinoma cell lines, *Cancer Res.,* 45, 3002, 1985.

23. **Inaba, M. and Johnson, R. K.,** Decreased retention of actinomycin D as the basis for cross-resistance in anthracycline resistant sublines of P388-leukemia, *Cancer Res.,* 37, 4629, 1977.

24. **Skovsgaard, T.,** Mechanisms of resistance to daunorubicin in Ehrlich ascites tumor cells, *Cancer Res.,* 38, 1785, 1977.

25. **Ueda, K., Cornwell, M. M., Gottesman, M. M., Pastan, I., Roninson, I. B., Ling, V., and Riordan, J. R.,** The *mdr*1 gene, responsible for multidrug-resistance, codes for P-glycoprotein, *Biochem. Biophys. Res. Commun.,* 141, 956, 1986.

26. **Ling, V., Kartner, N., Sudo, T., Siminovich, L., and Riordan, J. R.,** Multidrug resistance phenotype in Chinese ha..ster ovary cells, *Cancer Treat. Rep.,* 67, 869, 1983.

27. **Klohs, W. D., Steinkampf, R. W., Besserer, J. A., and Fry, D. W.,** Cross resistance of pleiotropically resistant P388 leukemia cells to the lipophilic antifolates trimetrexate and BW301U, *Cancer Lett.,* 31, 253, 1986.

28. **Houghton, J. A., Williams, L. G., Torrance, P. M., and Houghton, P. J.,** Determinants of intrinsic sensitivity to Vinca alkaloids in xenografts of pediatric rhabdomyosarcomas, *Cancer Res.,* 44, 582, 1984.

29. **Horton, J. K., Houghton, P. J., and Houghton, J. A.,** Relationship between tumor responsiveness, vincristine pharmacokinetics and arrest of mitosis in human tumor xenografts, *Biochem. Pharmacol.,* 37, 3995, 1988.

30. **Houghton, J. A., Meyer, W. H., and Houghton, P. J.,** Scheduling of vincristine: drug accumulation and response of xenografts of childhood rhabdomyosarcoma determined by frequency of administration, *Cancer Treat. Rep.,* 71, 717, 1987.

31. **Houghton, J. A., Williams, L. G., Dodge, R. K., George, S. L., Hazelton, B. J., and Houghton, P. J.,** Relationship between binding affinity, retention and sensitivity of human rhabdomyosarcoma xenografts to vinca alkaloids, *Biochem. Pharmacol.,* 36, 81, 1987.

32. **Fojo, A. T., Ueda, K., Slamon, D. J., Poplack, D. G., Gottesman, M. M., and Pastan, I.,** Expression of a multidrug-resistance gene in human tumors and tissues, *Proc. Natl. Acad. Sci. U.S.A.,* 84, 265, 1987.

33. **Bell, D. R., Gerlach, J. H., Kartner, N., Buick, R. N., and Ling, V.** Detection of P-glycoprotein in ovarian cancer: a molecular marker associated with multidrug resistance, *J. Clin. Oncol.,* 3, 311, 1985.

34. **Gerlach, J. H., Bell, D. R., Karakousis, C., Slocum, H. K., Kartner, N., Rustum, Y. M., Ling, V., and Baker, R. M.,** Detection of P-glycoprotein in human sarcomas by two monoclonal antibodies, *Proc. Am. Assoc. Cancer Res.,* 28, 229, 1987.

35. **Chan, H. S. L., Thorner, P., Haddad, G., Gallie, B. L., and Ling, V.,** Immunohistochemically identified P-glycoprotein correlates with adverse outcome in childhood soft tissue sarcoma, *Proc. Am. Assoc. Cancer Res.,* 30, 510, 1989.

36. **Horton, J. K., Houghton, J. A., and Houghton, P. J.,** Selection of primary resistance to melphalan (L-PAM) confers a multidrug resistant (MDR) phenotype not reversible by verapamil, *Proc. Am. Assoc. Cancer Res.,* 30, 524, 1989.

37. **Elliott, E. M. and Ling, V.,** Selection and characterization of Chinese hamster ovary cell mutants resistant to melphalan (L-phenylalanine mustard), *Cancer Res.,* 41, 393, 1981.

38. **Schabel, F. M., Jr., Skipper, H. E., Trader, M. W., Laster, W. R., Griswold, D. P., Jr., and Corbett, T. H.,** Establishment of cross-resistance profiles for new agents, *Cancer Treat. Rep.,* 68, 453, 1984.

39. **Brent, T. P., Houghton, P. J., and Houghton, J. A.,** O⁶-alkylguanine-DNA alkyltransferase activity correlates with the therapeutic response of human rhabdomyosarcoma xenografts to MeCCNU, *Proc. Natl. Acad. Sci. U.S.A.,* 82, 2985, 1985.

40. **Brent, T. P.,** Suppression of cross-link formation in chloroethylnitrosourea-treated DNA by an activity in extracts of human leukemic lymphoblasts, *Cancer Res.,* 44, 1887, 1984.

41. **Smith, D. G. and Brent, T. P.,** Response of cultured human cell lines from rhabdomyosarcoma xenografts to treatment with chloroethylnitrosoureas, *Cancer Res.,* 49, 883, 1989.

42. **Von Wronski, M., Brent, T. P., Pegram, C. N., and Bigner, D. D.,** Monoclonal antibodies against human O⁶-alkylguanine-DNA alkyltransferase, *Proc. Am. Assoc. Cancer Res.,* 30, 486, 1989.

Chapter 11

CHEMOTHERAPY FOR PREVIOUSLY UNTREATED PATIENTS WITH RHABDOMYOSARCOMA

Harold M. Maurer and William Crist

TABLE OF CONTENTS

I. INTRODUCTION

Chemotherapy is an essential component of the multidisciplinary management of childhood rhabdomyosarcoma (RMS) along with surgery and radiation therapy. The benefit of adjuvant combination chemotherapy was definitively demonstrated by Heyn and associates. In this study, 42 children with completely resected localized disease were given postoperative radiation and then randomly assigned to receive either chemotherapy or no further treatment.[1] One year of therapy with actinomycin D and vincristine resulted in relapse-free survival in 24 out of 28 patients (survival rate 85.7%) for periods of greater than 2 years after initial treatment. This result was compared to a survival rate of only 47% (survival in 7 of 15 patients) in the control group who received no chemotherapy. The benefit of chemotherapy also was demonstrated by Wilbur who showed that more intensive chemotherapy renders more extensive lesions amenable to control by resection or radiation therapy.[2]

It is generally agreed that chemotherapy should be used in treatment of all newly diagnosed patients with RMS, extraosseous Ewing's sarcoma, and undifferentiated sarcoma. The chief role of chemotherapy is to eradicate microscopic deposits of tumor. It also can be used to shrink large tumor masses to an operable size and to reduce the volume of tissue requiring radiation therapy. The use of chemotherapy as primary treatment is desirable as a means for minimizing the need for surgery and radiation therapy. However, current regimens are not able to predictably achieve this goal with a high degree of long-term success. Where use of the early chemotherapy to shrink large tumor masses has been carefully evaluated, such as in localized lesions of the bladder and prostrate, treatment failures were primarily caused by failure of local or regional tumor control.[3]

II. ATTAINMENT OF COMPLETE RESPONSE

Complete response to treatment is required for long-term disease control and cure. Until recently, response was judged almost exclusively on the basis of clinical assessment and the results of imaging studies. Although evaluation of response has improved considerably with use of modern imaging techniques, complete response cannot be absolutely ascertained without pathologic confirmation. Patients who appear to have attained a complete response by clinical examination and diagnostic imaging may still have microscopic evidence of residual tumor on pathologic examination.[4] On the other hand, patients who appear by clinical and imaging evaluations to have attained a partial response, or even no response, on pathologic examination may show only fibrosis and no evidence of residual tumor. A typical example of this problem is in RMSs arising in the nasopharyngeal region.

III. TREATMENT POLICY

Since there is no single "magic bullet" for treatment of RMSs, multiagent combination chemotherapy should be given in a coordinated planned program, along with surgery and radiation therapy.[5-7] Maximum tolerated doses of the various drugs are recommended in order to achieve maximum survival benefit. Chemotherapy should begin as soon as possible after biopsy or surgical resection of the tumor, when the extent or stage of the tumor has been determined. The Intergroup Rhabdomyosarcoma Study (IRS) clinical grouping classification is the most widely used staging scheme, consisting of groups I to IV. However, this classification suffers from the fact that it is based heavily on the extent of surgery employed.[8] Pretreatment staging, using the TNM (tumors, nodes, metastases) staging classification, is preferred and employed by members of the International Society of Pediatric Oncology (SIOP).[8] A new pretreatment staging classification, which is TNM-based, will be used for future IRS trials starting with IRS-IV.[9] This system will also be used by our European colleagues.

At the time of initial diagnosis, the sensitivity of tumor tissue to cytotoxic agents is greatest and there is also the greatest opportunity for cure. Thus, the most active agents should be used in combinations and in maximum dosages tolerated for front-line (initial) treatment. Holding highly active agents in reserve for treatment of potential relapse should be avoided. Clones of cells resistant to the "reserved" drugs are likely to emerge anyway when the tumor recurs, because of the phenomenon of multidrug resistance. A recent treatment concept which deserves attention advocates the use of alternating combinations of noncross-resistant drugs to prevent the emergence of resistant cell clones.[10] Unfortunately, evidence from studies of human RMSs xenografted into immunodeprived mice does not support this concept. These murine studies suggest that exposure to many of the active drugs currently used for initial treatment of RMS leads to cross-resistance to each other as well as to newer agents.[11]

IV. "STANDARD" CHEMOTHERAPY REGIMENS

The standard chemotherapeutic agents used for RMS, extraosseous Ewing's sarcoma, and undifferentiated sarcoma are vincristine, actinomycin D, cyclophosphamide, and adriamycin (doxorubicin) used in combinations of two, three, or four drugs.[5,6] The more intensive therapy is used for more advanced neoplastic disease. The two conventional regimens that are most often used are (1) intensive vincristine and actinomycin D, termed "intensive VA", and (2) the combination of vincristine, actinomycin D, and cyclophosphamide, termed "pulse VAC". When adriamycin was substituted for actinomycin D or added to these regimens, no additional gain in survival was seen, although adriamycin is an active agent when used alone.[5,6] Current IRS studies are evaluating the addition of cisplatin and etoposide (VP-16) to the VA and VAC regimens.[7]

A. INTENSIVE VA

This regimen consists of (1) actinomycin D, 0.015 mg/kg/day intravenously for 5 days (maximum single dose, 0.5 mg) starting on day 0, and (2) vincristine, 2 mg/m² intravenously weekly for six doses (maximum single dose, 2 mg) starting on day 21. Drug dosages are reduced by 50% in children less than 1 year of age. If the drugs are tolerated, the doses are increased to 75% and then to 100%. This two-drug regimen is repeated every 9 weeks for a total of six courses given in 53 weeks. If postoperative radiation is to be given, it should begin concomitantly with the first course of chemotherapy.

There is extensive experience with this two-drug regimen. It was first used by Children's Cancer Study Group and then in IRS I to III. At the present time, it is the IRS "standard" therapy for patients with nonalveolar tumors who are classified as clinical group I (localized disease, completely resected, nodes negative) and clinical group II (regional disease, grossly resected, nodes positive or negative). Disease-free survival is approximately 85% for clinical group I and 70% for clinical group II patients at 5 years. Tumor recurrences are equally divided between local/regional and metastatic sites.

B. PULSE VAC

Details of this regimen are outlined in Table 1. This regimen has been used extensively in the IRS studies for RMS patients with clinical group III (gross residual disease after surgery) and group IV (metastatic disease at diagnosis). The complete remission rate with this therapy is approximately 50 to 70%, and an additional 20% of patients attain a partial response. The median time to complete response is 12 to 16 weeks, although it may take as long as a year to attain such a response. About one-third of patients achieve a complete response prior to the administration of radiation therapy at week 6. Adriamycin and actinomycin D are equally effective in inducing a remission with this regimen. As expected,

TABLE 1
Outline of the Pulse VAC Regimen for Chemotherapy of Rhabdomyosarcoma

Vincristine, 2 mg/m^2, intravenously weekly for 13 doses (covering 12 weeks) starting on day 0 (maximum single dose, 2 mg), followed by a dose at week 16

Actinomycin D, 0.015 mg/kg/day, intravenously weekly for 5 days starting on day 0, day 84 (week 12), and day 112 (week 16) (maximum single dose, 0.5 mg)

Cyclophosphamide, 10 mg/kg/day, intravenously for 3 days starting on day 0, day 84 (week 12), and day 112 (week 16), and then one dose of 20 mg/kg intravenously is given on days 21, 42, and 63; however, cyclophosphamide should be omitted on days 42 and 63 in children who have the urinary bladder included in the radiation portal or who will have large volumes of bone marrow irradiated, such as irradiation to the whole abdomen, including the pelvic bones

Radiotherapy is given to the tumor bed as well as to any sites of metastases starting on day 42 (week 6); starting at week 20, the following course is repeated every 4 weeks through week 104

Vincristine, 2 mg/m^2, intravenously, on days 0 and 4 (maximum single dose, 2 mg)

Actinomycin D, 0.015 mg/kg/d intravenously for 5 days starting on day 0 (maximum single dose, 0.5mg)

Cyclophosphamide, 10 mg/kg/day intravenously for 3 days starting on day 0

Drug dosages are reduced by 50% in patients under 1 year of age; if the drugs are tolerated, doses are increased to 75 and then 100%.

TABLE 2
Recommended Doses for Triple Intrathecal Chemotherapy for Patients with Parameningeal Rhabdomyosarcomas. Drug Dosages and Total Volume Injected (Drug Plus Diluent) Is Given for Each Age Group

	Age			
Drug	Up to 1 year (4 ml)	2 years (6 ml)	3 years or older (8 ml)	9 years or older (10 ml)
Methotrexate,[a] mg	6	9	12	12
Hydrocortisone, mg	6	9	12	15
Cytosine arabinoside, mg	12	18	24	30

[a]   Calcium leucovorin is given as a single oral or intravenous dose 24 h after giving triple intrathecal chemotherapy, in the same dosage as the intrathecal methotrexate.

outcome is better for patients in group III than for group IV patients. At 5 years, the rate of disease-free survival is 69% and survival is 64% for group III patients as compared to disease-free survival of 38% and survival of 30% for group IV patients. Tumor recurrences are equally divided between local/regional and distant metastatic sites. Adding adriamycin to this regimen has not improved the outcome.

Patients with clinical group III or IV disease may present with cranial parameningeal sarcoma with tumors originating in nasopharynx, nasal cavity, nasal sinus, middle ear-mastoid region, or in the pterygopalatine and infratemporal fossae. These patients have a high risk of developing intracranial tumor by direct extension.[12] High risk patients are those with bone erosion at the base of the skull, cranial nerve palsy, and, of course, those who already show intracranial tumor at the time of diagnosis.[13] In addition to radiation therapy, patients at high risk of meningeal extension should receive intrathecal chemotherapy at weeks 0, 6, 12, and 20. Those patients with evidence of intracranial tumor should continue to receive intrathecal chemotherapy beyond week 20, with doses given every 8 weeks for up to 2 years from the date of the start of treatment. The dosages for triple intrathecal chemotherapy are listed in Table 2.

Primary repetitive pulse VAC therapy has also been given to patients with localized tumors arising in the bladder, prostate, vagina, or uterus.[3] However, this therapy does not provide durable bladder salvage, although survival is similar to that of patients treated with primary surgery. The 5-year survival rate with either approach (pulse VAC or primary

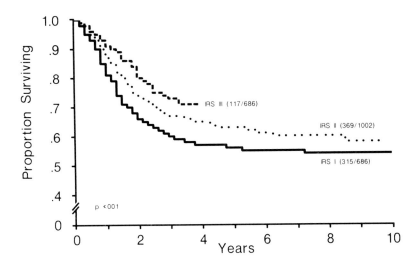

FIGURE 1. Comparison of the overall survival curves for all eligible patients entered on
IRS-I (1972—1978), IRS-II (1978—1984), and IRS-III (1984—1988). Numbers in parentheses represent deaths/total patients.

surgery) is approximately 70%, and approximately 25% of the bladders are retained at 3
years.

Patients with clinical groups I and II alveolar RMSs, particularly those with extremity
tumors, require more intensive therapy than their nonalveolar counterparts.[14] These patients
should receive the regimen of repetitive pulse VAC therapy as recommended for clinical
group III patients, but treatment may be stopped after 1 year of chemotherapy. Using this
strategy, disease-free survival is 69% and survival is 77% for these patients at 5 years.

V. CHEMOTHERAPY STRATEGIES IN IRS-III

The impact of the IRSs on patient survival has been significant since the start of these
studies in 1972. For the pre-IRS period 1963—1972, the End Results Program of the National
Intitutes of Health reported a 5-year survival rate of 28% for patients in all stages of RMS
combined, 54% survival for localized disease, 22% for regional disease, 8% for metastatic
disease, and 13% for unknown disease stage. Since the IRS registers approximately three
quarters of the cases of RMS that occur in the U.S., the accomplishments of the IRS have
had a very favorable impact on a large segment of patients with this tumor. In addition,
there has been diffusion of IRS therapy programs to nonparticipating patients in the U.S.
and to oncologists and their patients elsewhere in the world.

IRS-III began in 1984 and was closed to entry for all but a few strata of patients in
1988.[7] Patient follow-up is too short to report any results other than overall outcome. At 3
years, the overall survival rate of 73% is superior to that of IRS-II, in which there was a
survival rate of 67%, and IRS-I, with survival of 60%, ($p < 0.001$) (Figure 1). The same
relationship between IRS-III and the earlier IRS results is true for rate of prolonged complete
remission. The rate of prolonged complete remission (at 3 years) was 76% for IRS-III vs.
69% for IRS-II vs. 64% for IRS-I ($p < 0.001$) (Figure 2). The major improvement is in
group III which comprises 53% of all patients on study. Overall survival in group III is
80%, as compared to a survival rate of 69% in IRS-II and 57% in IRS-I ($p < 0.001$) (Figure
3). Combining all nonmetastatic patients (groups I, II, and III), the results show a definite
improvement in survival and complete response duration in IRS-III compared to IRS-II and
IRS-I. However, group IV patients given IRS-III therapy showed no improvement in outcome
compared to similar patients in IRS-II.

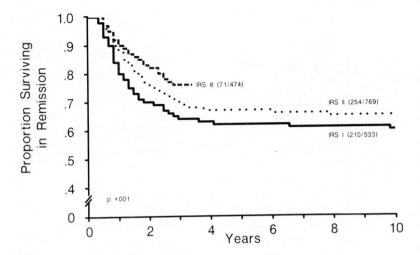

FIGURE 2.   Comparison of the complete remission duration curves for all eligible patients entered on IRS-I (1972—1978), IRS-II (1978—1984), and IRS-III (1984—1988). Numbers in parentheses represent treatment failures/total patients.

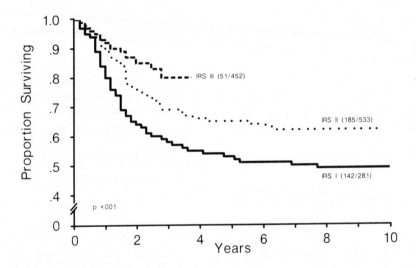

FIGURE 3.   Comparison of the overall survival curves for all eligbile clinical group III patients entered on IRS-I (1972—1978), IRS-II (1978—1984), and IRS-III (1984—1988). Numbers in parentheses represent deaths/total patients.

Treatments consisted of two to seven drugs given in combination, radiation therapy in all but group I patients with nonalveolar histology, second and third surgical operations (to document response and to excise residual disease), and intensification chemotherapy for patients who show partial response. Drugs used were combinations of vincristine, actinomycin D, cyclophosphamide, adriamycin, cisplatin, etoposide, and DTIC, which were given for 1 to 2 years. Treatments were assigned or randomized according to clinical group, histology, and primary site of tumor. IRS-III treatment protocols are more intensive than prior IRS regimens, and include multiple chemotherapeutic agents given at maximum tolerated doses, plus radiation therapy and additional surgical operations. Although more intensive, the 2% fatality rate due to drug toxicity in IRS-III was identical to that in IRS-I and II.

Details of the therapeutic strategies underscore the complex nature of this tumor. Clinical group I patients with nonalveolar tumors receive the intensive vincristine and actinomycin D (VA) regimen for 1 year without radiation therapy. Group II patients with nonalveolar tumors received postoperative irradiation and intensive VA with or without adriamycin an a randomized trial. Group II patients with paratesticular primary lesions are an exception and receive only the two-drug regimen (vincristine and antinomycin D) because their prognosis is quite favorable (85% 5-year survival). Group I and II patients with alveolar tumors receive postoperative radiation therapy, together with repetitive courses of pulse VAC plus adriamycin plus cisplatin for 1 year.

Clinical group III patients, excluding those with nonalveolar tumors of the orbit, scalp, cheek, oral cavity, parotid, larynx, and oropharynx, are randomized to receive either repetitive pulse VAC or the same agents along with adriamycin and cisplatin, or with adriamycin, cisplatin, and etoposide. All of these patients receive postoperative radiation therapy beginning at week 6. Second-look surgery is done at week 20 to document response and remove residual neoplastic disease. If patients are still in partial response after surgery, they receive "intensification" with either adriamycin plus DTIC, with actinomycin D plus etoposide, or with actinomycin D plus DTIC, depending upon which drugs they had received initially. A third surgical operation may be done after this course of therapy. Initial therapy is then continued to complete a period of 2 years from the start of chemotherapy. Group III patients with nonalveolar tumors of the head are treated with postoperative radiation and the intensive VA regimen for 1 year because of their more favorable prognosis as compared to other group III patients. Clinical group IV patients are treated like group III patients, except that there are no exclusions. Patients with cranial parameningeal RMSs are treated with radiation therapy and triple intrathecal chemotherapy as described above, in addition to being given their systemic chemotherapy.

Patients with localized tumors of the dome of the bladder, uterus, and vagina are treated differently than patients with localized tumors of the bladder neck or prostate. The former group (those with tumors of the bladder dome, uterus, and vagina) receives primary chemotherapy consisting of repetitive courses of pulse VAC plus adriamycin and cisplatin. Radiation therapy and surgery are reserved for cases with residual neoplastic disease. In the group with tumors of the bladder neck and prostate, radiation therapy is routinely given beginning at week 6 and surgery is used as needed for removal of residual disease. "Intensification" chemotherapy with two additional drugs is used in either case for patients who attain only a partial response. Patients with lesions of the bladder neck and prostate tend to fail with the primary chemotherapy approach and lose their bladders because of locally persistent or recurrent tumors. Thus, radiation therapy is incorporated in the treatment program for all patients with tumors originating at these primary sites.

VI. CHEMOTHERAPY STRATEGIES IN IRS-IV

Since the results of IRS-III are too early to be considered mature and stable, it is not possible to build a new study on the basis of IRS-III data. Thus, IRS-IV will take a different approach. IRS-IV will study promising "new" drugs given in combinations, use of hyperfractionated radiation therapy, and a new pretreatment staging classification which is based on the TNM system.

The "new" cytotoxic drugs that will be used are ifosfamide, etoposide, and melphalan.[15-17] Attractive combinations to be studied are ifosfamide plus etoposide, ifosfamide plus adriamycin, and melphalan plus vincristine. Ifosfamide, etoposide, and melphalan were shown to be highly active agents in the murine xenograft model as well as in clinical trials. The combination of ifosfamide and etoposide has been highly effective when given to previously treated patients, producing three complete responses and six partial responses in a group of 13 patients.[17] Other studies suggest that ifosfamide is superior to cyclophosphamide in treatment of some cyclophosphamide-resistant tumors.[18]

The overall strategy in IRS-IV for patients with tumor classified as pretreatment TNM stages 1, 2, and 3 will be a comparison of the following drug combinations: (1) VAC; (2) vincristine, actinomycin D, and ifosfamide (VAI); and (3) vincristine, ifosfamide, and etoposide (VIE). The trial will provide information comparing the efficacy of cyclophosphamide and ifosfamide, as well as comparing the efficacy of ifosfamide vs. the combination of ifosfamide and etoposide.

Since progress in treatment of patients with stage 4 (metastatic) RMSs has been minimal at best, an entirely new approach will be taken for treatment of this group. These patients will be treated initially with various two-drug regimens in a fashion resembling a phase II trial. After 12 weeks, they will be switched to a regimen consisting of repetitive courses of pulse VAC for the remainder of their chemotherapy. A comparison of the efficacy of the initial therapies will be made followed by efforts to detect clinical cross-resistance to subsequent therapy with pulse VAC. The two-drug regimens to which patients will be randomized are melphalan-vincristine, ifosfamide-etoposide, and ifosfamide-adriamycin. At the end of this trial, it is hoped that the relative effectiveness of these combinations will be apparent in rank order. A subsequent trial will use this information to possibly construct a more effective treatment plan than has been available heretofore for these patients with advanced disease.

VII. OTHER CHEMOTHERAPY STRATEGIES

The authors' European colleagues have been actively engaged in chemotherapeutic trials that are described in detail elsewhere in this book. The SIOP has been evaluating vincristine, antinomycin D, and ifosfamide, referred to as the IVA regimen, as initial therapy for patients in TNM stages 1 to 3 in a nonrandomized study.[19,20] The doses of drugs given are less intense than those in the proposed IRS-IV study and radiotherapy is not included routinely. Early results suggest an excellent complete response rate of 89%, including a response rate of 64% after giving the IVA regimen alone. However, the relapse rate is high, with only 54% of patients being in continuous remission at 2 years. Local recurrence is the chief problem in patients not receiving radiation therapy. Intensification of the IVA chemotherapy regimen is proposed in the successor study.

In the current German study, CWS-86, adriamycin is added to the IVA regimen in a nonrandomized trial. In this study the complete response rate after 7 weeks of treatment is used as a prognostic factor, with subsequent altering of therapy in patients showing poor responses.[21,22] The results of the trial are too early to report.

Investigators at the National Cancer Institute (NCI) studied high risk patients, defined as group III patients with primary tumors of the chest wall, retroperitoneum, perineum, and extremity, and group IV patients. These patients were treated with intensive courses of vincristine, adriamycin, and cyclophosphamide given in combination with radiation therapy, followed by a total body irradiation and autologous bone marrow replacement for those patients achieving a complete response.[23] The actuarial overall survival rate at 24 months was 68% and the disease-free survival rate was 48%. IRS-II treatment is at least as effective without being as intensive.

The SIOP is undertaking a new study of patients with clinical group IV RMSs, using carboplatin, epirubicin, ifosfamide, and actinomycin D in combination.[24] Patients attaining only a partial response will receive autologous bone marrow transplantation as additional induction therapy.

Investigators at Memorial Sloan-Kettering Cancer Center have reported preliminary results using alternating combination chemotherapy and hyperfractionated radiation therapy for patients with group III or group IV disease.[25] Induction therapy consisted of two cycles of VAC plus adriamycin, bleomycin, and methotrexate; the maintenance program included the same drugs given at reduced dosages. Radiation was delivered to the primary site twice a day in two separate courses during the period of induction therapy. The local control rate was 83% (10 out of 12 patients) and the overall survival was 58% (7 of 12 patients) at a median follow-up of 25 months. Compliance with the protocol was significantly improved over that of previous protocols in which concomitant chemotherapy and radiation therapy were given.

VIII. CONCLUSIONS

Significant progress has been made in the chemotherapy of nonmetastatic RMS, extraosseous Ewing's sarcoma, and undifferentiated sarcoma. However, metastatic disease, which is present in approximately 18% of the patients, continues to resist long-term control by current chemotherapy regimens. Treatment programs using newer agents, new combinations of drugs and novel strategies, or higher doses of existing effective agents are being tried. Also, these new chemotherapy regimens, when combined with the administration of hematopoietic growth factors, such as G-CSF or GM-CSF, and bone marrow transplantation, are potential therapies which may improve the outcome for these patients. An additional challenge will be the survival of these patients without late complications of therapy. With intensive research efforts underway internationally, these challenges may be met.

ACKNOWLEDGMENTS

This work was supported in part by the Department of Health and Human Services, Bethesda, MD, USPHS Grants CA-24507, CA-30138, CA-30969, CA-29139, and CA-13539, and the American Lebanon Syrian Associated Charities (ALSAC), Memphis, TN.

REFERENCES

1. **Heyn, R., Holland, R., Newton, W. A., et al.,** The role of combined chemotherapy in the treatment of rhabdomyosarcoma in children, *Cancer,* 34, 2128, 1974.
2. **Wilbur, J. R.,** Combination chemotherapy of embryonal rhabdomyosarcoma, *Cancer Chemother. Rep.,* 58, 281, 1974.
3. **Raney, R. B., Gehan, E. A., Hays, D. M., et al.,** Primary chemotherapy with or without radiation therapy and/or surgery for children with localized sarcoma of the bladder, prostate, vagina, uterus, and cervix: comparison of results in Intergroup Rhabdomyosarcoma Studies I and II, *Cancer,* 66, 2072, 1990.
4. **Weiner, E. S., Hays, D. M., Lawrence, W., et al.,** Second-look operations in children with groups III and IV rhabdomyosarcoma, *Proc. Am. Soc. Clin. Oncol.,* 8, 301, 1989.
5. **Maurer, H. M., Beltangady, M., Gehan, E. A., et al.,** The Intergroup Rhabdomyosarcoma Study-I: a final report, *Cancer,* 61, 209, 1988.
6. **Maurer, H. M., Gehan, E. A., Beltangady, M., et al.,** The Intergroup Rhabdomyosarcoma Study-II, *Cancer,* in press.
7. **Maurer, H. M., Gehan, E. A., Crist, W., et al.,** Intergroup Rhabdomyosarcoma Study-III. A preliminary report of overall outcome, *Proc. Am. Soc. Clin. Oncol.,* 8, 296, 1989.
8. **Lawrence, W., Gehan, E. A., Hays, D. M., et al.,** Prognostic significance of staging factors of the UICC staging system in childhood rhabdomyosarcoma: a report of the Intergroup Rhabdomyosarcoma Study-III, *J. Clin. Oncol.,* 5, 46, 1987.
9. **Gehan, E. A., Lawrence, W., Hays, D. M., et al.,** Pre-treatment staging system for pediatric rhabdomyosarcoma patients, *Proc. Am. Soc. Clin. Oncol.,* 7, 255, 1988.
10. **Goldie, J. H., Coldman, A. J., and Gudauskas, G. A.,** Rationale for use of alternating noncross resistant chemotherapy, *Cancer Treat. Rep.,* 6, 439, 1982.
11. **Horton, J. K., Houghton, P. J., and Houghton, J. A.,** Reciprocal cross-resistance in human rhabdomyosarcomas selected in vivo for primary resistance to vincristine or L-phenylalanine mustard, *Cancer Res.,* 47, 6288, 1987.

12. **Tefft, M., Fernandez, C., Donaldson, M., et al.,** Incidence of meningeal involvement by rhabdomyosarcoma of the head and neck in children. A report of the Intergroup Rhabdomyosarcoma Study, *Cancer,* 42, 253, 1978.

13. **Raney, R. B., Tefft, M., Newton, W. A., et al.,** Improved prognosis with intensive treatment of children with cranial soft tissue sarcomas arising in non-orbital parameningeal sites: a report from the Intergroup Rhabdomyosarcoma Study, *Cancer,* 59, 147, 1987.

14. **Heyn, R., Beltangady, M., Hays, D. M., et al.,** Results of intensive therapy in children with localized alveolar extremity rhabdomyosarcoma: a report from the Intergroup Rhabdomyosarcoma Study, *J. Clin. Oncol.,* 7, 200, 1989.

15. **Horowitz, M., Etcubanas, E., Christensen, M. L., et al.,** Phase II testing by melphalan in children with newly diagnosed rhabdomyosarcoma: a model for anticancer drug development, *J. Clin. Oncol.,* 6, 308 1988.

16. **Pratt, C. B., Douglass, E., Etcubanas, E., et al.,** Clinical studies of ifosfamidel/mesna at St. Jude Children's Research Hospital, 1983—1988, *Sem. Oncol.,* 16, 51, 1989.

17. **Miser, J. S., Kinsella, T. J., Triche, T. J., et al.,** Ifosfamide with mesna uroprotection and etoposide: an effective regimen in the treatment of recurrent sarcomas and other tumors of children and young adults, *J. Clin. Oncol.,* 5, 1191, 1987.

18. **Hilgard, P., Herdrich, K., and Brade, W.,** Ifosfamide; current aspects and perspectives, *Cancer Treat. Rev.,* 10, 183, 1983.

19. **Otten, J., Flamant, F., Rodary, C., et al.,** Treatment of malignant mesenchymal tumors of childhood with ifosfamide + vincristine + actinomycin D (IVA) as front-line therapy. A report on a study by the International Society of Pediatric Oncology, *Proc. Am. Soc. Clin. Oncol.,* 6, 223, 1987.

20. **Rodary, C., Rey, A., Olive, D., et al.,** Prognostic factors in 281 children with non-metastatic rhabdomyosarcoma at diagnosis, *Med. Pediatr. Oncol.,* 16, 71, 1988.

21. **Treuner, J., Suder, J., Keim, M., Kaatsch, P., and Neithammer, D.,** The predictive value of initial cytostatic response in primary unresectable rhabdomyosarcoma in children, *Acta Oncol.,* 28, 67, 1989.

22. **Treuner, J., Koscielnia, E., Snyder, J., et al.,** Results of the German Rhabdomyosarcoma Study (CWS-81). Analysis according to the international agreement on common description of the tumor, in *Proc. Int. Soc. Pediatric Oncology,* Jerusalem, Israel, September 13, 1987, 47.

23. **Kinsella, T. J., Miser, J. S., Triche, T. J., et al.,** Treatment of high risk sarcomas in children and young adults: analysis of local control using intensive combined modality therapy, *Natl. Cancer Inst. Monogr.,* 6, 291, 1988.

24. **Treuner, J., Carli, M., Flamant, F., et al.,** Outline of the SIOP European study on metastatic rhabdomyosarcoma in children, presented at the meeting of the Int. Soc. Pediatric Oncology, Trondheim, Norway, August 26, 1988.

25. **Mandell, L. R., Ghavimi, F., Exelby, P., et al.,** Preliminary results of alternating combination chemotherapy and hyperfractionated radiotherapy in advanced rhabdomyosarcoma, *Int. J. Radiat. Oncol. Biol. Phys.,* 15, 197, 1988.

Chapter 12

DISSEMINATED INTRAVASCULAR COAGULOPATHY, HYPERCALCEMIA, AND HYPERURICEMIA IN RHABDOMYOSARCOMA

Frederick B. Ruymann and Paul Thomas

TABLE OF CONTENTS

I. INTRODUCTION

The complications of disseminated intravascular coagulation (DIC) and hypercalcemia in rhabdomyosarcoma (RMS) occur most commonly in patients with a large tumor burden. These complications are underreported in the medical literature and they are taken in stride by most pediatric oncologists.

Massive tumor cell kill and the body's consequent response represent the Scylla and Charybdis (perilous channel) through which the patient must safely pass if he or she is to survive the malignancy. It is patients with metastatic RMS who are at greatest risk to develop DIC and hypercalcemia.

II. DISSEMINATED INTRAVASCULAR COAGULOPATHY

A. DESCRIPTION IN RHABDOMYOSARCOMA

In a review of 30 cases of RMS with bone marrow metastases at diagnosis treated on Intergroup Rhabdomyosarcoma Study-I, 3 were found to have had a major problem with DIC.[1] Alveolar histology was present in two of the patients. Bone metastases, as well as bone marrow metastases, were present in all three of the cases. The three patients with DIC came from a group of five who presented with a hemoglobin level of less than 11 g/dl and a platelet count of under 50,000/mm³. Petechiae and bleeding were present in three and two of the patients developed shock due to hypovolemia. Cancer chemotherapy was continued in all instances. Supportive care with platelet and red cell transfusions was the standard therapy used. One patient required transfusion of whole blood and fresh frozen plasma. Heparin was not utilized in any of the patients. Resolution of the DIC occurred gradually over a period of 1½ to 4 weeks, as the tumors went into remission with continued chemotherapy.

Twelve cases of DIC in patients with RMS, including the three just mentioned, were reported from 1952 to the present.[1-8] Ten of these cases with adequate data are summarized in Table 1.[1,2,4-8] The authors are aware of many other instances in their own experience and those of their colleagues which have not been reported. Investigators from the Institut Gustave-Roussy passingly mentioned five cases of DIC which occurred in association with metastatic RMS in a discussion of hypercalcemia in pediatric solid tumors.[9] Several of the early cases of DIC were probably not recognized as being related to a consumptive coagulopathy since the pathophysiology of this entity was identified only relatively recently.

B. PATHOPHYSIOLOGY

Traditionally, the occurrence of DIC in solid tumors has been attributed to tumor cell embolization or destruction of endothelium due to tumor invasion.[10-12] Findings in the reported cases of RMS and DIC support this mechanism. Bone marrow metastases were documented in half of the patients with DIC and RMS. Bone marrow metastases are present at the time of diagnosis in about one third of patients with metastatic disease.[1] Metastases to some locations are present in about one fifth of patients diagnosed with RMS registered on IRS-I and IRS-II.[13,14] Therefore, the expected incidence of overt bone marrow metastases in newly diagnosed patients with RMS is 1 in 15 or about 7%.

Circulating rhabdomyoblasts occur more commonly in patients with bone marrow metastases and were identified in case 7. Obstruction of the dural veins by tumor cells and subsequent DIC has been the mechanism proposed for the subdural hematoma in case 9.[8] Review of five additional cases of subdural hematoma in adults with metastatic solid tumors showed microscopic invasion of the dural veins by tumor cells. Patients with RMS who have either meningeal metastases or central nervous system extension from a parameningeal site are at increased risk to develop a subdural hematoma by this mechanism.

TABLE 1
Disseminated Intravascular Coagulation in Patients with Rhabdomyosarcoma

Case #	Age/Sex	Histology	Site	Metastatic sites	Initial laboratory studies						Signs of bleeding	Chemotherapy	Transfusion support	Heparin	Steriod	Recovery from DIC	Ref.
					Platelet (× 10³/μl)	Hgb (g/dl)	PT (s)	PTT (s)	Fibrinogen (mg/dl)	FDP (μg/ml)							
1	64 years/male	Embryonal by description	Rectus-abdominus	Liver, mesenteric bowel	—	8—9 g	—	—	—	—	Melena	None recorded		No	No	No	2
2	44 years/male	Alveolar	Retroperitoneal psoas	Diffuse abdominal involvement, chest, bones	60	7.9	47	39	215	160	Hematomas, melena	Cyclophosphamide	RBC, platelet	Yes	Yes	No	4
3	14 years/male	Embryonal	Gluteal	Bone marrow	3.0	8.8	26 (12.9)	132 (35.2)	40	328		Actinomycin, vincristine	Platelet	No	No	Yes—recovery in 6 days with remission of tumor	6
4	4 months/male	Embryonal	Flank (huge primary)	None at diagnosis (mets 3 months later)	471—3.0	—	26.3 (9.3)	90.4 (41.0)	115	40	Hemorrhagic, pleural effusion, petechiae	Actinomycin, vincristine	Not stated	No	No	Yes—recovery in 3 weeks with remission of tumor	6
5	8 years/male	Embryonal	Pharyngeal	Base of skull, lymph nodes	180 (150—400)	8.5	16 (60—120)	55 (30—50)	5.0 (2—4)	36	None	VADRC initially, no actinomycin	No	No	No	Chronic DIC, no bleeding	5
6	18 years/male	Alveolar	Maxillary sinus	Bone marrow, CNS, extension, lymph node	140	26.3 (Hct)	164 (11—14)	27 (27—39)	240	32	Epistaxsis, ecchymosis	Yes	Yes	No	No	Yes	7
7	17 years/female	Suspect embryonal	Buccal	Bone marrow, bone (meningeal)	19	9.2	14.5 (11.8)	46.9 (42.7)	298	40	Petechiae	Yes	Yes	Yes	No	Yes	8
8	11 years/male	Embryonal	Parotid	Bone marrow, bone	18	8.0					Petechiae, shock	VAC + ADR	RBC	No	No	Yes—recovery on day 26 with partial remission of tumor	1
9	15 years/female	Alveolar	Maxillary sinus	Bone marrow, bone, lymph node	48	8.8					Petechiae bleeding shock	VAC + ADR	RBC, platelet, whole blood, FFP	No	No	Yes	1
10	17 years/female	Alveolar	Retroperitoneal	Bone marrow, bone	21	9.5					Petechaie, hematuria	VAC + ADR	RBC, platelet	Yes	Yes	Yes—recovery on day 10 with partial remission of tumor	1

The balance between the production and consumption of coagulation factors in the patient with cancer is altered by cancer chemotherapy.[3,6,11,12] Not surprisingly, the 12 reported patients were initially made worse by chemotherapy. Thrombocytopenia, one of the hallmarks of DIC, was absent in case 6, but with the initiation of vincristine and actinomycin D the platelet count plummeted from 417,000 to 3000/mm^3. In case 7, there was a chronic DIC state, without overt bleeding, manifested by a shortened prothrombin time and increased fibrinogen catabolism, as shown by studies using I^{131}-labeled fibrinogen.[5] Since fibrinogen turnover studies are so infrequently done, chronic DIC may be more common than this single case would suggest. Increased fibrinogen production to five times normal has been documented in experimentally induced chronic DIC in mice following implantation of a plasma cell tumor.[15]

In screening for DIC, attention is often given to the prolonged prothrombin (PT) and partial thromboplastin (PTT) times. The most common hemostatic finding, however, in 50 adult patients with disseminated malignancy was a hypercoagulable state, which was manifested by a shortened bleeding time, coagulation time, and PTT.[11] Increased production of clotting factors with consequent shortening of the prothrombin time and PTT are probably triggered by both the release of thromboplastic substances by the tumor and increased endothelial injury resulting from hematogenous metastases or direct tumor extension. An extract of neuroblastoma tissue, which had caused DIC in a 4-year-old child, was tested in a thromboplastic activity assay.[16] The neuroblastoma extract had thromboplastic activity as potent as brain tissue, while extracts of normal adrenal gland had hardly any influence on the recalcification time.

Tumor progression has been associated with an increase in the levels of factor VIII antigen and factor VIII coagulant activity, as well as an increase in the ratio of ristocetin cofactor to factor VIII antigen.[16] In case 6, a unique factor VIII antigen was observed to be associated with DIC.[7] A slow-moving factor VIII antigen seen on crossed immunoelectrophoresis occurred in the presence of overt tumor, which disappeared during remission. An altered factor VIII molecule, or a phenomenon related to the DIC itself, was probably not the source of this slow-moving factor VIII antigen. The formation of a factor VIII antigen by a tumor product, or by synthesis of a neofactor VIII antigen by the tumor, are two proposed explanations.[7] These observations require confirmation and may lead to a more precise explanation of the pathophysiology of DIC in RMS.

C. MANAGEMENT

The successful management of DIC in a patient with RMS demands continued treatment of the underlying malignancy. The process of intravascular coagulation may initially be aggravated by chemotherapy. However, the continuity of cancer chemotherapy should be maintained, since it is the only approach which will, in the short run, stop the thromboplastin-generating malignancy, and in the long run, cure the patient. In discussing the management of DIC in patients with disseminated cancer, one author stated: "Therapy of the defibrination syndrome may be that of the underlying disease (if this is possible) or of the thrombotic state which complicates it."[3]

This same principle of treating the underlying disease has been affirmed in investigations on DIC in septicemia.[18] Septicemia often complicates advanced malignancy in children and should be considered in the differential diagnosis of a microangiopathic, hemolytic anemia. Supportive transfusions with platelets, fresh frozen plasma, and red cells are necessary to maintain capillary integrity, normal levels of circulating clotting factors, and an adequate blood volume.

Heparin may play a role in the treatment of tumor-associated DIC, but use of heparin is a distant third in priority behind cancer chemotherapy and supportive transfusion therapy. In the authors' experience, a low dose continuous infusion of heparin at 10 to 15 units/kg/h, as recommended for use in newborns, has been effective in managing otherwise uncontrollable DIC in childhood malignancies.[19] An initial bolus of heparin at 25 to 35 units/kg may be given prior to starting the low dose continuous infusion. A low dose infusion will minimize the prolonged heparin half-life associated with renal insufficiency. A continuous infusion avoids the antithrombin surge of a high dose heparin bolus which may precipitate new bleeding. Care must be taken to maintain platelet levels and clotting factors at adequate levels during heparin therapy, so as not to taunt hemorrhage. Massive hemorrhage occurred in case 10 when heparin was administered for a presumed renal vein thrombosis. Bleeding continued in spite of giving more than 20 units of platelets in 24 h. A subdural hemorrhage, such as occurred in case 9, will usually require surgical intervention.[8]

In summary, patients at high risk for DIC with RMS are older. They have metastatic disease with bone marrow or bone metastases, anemia, thrombocytopenia, and microangiopathic changes of red cells on the peripheral blood smear. Circulating rhabdomyoblasts may also be seen. If petechiae, bleeding, or ecchymoses are present in this context, DIC is well under way. Screening with the prothrombin time and PTT time is indicated in all patients with massive tumor burden. However, these tests may be shortened, normal, or only minimally prolonged. Evaluation of fibrinogen and fibrin degradation products is also useful.

Prolonged PT and PTT times, in the absence of liver disease, usually represent the failure of compensatory clotting factor overproduction to keep ahead of consumption of clotting factors. A worsening of clotting studies in such patients can be expected when chemotherapy is initiated. Continued administration of cancer chemotherapy and supportive transfusion therapy are the mainstays of patient care. Use of heparin should be reserved for cases in which the application of supportive measures does not maintain normal hemostasis.

III. HYPERCALCEMIA

A. DESCRIPTION IN RHABDOMYOSARCOMA

Hypercalcemia is an uncommon finding in a child presenting with a solid tumor. In a review of 2400 children with solid tumors from the period 1976 to 1982 treated at the Institut Gustave-Roussy, only 17 (0.7%) had hypercalcemia.[9] In 915 eligible cases with RMS entered on IRS-III, only 4 (0.4%) were identified as having serum calcium levels higher than 11.0 mg/dl. Eight cases of major hypercalcemia in children with RMS have been adequately described.[9,20-23] The major features of these cases are reviewed in Table 2; all calcium values have been converted to milligrams per deciliter for comparability. A ninth case of the authors is presented here.

B. REPORT OF A CASE

A 13-year-old boy presented at the referring hospital with a rapidly enlarging left testicle. At surgery, a large paratesticular mass was identified and a radical orchiectomy was performed. At this time, all laboratory evaluations, including calcium, BUN, and uric acid, were reported as normal. Three days after the orchiectomy, a scalp nodule was biopsied. Histologically, both the paratesticular mass and the scalp nodule were consistent with alveolar RMS. On admission, the patient was a moderately lethargic adolescent who complained of nausea. Apart from the well-healed surgical scars and absence of the left testicle, the physical examination was unremarkable.

Initial chest X-ray demonstrated lytic lesions in the metaphyseal area of both proximal humeri, with no pulmonary metastases. Laboratory studies revealed a normal routine blood count and urinalysis. The serum chemical determinations showed: calcium, 17.8 mg/dl; phosphorus, 3.8 mg/dl; uric acid, 16.2 mg/dl; BUN, 43 mg/dl; and creatinine, 2.1 mg/dl. An electrocardiogram was normal. A metastatic bone survey showed multiple lucencies in virtually all metaphyseal areas, including the pelvic bones. A bone scan was initially reported

TABLE 2
Rhabdomyosarcoma with Hypercalcemia

Case #	Age/sex	Histology	Site	Metastatic site	Serum calcium (mg/dl)	Creatinine	Treatment	MECH PTH ↑	Chemotherapy	Best tumor response	Hypercalcemia response	Survival (month)	Other	Ref.
1	15/female	Alveolar	Perineal	BM with delayed bone	xr13.8	1.7	Saline, furosemide, calcitonin, mithramycin	Yes	Extensive then PD	Minimal	Transient lowering	5		20
2	12/female	Embryonal	Oropharyngeal	Bone, BM	xr15.0	3.0	Saline, furosemide, prednisone, calcitonin	Yes	Extensive	Stable then PD	Transient lowering	A few months		20
3	15/female	Alveolar	Perianal	Pleura, peritoneum, bone	xr18.0	—		No	Extensive/and XRT	PD	Transient lowering	16	Increased, prostaglandin, E$_2$ mouse model	21
4	16/male	Undifferentiated	Paratesticular	Lung, LN; bone, BN	xr16.4	6.8	Saline, calcitonin, mithramycin, indomethacin	Yes	VC, ADR, VAC	Stable then PD	Decreased when	12	Increased, osteoclasts	22
5	12/male	Alveolar	Calf	Bone, BM, breast, LN	xr12.8	—		—	VAC, ADR	PD	Transient lowering	3		9
6	14/female	Alveolar	Forearm	Bone, BM, LN, breast	xr14.8	—		—	VAC, ADR	CR		17		9
7	13/female	Embryonal	Shoulder	Bone, BM; BM; LN; breast	xr15.1	—		—	VAC, ADR	CR		12	Associated, DIC at diagnosis	9
8	13/female	Embryonal	Breast	Bone, BM; epidural	xr13.3	—		—	VAC, ADR	PD	Transient lowering	2		9
9	13/male	Alveolar	Paratesticular	Bone	xr17.8	2.1	Saline, allopurinol, furosemide, dexamethasone, calcitonin, mithramycin	—	VAC/XTR/autologous BMT	CR		60	Increased, osteoclasts	This report, 1990

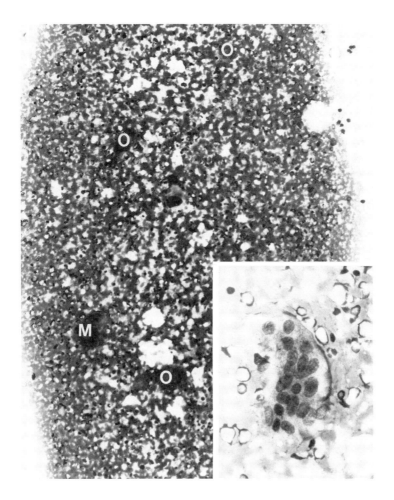

FIGURE 1.   Four osteoclasts (O) and a megakaryocyte (M) in one area of the bone marrow biopsy touch prep. (Wright-Giemsa; magnification × 150.) Inset: osteoclast detail. (Wright-Geimsa; magnification × 900.)

as being normal. However, when the bone scan was compared with the metastatic bone series, the findings were compatible with the presence of multiple, symmetrical areas of increased radionuclide uptake in the mataphyses. There was a marked increase in the number of osteoclasts seen on touch preparations of the bone marrow biopsy (Figure 1). Touch preps contained one to six osteoclasts per low power field. Both the bone marrow aspirate and the biopsy were free of tumor cells.

The early course of therapy for this patient is shown in Figure 2. Initially a high fluid load with normal saline at 4500 ml/m^2/24 h was given, in combination with furosemide, 0.5 mg/kg every 6 h, and dexamethasone, 5 mg/m^2 every 8 h, both intravenously. After 20 h, the serum calcium level was still elevated (17.9 mg/dl). A dose of 25 units of calcitonin was given intravenously at this time with a resultant lowering of the serum calcium to 14.4 mg/dl at 44 h. A dose of mithramycin, 1.0 mg (0.025 mg/kg), was given intravenously at approximately 48 h. A regimen of pulse VAC chemotherapy (consisting of vincristine, actinomycin D, and cyclophosphamide) in accordance with the IRS protocol, was started at 85 h. The patient also received allopurinol, 100 mg orally every 8 h.

Ionized calcium levels were not determined. During the entire course, the levels of serum albumin, phosphorous, and electrolyses were within normal limits. By day 9, the

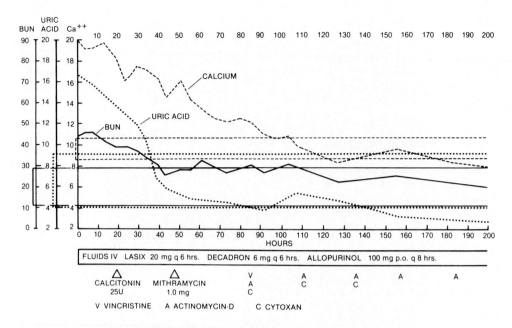

FIGURE 2.   Graph demonstrating the relationship of serum BUN, uric acid, and calcium (Ca²⁺) to treatment during the first 200 h. The normal range of values is indicated on each vertical axis and the boundaries are extended to identify the times during which the patient's values were normal.

serum calcium level had decreased to 7.9 mg/dl. Oral calcium gluconate was started at a dose of 1 g every 6 h for a total of 10 days to correct the hypocalcemia. The serum calcium level returned to normal during the remainder of the hospitalization. Several electrocardiograms performed during the course of therapy were all interpreted as being within normal limits.

The patient subsequently received additional courses of pulse VAC chemotherapy, bone marrow harvesting, whole body irradiation of 500 cGy administered in two half-body fractions, followed by autologous bone marrow transplantation. Reduced maintenance chemotherapy was then given for 2 years. Repeated bone marrow biopsies, while the serum calcium was normal, did not show increased numbers of osteoclasts. Follow-up radiographs showed complete healing of the lytic bone lesions, except for minimal sclerotic changes in the left proximal femur. The patient was free of disease until 4 years from diagnosis, when RMS and hypercalcemia recurred. In spite of extensive chemotherapy and radiotherapy, the patient expired 5 years from initial diagnosis.

The nine reported patients with hypercalcemia and RMS were all teenagers with bone metastases. Seven of the nine also had bone marrow metastases. A female predominance is evident.[9] Alveolar histology was also predominant. In all cases, the most effective treatment in lowering the serum calcium was active chemotherapy directed at the metastatic RMS. A rising or persistently elevated serum calcium always correlated with nonresponsive, progressive, or recurrent RMS. Patient 7 in this series was noted incidentally to also have DIC.

C. PATHOPHYSIOLOGY

Two mechanisms for hypercalcemia have been proposed in patients with RMS. In cases 1 and 2, serum parathyroid hormone (PTH) levels were elevated relative to the serum calcium levels. Although the absolute PTH values never exceeded the normal range, in view of the elevated serum calcium values there was a 96% or greater probability that the PTH levels were increased. In case 4, PTH levels were more than twice normal at diagnosis when the patient presented in renal failure. Temporary improvement in the serum calcium level occurred following chemotherapy, but not with administration of indomethacin alone. Hypercalcemia and elevated PTH values returned when the tumor recurred and became resistant to all therapy.

In case 3, the patient's parathyroid hormone levels were normal. When the patient's RMS was implanted into nude mice, the mice developed hypercalcemia together with prostaglandin E_2 values that were 15 times normal. When indomethacin, a prostaglandin E_2 inhibiter, was given to the mice the serum calcium and prostaglandin E_2 levels were reduced to normal. Both parathyroid hormone and 1 α,25-dihydroxy vitamin D were normal in the serum of tumor-bearing mice. These findings suggested that the elevated prostaglandin E_2, in the absence of any bony metastases, was the cause of the hypercalcemia.

Increased numbers of osteoclasts in the bone marrow aspirate and biopsy were present in cases 4 and 9. The observation of increased osteoclasts in the bone marrow should prompt the performance of a serum calcium level in any patient with a malignant neoplasm.

An increase in PTH of tumor origin was identified as the cause of hypercalcemia in a 6-month-old infant with a localized rhabdoid Wilms' tumor of the kidney and no bony metastases.[23] Raised levels of immune reactive PTH were demonstrated by immunoperoxidase staining in this histologically unique rhabdoid Wilms' tumor.[23] At least six other cases of hypercalcemia with nonmetastatic rhabdoid Wilms' tumors have been reported.[9,24] Since rhabdoid tumors of the kidney comprise less than 2% of Wilms' tumors (8 out of 427 cases) the association with hypercalcemia may be a distinctive feature in this rhabdomyosarcomatous renal malignancy.[25-27]

IV. HYPERURICEMIA

Elevation of the serum uric acid level above 7.0 mg/dl occurred in 47 out of 915 (5%) eligible IRS-III patients registered through August 31, 1989. Of the patients with hyperuricemia, six had values greater than 10 and less than 17 md/dl. These figures are probably underestimates of the incidence of hyperuricemia occurring at the start of the treatment, since in 237 (26%) of the 915 patients registered there was no record of the serum uric acid level.

V. MANAGEMENT OF HYPERCALCEMIA AND HYPERURICEMIA

The incidence of hypercalcemia[28-30] and hyperuricemia[31,32] is higher in an acute lymphoblastic leukemia and non-Hodgkin's lymphoma than in RMS. The management in sarcomas is simplified by the absence of renal infiltration, which occurs so commonly with lymphoid malignancies.[33] An initial and ongoing assessment of renal function, serum electrolytes, serum calcium, phosphorous, and magnesium is basic. A radiographic bone scan, done as part of a metastatic evaluation, will usually be positive in RMS if hypercalcemia is present. Baseline EKG and cardiac monitoring is desirable.

Vigorous hydration with 3000 to 4500 ml/m² of normal saline or 0.45 normal saline in D5W (5% dextrose in water) was used in most of the reported cases. However, caution needs to be taken in the presence of oliguria and renal failure in order to avoid overhydration. Furosemide in a dose of 0.5 mg/kg every 6 h will help maintain an adequate and more predictable urinary output. If shock is present, diuretics should be used with great caution and only with central venous monitoring in an intensive care unit. Intravenous sodium bicarbonate at 3 mEq/kg/d should be given to alkalinize the urine to a Ph of 7.0 to 7.5, provided hyperphosphatemia is not present. If there is evidence of DIC, the maintenance of an adequate blood volume and normal levels of clotting factors will minimize prerenal azotemia and lessen the chance of bleeding. Allopurinol in a dose of 400 mg/m²/day orally or intravenously in three divided doses should be started immediately. The intravenous form of allopurinol is still investigational in the U.S., but can usually be obtained overnight in an emergency by contacting the Burroughs-Wellcome medical representative.

Mithramycin has been slightly more effective than calcitonin in the treatment of hypercalcemia in RMS. If mithramycin is to be given, however, any evidence of renal insufficiency should be resolved. Unquestionably, the most effective means of lowering serum calcium in RMS is by giving multiagent chemotherapy, such as vincristine, actinomycin D, and cyclophosphamide (VAC). Many of the newer chemotherapy regimens contain cisplatin (CPDD) which has significant toxicity for the renal tubule. Presence of renal insufficiency precludes the safe use of this agent. Since multiagent chemotherapy will create a flood of nucleic acid due to rapid breakdown of the targeted sarcoma, it is prudent to wait at least 48 h after starting allopurinol to initiate chemotherapy. A serum uric acid level of less than 6.0 mg/dl is a reasonable goal at which cancer chemotherapy can be initiated.

Obviously, many circumstances could alter these general guidelines. The complications of hypercalcemia and hyperuricemia in RMS may require consultation with a pediatric nephrologist, cariologist, or intensivist, either individually or in combination. Several recent reviews on the management of the tumor lysis syndrome have been published and should serve as basic references.[34-36]

VI. SUMMARY

DIC is associated with bone and bone marrow metastases in RMS and is usually aggravated initially by chemotherapy. The presence of anemia and thrombocytopenia will often identify those at greatest risk for DIC. Hypofibrinogenemia or a prolonged PTT time is associated with ongoing DIC. Treatment of the underlying RMS with the maintenance of platelets, hemoglobin, and circulatory clotting factors is usually adequate to control DIC.

Hypercalcemia and hyperuricemia, like DIC, are associated with metastatic RMS. Tumor-associated parathormone or prostaglandin E_2 may mediate hypercalcemia. The presence of increased osteoclasts on a bone marrow aspirate should prompt evaluation of the serum calcium and a nucleide scan to identify bone metastases. Treatment of the underlying malignancy, hydration, and use of the xanthine oxidase inhibitor, allopurinol, are critical to the successful management of hypercalcemia and hyperuricemia in childhood RMS.

ACKNOWLEDGMENT

The authors are grateful to Miss Dawn Anderson for her assistance in preparing this manuscript and to Dr. Nili Peylan-Ramu for reading the manuscript and offering helpful suggestions.

REFERENCES

1. **Ruymann, F. B., Newton, W. A., Ragab, A. H., Donaldson, M. H., and Foulkes, M.,** Bone marrow metastases at diagnosis in children and adolescents with rhabdomyosarcoma: a report from the Intergroup Rhabdomyosarcoma Study, *Cancer,* 53, 368, 1984.
2. **Lechner, F. C. and Moran, T. J.,** Rhabdomyosarcoma with fetal haemorrhage from intestinal metastases: case report with autopsy, *Am. J. Clin. Pathol.,* 22, 461, 1952.
3. **Merskey, C. and Johnson, A. J.,** Diagnosis and treatment of intravascular coagulation: pathogenesis and treatment of thromboemolic diseases, *Thromb. Diath. Haemorrh.,* 21, 55, 1966.

4. **Eldor, A., Naparstek, E., Boss, J. H., and Brian, S.,** Alveolar rhabdomyosarcoma presenting as sub-acute intravascular coagulation, *J. Clin. Pathol.,* 30, 661, 1977.

5. **Goldschmidt, B. and Koòs, R.,** Low intensity intravascular coagulation in rhabdomyosarcoma, *Orv. Hetil.,* 121, 905, 1980.

6. **Sills, R. H., Stockman, J. A., Miller, M. L., and Stuart, M. J.,** Consumptive coagulopathy: a complication of therapy of solid tumors in childhood, *Am. J. Dis. Child.,* 132, 870, 1978.

7. **Butler, W. M., Scialla, S. J., and Taylor, H. G.,** Alveolar rhabdomyosarcoma associated with disseminated intravascular coagulation and a unique factor VIII antigen, *Arch. Intern. Med.,* 142, 1379,1982.

8. **Furui, T., Ichihara, K., Ikecla, A., Inao, S., Hirai, N., Yoshida, J., and Kageyama, N.,** Subdural hematoma associated with disseminated intravascular coagulation in patients with advanced cancer, *J. Neurosurg.,* 58, 398, 1983.

9. **Leblanc, A., Cailland, J. M., Hartmann, O., Kalifa, C., Flamant, F., Patte, C., Tournade, M. F., and Lemerle, J.,** Hypercalcemia referentially occurs in unusual forms of childhood non-Hodgkin's lymphoma, rhabdomyosarcoma, and Wilms' tumor, *Cancer,* 54, 2132, 1984.

10. **Cohan, M., Pittman, G., and Hoffman, G. C.,** Hemolytic anemia tumor cell emboli and intravascular coagulation, *Arch. Pathol. Lab. Med.,* 93, 305, 1972.

11. **Miller, S. P., Sanchez-Avalos, J., Stefanski, T., et al.,** Coagulation disorders in cancer. Clinical and laboratory studies, *Cancer,* 20, 1452, 1967.

12. **Peck, S. D. and Reiquam, C. W.,** Disseminated intravascular coagulation in cancer patients: supportive evidence, *Cancer,* 31, 1114, 1973.

13. **Maurer, H. M., Beltangady, M., Gehan, E. A., Crist, W., Hammond, D., Hays, D. M., Heyn, R., Lawrence, W., Newton, W., Ortega, J., Ragab, A. H., Raney, R. B., Ruymann, F. B., Soule, E., Tefft, M., Webber, B., Wharam, M. D., and Vietti, T. J.,** The Intergroup Rhabdomyosarcoma Study-I: a final report, *Cancer,* 61, 209, 1988.

14. **Maurer, H. M., Gehan, E. A., Beltangady, M., Crist, W., Dickman, P. S., Donaldson, S. S., Fryer, C., Hammond, D., Hays, D. M., Morris-Jones, P., Lawrence, W., Newton, W., Ortega, J., Ragab, A. H., Raney, R. B., Ruymann, F. B., Soule, E. H., Tefft, M., Webber, B., Weiner, E., Wharam, M., and Vietti, T.,** The Intergroup Rhabdomyosarcoma Study-II, *Cancer,* in press.

15. **Laki, K.,** Fibrinogen and metastases, *J. Med.,* 5, 23, 1974.

16. **Berglund, G.,** Three cases of disseminated intravascular coagulation, *Acta Paediatr.,* 59, 664, 1970.

17. **Scialla, S. J., Barr, C. F., Waldorf, M. A., et al.,** Factor VIII complex in cancer patients, abstracted, *Clin. Res.,* 26, 441, 1978.

18. **Corrigan, J. J., Ray, W. L., and May, N.,** Changes in the blood coagulation system associated with septicemia, *N. Engl. J. Med.,* 279, 851, 1968.

19. **Hathaway, W. E. and Bonnar, J.,** *Perinatal Coagulation,* Grune & Stratton, New York, 1978.

20. **Hutchinson, R. J., Shapiro, S. A., and Raney, R. B.,** Elevated parathyroid hormone levels in association with rhabdomyosarcoma, *J. Pediatr.,* 92, 780, 1978.

21. **Takeuchi, T., Takeuchi, H., Hoshino, R., and Ohmi, K.,** Rhabdomyosarcoma-induced hypercalcemia in a nude mouse, *Cancer,* 50, 94, 1982.

22. **Elomaa, I., Lehto, V., and Selander, R.,** Hypercalcemia and elevated serum parathyroid hormone level in association with rhabdomyosarcoma, *Arch. Pathol. Lab. Med.,* 108, 701, 1984.

23. **Mayes, L. C., Kasselberg, A. G., Roloff, J. S., and Lukens, J. N.,** Hypercalcemia associated with immunoreactive parthyroid hormone in a malignant rhabdoid tumor of the kidney (rhabdoid Wilms' tumor), *Cancer,* 54, 882, 1984.

24. **Rousseau-Merck, M. F., Boccon-Gibod, L., Nogues, C., et al.,** An original hypercalcemic infantile renal tumor without bone metastases: heterotransplantation to nude mice. Report of two cases, *Cancer,* 50, 85, 1982.

25. **Beckwith, J. B. and Palmer, N. F.,** Histopathology and prognosis of Wilms' tumor: results from the First National Wilms' Tumor Study, *Cancer,* 41, 1937, 1978.

26. **Palmer, N. F., Beckwith, J. B., Sutow, W. W., and Meyer, J. A.,** Rhabdoid tumor of kidney (RTK): clinical results, *Proc. AACR ASCO,* 21 (Abstr.), 386, 1980.

27. **Haas, J. E., Palmer, N. F., Weinberg, A. G., and Beckwith, J. B.,** Ultrastructure of malignant rhabdoid tumor of the kidney, *Hum. Pathol.,* 12, 646, 1981.

28. **Weeks, D. A., Beckwith, J. B., Mierau, G. W., and Luckey, D. W.,** Rhabdoid tumor of the kidney: a report of 111 cases from the National Wilms' Tumor Study Pathology Center, *Am. J. Surg. Pathol.,* 13, 439, 1989.

29. **Stein, R. C.,** Hypercalcemia in leukemia, *J. Pediatr.,* 78, 861, 1971.

30. **Stapleton, F. B., Lukert, B. P., and Linshaw, M. A.,** Treatment of hypercalcemia associated with osseous metastases and lymphoma, *J. Pediatr.,* 89, 1029, 1976.

31. **Speigel, A., Green, M., McGrath, I., et al.,** Hypercalcemia with suppressed parathyroid hormone in patients with Burkitt's lymphoma, *Am. J. Med.,* 64, 691, 1978.

32. **Reiselbach, R. E., Bentzel, C. J., Cotlove, E., et al.,** Uric acid excretion and renal function in the acute hyperuricemia of leukemia, *Am. J. Med.,* 37, 872, 1964.
33. **Kyellstrand, C. M., Cambell, D. D., von Hartitzsch, B., et al.,** Hyperuricemic acute renal failure, *Arch. Intern. Med.,* 133, 349, 1974.
34. **Lundberg, W. B., Codman, E. D., Finch, S. C., et al.,** Renal failure secondary to leukemic infiltration of the kidneys, *Am. J. Med.,* 62, 636, 1977.
35. **O'Connor, N. T., Prentice, H. G., and Hoffbrand, A. V.,** Prevention of urate nephropathy in the tumour lysis syndrome, *Clin. Lab. Haematol.,* 11, 97, 1989.
36. **Stokes, D. N.,** The tumour lysis syndrome. Intensive care aspects of paediatric oncology, *Anesthesia,* 44, 133, 1989.
37. **Silverman, P. and Distelhorst, C. W.,** Metabolic emergencies in chemical oncology, *Semin. Oncol.,* 16, 504, 1989.

Chapter 13

RESULTS OF TREATMENT OF RHABDOMYOSARCOMA IN THE EUROPEAN STUDIES

Joern Treuner, Francoise Flamant, and Modesto Carli

TABLE OF CONTENTS

I. INTRODUCTION

The only way in which the value of chemotherapy, surgery, radiotherapy, or a combination of these modalities can be assessed is by clinical therapeutic studies. This is especially true in the case of a rare tumor like rhabdomyosarcoma (RMS). By study of a reasonable number of patients treated according to a standard protocol, with use of thorough documentation, together with careful statistical analysis of the data collected, answers to several of the open questions on therapy can be found. In this way, the treatment of the majority of childhood malignancies could be fundamentally improved, which, in turn, would surely lead to better treatment results. A multicenter study is particularly advantageous in evaluating the treatment of soft tissue sarcomas, especially in the case of RMS.

Although cooperative studies on therapy of childhood malignancies began in the 1960s in the U.S., this method of clinical research gained real popularity only in the 1970s and early 1980s. Pioneer work in this field was done by the Intergroup Rhabdomyosarcoma Study (IRS) which began in 1972 after three American groups fused together.[1] The lead was thus set for researchers who were striving to improve the treatment of soft tissue sarcomas in children and adolescents in Europe. Many elements in the IRS were borrowed by some of the European counterparts and some countries even took the treatment design over completely.[2]

In addition, the direction which the European studies took was also greatly influenced by the vast experience of the IRS.

A comparison of the results of the European studies and the IRS studies would show only minor differences. One such difference is that the European groups attempted to individualize treatment as far as possible, by carefully considering the various risk factors that are evident at the time of diagnosis or which arise in the course of treatment.

The last 15 years have seen the founding of the three major study groups for the treatment of childhood soft tissue sarcomas in Europe. Chronologically, the therapy studies of the Société Internationale d'Oncologie Pédiatrique (SIOP), headed by Francoise Flamant from France, came first.[3] The Gruppo Cooperativo Italiano, founded by Modesto Carli in Padua, Italy followed.[4] Then came the studies of the Deutsche Gesellschaft fuer Paediatrische Onkologie, which are better known as the German Cooperative Soft Tissue Sarcoma (CWS) studies headed by Joern Treuner.[5]

Among the European studies, the SIOP group has the largest case material and the longest experience. Still, the European groups have comparatively less experience than the IRS. However, the European study groups have not only attained their own standing, but have also contributed to the improvement in the treatment of soft tissue sarcomas in children and adolescents. All three groups enjoy a very close cooperation with each other as well as with the IRS study group.

On the whole, the individual study designs of the European groups do not differ from each other. While the Italian and German studies are based on the IRS grouping system, the main staging criterion used in the SIOP studies is local tumor extension according to the TNM (tumor, nodes, metastases) classification.

By sharing their experience, the European groups have arrived at common definitions and criteria for evaluation. Their joint efforts have led to an exchange of valuable information which, in turn, has led to improvements in the various study designs. The fact that the European groups can now easily compare their data has raised the hope that important questions can be answered in a shorter time. Furthermore, interaction is the first step in setting up a standard study on a European level. This chapter outlines the genesis of the three main groups, as well as presenting their latest results.

TABLE 1
Results of the First International Society of Pediatric Oncology (SIOP) Study

3-year survival rate of 40% using VAC-VAD chemotherapy in RMS stage III patients.
Protochemotherapy instead of primary extensive surgery did not improve the survival in stage III RMS patients.
Primary chemotherapy with complementary surgery or radiotherapy reduced the importance of sequelae except
  patients with prostatic RMSs.

II. THE FIRST SIOP STUDY

In 1975, SIOP started a sequential trial in which treatment centers from Holland, Belgium, Sweden, Switzerland, France, and the U.K. (only until 1978) participated.[3] By 1983, there were 81 RMS patients registered. Only patients with tumors extending into adjacent tissues, and in whom a complete excision of the tumor could not be achieved at initial surgery (stage III according to the IRS criteria) were selected (Table 1).

Chemotherapy, according to the VAC regimen, consisted of vincristine (2 mg/m^2 on days 1 and 14), dactinomycin (15 µg/kg/day from days 1 to 5), and cyclophosphamide (200 mg/m^2/day from day 1 to day 5). Following a course of this chemotherapy regimen, the patients were randomly assigned to arm A or arm B. Arm A consisted of alternately VAC and VAD (vincristine and adriamycin), until maximum reduction of the tumor volume was achieved. Repeat (second-look) surgery or radiotherapy (RT) or both, to the residual tumor, then followed. In maintenance chemotherapy, VAC and VAD were given alternatingly. Arm B consisted of extensive surgery (on bladder/prostate sites) or irradiation with 4500 cGy to the initial tumor volume, or both, followed by the same maintenance chemotherapy. The patients were paired according to the primary site and the results of each pair were assessed after three years. Preference was then given to the treatment which gave the best results.

Only 63 out of the 81 registered patients could be analyzed. There were 32 treated in arm A and 31 in arm B. No significant differences were observed between the two arms: the same number of local recurrences, failures to gain local control, and more importantly, the same number of cases of secondary meningeal involvement in the head and neck sites were observed. The overall 3-year survival rate of 40% in both groups was low. However, patients treated according to arm A, who received presurgical chemotherapy, had less sequelae from surgery or radiotherapy.

It must be mentioned that in the group of patients with prostatic tumors no complete remissions were achieved. These patients underwent complementary anterior exenteration.

III. THE SIOP MMT-84 STUDY

The second study of the SIOP was conducted from 1984 until 1988. The goal was to study all cases of malignant mesenchymal tumors (MMT) in children and adolescents which the group registered.[6] Once again, the objective was to apply an intensification of initial chemotherapy so that patients who achieved complete remission (CR) through chemotherapy would need less complementary local treatment in the form of surgery, irradiation, or both. Another aim was to avoid, as far as possible, the adverse consequences of therapy.

It was decided to use ifosfamide in the chemotherapy combination instead of cyclophosphamide. This decision was based on pilot studies conducted by the Amsterdam group, as well as by the SIOP group in Villejuif. Studies showed that, in terms of CR, the combination of ifosfamide, vincristine, and dactinomycin (actinomycin D) (IVA) was superior to the regimen consisting of vincristine, dactinomycin, and cyclophosphamide (VAC).[7] The IVA combination was given as follows: ifosfamide (3 g/m^2 on days 1 and 2), vincristine (1.5 mg/m^2 on day 1), and dactinomycin (900 µg/m^2 on days 1 and 2). Three to 10 courses

TABLE 2
SIOP-Malignant Mesenchymal
Tumor (MMT)-84 Study:
Nonmetastatic
Rhabdomyosarcoma

Response to therapy	%
3-year survival	72
3-year EFS	53
Local failures	30
CR (including stages III and IV)	83

of IVA were given, depending on the stage of the tumor and the response achieved. Post-surgical IVA chemotherapy was given after an initial biopsy was done, even with tumors classified as stage pT1 or pT2a.

As mentioned earlier, patients who achieved CR (preferably proved by biopsy) with chemotherapy did not receive complementary local treatment in the form of surgery or irradiation. In the case of partial remission (PR), either limited surgery was performed or radiotherapy given, or second line chemotherapy (100 mg/m^2 of cisplatinum, and 60 mg/m^2 of adriamycin) administered every 21 days, followed by surgery or radiotherapy to the residual tumor.

To avoid adverse effects of radiotherapy on the brain in children under 5 years of age, patients with parameningeal RMSs who had achieved CR following initial chemotherapy were randomized. In this randomization IVA was continued in certain patients, while in others consolidation was applied either by means of heavy chemotherapy and by use of the technique of bone marrow rescue. However, parameningeal tumors with intracranial extension in patients older than 5 years of age were irradiated after three courses of IVA. Patients who reached CR only after being given second-line chemotherapy received heavy chemotherapy and bone marrow rescue.

The CR rate 12 months before the follow-up period was completed was 83% (including stage IV patients). In patients with measurable tumor in whom complete remission was achieved through use of IVA chemotherapy alone, the CR rate is 58%. This rate is higher than that of those who reached CR through use of the VAC regimen (25%) in the first SIOP trial (Table 2).

The SIOP MMT-84 study registered 593 cases, of which only 406 patients were eligible for analysis. Among them were 283 RMSs (70%), 109 nonrhabdomyosarcomatous MMTs (27%), and 14 others. The median follow-up period for the RMS patients was 3 years; the 3-year survival rate was 66%, as compared with a survival rate of only 53% in the previous SIOP study. The event-free survival rate (EFS) was 47%, compared to a rate of 47% in the 1975 study. The 243 nonmetastatic patients had a 3-year survival rate of 72% and an EFS rate of 53%, compared with rates of 56 and 50%, respectively, in the previous study.

Among 164 nonmetastatic patients who had follow-up for more than 2 years, 153 are in CR. Patients who achieved CR through surgery alone (14%) had an EFS rate of 82%. In patients with chemotherapy-induced CR (58%), the EFS rate was 49%. Those who reached CR through chemotherapy combined with surgery, with or without radiotherapy for eradication of a small residue (10%), had an EFS rate of 42%. In all, 18% of the patients achieved a CR after chemotherapy plus radiotherapy on the initial tumor volume, extensive surgery, or both. In other words, only 18% of the patients achieved CR as a result of aggressive local treatment (Table 3).

TABLE 3
SIOP-Malignant Mesenchymal Tumor
(MMT)-84 Study; Nonmetastatic
Rhabdomyosarcomas

Therapy to obtain CR	CR rate (%)	EFS[a] rate (%)
Surgery (S)	14	82
Chemotherapy (CT)	58	49
CT + S + radiotherapy	10	42
Aggressive local treatment	18	78

[a] EFS = event-free survival.

TABLE 4
SIOP-84 MMT Study: Nonmetastatic Patients, Survival by Site

Primary site	Number	3-year survival %	(SE)	3-year EFS %	(SE)
Orbit	26	94	(6)	70	(10)
Nonparameningeal head/ neck	38	66	(9)	45	(9)
Parameningeal	33	61	(11)	48	(10)
Genitourinary					
Bladder-prostate	21	84	(11)	65	(12)
Vagina, paratesticular	41	85	(9)	76	(10)
Limbs	30	73	(10)	40	(10)
Other	54	55	(8)	40	(8)
Total	243	72	(4)	53	(4)

Note: SE = standard error.

The SIOP MMT-84 study for MMTs showed an excellent CR rate of 93% for non-metastatic RMSs and it also achieved its aim of using less aggressive methods of local treatment (Table 4). The rate of overall survival after 3 years is higher in this study than in the previous study, but the follow-up is too short yet to make a definitive comparison. It must be mentioned, however, that about half of the patients who relapsed went into second remission and were still disease free after 18 months of follow-up.

IV. THE SIOP MMT-89 STUDY

SIOP's latest study is based on the prognostic factors which emerged from the earlier studies.[8] As a result, patients are divided into five prognostic groups. The stratification of the risk groups is done according to the site and degree of local extension of the primary tumor.[9]

The first prognostic group is group A, which comprises all patients with tumors at any site which have been completely excised, that is stage IpT1, N0 M0 according to the TNM classification. From the prognostic point of view, this is the most favorable group. The treatment plan for group A (9% of the cases) after initial tumor resection calls for two courses of chemotherapy. The chemotherapy regimen excludes ifosfamide and cyclophosphamide but consists of vincristine and dactinomycin given at 3-week intervals.

Group B comprises patients with tumors classifed as stage IIpT2 or IpT3abc (N0 M0), the tumors being located only in the following sites: vagina, paratesticular, orbit, nonparameningeal head and neck, bladder, prostate. In this group, which comprises 15% of the patients, chemotherapy is started after initial surgery or biopsy. The four courses of chemotherapy consist of the following: ifosfamide (3 g/m^2 on days 1, 2, and 3), vincristine (1.5 mg/m^2 weekly for five doses and on day 1 of the last course), and dactinomycin (1.5 mg/m^2 on day 1 of each of the four courses). The first assessment is made 20 days after the first course. If the tumor shows progression, change to second-line regimen of chemotherapy is made. A second assessment is done after two courses of chemotherapy. If the tumor shows a regression of less than 50%, biopsy or exploratory surgery is attempted; if the tumor or its residue cannot be removed without undue mutilation of the patient, a second line chemotherapy regimen is given. If there is no residual tumor evident after the third and fourth course of initial chemotherapy is given, treatment is discontinued. The third assessment is done after four courses of chemotherapy. If only a PR is obtained, surgical resection is performed, followed by radiotherapy if incomplete. If surgery is impossible, radiotherapy alone is planned.

Group C in the SIOP classification system includes patients who fulfill the following criteria: stage IpT3abc, N0 M0, and sites other than those in group B; stage II (T2 N0 M0); and stage III (T1 T2 N1 M0). This group has the same chemotherapy schedule as the group B patients after biopsy or surgery. Not more than six courses are given. If there is residual tumor evident after chemotherapy and surgery, radiotherapy is given during the fifth or sixth courses of chemotherapy. A fourth assessment is done after 4.5 months or after six courses of IVA chemotherapy in patients who show evidence of continued improvement at the third assessment.

Group D in the SIOP classification system includes patients older than 3 years of age who have parameningeal involvement by tumor. Radiotherapy and chemotherapy are given simultaneously. The radiotherapy is directed to the base of the skull and to the area comprising the intracranial tumor (with 2-mm margins) and whole brain irradiation is avoided.

Group E patients have distant metastases and are treated according to the new European stage IV RMS protocol.

In summing up, it could be said that the SIOP study design for the treatment of MMTs in childhood and adolescents tried to avoid radical surgery by using chemotherapy instead. An effort was made to use radiotherapy only when it was unavoidable. This has been SIOP's basic treatment policy from the beginning and has been applied consistently in all of their studies.

V. THE ITALIAN EXPERIENCE

From October 1979 to December 1986, 160 RMS patients entered the first Italian study for the treatment of childhood soft tissue sarcomas.[4] The patients were staged according to the IRS grouping system. The main objectives of the study were to provide homogeneous treatment of RMS in children on a national basis and to improve the survival rate as well as the quality of life of these patients.

The therapeutic protocol called for primary chemotherapy in stage III patients, followed by irradiation of residual tumor in an attempt to avoid radical surgery in unresectable tumors. Patients received either a combination of vincristine, dactinomycin, and cyclophosphamide (VAC) or the same combination of drugs was administered together with a single large dose of 1.7 mg/m^2 of dactinomycin (VAC-M). The maintenance chemotherapy consisted of alternate courses of VAC and VAC-M (Figure 1).

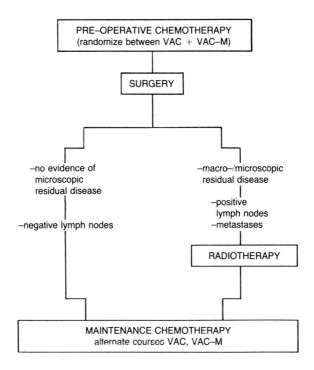

FIGURE 1. Design of the Italian soft tissue sarcoma study RMS-79.

TABLE 5
Italian Soft Tissue Study-79: Survival
of Rhabdomyosarcoma Patients

Stage	Number	5-year survival rate (%)
I	27	83
II	14	72
III	65	63
IV	12	33

There were 27 patients with stage I tumors, of whom 20 are in CR, and the 5-year survival rate for this group is 83%. There were only seven treatment failures, all of them with only local recurrence of tumor. Of the 14 patients in stage II, 11 achieved complete remissions and 3 had recurrence of tumor (2 relapsed locally and 1 showed distant metastases). The survival rate for stage II patients was 72% (Table 5).

Two regimens of chemotherapy were randomly assigned in stage III patients: dactinomycin was given either in a single dose or in repeated doses over 5 days. However, no difference in the outcome could be observed between the VAC and VAC-M regimens.[10] There were 65 stage III patients, of whom 34 survived, while 18 relapsed locally, 5 developed metastases, and 30 failed to respond to chemotherapy. Among the patients who developed metastases, three had both local and systemic metastases and two died of toxic complications. The 5-year survival rate for this group was 63%.

In group IV, 12 patients with disseminated RMS were registered, 8 of whom failed to respond to chemotherapy, 4 due to tumor progression, and 4 due to new metastatic lesions. The 5-year survival rate was 33% for this group.

TABLE 6
Italian Soft Tissue Sarcoma Study; Survival of
Rhabdomyosarcoma Patients

Tumor site	Number	5-year survival rate (%)
Orbit	21	100
Genitourinary	29	88
Head/neck (nonparameningeal)	10	63
Head/neck (parameningeal)	22	48
Limbs	20	54

One of the findings of the Italian study concerned the tumor site. The best prognosis was seen in orbital RMS, which had a 5-year survival rate of 100%. Tumors of the genitourinary tract (including paratesticular RMSs) came next, with a survival rate of 88%, while nonparameningeal RMSs of the head and neck region had a survival rate of 63%. The 5-year survival rate for patients with parameningeal RMS was 48%, while in patients with these tumors of the extremities it was 54% (Table 6). A significant difference in the survival rate of patients with the embryonal type of RMS (74%) and that of the alveolar type (42%) could be observed.

A very important analysis was done by the Italian group on the correlation between the findings on clinical and histopathological examination of lymph nodes in soft tissue sarcomas. Although a positive correlation between clinical and histopathological findings was observed, the results are very uncertain when the clinical findings in a given case are negative.[11]

The 1979 Italian study also investigated the question as to whether lymph nodes were a prognostic factor.[12] It turned out that lymph node involvement could only be associated with more advanced neoplastic disease, and there was no difference between lymph node involvement and histological subtype of the tumor. A high rate of lymph node involvement was found in children with RMSs originating in the retroperitoneum, in an extremity, or in the head/neck area. Presence of lymph node involvement was also shown to be an unfavorable prognostic factor in cases with nonmetastatic RMSs.

VI. THE NEW ITALIAN STUDY (RMS-87)

The present and ongoing Italian study began in 1987. It was based not only on the results of the previous Italian study, but also on the findings of the IRS III, the SIOP MMT-84, and the German CWS-81 studies.

In this Italian study, the patients are staged only after initial surgery, following which chemotherapy is planned. Patients in whom the primary tumor is completely removed, the intensity of the chemotherapy to be given depends on whether the histology is classified as favorable or unfavorable. If the tumor is primarily inoperable (stage III according to the IRS staging criteria), preoperative chemotherapy lasting 9 weeks is given, then the patients are stratified according to the degree of response to chemotherapy. Patients who achieve CR after 9 weeks of chemotherapy are explored surgically, with histological examination of any remaining tumor. Local radiotherapy is not given in patients whose tumors have favorable histology and who also have a histologically proven remission. Chemotherapy, however, is continued.

When surgical intervention is difficult (such as in orbital tumors) a surgical exploration is not done. Instead, hyperfractionated radiotherapy is given in addition to chemotherapy. In patients who respond well (showing greater than $2/3$ regression of tumor size) during the initial cycle of chemotherapy, an attempt is made to remove the residual tumor without damaging the affected organ or its function. However, if it is clear that surgical intervention would entail serious damage to normal tissues and organs, the patient is given chemotherapy and radiotherapy simultaneously.

In nonresponders and in patients who show a response of less than $^2/_3$ regression of tumor size after the first chemotherapy cycle, the chemotherapy regimen is changed and radiotherapy is given simultaneously. This regimen is continued until a satisfactory tumor reduction is achieved. If the tumor does not respond, an attempt is made to radically resect it.

In cases in which the tumor is resected at the initial operation and where histology is favorable, the chemotherapy regimen of dactinomycin and vincristine is given over 20 weeks. However, for tumors resected at the initial operation but having histology that is unfavorable, ifosfamide is added to the chemotherapy regimen, which is then given over a period lasting 26 weeks.

Primary inoperable tumors are treated with an initial chemotherapy regimen consisting of vincristine, dactinomycin, ifosfamide, and adriamycin (VAIA). Unlike the dosage scheme used in the German CWS-86 study, in which 3 g/m² of ifosfamide is given over 2 days, the Italian group gives 1.5 mg/m² of this drug over 5 days. Therefore, it will be interesting to compare the results in patients given the different ifosfamide dosages in the German and Italian studies.

VII. THE FIRST GERMAN STUDY (CWS-81)

At the time when the first West German multicenter study was drafted, chemotherapy was considered to be an essential part of cancer treatment. Starting in 1981, the CWS-81 study attempted to use chemotherapy as a means of gaining and maintaining local tumor control. The study was also designed to provide therapy adapted to the risk of tumor recurrence (risk-adapted therapy) in patients with tumors that are inoperable at initial surgery.

Between 1981 and 1985, the CWS-81 study registered 352 patients, whose clinical and laboratory data were sent in from 50 hospitals located in West Germany and Austria. Of the 352 patients, there were 287 with tumors sensitive to chemotherapy (group A), including RMSs, synovial sarcomas, and undifferentiated sarcomas. Only 240 of these patients were treated strictly according to the CWS-81 protocol, and 153 of these were patients with RMSs.[13]

Using the IRS classification system, four groups of patients were created. During the first 7 weeks, all patients in stages I and II were given a combination of vincristine, dactinomycin, cyclophosphamide, and adriamycin (VACA). Those in stage IV received a modified chemotherapy regimen in which cyclophosphamide was replaced by ifosfamide (VAIA). Poor and nonresponders to the first course of VACA were also given the VAIA regimen.[14]

Adjuvant chemotherapy lasting 36 weeks was given to patients in stages I and II, while patients in stages III and IV received a total of 16 weeks of preoperative chemotherapy. All patients underwent a second-look operation during week 16, after which a decision was made as to whether radiotherapy would be given. In other words, there was no radiotherapy planned in patients who showed absolutely no evidence of residual tumor after the second-look operation (stage Ipc). However, a dose of 4000 cGy was given to patients who had microscopic residual tumor (stage IIpc), and a dose of 5000 cGy was given to those with gross residual tumor (stage IIIpc) (Figures 2 and 3).

The biggest problem that the German CWS study group faced in its first study was local relapse. If, for example, the number of local relapses was excluded from the calculations, successful treatment in 87% of the patients could be claimed. The updated analysis of the

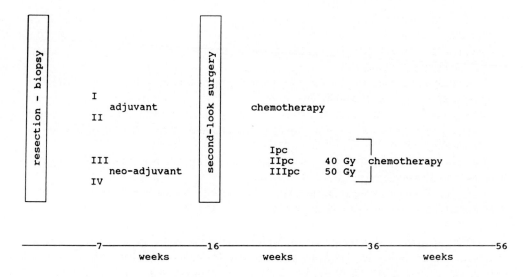

FIGURE 2.   Design of the German soft tissue sarcoma study CWS-81.

results of the CWS-81 study, however, showed that 20% of the patients had local relapses, with 10% of patients having initial tumor progression which could not be arrested. Only 5 to 10% developed metastases.

The EFS of the group A protocol patients was 70% and the overall survival rate was 65%, which included only those with tumors sensitive to chemotherapy. However, for the patients with nonmetastatic RMSs in this group, the EFS rate was 63% and overall survival was 69%. Therefore, it could be extrapolated that the CWS group had to impose a curative regimen of therapy for a second time, because of a local relapse, in only about 6% of the RMS patients. Observed over a period of 96 months and according to stage, the EFS rate of the 1981 study of nonmetastatic RMS patients was as follows: stage I, 81%; stage II, 68%; and stage III, 56% (Figure 4).

The type of local tumor treatment given to patients was stratified according to degree of response during the 16th week of therapy. However, there was no parallel change between the survival rates of the three postchemotherapy groups (stages Ipc, IIpc, and IIIpc) and the initial stage III patients. This finding could be attributed to the fact that the efforts for local tumor control were applied too late.

The German CWS study group found a correlation between chemotherapy and prognosis as early as week 7 to 9, that is, after the first cycle of chemotherapy.[15] Multivariate and univariate analyses confirmed that the initial response to chemotherapy by weeks 7 to 9 was of great prognostic value. The next most important prognostic factor was the size of the tumor, followed by the degree of tumor extension (TNM classification) (Figure 5).

The rate of tumor shrinkage in response to initial chemotherapy was shown to be an early prognostic factor in primarily unresectable tumors. This fact was then used as the basis for the next CWS study.

VIII. THE CWS-86 STUDY

Drawing from the results of the CWS-81 study, the German CWS study group planned a sequel study starting in 1986. It was decided to reduce the radiotherapy dose to 3200 cGy in patients who were good responders, as well as to give irradiation in hyperfractionated doses during weeks 7 to 12. Poor responders receive 5400 cGy. The radiotherapy and chemotherapy are given simultaneously. Through these changes in the treatment program, the CWS group hopes to attain better local tumor control (Figure 6).

V A C A

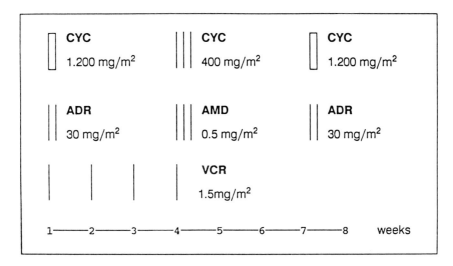

V A I A II

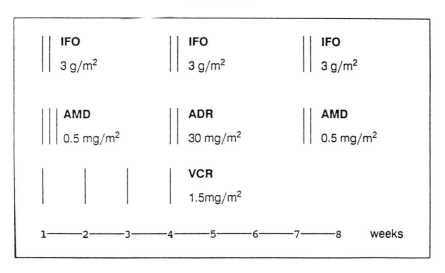

FIGURE 3.   Chemotherapy schedules of the CWS studies. CYC = cyclophosphamide; ADR = adriamycin/doxorubicin; AMD = actinomycin D; VCR = vincristine; IFO = ifosfamide.

The chemotherapy regimen was also changed, with the objective of improving the response to initial chemotherapy: in the CWS-86 protocol, ifosfamide has replaced cyclophosphamide. Preliminary results of the second German study indicate that this change has produced improved results, since there are clearly more good responders to initial chemotherapy (among stage III patients, for instance) than in the previous study (Figure 7).

It has not been fully possible to solve the problem of local relapse in the new study. However, it is clear that relapses mainly occur in patients with tumors in the head and neck area, in the urogenital/prostate area, in the retroperitoneum, and in the extremities. Since the second study is not yet complete, it is not possible to predict if the results will be better than those of the previous study. It also remains an open question as to whether patients who initially respond better do, in fact, continue to benefit from this treatment in the long term.

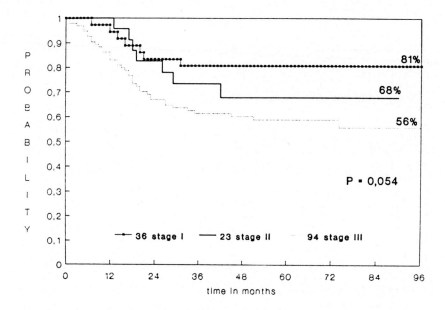

FIGURE 4. Event-free survival (EFS) rate of RMS protocol patients treated according to stage (CWS-81 study).

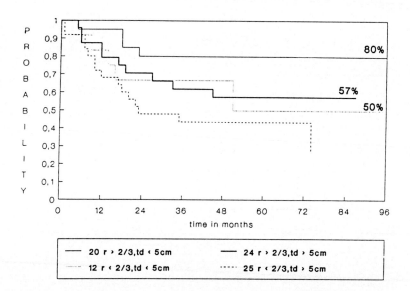

FIGURE 5. Event-free survival (EFS) rate of RMS protocol patients treated according to tumor diameter and response at week 7 (CWS-81 study): r = regression of; >2/3 = more than two thirds the original tumor volume remaining after 7 weeks of chemotherapy; <2/3 = less than two thirds the original tumor volume remaining after 7 weeks of chemotherapy; td = tumor diameter.

The German studies have shown that therapy adapted to the risk of tumor recurrence (risk-adapted therapy) is possible and can be successful. However, the role of radiotherapy in the German CWS-81 study remains unclear, although use of the reduced dose of 3200 cGy for good responders seems to be justified in the CWS-86 study. Among the problems that continue to face the CWS group are local relapses (10 to 20% in both studies) and the salvage therapy for poor responders and nonresponders. These patients still face a high risk of metastasis despite radical surgery.

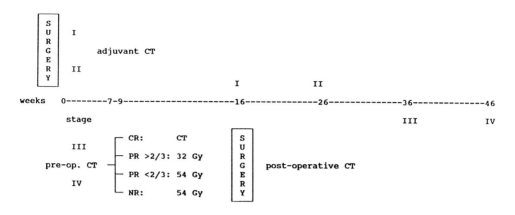

FIGURE 6.   Design of the German CWS-86 study.

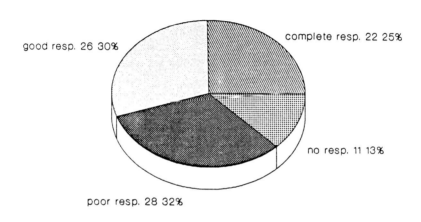

A

B

FIGURE 7.   (A) Response to initial chemotherapy in the CWS-81 study; (B) response to initial chemotherapy in the CWS-86 study.

IX. PROSPECT OF A UNIFIED EUROPEAN STUDY

As there are very many similarities between the current European studies, the hope for a common study design in the near future could easily be realized. In fact, a first step in this direction was taken in 1989, when it was decided to treat all primarily disseminated soft tissue sarcomas uniformly in Europe, through the three groups: the SIOP, and the German and the Italian groups.

X. SUMMARY

This chapter describes the results achieved by the European therapy studies on the treatment of childhood soft tissue sarcoma. It also presents the study designs of the current European studies.

There are three main study groups in Europe: the SIOP group in France, the Italian group, and the German group. A total of four studies have already been completed: two of them by the SIOP (the SIOP-75 and the MMT-84), and the other two; the Italian-79 study and the German CWS-81 study. The current studies being conducted are the SIOP MMT-89, the Italian ISS-87, and the German CWS-86.

Up to now, the results of these studies have been identical to a great extent. The therapy strategy shared by all of the European studies is that therapy should be adapted to as great an extent as possible to the individual risks (risk-adapted therapy). The SIOP studies individualize therapy by following the TNM classification which is based on the primary post-surgical stage. The Italian and German studies have based their staging system on the lines of the IRS grouping scheme. That is, patients are grouped after initial surgery. These latter two studies regroup the patients after measuring the response to initial chemotherapy and repeat (second-look) surgery. One conspicuous element of the European studies is that radiotherapy is not used to a great extent. Instead, intensive chemotherapy is given. The main problem that the European studies face is the problem of local (rather than systemic) relapse. On the whole, the results of the European studies — in terms of primary stage and tumor site — are comparable to those of the IRS. The survival rate of the completed studies ranges from between 50 and 80%, depending on the tumor site.

The current three studies in Europe share similarities in their designs. The standard chemotherapy combinations also comprise the same drugs, namely, vincristine, adriamycin, ifosfamide, and dactinomycin. The differences are only in dosage.

In 1989, a European study was started in which several countries began to treat patients with primary, disseminated soft tissue sarcoma uniformly. In the near future, it is hoped to set up a study on localized soft tissue sarcomas.

ACKNOWLEDGMENT

The authors would like to thank Ms. Priscilla Herrmann for her invaluable assistance in the preparation of this chapter.

REFERENCES

1. **Maurer, H. M.,** The Intergroup Rhabdomyosarcoma Study (NIH); objectives and clinical staging classifications, *J. Pediatr. Surg.,* 10, 977, 1975.
2. **Carli, M., De Bernardi, B., Castello, M., et al.,** Long-term results in childhood rhabdomyosarcoma; a retrospective study in Italy, *Pediatr. Hematol. Oncol.,* 3, 371, 1986.

3. **Flamant, F., Rodary, C., Voute, P. A., and Otten, J.,** Primary chemotherapy in the treatment of rhabdomyosarcoma in children: trial of the International Society of Pediatric Oncology (SIOP) preliminary results, *Radiother. Oncol.,* 3, 227, 1985.

4. **Carli, M., Perilongo, G., Guglielmi, M., et al.,** Rhabdomyosarcoma in childhood: a report from the Italian Cooperative Group, in Proc. 17th SIOP Meeting, Venice, 1985, 89.

5. **Treuner, J., Kaatsch, P., Anger, Y., et al.,** Ergebnisse der Behandlung von Rhabdomyosarkomen (RMS) bei Kindern. Ein Bericht der Cooperativen Weichteilsarkomstudie (CWS-81) der Gesellschaft für Pädiatrische Onkologie, *Klin. Paediatr.,* 198, 208, 1986.

6. **Flamant, F., et al.,** Results of the SIOP MMT-84 Study, Abstract, SIOP 21 Meeting, Prague, Czechoslovakia, September 18 to 22, 1989.

7. **De Kraker, J. and Voute, P. A.,** The role of ifosfamide in paediatric soft-tissue sarcoma, in Proc. 17th SIOP Meeting, Venice, 1985, 104.

8. **Rodary, C., Rey, A., Olive, D., et al.,** Prognostic factors in 281 children with non-metastatic rhabdomyosarcoma (RMS) at diagnosis, *Med. Pediatr. Oncol.,* 16, 71, 1988.

9. **Rodary, C., Flamant, F., and Donaldson, S. S.,** (For the SIOP-IRS Committee): an attempt to use a common staging system in rhabdomyosarcoma; a report of an international workshop initiated by the International Society of Pediatric Oncology (SIOP), *Med. Pediatr. Oncol.,* 17, 210, 1989.

10. **Carli, M., Pastore, G., Perilongo, G., et al.,** Tumor response and toxicity after single high-dose versus standard five-day divided-dose dactinomycin in childhood rhabdomyosarcoma, *J. Clin. Oncol.,* 6(4), 654, 1988.

11. **Carli, M., Pastore, G., De Bernardi, B., et al.,** Correlation between clinical and pathological examination of regional lymph nodes in childhood soft-tissue sarcomas (STS). A report from the Italian Cooperative Study RMS-79, Abstract, SIOP 19th Meeting, Jerusalem, Israel, September 13 to 18, 1987.

12. **Carli, M., Pastore, G., Guglielmi, G., et al.,** Lymph-node invasion and prognosis in childhood rhabdomyosarcoma. A report from the Italian Rhabdomyosarcoma Cooperative Group, SIOP 16th Meeting, Barcelona, Spain, September 17 to 21, 1984.

13. **Treuner, J.,** (For the CWS Group): updated results of the CWS-81 study, in Proc. Annu. Meeting of the German Cooperative Study, Stuttgart, West Germany, October 1989.

14. **Treuner, J., Koscielniak, E., and Keim, M.,** (For the CWS group): comparison of the rates of response to ifosfamide and cyclophosphamide in primary unresectable rhabdomyosarcomas, *Cancer Chemother. Pharmacol.,* 24(Suppl.), 48, 1989.

15. **Treuner, J., Suder, J., Keim, M., et al.,** The predictive value of initial cytostatic response in primary unresectable rhabdomyosarcoma in children, *Acta Oncol.,* 28, 67, 1989.

Chapter 14

NOVEL THERAPEUTIC STRATEGIES FOR THE TREATMENT OF RHABDOMYOSARCOMA AND SOFT TISSUE SARCOMAS: OBSERVATIONS WITH ARTERIAL INFUSION CHEMOTHERAPY

Norman Jaffe, Ya-Yen Lee, Marija Auersperg, Marija Us-Krasovec, Olga Porenta, W. Gohde, and Janez Lanovec

TABLE OF CONTENTS

I. INTRODUCTION

Major advances have been achieved in the management of malignant tumors in childhood.[1-18] These advances are evident, particularly in bone and soft tissue sarcomas, and may be attributed to the accelerating deployment of multidisciplinary treatment strategies. Thus, combinations of surgery, radiation therapy, and chemotherapy have yielded improved survival, avoided the necessity for amputation, enhanced the incidence of organ and limb preservation, and provided forms of useful palliation. A fundamental component of this strategy was the application of chemotherapy, with the use of agents with different mechanisms of action and minimal overlapping toxicity.

Successes achieved in the soft tissue sarcomas, particularly in rhabdomyosarcoma (RMS) appear to be approaching a plateau. Review of the experience in the first and second intergroup Rhabdomyosarcoma Studies (IRS-I and -II) does not reveal any significant advances during the past decade.[17] A recent report suggests improvements in results of therapy may be emerging in IRS-III. However, the results are preliminary and appear to have been attained at the cost of an increase in toxicity.[18] Additional follow-up will be required before any durable improvement in response may be appreciated.

As a consequence of the above circumstances, alternate forms of treatment utilizing newer agents and/or different strategies, or different strategies with existing agents, constitute an important part of any therapeutic investigation. In this chapter, the authors will report the preliminary results of studies utilizing intra-arterial chemotherapy for the treatment of the primary tumor and will outline tactics and strategies of its implementation. They also present preliminary data on chemotherapeutic manipulation of the cell cycle monitored by cytophotometric DNA measurements and cytomorphology.

II. MATERIALS AND METHODS

A. M. D. ANDERSON CANCER CENTER

Intra-arterial *cis*-diamminedichloroplatinum-II (CDP) or cisplatin has been utilized at the M. D. Anderson Cancer Center as a major component of the treatment of osteosarcoma.[1] It has also been investigated in several patients with inoperable soft tissue sarcomas as a potential means for facilitating surgical extirpation or to improve the therapeutic efficacy of radiation therapy. To date, eight such patients have been treated (Table 1). Seven had previously received or were receiving established chemotherapeutic regimens known to be effective in soft tissue sarcomas. In three patients, the tumors were considered resistant to chemotherapy because of recurrence of tumor or failure to respond. In two patients, intra-arterial cisplatin was interposed between seemingly effective courses of vincristine, actinomycin-D, and cyclophosphamide (the VAC regimen), in an effort to obtain maximum tumor reduction prior to an attempt at definitive surgery or radiation therapy. The tumors in intracranial and parameningeal sites were considered inoperable, or if they were operated upon, would be attendant with unacceptable mutilation. They were retrospectively classified as stage III according to criteria of the IRS.[7]

Treatment with intra-arterial cisplatin commenced with an intravenous infusion of 5% dextrose in 0.5% saline in order to provide 12 to 24 h of prehydration at a rate of 3000 ml/m^2/24 h. Eight hours prior to the intra-arterial infusion, the fluid intake was augmented to deliver 2000 ml of 5% dextrose in 0.5% saline (Figure 1). This was followed by 500 ml of the same fluid given in the ninth hour. Immediately prior to the infusion of cisplatin, 50 ml of 20% mannitol was administered intravenously over 15 min. Intra-arterial cisplatin was then initiated and administered over 2 h for extremity lesions and for 1 h for head and neck tumors. The dose was 150 mg/m^2 (dissolved in 300 ml of normal saline) for extremity lesions and 100 mg/m^2 (dissolved in 200 ml of normal saline) for tumors of the head and

TABLE 1
Patient Characteristic Treatment and Results

Patient	Age (years)	Diagnosis	Site	Metastases	Previous therapy	Current therapy	Response	Comment
1	11½	RMS	Infratemporal fossa with intracranial extension		A-VAC, XRT	I-A CDP × 6 (PR)	Marked regression	Refused further therapy lost to follow-up
2	4½	RMS (recurrent)	Middle ear, infratemporal fossa, and pteryoid		VAC	I-A CDP × 6	Marked regression (PR)	Response followed by XRT Alive and well 6+ years
3	3	RMS	Infratemporal fossa with intracranial extension		A-VAC	VAC interposed with I-A CDP × 7	Marked regression after five courses (PR) Tumor escape suspected after the sixth course and confirmed after the seventh course	XRT administered when tumor escape confirmed Surgical resection after XRT and additional VAC Alive and well 5+ years
4	13	RMS (recurrent)	Parapharynx and intracranial		A-VAC, XRT	I-A CDP × 1 CDP (intravenous) × 2	Mild regression after CDP × 1 (PR)	Stricture branch of external carotid artery preventing additional I-A CDP; died of progressive local disease
5	3	RMS	Nasopharynx, middle ear, and intracranial extension		A-VAC	I-A CDP × 3	NR	No response to intravenous CDP Died of local progressive disease

TABLE 1 (continued)
Patient Characteristic Treatment and Results

Patient	Age (years)	Diagnosis	Site	Metastases	Previous therapy	Current therapy	Response	Comment
6	12	RMS	Maxilla, infra-temporal fossa	Lungs	A-VAC XRT CDP 5-FU	I-A CDP × 4	NR	No change in primary tumor or metastases during I-A CDP; lost to follow-up
7	9	Hemangiopericytoma	Axilla			I-A CDP × 1	No change in size	Radiation therapy followed by surgical excision Alive 6+ years
8	13 1/2	Malignant fibrous histiocytoma (radiation induced)	Maxilla	Humerus	VAC	I-A CDP × 3	Reduction in tumor size after first course Subsequent progression after second and third course	Died of local progressive disease No change in metastases
9	10	RMS	Temporal fossa and local parameningeal area	Regional nodes XRT	A-VAC bleomycin MTX	First course velban CDP, MTX	Regression in tumor size with first course Cytology III[a] Shift in DNA curve[b]	Died 4 months with local and meningeal extension
						Second course: velban I-A (aborted) followed by XRT	— No response to aborted second course of velban	

| 10 | 12 | Malignant schwannoma | Thigh | First course velban, CDP bleomycin adriamycin
Second course CDP, velban bleomycin 5-FU, adriamycin | No clinical response
Cytology evaluation not possible
Increased number of mitoses in histology | Died of pulmonary metastases 2 years after diagnosis |

Note: Patients 1 to 8 were treated at M. D. Anderson Cancer Center, Houston, Texas. Patients 9 and 10 were treated at the Onkoloski Institut, Ljubljana, Yugoslavia.

Abbreviations: VAC = vincristine, actinomycin D, and cyclophosphamide; A-VAC = vincristine, actinomycin D, cyclophosphamide, and adriamycin; CDP = *cis*-diamminedichloroplatinum-II (*cis*-platin); MTX = methotrexate; IA = intra-arterial administration; XRT = radiation therapy.

a   See text for cytology parameters of response.
b   See text for DNA changes.

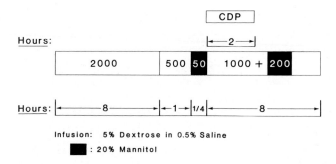

FIGURE 1.   Schedule for intra-arterial *cis*-diamminedichloroplatinum-II (CDP). Patients received a maintenance intravenous infusion of 3000 ml/ m^2 of 5% dextrose in 0.5% saline solution. The infusion was interrupted for $9\frac{1}{4}$ h to permit administration of the following: 500 ml of 5% dextrose in 0.5% saline (1 h), 50 ml of 20% mannitol ($\frac{1}{4}$ h), and 200 ml of 50% mannitol dissolved in 1000 ml of 5% dextrose in 0.5% saline (8 h). Intra-arterial cisplatin (CDP) was administered over a period of 2 h for extremity tumors and for 1 h for head and neck tumors. The maintenance infusion (1000 ml of 5% dextrose in 0.5% saline with 10 cc of 10% calcium gluconate, 10 meq of magnesium sulfate, and 20 meq potassium chloride) was then reinstated. Cisplatin was dissolved in 300 ml of normal saline for extremity tumors and in 200 ml of normal saline for head and neck tumors. A dose of 3000 IU of heparin was also added. The depicted volumes of 20% mannitol (50 ml 10 g and 200 ml, 40 g, respectively) were utilized for patients with a surface area of 1 to 1.5 m^2. Appropriate adjustments were made for children with smaller surface areas (see text).

neck. Sodium heparin as an anticoagulant, at a dose of 1500 to 3000 IU according to age, was also added. Concurrently, the intravenous infusion was altered to 1000 ml of 5% dextrose in 0.5% saline plus 200 ml in 20% mannitol for delivery over 8 h. In the ninth hour, this infusion was replaced by 1000 ml of 5% dextrose in 0.5% saline together with 10 ml of 10% calcium gluconate, 10 meq of magnesium sulfate, and 20 meq of potassium chloride for administration as 3000 ml/m^2 for 24 h.

Intra-arterial infusions required insertion of a catheter percutaneously by means of the Seldinger technique through the brachial or femoral artery under anesthesia. The tip of the catheter was positioned under fluoroscopic guidance into the appropriate vessel supplying the neoplasm. A Sigma motor volumetric infusion pump, primed with 150 ml of saline and 2000 IU of heparin, was then attached to the catheter and the infusion initiated at 120 ml/ h in preparation for giving cisplatin. During and after the infusion, the affected limb and insertion site were inspected at half-hour intervals. After removal of the catheter, pressure was applied over the insertion site for 5 min. The peripheral pulses distal to the insertion site and affected limb were then monitored at 2-h intervals for 24 h.

Prerequisites for treatment included a creatinine clearance of over 60 ml/min/m^2 and normal values of the serum electrolytes, creatinine, calcium, phosphorus, magnesium, liver function studies, and hemogram. Results of these tests (except creatine clearance) were obtained daily. Hospitalization was required for 48 to 72 h, during which fluid and electrolytes were monitored daily and antiemetics were administered as required. The intra-arterial infusions were repeated at 2-week intervals for a total of seven courses.

B. INSTITUTE OF ONCOLOGY (ONKOLOSKI INSTITUT), LJUBLJANA, YUGOSLAVIA

Intra-arterial chemotherapy was investigated initially at the Onkoloski Institute, Ljubljana in the early 1970s predominantly for head and neck tumors.[19-22] It was eventually adopted as individualized infusional treatment for inoperable tumors and high risk patients. In addition, cytomorphological studies and cytophotometric DNA measurements of tumor cells were introduced for early prediction of efficacy and rational timing of drugs in chemotherapeutic schedules.[19,23-29] These investigations were conducted on fine-needle aspiration biopsies (FNAB) of tumors taken before, during, and after chemotherapy. Single cell DNA measurements using a Feulgen staining procedure with acid hydrolysis in 4 NHCl at 28°C for 60 min were carried out on a Vickers 85 cytophotometer.[21,24,27] Commencing in 1988 DNA measurements were performed on a flow cytophotometer (PAS II, Partec, Munster, Germany).

C. CYTOMORPHOLOGICAL EVALUATION

The effect of chemotherapy was determined by changes in the tumor cell population. This included changes in the distribution pattern of tumor cells and degenerative changes, i.e., enlarged and/or bizarre-shaped cells, vacuolization of cytoplasm and nuclei, chromatin clumping, pyknosis, and disintegration. The effect of chemotherapy was classified according to the number of affected cells and the severity of changes as good (III), moderate (II), and poor or no effect (I). This was categorized as follows: good effect — severe changes in majority of tumor cells; moderate effect — approximately 50% of damaged cells; poor effect — less than 50% damaged cells.[28]

D. HISTOLOGICAL CLASSIFICATION — THE EFFECT OF CHEMOTHERAPY

The same principle as in evaluation of the effect of osteosarcoma was adopted.[30] This was based on the extent of necrosis of the resected specimen.

E. CHEMOTHERAPY

Low doses of vinblastine (VLB), 2 mg in 12 to 24 h infusion, or CDP, 50 mg/m^2 in 8 to 24 h infusion, were used as modulators of cellular kinetics (monitored by DNA measurements). Changes in DNA distribution pattern induced by VLB or CDP were used for timing of drugs in combined chemotherapy schedules, i.e., drugs predominantly active in S or G$_2$ + M phases were infused after VLB or CDP when the accumulation of cells in the respective phases of the cell cycle was demonstrated in the DNA histogram. Also, VLB, CDP, adriamycin (ADR), bleomycin (Bleo), and methotrexate (MTX) were used in combination chemotherapy. The duration of infusions, as well as the intervals between infusions, were individualized and planned according to the results of DNA measurements after test doses of VLB and CDP. Courses of chemotherapy, based on the results of DNA measurements and cytomorphologic effect, were repeated at 2-week intervals. Treatment was maintained until the tumor was deemed suitable for surgery and/or it appeared that additional benefit would not accrue.

Six adult patients (to be reported separately) and two pediatric patients were entered in the study of individualized intra-arterial infusional chemotherapy. One had an inoperable RMS of the infratemporal fossa and the second a malignant schwannoma of the thigh. Percutaneous cannulation of the artery utilizing the Seldinger technique was used in one and operative cannulation in the other. The position of the catheter was checked by dye injection (patent blue) and infusion of 99 mTc MAA (macro aggregated albumin) as described previously.[19,22] To outline the components of this novel therapeutic approach, the treatment of one of the patients will be described in detail.

Patient 9 (Table 1) was a 10-year-old boy who developed a RMS of the right infratemporal region. He responded initially to conventional treatment with VAC, ADR, Bleo, and MTX and radiation therapy (5600 cGy) but developed a local regional recurrence several months later. At the time of initiation of intra-arterial chemotherapy, the tumor measured 5.0 × 5.0 × 5.0 cm, involved the temporal and zygomatic region, and extended to the

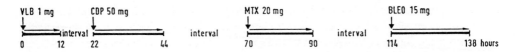

FIGURE 2.   Schedule of chemotherapy for intra-arterial treatment of RMS (Onkoloski Institut). Abbreviations: VLB = velban, CDP = *cis*-diamminedichloroplatinum-II (cisplatin), MTX = methotrexate, and Bleo = bleomycin.

lateral border of the right orbit. It was fixed to the temporal muscle and underlying bone and was accompanied by a diffuse tumorous infiltration measuring approximately 6.0 × 6.0 × 4.0 cm in the submandibular area. Cure with the most aggressive form of surgery was unrealistic and individualized intra-arterial chemotherapy as a potential method of salvage was proposed.

The usual access to the external carotid by the superficial temporal artery was impossible because of the overlying tumor. Consequently, the external carotid artery was cannulated via the superficial thyroid artery under general anesthesia. A metastatic lymph node removed to access the artery confirmed the presence of recurrent RMS. An excellent distribution of the infused material in the tumor region was achieved as demonstrated by dye injection (patent blue) and 99m TcMAA. Chemotherapy was comprised of VLB, CDP, MTX, and Bleo (Figure 2). The selection of chemotherapy was based on previous experiences, results of serial FNAB DNA measurements, and morphologic observations similar to those performed in adults.[25] Treatment achieved a distinct response (*vide infra*).

Fourteen days after the first course of intra-arterial chemotherapy there was a suggestion of tumor escape. A second course of treatment was therefore initiated, but the patient inadvertently removed the arterial catheter during the VLB infusion. He was immediately taken to the operating room for revision and the wound was opened and rinsed with isotonic saline. Reinsertion of the catheter was then attempted. However, it was impossible to achieve good distribution of the injected dye and the catheter was removed with ligation of the superior thyroid artery. In the second course, because of this complication, only 0.3 mg of VLB was administered.

Surgery was performed 11 days after the second course. Resection of the primary tumor together with the overlying skin, underlying temporal muscle, partial temporal zygomatic bone, and parotid gland (with conservation of the facial nerve) was accomplished. Destruction of the squamous part of the temporal bone measuring approximately 2.0 cm was observed. It was impossible to achieve free margins as the tumor protruded through the eroded bone to dura. However, submandibular lymph node dissection and extirpation of the salivary gland were performed. This was followed by additional radiation therapy (3600 cGy). During radiation, VLB, 1.0 mg over 12 h, and CDP, 20.0 mg, were administered by intravenous infusion at weekly intervals with minimal response. MTX was also administered intrathecally. Despite this aggressive approach, the patient died 4 months later of local recurrence and central nervous system involvement. (See Section III for more details.)

The second pediatric patient had a 14.0 × 10.0 cm inoperable malignant schwannoma of the thigh. A limb-sparing surgical procedure was impossible; and the tumor could only be removed by amputation, which was refused. She was consequently treated with two courses of intra-arterial chemotherapy comprised of VLB, Bleo, CDP, 5FU, and ADR. There was no apparent clinical response. After failure of intra-arterial chemotherapy consent for amputation was obtained and the operation performed.

III. RESULTS

A. M. D. ANDERSON CANCER CENTER
Four of six patients with intracranial RMSs responded to intra-arterial cisplatin. One

patient with a tumor in the middle cranial fossa achieved significant reduction following the fourth course of intra-arterial chemotherapy (patient 1, Table 1, Figure 3A to F). Additional treatment was refused. The second patient, who had a lesion of the middle ear, achieved a partial response after six courses. Radiation therapy was then administered and he has remained free of disease over 5 years (patient 2, Table 1, Figure 4A to C). The third patient, who had an infratemporal lesion, also achieved a partial response with seven courses of intra-arterial cisplatin interposed with VAC. The remission lasted approximately 6 months. During administration of the seventh course, the arteriogram suggested recurrence of tumor growth. The patient consequently received radiation therapy followed by surgical extirpation of the tumor. He also remained free of disease for over 5 years.

The fourth patient, who had a RMS in the parameningeal region, achieved stable disease lasting 2 months after the first course of therapy. The tumor was inoperable and additional intra-arterial therapy could not be administered because of arterial stricture. She later died of progressive local regrowth of tumor. Two patients failed to respond to three and four courses, respectively. The remaining two patients, one with a malignant hemangiopericytoma of the arm and one with a malignant fibrous histiocytoma of the neck, received only one course of intra-arterial therapy and were considered inevaluable.

B. ONKOLOSKI INSTITUT

Twenty-four hours after the first course of intra-arterial chemotherapy, clinical observation demonstrated rapid reduction of the size of the primary tumor as well as shrinkage of metastases in the patient with RMS in the infratemporal fossa. Six days after treatment, the primary tumor was reduced in size to $1.5 \times 2.0 \times 2.0$ cm, and the submandibular infiltration was noted to have shrunk to $1.5 \times 2.0 \times 2.0$ cm.

FNAB revealed an excellent effect of the velban infusion. All tumor cells seemed to be damaged. They were pyknotic and disintegrated (grade III). Velban also seemed to be more effective than cisplatin. However, 5 days after completion of treatment, cytological examination revealed rare viable cells. By the 14th day, FNAB demonstrated that as many as 30% of the cells were viable.

Single cell DNA measurements after velban (Figure 5) and cisplatin were similar (not shown in Figure 6). Histograms after completion of chemotherapy revealed a reduction in the number of cells with high DNA values when compared to those observed prior to treatment (Figure 6). Fourteen days later, however, the DNA histogram was very similar to the pretherapy baseline. This observation also correlated with cytomorphological findings, which demonstrated recurrence and proliferation of tumor cells. Histological examination after the second aborted course of chemotherapy still revealed evidence of response, with the presence of large necrotic areas within the primary tumor and residual viable cells close to the periphery.

In the patient with malignant schwannoma there was no clinical evidence of response. There was 40% tumor necrosis in the resected specimen and 10 times more mitoses than in the biopsy specimen examined prior to intra-arterial chemotherapy. Unfortunately DNA studies and cytomorphological examination to evaluate the effects of treatment were insufficient since an adequate number of malignant cells for measurement in FNAB specimens was not available. The patient died 30 months after diagnosis of pulmonary metastases. In an adult patient (to be reported separately) with similar histologic findings after intra-arterial chemotherapy there was a low percentage of necrosis and an increased number of mitoses. Further, DNA measurements also showed an important shift to the $G_2 + M$ compartment with a depletion of the G_1 peak. These findings suggested a block of cells in $G_2 + M$ phases and could also have been indicative of an effect of chemotherapy. Cytomorphological evaluation also showed damaged tumor cells which was also consistent with an effect induced by chemotherapy despite the 40% necrosis found on histology.

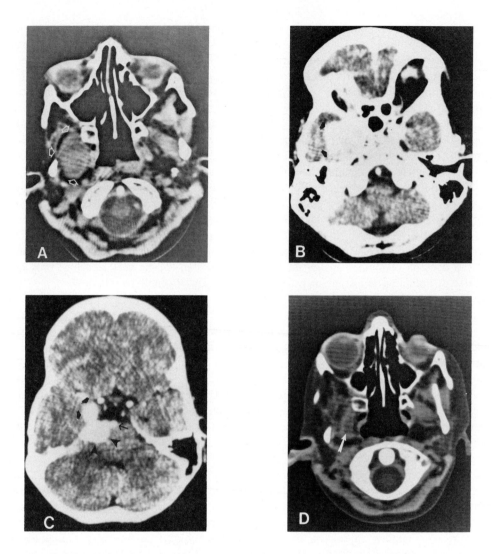

FIGURE 3.   Preinfusion computerized tomogram (CT) scan. (A) Recurrent RMS involving the right medial pterygoid muscle (white short arrows) is well demonstrated. (B) Direct intracranial extradural extension, through the floor of the middle cranial fossa, is readily appreciated in the medial aspect of the right middle cranial fossa (black short arrows) and the right anterolateral aspect of the posterior fossa (black arrowheads [C]). The tip of the basilar artery (black long arrow) is slightly displaced. (D) Postinfusion CT scan after four courses of intra-arterial *cis*-diamminedichloroplatinum-II into the right internal maxillary artery. The tumor in the right pterygoid region has significantly regressed with the demonstration of central necrosis (white long arrow). (E) The intracranial extension has completely disappeared and (F) the basilar artery (black long arrow) has returned to a normal position. (Reproduced from Jaffe, N. Cangir, A., Lee, Y., et al., *Regional Cancer Treatment*, Vol. 29, Aigner, K. R., Patt, Y. Z., Link, K. H., and Kreidler, J., Eds., S. Karger, Basel, 1988, 292. With permission.)

C. EFFECTS OF INTRA-ARTERIAL CHEMOTHERAPY ON DISTANT METASTASES

Only two patients in this series had pulmonary metastases which remained stable. The others did not have distant metastases, and none developed metastases during treatment. Therefore, this experience did not determine the effect of the systemic concentration of chemotherapy, if any, in prevention or eradication of metastases.

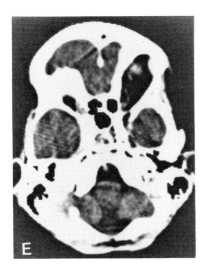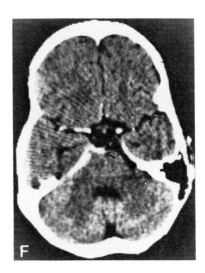

FIGURE 3 (continued)

D. TOXICITY

The toxicity of intra-arterial cisplatin consisted of nausea, vomiting, reduction of creatinine clearance, and auditory dysfunction. Local skin reactions manifested as pain, edema, discoloration, hyperpigmentation (particularly around the neck in head and neck tumors), and subcutaneous induration in the region of the tip of the catheter. The local reactions due to intra-arterial cisplatin, however, did not preclude performance of surgical procedures.

At the Onkoloski Institut, no toxicity with the intra-arterial chemotherapy was observed.

IV. DISCUSSION

VAC chemotherapy (vincristine, actinomycin D, and cyclophosphamide) is the most effective combination of chemotherapy for the treatment of RMS and soft tissue sarcomas in children.[8,9,13,14,17] Although adriamycin is an active agent and is useful in treating malignant soft tissue sarcomas in adults,[31] it has apparently not produced any additional benefit when added to the VAC regimen.[17] Promising agents for possible future study include etoposide (VP-16),[32] ifosfamide,[33] melphalan,[34] cisplatin,[32] and high dose methotrexate with citrovorum factor rescue.[35] These agents are all administered intravenously.

Intra-arterial chemotherapy, as opposed to the intravenous route, may improve the efficacy of an agent as a consequence of increased local tumoricidal concentrations of drug delivered to the tumor. This strategy increases the uptake of drug by tumor cells and relies essentially on a "first pass" effect. Thus, on first pass, there is high extraction of drug by the perfused tumor prior to clearance of the drug by various organs during subsequent passage through the systemic circulation. More extensive destruction of tumor is thereby achieved. This approach has been utilized in osteosarcoma[1] and sarcomas in adults.[36] As demonstrated in this study, intra-arterial chemotherapy appears to be effective in children: four out of six patients responded to cisplatin and one responded to the combination of velban, cisplatin, methotrexate, and bleomycin. Several favorable responses also occurred in patients who had relapsed following prior treatment with the conventional VAC regimen, or with VAC combined with adriamycin and radiation.

Factors responsible for the success of regional or intra-arterial chemotherapy include higher concentrations of the agent reaching the tumor, the duration of the intra-arterial treatment, dosage, schedule, effects on cell membrane transport and permeability, and tumor

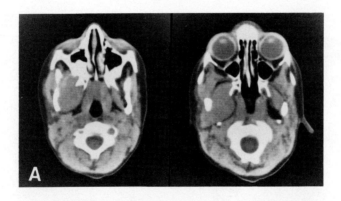

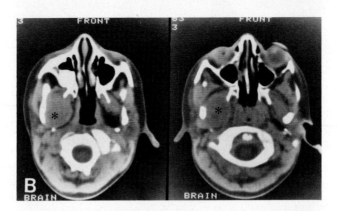

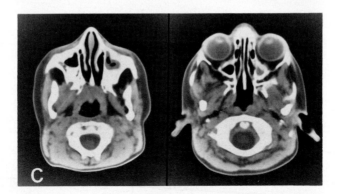

FIGURE 4. (A) Axial computerized tomography (CT) scans in a patient
with intracranial RMS before initiation of intra-arterial chemotherapy. There
is an expansile soft tissue mass arising from the right pterygoid muscle
extending into the right parapharyngeal space. (B) After six courses of
intra-arterial cisplatin (CDP), hypodensity of the tumor (asterisks) consistent with necrosis is present. The angiogram demonstrated disappearance
of neovascularity and stain (not shown). (C) Follow-up CT scan after
treatment with interarterial cisplatin and radiation therapy (1 month later)
resulted in complete disappearance of tumor. This CT scan was taken 2
years later and confirms the absence of tumor.

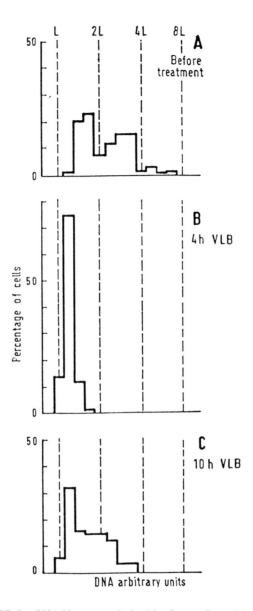

FIGURE 5. DNA histograms obtained by fine-needle aspirate biopsy (FNAB) in the patient with RMS of the infratemporal region. Velban, 1 mg, was administered intra-arterially over 12 h. (A) Wide distribution of DNA values indicates a multiclonal, rapidly proliferating tumor. In histograms (B) and (C), there are significant reductions in the number of cells with high DNA values. Some normal cells (macrophages) are probably present in the highest "near diploid" peak in (B).

sensitivity.[1,19] Higher local drug concentrations may be particularly advantageous if resistance to destruction of the tumor is due to inadequate drug exposure, that is, inadequate concentration of drug in the tumor. Some chemotherapeutic agents are also more effective when administered by prolonged infusions, as opposed to a bolus injection. There is currently no agreement in regard to the size of the dose and duration of intra-arterial treatment; doses and durations now used are based on animal studies and on limited clinical trials.[19]

If injected into arteries of a large caliber, the chemotherapeutic agent is rapidly diluted to concentrations approximating that produced by intravenous injection.[19] In order to obtain

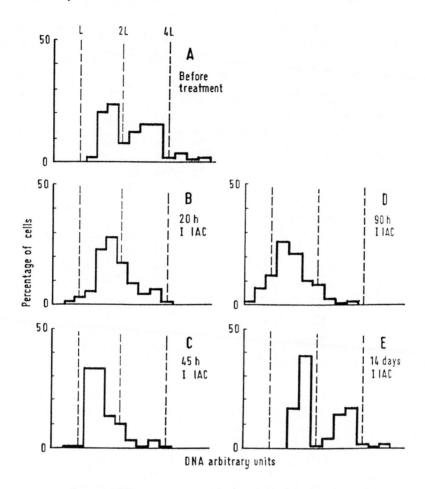

FIGURE 6.   DNA histograms after one course of intra-arterial chemotherapy as outlined in Figure 2. Reduction in the percent of cells with high DNA values is observed in (B), (C), and (D) in comparison with (A). Fourteen days after treatment (E), there is reappearance of cells with high DNA values consistent with presence of proliferating tumor. IAC = infusional intra-arterial chemotherapy.

the highest concentrations of drug at the tumor site, the arterial catheter should be correctly placed and major arterial side branches should be carefully obliterated or ligated. By this means, it is also possible to direct the flow of the chemotherapeutic agent predominantly to the tumor and reduce the infusion of drug into surrounding healthy tissues. The correct position of the catheter and the size of the infused region can be determined by injection of methylene blue or, preferably, TcMAA into the cannulated artery.[19,22]

The efficacy of intra-arterial chemotherapy may also be affected by vascular communications which develop during treatment due to rapid disintegration of perfused tissues. This tissue destruction in turn may cause release of histamine and allied substances which can effect the caliber of blood vessels. These microvascular changes were shown to occur by means of isotope studies; they manifested as "shunts" which anatomically in all probability appeared to be abnormally dilated capillaries.[19] In view of this finding, antihistaminics were occasionally administered prior to and during the course of intra-arterial chemotherapy.

Rapid intra-arterial injections may give rise to turbulence and thorough mixing of the chemotherapeutic agent and blood within the artery. This produces fairly uniform distribution of the mixture of blood and drug within vessels branching off near the tip of the catheter. Conversely, a very slow infusion may produce laminary flow and an uneven distribution of drug into the immediate branches. Peripherally, the localized high concentration of drug may produce areas of induration and ulceration. A recent attempt to avoid the problem of uneven distribution of injected drugs involved the use of a pulsatile pump.[37]

In most intra-arterial infusions, performed without tourniquet occlusion, the drug enters the systemic circulation and toxicity is not reduced. Thus, it may also still provide an effect against micrometastases. The ability of the drug to destroy disseminated metastases will ultimately be influenced by systemic concentrations of the drug and the duration of exposure of tumor cells to the drug. In contrast, in isolation perfusion, a high local drug level in blood and soft tissues is achieved with minimal leak of drug to the systemic circulation.

Unfortunately, intra-arterial chemotherapy is very complex. In children it requires general anesthesia and is labor intensive. Because of this problem, there are few reports on the use of intra-arterial chemotherapy in pediatrics. It has been used extensively in osteosarcoma with excellent results. Further, in another reported study, two RMSs and one juvenile fibrosarcoma in advanced stages were rendered operable by intra-arterial adriamycin and actinomycin-D.[38]

In evaluating response, discrepancies may exist in assessing the clinical, cytological, and histological effects of chemotherapy.[39] The conventional method of measuring the diameter of the tumor may also not be an accurate index of the effect of therapy. Damaged necrotic tumor can persist for a prolonged period; consequently, tumor measurements may remain unchanged and lead to an incorrect judgment that the chemotherapy is ineffective. To some extent, this perception may be avoided by examining changes in the character of the tumor by CT scan or ultrasound.[40] This tactic was also employed, in part, in patient 2 (Figure 4).

Also, there is no universally accepted method for assessing effects of chemotherapy on soft tissue sarcomas by histologic criteria. At the Onkoloski Institut, assessment of effect of chemotherapy was based principally upon occurrence of necrosis. For this purpose, aspiration biopsy and cytologic examination were used to demonstrate the necrotic changes following chemotherapy. This approach permitted assessments to be made with a minimum of discomfort and without exposing the patient to major risk. During the course of treatment, degenerative changes of the malignant cells reflecting the effects of chemotherapy were also observed. Cytologically, early damage can be detected within 24 h, whereas clinical response may only be observed later.[19,22,41]

It is logical to assume that necrosis of 60% of tumor in a surgical specimen could indicate major sensitivity of tumor to the drug and a pronounced effect of intra-arterial treatment.[30] However, evaluation of the effect of chemotherapy by pathological studies is difficult and may be unreliable because of heterogeneity of response within the tumor. There may also be discrepancies of interpretation in comparing the extent of necrosis in a small prechemotherapy biopsy with that of specimens obtained from later resection of the tumor. An additional drawback is evaluation of a static situation, that is, a situation where the drug therapy produces no change in the tumor.

In spite of the above problems, repeated cytological studies provide an opportunity to follow the evolution of drug-induced changes in tumor cells.[42] This method also recognizes the possibility that the tissue aspirate may contain tumor with different cell populations and yield a false interpretation. Another problem is the natural heterogeneity of soft tissue sarcomas and the lack of experience by pathologists in evaluating chemotherapy-related changes in these tumors. While these caveats were recognized, it was felt that they were minimized with concurrent DNA measurements.

Many chemotherapeutic agents are phase specific, that is, they act only on cells in specific phases of the mitotic cycle. Furthermore, because tumor cells are generally in different phases of cycle at any given time, a phase specific agent can only affect a fraction of the tumor cell population. Therefore, the effect of a particular agent is usually limited.

Moreover, only a small fraction of the cell population takes part in the cell cycle while the remainder are "dormant" and are not affected by most agents.

DNA measurements were found to be useful in addressing the problem of tumor cells being present in different phases of the growth cycle, and in planning rational approaches to destroy these cells by chemotherapy.[24-27] The method of DNA measurement was objective and reproducible and the findings were independent of the examiner's experience. In combination with cytomorphologic studies, DNA measurement was shown to yield useful information on the efficacy and timing of chemotherapy. Thus, in early studies, a therapeutic advantage was induced by synchronization of cells in their growth cycle, simultaneous passage of more than the average number of tumor cells through various phases of the cell cycle, and use of phase specific drugs.[43] This appropriate timing of chemotherapy was probably responsible for the favorable effects of therapy observed in the patient with infratemporal RMS treated at the Onkoloski Institut.

Additional numbers of patients treated in this way, together with clinical follow-up, are needed before definitive conclusions regarding the usefulness of changes in DNA distribution pattern and manipulation of the cell cycle can be made. However, studies performed thus far demonstrate that endoreduplication of DNA or shifts of cells to S and G_2 to M compartments of the growth cycle suggest a good chemotherapeutic effect. This concept may help explain some of the remarkable successes achieved with individualized infusional therapy in several patients.[24-27]

V. CONCLUSIONS

The known limitations in tumor destruction of strategies currently available for the treatment of soft tissue sarcomas necessitate investigation of alternate forms of therapy. This chapter has outlined two possible additional approaches: (1) intra-arterial (individualized) administration of chemotherapy and (2) DNA manipulation of the cell cycle. The experience reported in this chapter with two patients at the Onkoloski Institut indicates that DNA manipulation of cells in the growth cycle and timing of chemotherapy are practical and feasible. Further trials with both strategies, particularly in primary inoperable tumors, appear to be warranted.

ACKNOWLEDGMENT

This work is supported in part by a Fulbright Scholarship, 1989 and 1990.

REFERENCES

1. **Jaffe, N., Knapp, J., Chuang, V. P., et al.,** Osteosarcoma: intra-arterial treatment of the primary tumor with cis-Diamminedichloroplatinum-II (CDP), angiographic, pathologic and pharmacologic studies, *Cancer,* 51, 402, 1983.
2. **Goorin, A., Perez-Atayde, A., Gibhardt, M., et al.,** Weekly high dose methotrexate and doxorubicin for osteosarcoma. The Dana Farber Cancer Center/The Childrens Hospital Study III, *J. Clin. Oncol.,* 5, 1178, 1987.
3. **Rosen, G., Caparros, B., Huvos, A. G., et al.,** Preoperative chemotherapy for osteosarcoma. Selection of post-operative adjuvant chemotherapy based upon response of the primary tumor to preoperative chemotherapy, *Cancer,* 49, 1221, 1982.
4. **Jurgens, H., Exner, U., Gradner, H., et al.,** Multidisciplinary treatment of primary Ewing's sarcoma of bone, *Cancer,* 61, 23, 1988.

5. **D'Angio, C. J., Evans, A. E., Breslow, N., et al.,** The treatment of Wilms' tumor. Results of the Second National Wilms' Tumor Study, *Cancer,* 47, 2304, 1981.
6. **D'Angio, C. J., Breslow, N., Beckwith, B., et al.,** Treatment of Wilms' tumor. Results of the Third National Wilms' Tumor Study, *Cancer,* 64, 349, 1989.
7. **Maurer, H. M., Beltangady, M., Gehan, E. A., et al.,** The intergroup rhabdomyosarcoma study-I, *Cancer,* 61, 209, 1988.
8. **Raney, R. B., Tefft, M., Newton, W. A., et al.,** Improved prognosis with intensive treatment of children with cranial soft tissue sarcomas arising in nonorbital parameningeal sites, *Cancer,* 59, 147, 1987.
9. **Hays, D. M., Shimada, H., Raney, R. B., Jr., et al.,** Sarcomas of the vagina and uterus: the intergroup rhabdomyosarcoma study, *J. Pediatr. Surg.,* 20, 718, 1985.
10. **Bell, J. Averette, H., Davis, J., and Toledaro, S.,** Genital rhabdomyosarcoma: current management and review of the literature, *Obstet. Gynecol. Surv.,* 41, 257, 1986.
11. **Kinsella, T. J., Miser, J. J., Trechi, T. J., et al.,** Treatment of high risk sarcomas in children and young adults. Analysis of local control using intensive combined modality therapy, *NCI monogr.,* No. 6, 291, 1988.
12. **Hays, D. M., Raney, B., Jr., Lawrence, W., Jr., et al.,** Bladder and prostatic tumors in the intergroup rhabdomyosarcoma study (IRS-I). Results of therapy, *Cancer,* 50, 1472, 1982.
13. **Jaffe, N., Murray, J., Traggis, D., et al.,** Multidisciplinary treatment for childhood sarcoma, *Am. J. Surg.,* 133, 405, 1977.
14. **Loughlin, K. R., Retig, A. B., Weinstein, H. J., et al.,** Genitourinary rhabdomyosarcoma, in *Recent Concepts in Sarcoma Treatment,* Ryan, J. R. and Baker, L. O., Eds., Kluwer Academic Publishers, Dordrecht, 1988, 136.
15. **Wharam, M. D., Foulkes, M. A., Lawrence, W., Jr., et al.,** Soft tissue sarcoma of the head and neck in childhood. Nonorbital and nonparameningeal sites. A report of the intergroup rhabdomyosarcoma study (IRS)-1, *Cancer,* 53, 1016, 1984.
16. **Raney, R. B., Jr., Tefft, M., and Maurer, H. M.,** Disease patterns and survival rate in children with metastatic soft tissue sarcoma. A report from the intergroup rhabdomyosarcoma study (IRS)-1, *Cancer,* 62, 1257, 1988.
17. **Maurer, H. M.,** Pediatric experience in rhabdomyosarcoma, in *Recent Concepts in Sarcoma Treatment,* Ryan, J. R. and Baker, L. O., Eds., Kluwer Academic Publishers, Dordrecht, 1988, 136.
18. **Maurer, H., Gehan, E., Crist, W., et al.,** Intergroup rhabdomyosarcoma study (IRS)-III. A preliminary report of overall outcome, *Proc. ASCO,* 8, 1154, 1989.
19. **Auersperg, M., Erjavec, M., Obrez, I., and Us-Krasovec, M.,** Experience gained during the introduction and development of intra-arterial chemotherapy of the head and neck tumors, *Radiol. Iugosl. 4 Fosc.,* 3, 27, 1970.
20. **Auersperg, M., Furlan, L., Maroll, K., and Jereb, B.,** Intra-arterial chemotherapy and radiotherapy in locally advanced cancer of the oral cavity and oropharynx, *Radiat. Oncol. Biol. Phys.,* 4, 273, 1978.
21. **Auersperg, M., Soba, E., and Vrasper-Porenta, O.,** Intravenous chemotherapy with synchronization in advanced cancer of oral cavity and oropharynx. III, *Krebsforsch,* 90, 149, 1977.
22. **Erjavec, M., Auersperg, M., and Obrez, I.,** Isotope scanning in intra-arterial infusion chemotherapy, *Invest. Radiol.,* 5, 122, 1970.
23. **Auersperg, M., Erjavec, M., and Us-Krasovec, M.,** Accumulation of 99m-Tc bleomycin in human squamous cell carcinoma in vivo after synchronization by vinblastine, *IRCS,* 3, 560, 1975.
24. **Auersperg, M., Porenta, O., Us-Krasovec, M., et al.,** Cytophotometric DNA studies in human head and neck tumors after cis-platinum infusion, in Proc. 13th Int. Congr. of Chemotherapy, Spitzy, K. H. and Karrer, K., Eds., Vienna, 1983, 280/8.
25. **Auersperg, M., Zorc, R., Us-Krasovec, M., et al.,** DNA measurements used for planning of multimodal treatment in sarcomas, in *Abstracts of Lectures, Symposia and Free Communications,* Vol. 2, S. Karger, Basel and Akademiai Kiado, Budapest, 1986, 637.
26. **Auersperg, M., Pompe, F., and Bergent, D.,** Cis-platinum-based combined intra-arterial chemotherapy of head and neck tumors, in *Advances in Regional Cancer Therapy,* Kreidler, J., Link, K. H., and Aigner, K. R., Eds., S. Karger, Basel, 1988, 105.
27. **Auersperg, M., Zorc, R., Us-Krasovec, M., et al.,** Chemotherapy for Hürtlle cell carcinoma based on sequential DNA measurements, *Radiol. Iugosl.,* 22, 269, 1988.
28. **Us-Krasovec, M.,** Changes in Malignant Cells under the Influence of Chemotherapy, Doctors thesis, Medicinska Fakulteta, Ljubljana, 1972 (Slovene, summary in English).
29. **Us-Krasovec, M. and Auersperg, M.,** Effect of intra-arterial chemotherapy on tumor cells, *Panminerva Med.,* 13, 261, 1971.
30. **Ayala, A. G., Mackay, B., Jaffe, N., et al.,** Osteosarcoma: the pathological study of specimens from en bloc resection in patients receiving pre-operative chemotherapy, in *Status of Curability of Childhood Cancers,* van Eys, J. and Sullivan, M. P., Eds., Raven Press, New York 1980, 111.

31. **Antman, K. H. and Elias, A. D.,** Chemotherapy of advanced soft tissue sarcomas, *Semin. Surg. Oncol.,* 4, 53, 1988.
32. **Carli, M., Perilongo, G., Montezesnolo, L., et al.,** Phase II trials of cis-platinum and VP-16 in children with advanced soft tissue sarcomas: a report from the Italian Cooperative Rhabdomyosarcoma Group, *Cancer Treat. Rep.,* 71, 525, 1987.
33. **Pratt, C. B., Horowitz, M. E., Meyer, W. N., et al.,** Phase II trial of ifosfamide in children with malignant solid tumors, *Cancer Treat. Rep.,* 71, 131, 1987.
34. **Horowitz, M. E., Etcubanas, E., and Christensen, M. L.,** Phase II testing of melphalan in children with newly diagnosed rhabdomyosarcoma: a model for anticancer drug development, *J. Clin. Oncol.,* 6, 308, 1988.
35. **Bode, U.,** Methotrexate as relapse therapy for rhabdomyosarcoma, *Am. J. Pediatr. Hematol. Oncol.,* 8, 70, 1986.
36. **Bramwell, V. H. C.,** Intra-arterial chemotherapy of soft tissue sarcoma, *Semin. Surg. Oncol.,* 4, 66, 1988.
37. **Wright, K. C., Wallace, S., Kim, E., et al.,** Pulsed arterial infusions chemotherapeutic implications, *Cancer,* 57, 1952, 1986.
38. **Hatae, Y., Takeda, T., Nakadate, H., et al.,** Intra-arterial chemotherapy of soft tissue sarcoma in children, *Gon To Kageku Ryoho,* 13, 3271, 1986.
39. **Azzarelli, D., Quagliuolo, V., Colella, G., et. al.,** *Abstracts 4th Int. Conf. on Advances in Regional Cancer Therapy,* ICRCT, Berchtesgaden, 1989, 62.
40. **Shimizu, H., Jaffe, N., and Eftekhari, F.,** Massive Wilms' tumor: sonographic demonstration of therapeutic response without alteration in size, *Pediatr. Radiol.,* 17, 493, 1987.
41. **Auersperg, M. and Us-Krasovec, M.,** In vivo sensitivity test for guided chemotherapy of malignant tumors, in *Proc. 6th Int. Cong. of Chemotherapy,* Vol. 2, University of Tokyo Press, Tokyo, 1970, 535.
42. **Us-Krasovec, M. and Auersperg, M.,** Effect of intra-arterial chemotherapy on tumor cells, *Minerva Chir.,* 24, 1084, 1969.
43. **Van Putten, L. M., Keizer, J. H., and Mulder, J. H.,** Perspective in cancer research. Synchronization in tumor chemotherapy, *Eur. J. Cancer,* 12, 79, 1976.

Chapter 15

PATTERNS OF TREATMENT FAILURE AND THE MEANING OF COMPLETE RESPONSE IN RHABDOMYOSARCOMA

Modesto Carli and Giorgio Perilongo

TABLE OF CONTENTS

I. INTRODUCTION

Despite the advances in treatment of childhood rhabdomyosarcoma (RMS) achieved in the last two decades, about 30% of patients who achieve a complete response (CR) will have recurrence of the tumor.[1] This event almost always indicates a dismal prognosis.[2] Analysis of the pattern of recurrence of RMS and the biological and clinical characteristics of the relapsing tumors can give important clues for understanding the natural history of these neoplasms in relation to the therapy used. This information can be critical for improving therapeutic strategies and, hopefully, for reducing the relapse rate of children with this tumor.

The 1988 International Workshop on Childhood Rhabdomyosarcoma defined "complete remission" as follows: "There is disappearance of all clinical signs of disease or tumor residual (partial remission) persisting over a 6 month period of time".[3] "Local relapse" was defined as the reappearance of tumor in the original site of the primary tumor in patients who achieved CR. "Regional failure" was defined as recurrence of tumor in adjacent tissues or regional lymph nodes; and "metastases" were defined as the distant appearance of new lesions. These definitions will be used in this chapter.

II. PATTERNS OF RECURRENCE OF TUMOR

Lack of local tumor control is the major reason for treatment failure. In fact, the first recurrence of a RMS takes the form of an isolated local or regional relapse in 50 to 60% of cases. Recurrence is manifested as a distant lesion in 20 to 30%, and there is a combined distant and local relapse in the remaining 10 to 20%.[2] The relevance of local tumor failure in progression of RMS has been confirmed. Thus, in a study of 236 tumor deaths due to RMS, almost 70% of the cases had local tumor progression or local extension of the tumor, which was associated with metastases in 54% of cases.[4]

The lungs are by far the most frequent sites of metastases, followed by soft tissues, regional and distant lymph nodes, bone, liver, and the brain.[4] Specific patterns of tumor progression are associated either with certain histological subtypes or with locations of the primary tumor.

The disease-free survival curve for childhood RMS seems to plateau in 6 years.[1] Thus, if later recurrences cannot be ruled out, the time risk for recurrence of this tumor probably is 6 years. In the Intergroup Rhabdomyosarcoma Study-I (IRS-I) experience, the median duration of complete remission for patients with relapses in regional or distant sites was 43 weeks, with a range between 8 and 156 weeks. On the other hand, for patients with local tumor recurrence, the median duration of remission was 36 weeks, with a range of 4 to 190 weeks.[2] The vast majority of relapses in RMS occurs within the first 2 years from diagnosis.

A. EFFECT OF EXTENT OF TUMOR

Relapse rate increases according to the extent of the tumor at the time of presentation, as defined by the IRS staging system (Table 1). In fact, so far all studies on childhood RMS which adopted that system have confirmed the extent of the tumor (group) as the major prognostic factor for determining overall and disease-free survival. For group I patients, the first tumor relapse takes the form of local relapse in the majority of cases. In the Italian Study (RMS-79), all of the seven patients who relapsed had a local failure.[5] Likewise, 4 out of 7 in the German study (CWS-81)[6] and 18 out of 22 in IRS-II showed local recurrence.[7]

On the other hand, the frequency of distant metastases increases from group I to group IV. However, it must be noted that many studies do not report different rates of metastases between groups II and III. According to the IRS-I study, in group IV patients, tumor recurrence takes the form of metastases in previously uninvolved locations in almost half

TABLE 1
Relation of Relapse Pattern and Clinical Group at Diagnosis

Group/ study	Number of patients in CR	LR + R	LR + Mets	Mets	UK	RR (%)
Group I						
CWS-81	36	4	1	2	—	19
RMS-79	29	7	—	—	—	24
IRS-I	86	6	—	10	—	19
IRS-II	103	18	—	4	1	22
Group II						
CWS-81	23	5	1	1	—	30
RMS-79	20	4	1	1	—	30
IRS-I	177	12	2	35	—	28
IRS-II	131	19	3	7	3	32
Group III						
CWS-81	94/79	18	4	2	—	25
RMS-79	76/61	17	2	4	—	37
IRS-I	280/194	27	4	41	1	37
IRS-II	408/295	49	15	18	8	27
Group IV						
CWS-81	37/18	7	3	5	—	83
RMS-79	18/8	—	1	3	—	50
IRS-I	129/65	9	4	31	—	68
IRS-II	171/89	18	7	27	—	52

Abbreviations: CWS-81 = West German Soft Tissue Sarcoma Study, 1981; RMS-79 = Italian Rhabdomyosarcoma Study, 1979; IRS-I = Intergroup Rhabdomyosarcoma Study I; IRS-II = Intergroup Rhabdomyosarcoma Study II; CR = complete remission; Mets = distant metastases; UK = unknown site; RR = relapse rate at 5 years; LR + R = local + regional recurrence.

of the cases, chiefly in bone and CNS. Tumor recurrence is seen in the site (sites) of previous metastatic disease in more than 30%, and only 20% of the relapsing patients had either local or regional extension of the tumor at the time of first relapse.[8]

Raney analyzed the time of relapse according to the type of recurrence and the clinical stage at presentation. The median duration of CR for patients with a local recurrence did not show any relationship with tumor stage,[1] being for group I 37 weeks, group II 12 weeks, group III 57 weeks, and for group IV 16 weeks. On the other hand, for children with distant metastases, the median duration of CR decreases according to the extent of disease at presentation. In fact, the duration of CR was 70 weeks for group I, 37 weeks for group II, 39 weeks for group III, and 28 weeks for group IV. It was also reported that all but 3 of the 108 group IV patients of the IRS-I study who relapsed had the recurrence detected within 2 years from diagnosis.[8]

The International Society of Pediatric Oncology (SIOP) has adopted a presurgical clinical staging system defining tumor extension according to tumor dimensions, involvement of adjacent organs, lymph node involvement, and the presence of metastases. This is called the TNM (tumor, nodes, metastases) staging system.[9] Also, according to this staging system, an increase in relapse rate can be documented along with increased tumor extension at presentation (Table 2).[10] No difference in the rate of local recurrence is evident among different stages of the tumor, while an increased rate of metastases is clearly evident as one goes from stage I to stage III.

B. EFFECT OF HISTOLOGIC SUBTYPE

All series of childhood RMS uniformly report a higher relapse rate for alveolar RMS (A-RMS) than for the other histologic subtypes, considered either alone or in combination.

TABLE 2
Relation of Relapse Pattern and TNM
Stage at Diagnosis

TNM stage	Number of patients	LR (%)	Mets (%)
I	85	35	1
II	133	35	6
III	29	33	15

The relapse rate for the alveolar variant ranges from 58 to 71% according to various reports.[5-7,10] A-RMS tends to recur locally as well as to metastasize. In the Italian experience, 11 out of 15 patients with A-RMS (stage I or II) who relapsed showed a local recurrence, 2 had isolated metastases, and 2 had combined local and distant relapse as the first evidence of tumor failure.[5] A similar prevalence of local recurrence, associated or not with distant metastases, was reported by SIOP.[10] In any case, it has been reported that A-RMSs had the highest frequency of metastases (alone or with local progression) at the time of death among the various histologic subtypes of this tumor (94%). On the other hand, death due to local progression alone from the primary lesion was the lowest, occurring in only 6% of cases of A-RMS.[4] This means that, regardless of the initial manifestation of tumor failure, A-RMSs are at high risk of dissemination.

As mentioned before, different patterns of tumor dissemination according to the histologic sub-type have been proposed. According to one report, the sites of distant metastases for A-RMSs were bones, regional lymph nodes, and lung, in terms of frequency, while for the embryonal type (E-RMS) the lungs were the most frequent site of distant dissemination.[11] Another study reported that at the time of death, A-RMS has the highest rate of regional lymph node involvement.[4]

It is worthwhile to note that the breast is a rare site of metastases for A-RMS. In a study of 108 consecutive RMS patients seen in one institution, there were only 7 cases that developed metastatic tumor to the breast. Four of them occurred in females; six of the seven were A-RMSs, and all of them originated on an extremity or a buttock.[12] In a more recent report, three cases of breast metastases were observed among eight cases of A-RMS of the female genitalia.[13] Interestingly, these cases occurred in adolescent girls undergoing breast development. Breast localization, other than with the alevolar subtype, has also been connected with the physiologic state. According to one author, there are no cases of A-RMS metastatic to the breast in women.[14] Finally, there were no cases of breast metastases among the 47 children and adolescents with primary E-RMS of the female genital tract enrolled in IRS-I and IRS-II.[15] Only rare cases of A-RMS originating in the breast are reported.[16]

Efforts to further identify those histologic variants of childhood RMS which are associated with different relapse rates, and consequently have a different prognosis, have not yet been concluded. Within the "favorable" and the "unfavorable" histology groups, new subtypes other than the classic aveolar and embryonal variants have been recently added. These subtypes include the solid alveolar variant and the anaplastic and monomorphous variants in the poor prognosis group,[17] and the leiomyomatous variant in the good prognosis group.[18] Understanding of the biological behavior as well as the relapse pattern of these histologic subtypes deserves additional and more extensive clinical investigation.

C. EFFECT OF LOCATION OF TUMOR

The biological behavior of RMSs in children is greatly influenced by the anatomic location of the tumor. In fact, the primary site of the tumor is an important prognostic factor since tumors in different locations have different relapse rates.[1] The highest relapse rate is

TABLE 3
Relation of Relapse Rate and Primary Site

Stages I to III

Group/ study	Number of patients in CR	LR + R	LR + Mets	Mets	RR (%)
Orbit					
CWS-81	18/17	4	—	—	23
RMS-79	23/21	6	—	—	28
SIOP-84[a]	26/26	29%	—	—	—
Head/neck nonparameningeal					
CWS-81	11/11	4	—	—	36
RMS-79	10/9	3	—	1	44
SIOP-84	24/27	43%	—	7%	—
Head/neck parameningeal					
CWS-81	33/26	7	1	—	30
RMS-79	20/12	2	—	1	25
SIOP-84	44/39	43%	—	5%	—
Genitourinary bladder-prostate					
CWS-81	18/14	2	—	2	28
RMS-79	11/11	2	—	—	18
SIOP-84[a]	22/21	30%	—	—	—
Genitourinary nonbladder-prostate					
CWS-81	27/27	1	1	1	0.07
RMS-79	19/19	—	—	1	0.05
SIOP-84[a]	47/45	11%	—	10%	—
Extremity					
CWS-81	23/21	6	2	3	52
RMS-79	16/14	6	—	1	50
SIOP-84[a]	31/28	38%	—	10%	—
Others					
CWS-81	23/22	3	1	1	22
RMS-79	29/22	9	2	2	59
SIOP-84[a]	51/44	44%	—	4%	—

[a] Relapse rate at 3 years.

Abbreviations: CWS-81 = West German Soft Tissue Sarcoma Study, 1981; RMS-79 = Italian Rhabdomyosarcoma Study, 1979; SIOP-84 = International Society of Pediatric Oncology Study, 1984; LR + R = local + regional recurrence; Mets = metastases; RR = relapse rate at 5 years.

in patients whose tumor arises in the retroperitoneum, pelvis, extremities, perineum-anus, and gastrointestinal tract.[2] Orbit, head-neck (nonparameningeal), and genitourinary RMSs have the lowest incidence of tumor recurrence.[4,19,20] Orbit, head-neck, retroperitoneal, and genitourinary tumors have a tendency to disseminate locally and regionally.

Tumors originating in cranial-parameningeal locations have a high propensity to disseminate within the CNS.[20] Head-neck, nonparameningeal RMSs have shown an equal tendency to recur both locally and distantly (particularly for primary neck tumors).[21] Extremity tumors have a strong tendency to produce distant metastases, with or without local progression at the time of tumor recurrence (Table 3). Nonpulmonary metastases are frequently associated with primary tumors of an extremity.[22] At death, a relatively high frequency of liver metastases was found among patients with tumors arising in primary sites below the diaphragm, such as retroperitoneum and genitourinary tract tumors. Tumors arising in these sites had liver metastases in 38% (retroperitoneum) and 41% (GU) of cases. Brain metastases, present in 20% of cases overall, are more frequently found in extremity tumors, occurring in 37% of cases.[4,21]

Differences in primary sites according to histologic subtypes have been documented in childhood RMSs. Parameningeal and orbital RMSs have a high incidence of the embryonal type (76%), while tumors of the extremities and perineum and anus have the highest proportion of the alveolar type (48%).

A multivariate analysis was done to evaluate the magnitude of the role a particular site or histologic type plays in the pattern of tumor progression.[4] It was demonstrated that although the association of both the histology and primary site with the pattern of tumor progression at death was statistically significant, the relationship between primary site and tumor spread was stronger. Specifically, the parameningeal sites showed a much stronger influence in determining local progression than did the embryonal histologic subtype. In addition, the extremity site was more strongly associated with the occurrence of distant metastases, with or without the presence of local progression at death. As noted before, the frequency of distant metastases alone at the time of death was much higher with the alveolar histologic subtype.

The poor prognosis of alveolar tumors of the extremity has already been documented by almost all cooperative studies on childhood RMS. The IRS-I and IRS-II experiences with A-RMSs of the extremity were recently reviewed.[20] Among the 74 patients studied, 31 suffered a tumor failure (42%). Eleven were local relapse, 8 were regional recurrences, 15 had distant metastases, and 1 showed both local recurrence and distant metastases. Interestingly, the 8 regional relapses occurred in the regional lymph nodes.

The propensity of regional lymph node spread of A-RMSs of the extremities has been known since the first definition of A-RMS in the 1950s.[22] The incidence of lymph node involvement for extremity primaries varies between 17 and 19%, according to different series. It is also worthwhile to note that metastatic locations for alveolar extremity RMSs of the IRS varies from lung (six cases), to soft tissue (4), lymph nodes (three), bone (one), bone marrow (one), and liver (one).

The presence of clinically or histologically proven positive regional lymph nodes at the time of presentation implies a more aggressive biological behavior and a higher tendency to recurrence.[25,26] The tendency for lymph node involvement at the time of initial presentation and at the time of tumor failure seems to be particularly relevant for specific locations. These tumor locations associated with lymph node spread include extremities, genitourinary tract, paratesticular and prostate, pelvis-retroperitoneum, and the thorax and abdomen. The overall incidence of lymph node involvement for these locations has been estimated to be extremities, 12%; genitourinary tract, 24%; paratesticular, 26%; prostate, 41%; pelvis-retroperitoneum, 23%; and thorax-abdomen, 25%.[25]

In the IRS-I and IRS-II experiences, 7 out of 79 patients with these localized paratesticular RMSs relapsed. Among these seven patients, seven showed regional lymph node recurrence, three in the groin and one in the lymph nodes both in the groin and retroperitoneum, and three had distant metastases.[27]

Furthermore, sex and age[28,29] do not seem to have an influence on the biological behavior of childhood RMSs, and consequently had no effect on the pattern of tumor recurrence. Nonetheless, it must be noted that a SIOP study indicated that female sex is a possible negative prognostic factor for these tumors.[29]

D. OTHER FACTORS AFFECTING PATTERNS OF TUMOR RECURRENCE

The relapse pattern of childhood RMS has been discussed by analyzing the clinical chracteristics of relapsing patients with this tumor. Hopefully, in the near future, molecular genetic studies will give us more insight into the biological behavior of these tumors, and will help us in identifying more precisely the different risk groups according to tendency for tumor relapse.

It seems already fairly clear that E-RMSs and A-RMSs have different and specific genetic abnormalities.[30] Loss of constitutional heterozygosity for loci on chromosome 11p has been consistently reported for E-RMSs. Also, a unique chromosomal translocation t(2;13) between chromosome bands 2q37 and 13q14 has been more frequently seen in association with the alveolar subtype. Whether these chromosomal abnormalities are critical for explaining the different biological behavior of these tumors is a matter for further investigation.

The likelihood and pattern of tumor recurrence are strongly influenced by therapy. Among the recent advances in the treatment of childhood RMSs, we can identify certain treatment refinements, other than more effective chemotherapy, which clearly modified the relapse pattern of these tumors. The most striking example is parameningeal RMSs, with increased risk of meningeal extension, which show improved survival following use of more intensive local radiotherapy.[18] In the past, 35% of these patients developed meningeal involvement and 90% died of this complication. In a recent study, large field radiotherapy was given early in the treatment program concurrently with a regimen of intensive systemic chemotherapy. With this treatment, the relapse rate dropped from 33 out of 65 in the historical control group to 11 out of 52 in the intensively treated (experimental) group. However, what was more remarkable was the difference in the site of recurrence. In the historical control group, 19 patients had a meningeal relapse, while in the intensively treated group none had secondary meningeal involvement. Eleven children in the earlier study had local/regional failure, while there were only three such failures in the recent study. The rates of distant metastases in the two studies were 3 out of 65 and 8 out of 52, respectively.[20]

A similar modification of the pattern of tumor failure is expected for "unfavorable histology" group I extremity RMSs.[22] Most of the current studies on these patients are incorporating more intensive systemic chemotherapy combined with local radiation therapy. In the past, these patients were treated with chemotherapy alone. Preliminary results seem to indicate a decrease in the rate of local recurrence and a lower incidence of metastases for these tumors.

III. DEFINING COMPLETE RESPONSE

High local relapse rate is the hallmark of the biological behavior of childhood RMS and underscores the difficulty in detecting "minimal residual disease" for these children. It could be argued that, in addition to technological problems, the failure to detect minimal residual disease is in part due to an unwillingness to aggressively look for it. In this regard, it is critical to clarify the term "CR" as applied to this tumor.

Achievement of the state of CR is a fundamental step toward actual cure. A retrospective analysis was done on 70 children with RMS treated in various Italian pediatric centers from 1968 to 1978. It was found that none of the patients whose maximum response was considered partial survived longer than 28 months, and in those whose response was less than partial, none survived longer than 9 months.[31] In addition, the authors analyzed survival data according to the maximum response to therapy in 142 evaluable patients enrolled in the prospective Italian cooperative RMS study from October 1979 to June 1986. In this analysis, they found the same trend: 85 of the 118 patients who achieved a CR were alive, with a median follow-up of 60 months, while the median survival time of 24 children who never achieved CR was only 7.5 months.[5]

The designation of CR may also influence treatment. In many studies, patients who achieve CR as a result of initial definitive surgery, or following chemotherapy for tumors in special locations such as those arising in the bladder, vagina, or orbit, do not receive radiotherapy.[23,33]

Recently, some investigators have noted that the rapidity of the tumor response and, particularly, the achievement of a CR is an important "dynamic" prognostic factor. It was

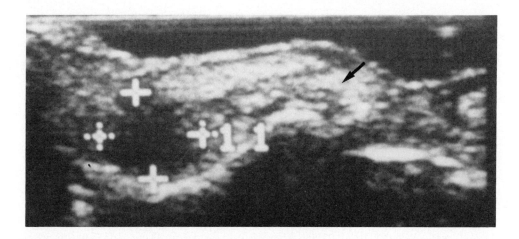

FIGURE 1.   Embryonal RMS in a 14-year-old boy. Longitudinal ultrasound scan of nasolabial fold shows a hypoechogenic mass adjacent to the alveolar process of the maxillary bone (arrow) after 8 months of therapy, including 400 cGy of radiotherapy. Second-look operation revealed persistent presence of viable tumor cells.

shown that with the new treatment program, patients found to have CR by week 7 have an excellent survival rate.[34] In addition, the time at which the statement "CR" is made is the starting time for calculation of "disease-free survival". Disease-free survival is the parameter frequently used to compare the results of different studies.

IV. CONCLUSIONS

It is evident that a large amount of information is needed to precisely determine the tumor response and, particularly, to establish the presence of CR. However, there is lack of uniform and standardized criteria for defining a CR. For example, in the clinical grouping system adopted by the IRS and also used in other European studies, the definition of CR for patients in group I is based on pathological criteria. On the other hand, group II patients are conventionally considered to be in CR, even if microscopic residual tumor is still present after attempted surgical resection of the tumor. The problem is more evident for group III and IV patients, for whom the achievement of CR is usually defined by clinical and laboratory examination. In fact, the anatomic location of the tumor (for example, parameningeal, orbital, or retroperitoneal-pelvic) often makes histologic assessment of tumor response difficult. In these cases, the evaluation of tumor response is based mainly on the results of noninvasive imaging and biochemical studies. The inadequacy of these tools in defining microscopic disease is obvious.

For patients in clinical groups III and IV, a peculiar aspect also emerges: evidence of residual tumor is often seen after completion of chemotherapy and radiotherapy. In these cases, it is often difficult to define whether the lesions observed are residual tumors or tissue alterations due to radiation therapy and chemotherapy, such as necrosis and fibrosis (Figures 1 to 3).

In such cases, the attitude of different investigators varies. The most common tendency is to arbitrarily consider the patient to be in complete remission after 6 months of stable partial response, as established in the International Workshop on Rhabdomyosarcoma (which was held in Paris, 1988). The empirical nature of this definition is evident.

However, the best available clinical evaluation of response may not correlate with histopathologic evidence of remission. In order to compare these two parameters, the role of the second-look operation was evaluated as a means of establishing the relationship between clinical and pathological responses in clinical group III and IV patients enrolled in

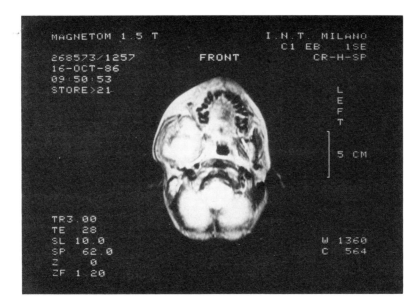

FIGURE 2. Embryonal RMS in a 14-year-old boy. Axial MRI scan demonstrated a huge tumor mass in the pterygomaxillary fossae which remained unchanged after 12 months of aggressive chemotherapy plus 5400 cGy of radiotherapy. Histological examination after radical surgical excision revealed the presence of only fibrotic tissue.

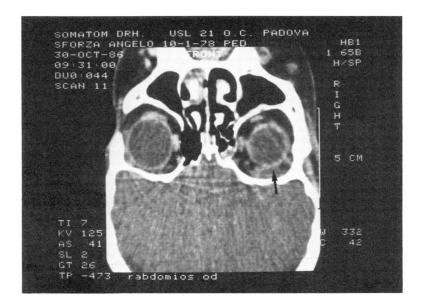

FIGURE 3. Alveolar RMS in an 8-year-old boy. Axial CT scan of the orbit demonstrated a persistent abnormality (isodense tissue) in the superior quadrant of the right orbit (arrow) after 12 months of chemotherapy plus 5400 cGy of radiotherapy. Second-look operation revealed the presence of only fibrotic tissue.

IRS-III. Complete histopathologic response was confirmed by second-look operations in 31 out of 45 patients who, according to clinical examination, were in CR. However, second-look operations resulted in upgrade to CR in 56 out of 85 patients with clinical partial response and in 23 out of 35 patients who were clinically considered as nonresponders.

Thus, these findings clearly indicate the poor correlation between clinical and pathological investigations in evaluating the quality or nature of tumor response.

In view of the many studies for improving therapy in childhood RMS and pooling the data derived from various studies, it is important to precisely determine the criteria used to define CR, and to evaluate patients for microscopic residual disease. For this purpose, the authors think that histological assessment of the tumor, rather than relying on clinical findings alone, is the more reliable standardized approach. They believe that an aggressive approach is still required for the majority of children with RMS. Improvement in surgical techniques and development of new technology may result in a notable reduction in the number of cases in which a pathological approach to identify CR is currently not feasible. These improvements would further reduce the margin of error related to the physician's assessment of the tumor and selection of treatment.

REFERENCES

1. **Maurer, H. M., Beltangady, M., Gehan, E. A., et al.,** The Intergroup Rhabdomyosarcoma I; a final report, *Cancer,* 61, 207, 1988.
2. **Raney, B., Crist, W., Maurer, H. M., et al.,** Prognosis of children with soft tissue sarcoma who relapsed after achieving a complete response; a report from IRS-I, *Cancer,* 52, 44, 1983.
3. Minutes of the 4th Int. Workshop on RMS, Paris, February 16, 1988.
4. **Shimada, H., Newton, W. A., Soule, E. D., et al.,** Pathology of fata rhabdomyosarcoma; report from the IRS-I & II, *Cancer,* 59, 459, 1987.
5. **Carli, M.,** (For the Italian Cooperative Study): updated results of the RMS-79 study, in *Proc. Annu.* Meeting of the Italian Cooperative Study, Padova, Italy, March 1990.
6. **Treuner, J.,** (For the CWS Group): updated results of the CWS-81 study, in *Proc. Annu.* Meeting of the German Cooperative Study, Stuttgart, West Germany, October 1989.
7. **Maurer, H. M., Gehan, E. A., Beltangady, M., et al.,** The Intergroup Rhabdomyosarcoma Study II, *Cancer,* submitted.
8. **Raney, B., Tefft, M., Maurer, H. M., et al.,** Disease pattern and survival rate in children with metastatic soft tissue sarcoma; a report from IRS, *Cancer,* 62, 1257, 1988.
9. **Harmer, M. H., Ed.** *TNM Classification of Pediatric Tumors,* UICC (Union International Contre le Cancer, Geneva, 1982, 23.
10. **Rodary, C. and Flamant, F.,** Data on SIOP study regarding relapse rate for stage and alveolar rhabdomyosarcoma, personal communication to the author, 1990.
11. **Hays, D. M., Newton, W. A., Soule, E. D., et al.,** Mortality among children with rhabdomyosarcoma of the alveolar histologic subtypes, *J. Pediatr. Surg.,* 18, 412, 1983.
12. **Howarth, C. B., Caces, J. N., Pratt, C. B., et al.,** Breast metastases in children with rhabdomyosarcoma, *Cancer,* 46 2520, 1980.
13. **Copeland, L. J., Sneige, N., Stringer, A., et al.,** Alveolar rhabdomyosarcoma of the female genitalia, *Cancer,* 56, 849, 1985.
14. **Lloyd, R. V., Hajdu, S. I., and Knapper, W. H.,** Embryonal rhabdomyosarcoma in adults, *Cancer,* 51, 557, 1983.
15. **Hays, D. M., Shimada, H., Raney, B., et al.,** Clinical staging and treatment result in rhabdomyosarcoma of the female genital tract among children and adolescents, *Cancer,* 61, 1893, 1988.
16. **Sugar, J. and Sapi, Z.,** Alveolar rhabdomyosarcoma: a case report, *Arch Geschwulstforsch.,* 58(6), 445, 1988.
17. **Palmer, H. and Foulkes, M.,** Histopathology and prognosis in the Second Intergroup Rhabdomyosarcoma Study (IRS-II), *Proc. Am. Soc. Clin. Oncol.,* 2, 897, 1983.
18. **Carli, M., Grotto, P., Cavazzana, A., et al.,** Prognostic significance of histology in childhood rhabdomyosarcoma; improved survival with a new histologic leiomyomatous subtype, *Proc. Am. Soc. Clin. Oncol.,* 9, 1153, 1990.
19. **Loughlin, K. R., Retik, A. B., Winstein, U. J., et al.,** Genitourinary rhabdomyosarcoma in children, *Cancer,* 63, 1600, 1989.
20. **Raney, B., Tefft, M., Newton, W., et al.,** Improved prognosis with intensive treatment of children with cranial soft tissue sarcoma arising in non-orbital parameningeal sites; a report from IRS, *Cancer,* 59, 147, 1987.

21. **Wharam, M. D., Foulkes, A., Lawrence, W., et al.,** Soft tissue sarcoma of the head and neck in childhood non-orbital and nonparameningeal sites; a report from the IRS-I, *Cancer,* 53, 1016, 1984.

22. **Heyn, R., Beltangady, M., Hays, D., et al.,** Results of intensive therapy in children with localized alveolar extremity rhabdomyosarcoma; a report from IRS, *J. Clin. Oncol.,* 7, 200, 1989.

23. **Sarno, J. B., Wiener, L., Waxman, M., and Kwee, J.,** Sarcoma metastatic to the central nervous system; a review of the literature, *Med. Pediatr. Oncol.,* 13(5), 280, 1985.

24. **Ripella, J. E. and Theriault, J. P.,** Sur unc forme nicconnve de sarcome des partics molles le rhabdomyosarcoma alveolaire, *Ann. Anat. Pathol.,* 1, 88, 1956.

25. **Lawrence, W., Hayes, D. M., Heyn, R., et al.,** Lymphatic metastases with childhood rhabdomyosarcoma; a report from IRS, *Cancer,* 60, 910, 1987.

26. **Pedrick, T. J., Donaldson, S. S., and Cox, R. S.,** Rhabdomyosarcoma; the Stanford experience using a TNM staging system, *J. Clin. Oncol.,* 4, 370, 1986.

27. **Raney, B., Tefft, M., Lawrence, W., et al.,** Paratesticular sarcoma in children and adolescence; a report form IRS I and II, 1973—1983, *Cancer,* 670, 2337, 1987.

28. **Ragab, A. H., Heyn, R., Tefft, M., et al.,** Infants younger than 1 year of age with rhabdomyosarcoma, *Cancer,* 58, 2606, 1986.

29. **Rodary, C., Rey, A., Olive, D., et al.,** Prognostic factors in 281 children with nonmetastatic rhabdomyosarcoma at diagnosis, *Med. Pediatr. Oncol.,* 16, 71, 1988.

30. **Scrable, H., Witte, D., Shimada, H., et al.,** Molecular differntial pathology of rhabdomyosarcoma, *Gene Chromosomes Cancer,* 1, 23, 1989.

31. **Carli, M., De Bernardi, B., Castello, M., et al.,** Long term results in childhood rhabdomyosarcoma: A retrospective study in Italy, *Pediatr. Hematol. Oncol.,* 3, 371, 1986.

32. **Voute, A., Vos, A., De Kraker, J., et al.,** Rhabdomyosarcoma: chemotherapy and limited supplementary treatment: program to avoid mutilation, *Natl. Cancer Inst. Monogr.,* 56, 121, 1981.

33. **Carli, M., Passcrini, G., Perilongo, G., et al.,** Is conservative treatment effective in the management of bladder, prostate and vagina rhabdomyosarcoma? Preliminary results of the Italian Cooperative Group. Proceedings of the XVII Societe International d'Oncologie Pediatrique (SIOP) Meeting, Venice, 1985, 128.

34. **Treuner, J., Suder, J., Kein, M., et al.,** The predictive value of mitral cytostatic response in primary unrectable rhabdomyosarcoma in children, *Acta Oncolog.,* 28, 67, 1989.

35. **Wiener, E., Hays, D., Lawrence, W., et al.,** For the IRS Committee–second-look operations are important for children in groups III and IV rhabdomyosarcoma, *Proc. Am. Soc. Oncol.,* 8, 1183, 1989.

Chapter 16

EVALUATION AND TREATMENT OF RELAPSED RHABDOMYOSARCOMA

James S. Miser

TABLE OF CONTENTS

I. INTRODUCTION

Although great progress has been made in the treatment of newly diagnosed rhabdomyosarcoma (RMS) in the last 20 years, a significant number of children and young adults continue to relapse and die of this tumor.[1-3] The results of the Intergroup Rhabdomyosarcoma Studies (IRS) indicate that approximately 15% of patients with group I tumors and 30% of patients with group II tumors will relapse in spite of having been given moderately aggressive chemotherapy.[4] Furthermore, 36% of patients with group III tumors (having gross residual macroscopic evidence of tumor at diagnosis) and 70% of patients with group IV tumors (with presence of distant metastases at diagnosis) can be expected to die by 5 years after the diagnosis.[4]

In general, the outcome of patients with recurrent RMS is quite poor. The largest series of patients who had recurrent RMS after having achieved an initial complete response (115 recurrences out of 341 patients achieving remission) was from the first IRS (IRS-I). This study demonstrated that although effective retrieval therapy could prolong survival, very few patients were cured. Only 2 of 12 patients (17%) with local recurrence and only 3 of 78 patients (4%) with metastatic recurrence remained free of subsequent relapse.[5] Furthermore, virtually all patients who did not achieve an initial complete response, being 82 out of 423 newly diagnosed patients, eventually died of progressive disease.[2-5] Thus, in spite of improvements in therapy of RMS, major challenges remain in both preventing and treating the recurrence of RMS.

II. CHARACTERIZING THE RELAPSE

In evaluating the patient with recurrent rhabdomyosarcoma, important characteristics of the relapse must be determined both to accurately assign prognosis and to plan appropriate therapy.

A. LOCAL RELAPSE VS. SYSTEMIC RELAPSE

Children with a recurrence of RMS only in the primary site have a better outcome than those who relapse with distant metastases; however, their outcome is still poor.[5] In the report from IRS-I, 2 of 12 patients (17%) with local recurrence, compared to only 3 out of 78 patients (4%) with metastatic recurrence, remained free of subsequent relapse.[5] An important factor that contributes to the poor prognosis of patients with local recurrences at the primary site is that these patients often have a tumor that has already undergone radiation therapy and is unresectable at the time of relapse. These patients frequently have uncontrolled tumor at this primary site for an extended period of time before relapsing systemically. Typically, such local relapses occur in the orbit, parameningeal, retroperitoneal, and prostatic sites.

An exception to the poor prognosis associated with relapses in the primary site is the local failure of patients with vaginal primary sites that were treated initially without surgery. These patients usually have tumors with embryonal, often botryoid, histology, they usually reachieve local control with surgery, and usually do not subsequently recur in metastatic sites. It is important to note, however, that local recurrences of RMS in other sites are very often associated with simultaneous or subsequent appearance of distant metastases.

Patients with systemic relapses have a higher rate of subsequent relapse than those who only show relapse in the primary site. In spite of receiving salvage chemotherapy, patients with relapses in metastatic sites usually fail again. They fail because of the inability of chemotherapy to control tumor in these known sites and because of inability to prevent subsequent metastases in other sites. Thus, the major problem in patients with a metastatic recurrence of RMS is the inability of chemotherapy to effectively prevent subsequent relapse. In contrast, in patients with relapses in the primary site, the major problem is often the inability to again control the local disease. Moreover, in cases of local failure chemotherapy intended to destroy the systemic metastases is often inadequate as well.

B. FAILURE ON THERAPY VS. FAILURE OFF THERAPY: RESISTANT VS. SENSITIVE RELAPSE

Patients who relapse while receiving chemotherapy are usually considered to be "resistant" to standard chemotherapy, although this oversimplifies the clinical situation. In IRS-I, only 2 out of 74 patients who relapsed while on chemotherapy remained disease-free after being given salvage chemotherapy. This was compared to 3 out of 16 patients who relapsed while not receiving chemotherapy and subsequently remained disease-free following salvage chemotherapy.[5] The chemotherapy used in the initial therapy and the actual mechanisms of tumor resistance are likely to be the most important factors in determining the subsequent response to retrieval therapy. Nevertheless, patients who relapse after having completed initial therapy do have a better outcome than those who relapse while receiving their initial chemotherapy regimen.

Much research remains to be done in determining the actual cause of relapse and the mechanism of drug resistance. Recently, one mechanism of resistance has been explored. Expression of the multidrug-resistant gene, P170, appears to play a major role in the emergence of resistant clones of RMS cells.[6] If this mechanism is shown to be the major mechanism of relapse in RMS, then treatment strategies aimed at overcoming or preventing the emergence of these resistant clones will be of utmost importance, if a successful outcome with initial and retrieval treatment is to be expected.

Patients who never achieve a complete remission on initial standard therapy, and patients who are primarily resistant to initial chemotherapy, have a lower response rate to retrieval therapy. These patients fare even more poorly than those who relapse after achieving a complete remission.

C. LIMITED VS. EXTENSIVE RELAPSE

In patients with newly diagnosed RMS, extent of the tumor is a major determinant of outcome.[2-4] Similarly, patients with a limited recurrence in one or two sites fare better in both the short term and long term than those patients with extensive tumor in one site or with tumors in multiple sites. Early discovery of relapse while the recurrent tumor is still limited in extent will often result in an improved response to retrieval therapy and a better outcome. This observation justifies the careful surveillance of patients with frequent follow-up imaging studies during and following initial treatment.

D. STAGE OF DISEASE AT ORIGINAL DIAGNOSIS

Patients with higher stage tumors at presentation have a higher rate of relapse than patients who had lower stage tumors. Similarly, patients with higher stage tumors at original diagnosis also have a worse prognosis when given salvage therapy after relapse than patients who had more limited tumors at original diagnosis. Specifically, patients with recurrent RMS who had metastatic tumors at diagnosis are likely to have tumors with a very different biology when compared to the biology of recurrent RMSs in patients who did not have metastases at the time of diagnosis. These biological differences in the tumor not only play a major role in the response to the original therapy, but they strongly affect the outcome of retrieval therapy as well.

E. ORGAN OF RELAPSE

Patients who relapse in bone and bone marrow generally fare worse than those who relapse in lung. In particular, patients with limited recurrence in lung fare considerably better than patients with limited metastases in bone or bone marrow. In contrast, patients with extensive lung involvement have a very poor prognosis. Patients with lymph node metastases at relapse have an intermediate but usually poor prognosis.

F. PREVIOUS TREATMENT

It is a general principle that the extent of previous chemotherapy is inversely related with the overall response rate and the chance of response to retrieval chemotherapy in an individual patient: the response rate to a specific chemotherapy regimen is lower in patients who have received a greater number of previous treatment regimens. However, this relationship has not been clearly established for RMS (see Section V.A). Furthermore, this relationship may not be true for all retrieval regimens; in particular, this relationship of response at relapse to the extent of previous chemotherapy does not appear to be true for the ifosfamide and etoposide regimen.

III. RELAPSE RELATED TO SITE OF ORIGINAL TUMOR

Not only is the propensity to relapse related to location of the original primary site of the RMS, but the type of the relapse is also related to location of the primary tumor. RMSs at different sites have different tumor biology and have different incidences of the alveolar histologic type. Moreover, histology and other biological factors are likely to be more important than the actual position or location of the tumor; however, either directly or indirectly the type of relapse is related to location of the initial primary site.

A. ORBITAL RMS

The prognosis for most newly diagnosed patients with orbital RMS is good.[2,3,7,8] The tumor is usually not metastatic at diagnosis, it does not involve regional lymph nodes, and it usually has embryonal histology. Although orbital RMSs can recur in distant metastatic sites, they often present first with a local recurrence in the orbit. Distant metastases may occur therafter, often in the lung. After biopsy to establish a diagnosis, many patients with orbital RMS are initially treated with chemotherapy and radiation. Thus, the outcome following a local relapse is ultimately related to the ability to surgically eradicate the locally recurrent lesion. Because systemic metastases do subsequently occur, effective systemic therapy is important to both reduce the size of the local tumor and to prevent further metastatic spread of the disease.

B. PARAMENINGEAL RMS

Patients with parameningeal RMS are usually treated initially with radiotherapy and chemotherapy; surgery usually plays only a limited role.[9] Recurrences of the tumor are often local or regional, involving the central nervous system (including the meninges) and regional lymph nodes.[9] Systemic metastases often follow local or regional recurrence; however, metastases may also occur either before local recurrence of the tumor or even without locally recurrent tumor. Recurrence in the central nervous system is often meningeal and is extremely difficult to eradicate permanently, although use of intrathecal cytosine arabinoside and methotrexate and craniospinal irradiation can induce remissions. Intrathecal administration of activated oxazaphosphorines may be more effective, since these agents are known to have significant activity against RMS when given systemically.

C. CHEST WALL RMS

RMSs that occur on the chest wall have an intermediate prognosis when treated with standard therapy.[10,11] RMSs occurring at this site are often initially treated with surgical excision, which is either followed or preceded by chemotherapy. Although local recurrences are not uncommon, of special concern are regional recurrent tumors on the pleural surface located outside the initial field of radiation therapy or outside the initial field of surgical excision. Systemic spread to lymph nodes, bone, bone marrow, and lung may also be seen.

D. ABDOMINAL AND RETROPERITONEAL RMS

RMSs that arise in the retroperitoneal and abdominal regions are often initially unresectable and, thus, they often will have been treated with radiation and chemotherapy.[12,13] Local recurrences and abdominal spread are as common as systemic recurrences in the liver, lung, and other sites.[12,13]

Regional abdominal and retroperitoneal recurrences are very difficult to eradicate because of the diffuse nature of the regional recurrence and because of inability to effectively incorporate high dose abdominal irradiation or surgery into the treatment plan. Use of radiation is a problem because the dose required to eradicate the tumor results in significant toxicity to the bowel and bone marrow. Toxicity to the bone marrow decreases the patient's tolerance to subsequent chemotherapy. Surgical excision of the tumor is often not possible or successful because of the diffuse nature of the recurrent abdominal or retroperitoneal tumor. Thus, out of necessity, there is often a great reliance upon systemic chemotherapy to control regional spread of the tumor. Unfortunately, this strategy is often unsuccessful.

E. GENITOURINARY RMS

Vaginal RMSs generally have a good prognosis.[2-4,14,15] The most common recurrence is at the primary site and is rarely accompanied by spread to lymph nodes or systemic metastases. These local recurrences can usually be extirpated surgically, with or without accompanying radiation therapy and with use of only limited chemotherapy.

Newly diagnosed prostatic RMSs have an intermediate prognosis.[2,3,12,16,17] Recurrences of prostatic RMS can be local, regional, or systemic. Because the initial therapy to the primary site is often radiation,[17] a local recurrence must be treated with surgery in most instances, usually after an attempt is made to reduce the tumor bulk at the primary site with aggressive chemotherapy. Innovative approaches to radiation therapy may also be of benefit.

When paratesticular RMSs recur, they often recur with regional and retroperitoneal nodal involvement.[18] Enlarged retroperitoneal lymph nodes due to metastases from a paratesticular RMS can actually present as a mass lesion simulating a primary tumor. The lungs are the most common metastatic site outside the pelvis and retroperitoneum. Local recurrences are less common. The initial treatment of the relapse usually is an aggressive chemotherapy regimen followed by irradiation or surgery in an attempt to eradicate residual metastases.

RMSs occurring at other genitourinary sites have an intermediate prognosis.[16,17] In cases where only limited surgery or no surgery is used to control the initial primary tumor, there is a high incidence of local recurrence.[16,17] In these cases, aggressive surgery is usually required to control the local recurrence. Unfortunately, local recurrences of tumors in these sites are often associated with regional nodal spread and distant metastases of the tumor. Thus, treatment of tumor recurrences in these patients should initially consist of an aggressive chemotherapy regimen followed by an attempt to eradicate the remaining local tumor with surgery. This strategy addresses the two important problems seen in this group of patients: the high rate of associated systemic metastases and the often extensive locally recurrent tumor.

F. EXTREMITY RMS

These tumors often occur in older children and young adults and have a much higher incidence of the alveolar histology compared to RMSs arising at other sites.[19,20] Recurrences following treatment of an extremity RMS are often regional to lymph node areas including the groin and axilla.[20] This pattern of regional spread is typical of the alveolar histologic subtype. Unfortunately, these tumors also commonly metastasize to lung, bone, soft tissue, and bone marrow. Rarely, metastases to the breast may also be seen, typically with tumors of alveolar histology. Local recurrences are less common. In light of the regional and systemic nature of the relapses, the most appropriate therapeutic approach is to begin with aggressive systemic chemotherapy. This is followed by radiation therapy or possibly surgery to eradicate residual tumor in regional sites. When these tumors recur, the prognosis is very grave.

IV. TREATMENT OF RELAPSED RMS

Because the prognosis of patients with relapsed RMS is usually very poor, the treatment approach must be an aggressive one. Nevertheless, a clear understanding of the pattern of metastases and an assessment of the prognosis of each patient should dictate the approach used to treat the recurrent tumor. A successful treatment approach should include a regimen of combination chemotherapy to which the individual patient's tumor is not resistant, given on a dose-intensive schedule. Innovative use of radiation and surgery, and the use of new modalities, such as bone marrow transplantation and intraoperative radiation, should be considered where appropriate.

Because there are many possible patterns of relapse, the treatment plan must first address the main problems at hand. Generally, chemotherapy should be administered first in order to (1) enhance control of the existing metastatic lesions or the recurrent primary lesion, and (2) to prevent the development of new metastases. Radiation therapy or surgery is then used as appropriate to eradicate residual tumor. The most important reason to administer chemotherapy first is to address the main problem: presence of overt or occult systemic metastases. Beginning the treatment of recurrent RMS with either surgery or radiation therapy will often treat the most apparent tumor, but surgery and radiotherapy will usually effect only a small portion of the tumor actually present. This approach will result not only in unnecessary delays in the implementation of chemotherapy, but also in unwanted complications due to overlapping adverse effects of chemotherapy, radiation, and surgery especially on the gastrointestinal tract and bone marrow.

In light of the adverse interactions between chemotherapy, radiation, and surgery, the timing of the integration of radiation, surgery, or both must be carefully considered in designing a treatment plan.

Finally, as in treatment of patients with newly diagnosed RMS, it is extremely important to pursue all avenues available in order to achieve a complete remission. Patients who achieve a second complete remission have the potential to remain disease-free for an extended period. Unfortunately, patients who achieve only a partial response to multimodality therapy survive only slightly longer than those who do not respond at all.

A. ROLE OF SURGERY

It is usually, but not always, necessary to document recurrence by histological examination. In most cases, a tissue specimen from a needle biopsy will suffice. When more sensitive and informative tests of tumor biology become available, however, more extensive evaluation of the tissue may be needed, thus requiring open biopsy.

For patients with local recurrences of tumor at the primary site, surgery is usually the most appropriate modality to be used. Surgery is used first if it is feasible, if it is ethically appropriate, and only if it can be undertaken without causing undo delay in chemotherapy. However, unless the recurrent tumor is very small, the surgical procedure is virtually without complications, and surgery does not result in a delay in implementing the chemotherapy, the planned surgical procedure should be postponed until after chemotherapy has been given. This policy should be used for most primary sites. However, local recurrences of vaginal primaries, which are virtually without risk of systemic spread following standard chemotherapy, can be resected initially if the recurrence is small.[14,15] With locally recurrent tumors, the advantages of beginning therapy with systemic chemotherapy are twofold: (1) most local recurrences are associated with a high incidence of systemic metastases, and (2) the chemotherapy will reduce the size of the recurrent primary tumor, potentially allowing the subsequent surgical procedure to be more effective and often less extensive.

For patients with systemic recurrences, the role of surgery must be individualized. Resection of residual responding systemic tumor is essential in order to achieve a complete remission. Unfortunately this is not possible in many cases. The timing of surgery must be also individualized, but should be delayed until the maximal chemotherapy effect has been achieved, which is usually after four to six cycles of chemotherapy. Furthermore, the surgical procedure or procedures should usually not be undertaken unless there is potential for complete eradication of all the apparent tumor. Surgical removal of progressive systemic metastases that are unresponsive to chemotherapy is usually not an effective strategy. Such surgery rarely results in cure or in a significant prolongation of disease-free survival.

B. ROLE OF RADIATION THERAPY

Radiation therapy plays an important role in managing many patients with recurrent RMS. It is rare for RMSs to present with an acute neurologic emergency as the first evidence of relapse. However, should this occur, radiation therapy, surgery, or both should be instituted immediately. In most other circumstances, radiation therapy should be delayed until an intensive chemotherapy regimen has been given and a response of the tumor achieved. In patients with local recurrences only, radiation therapy may be used depending on the site of the tumor and whether radiation had been used previously. Most often when repeat irradiation is required, chemotherapy is given first, residual tumor is grossly excised, and radiation is delivered in a limited dose and to a limited volume of tissue. If radiation has not been previously given to the site, then initial chemotherapy followed by gross total removal of tumor, followed by full dose radiation is the preferred sequence.

If a local recurrence is associated with systemic metastases, and if the only surgical approach to the recurrence at the primary site is an amputation or a major extirpative procedure, limited radiation may be required for local control while assessing the response of the systemic metastases. This approach avoids performing major surgical procedures on patients with metastases outside the surgical field.

In patients with systemic metastases, radiation therapy should almost never precede chemotherapy if a curative approach is being taken. Only in an emergency situation to control pain, to prevent a neurologic emergency, or to prevent obstruction of a hollow viscus should radiation be delivered first. This approach maximizes the benefit of chemotherapy and minimizes the potentiation of radiation toxicity by chemotherapy that frequently results in significant delays in treatment.

Following a response to chemotherapy, radiation is often delivered to sites of residual tumor, especially when tumor is present in a limited number of sites. Therapeutically, each site should be viewed as a new primary site, requiring full multimodality therapy to effect permanent control. Bone lesions, if limited in number and volume, should usually receive radiation therapy after at least four to six cycles of chemotherapy. If radiation to larger volumes is required, radiation should probably be delayed even longer, especially if a significant volume of bone marrow is included in the radiation field or fields. Bone lesions that respond to chemotherapy will frequently recur if consolidative radiation is not delivered. Metastases to soft tissue should receive radiation if surgery has not been utilized or if the tissue margins at surgery show presence of residual tumor. Furthermore, when surgery is not performed, radiation therapy should be delivered to the tumor bed, with a field including an adequate margin of surrounding tissue, even if there is no residual tumor apparent on imaging studies or by physical examination.

In patients with Ewing's sarcoma and Wilms' tumor, whole lung irradiation has demonstrated efficacy in the control of microscopic metastases.[21] In patients with RMS, however, efficacy of whole lung irradiation for control of occult pulmonary metastases has not been demonstrated. Because of lack of evidence to support the use of whole lung irradiation, this technique is not now advocated for patients with RMS. Similarly, although total body irradiation has shown efficacy in the treatment of Ewing's sarcoma,[22,23] TBI is not of proven benefit in the treatment of RMS.

C. ROLE OF CHEMOTHERAPY IN TREATMENT OF RELAPSED RMS

In almost all cases, except as noted above, patients with recurrent RMSs should be treated initially with an aggressive regimen of reinduction chemotherapy. Following four to six courses of this chemotherapy, radiation may be delivered to the tumor bed or to the residual tumor. Surgery may also be required to eradicate the residual tumor. However, early use of radiation and surgery for local control of the tumor will often cause decrease in the dose intensity of the chemotherapy, a reduction that will result in the failure of the overall therapeutic strategy.

At this time, the most common initial standard treatment regimens for newly diagnosed RMS utilize vincristine and dactinomycin, with or without cyclophosphamide and adriamycin depending on clinical staging. New regimens are being developed that will, of course, affect the way chemotherapy is used to treat recurrent RMS. Many chemotherapeutic agents, combinations of drugs, and regimens have been used to treat recurrent RMS. These include high dose methotrexate, melphalan, the combination of cisplatin and etoposide, and most recently the combination of ifosfamide and etoposide.[24-30]

1. Ifosfamide and Etoposide

Preliminary results from phase II studies of ifosfamide demonstrated antitumor activity of this agent against RMS (two out of nine patients responded partially). Phase II studies of etoposide also demonstrated activity against RMS. Based on these findings, ifosfamide and etoposide were combined in a phase II trial in an attempt to retrieve patients with recurrent solid tumors.[28-30]

Ifosfamide, an oxazaphosphorine, is a structural isomer of cyclophosphamide, with one chloroethyl group present on each of the nitrogen atoms.[30] Although the mechanisms of action and pharmacokinetics of these two agents are believed to be similar, it has become clear that there are certain clinical differences. Etoposide, an epipodophyllotoxin, has its primary mechanism of action through topoisomerase II.[29] The rationale for using the combination of these two agents was that both agents had significant antitumor activity when given individually, their nonhematopoietic toxicities did not overlap, the agents could be combined at "full phase II doses", and their mechanisms of antitumor activity were different.[30] A likely potential mechanism of interaction between the two agents is that etoposide may prevent the repair of ifosfamide-induced DNA damage through its interference with topoisomerase II, which is the enzyme mediating the resealing of double-strand DNA breaks.[30]

These two drugs are given according to the following schedule: ifosfamide (1800 mg/m^2/day for 5 days) with mesna (2880 mg/m^2/day for 5 days), and preceded each day by etoposide (100 mg/m^2/day). This regimen, delivered every 3 weeks for 12 cycles, has been very effective in the treatment of recurrent RMSs. Of 66 evaluable patients with recurrent RMS treated on this regimen, 9 achieved a complete response and 30 achieved a partial response with chemotherapy alone, for an overall response rate of 59%. After assessing the response to initial chemotherapy (usually four courses), multimodality therapy including either radiation or surgery or both was then delivered to achieve the best response. After obtaining the best possible response with multimodality therapy, chemotherapy was continued to complete the 12 cycles of treatment. With this approach the subsequent progression-free survival of those 46 patients who achieved either a complete response, partial response, or stable disease in response to chemotherapy was 20% at more than 2 years (Figure 1).[30]

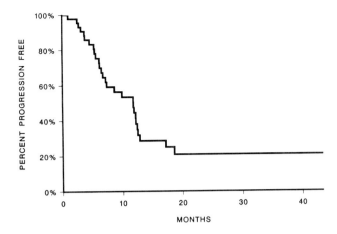

FIGURE 1. Curve showing progression-free survival for 46 patients who achieved either a complete response (9 patients), partial response (30 patients), or stable disease (7 patients). This response was observed in patients with relapsed RMSs following chemotherapy with ifosfamide and etoposide given according to the schedule indicated in the text.

With use of this combination of drugs, the number of previous regimens or the previous exposure to cyclophosphamide has not clearly correlated with outcome, even if the patient is known to be clinically resistant to cyclophosphamide or to multiple other chemotherapeutic regimens. However, prior exposure to renal toxic agents, specifically cisplatin, is associated with greater toxicity and probably causes a poorer response to ifosfamide and etoposide.[31] This finding is likely due to the fact that ifosfamide causes a certain degree of renal toxicity and the drug is primarily excreted by the kidney.[31]

In light of these good initial response rates and the significant but small number of long-term survivors, the combination of ifosfamide and etoposide should be the backbone of retrieval chemotherapy for patients with RMS who relapse during or after treatment with chemotherapy regimens consisting primarily of vincristine, adriamycin, dactinomycin, and cyclophosphamide, with or without cisplastin.

2. Other Chemotherapy Regimens

The combination of cisplatin and etoposide has a low degree of efficacy in the treatment of recurrent RMS and is associated with significant acute and chronic toxicity to organs other than the bone marrow.[21] Melphalan, although active in newly diagnosed patients when combined with vincristine, has a very low degree of activity in patients with recurrent tumors.[26] Methotrexate also has a limited degree of antitumor activity in RMS.[24] Retreatment of patients with recurrent tumors using drugs that they have previously been exposed to but at higher doses has been tried. Unfortunately, this approach has resulted in little lasting benefit, but has caused great toxicity.

3. Role of High Dose Therapy Followed by Bone Marrow Rescue

The role of high dose chemotherapy followed by bone marrow rescue in the treatment of patients with recurrent RMS is not yet established. It is intriguing to hypothesize that resistance of tumor could be prevented or overcome by the use of a combination of multiple drugs which have myelosuppression as the only toxicity. In fact, however, the efficacy and toxicity of this approach has only begun to be investigated in the setting of recurrent RMS.

Three major problems with this approach must be addressed and overcome if this therapeutic strategy is to be used successfully to treat recurrent RMS. First, it has not been demonstrated that systemic radiation therapy plays a role in the treatment of RMS in general or in the treatment of recurrent RMS in particular. Second, there is no obvious chemotherapeutic regimen with known efficacy and established toxicity that can be used. Finally, single courses of intensive chemotherapy regimens with or without systemic radiation have limited capability to eradicate RMSs. In light of these problems, the principal role for high dose chemotherapy, with or without total body irradiation, is in the treatment of patients who have achieved a second remission and have no overt residual tumor.

Carefully constructed pilot trials closely evaluating the feasibility of new high dose regimens should be carried out before high dose therapy with bone marrow rescue is investigated in randomized trials. Use of high dose therapy plus bone marrow rescue in patients with overt evidence of tumors, or who have tumors resistant to conventional retrieval chemotherapy, should be tried only in carefully monitored phase I and phase II trials.

V. TREATMENT APPROACH BY TYPE OF RECURRENCE

A. LOCAL RECURRENCE

As outlined in preceding sections, the treatment of patients with local recurrences of tumor must address two major problems. First, the locally recurrent tumor is often not reliably or easily eradicated with conventional radiation or surgery. The second problem is that the local recurrence is often accompanied by or followed by a systemic relapse. Chemotherapy addresses both of these problems by reducing the size of the primary lesion, thus potentially enhancing local control, and by treating the associated overt tumors as well as occult metastases. Thus, chemotherapy should usually be used first when treating patients who have locally recurrent tumors. Whether radiation, surgery, or both are subsequently used to treat the residual local tumors depends on the nature of previous therapy given to the primary tumor, as well as the site and size of the recurrent tumor. In most instances, use of radiation and surgery is delayed until at least 3 months after instituting the aggressive chemotherapy regimen. Following completion of the radiotherapy or surgery, additional adjuvant chemotherapy is required for at least 6 months unless high dose therapy with bone marrow rescue is substituted for this "continuation" chemotherapy.

B. LUNG RECURRENCE

Usually a solitary pulmonary nodule must be removed in order to establish that a relapse has occurred and to exclude an infectious etiology for the nodule. This procedure has therapeutic benefit as well, but does not allow assessing the response of the tumor to chemotherapy. Following resection of the solitary nodule, chemotherapy is administered for 6 to 9 months as adjuvant therapy.

When multiple pulmonary nodules are present, systemic chemotherapy is administered initially for at least 3 months. Surgical extirpation of responding residual tumor is then accomplished. Postoperative chemotherapy is administered for at least 6 months to prevent subsequent occurrence of systemic metastases. Occasionally radiation therapy is used to treat responding but unresectable residual tumors as well. However, use of whole lung radiation has not been shown to be effective in the treatment of recurrent RMS.

C. SOFT TISSUE RECURRENCE (INCLUDING BRAIN)

A very small recurrence in soft tissue can often be completely excised. Histologic examination of the excised tissue establishes that a relapse has occurred and at the same time the operation eliminates all visible evidence of tumor. Again, this approach does not permit assessing response to induction chemotherapy. Nevertheless, postoperative chemotherapy is given for 6 to 9 months even though antitumor response cannot be assessed. For soft tissue recurrences of any significant size, only a biopsy should be performed to establish the diagnosis. This is then followed by systemic chemotherapy. Chemotherapy is given for at least 3 months in order to assess the response to chemotherapy, to treat systemic metastases early, and to reduce the size of the soft tissue mass. At this point, surgery, radiation, or both should be used to eradicate at the soft tissue site of recurrent tumor. Chemotherapy is then continued for an additional 6 months.

D. BONE RECURRENCE

The approach to recurrences of RMS in bone relies almost completely on systemic chemotherapy because a recurrence in a bony site is an indication that widespread systemic metastases are present. If only a small number of bony metastases are present, radiation therapy should be delivered to the sites of bony metastases following initial systemic chemotherapy. If a large amount of bone marrow is included in the volume of tissue irradiated, then the radiation therapy should be delayed until at least 6 months of systemic chemotherapy have been given. Occasionally surgery is required if the recurrent tumor causes significant bony destruction and results in pathologic fracture.

E. OTHER RECURRENCES

The prognosis for patients with a bone marrow recurrence is very grave. The only effective therapy is chemotherapy. Unfortunately, these individuals usually do not tolerate aggressive chemotherapy well because they have reduced bone marrow function.

Combined relapses with metastases to multiple sites require combined therapeutic approaches as outlined above. However, treatment of combined relapse relies almost completely on chemotherapy.

VI. CURRENT CHALLENGES OF THERAPY

At the present time, the response rate to induction chemotherapy for recurrent RMS is at best 70%. This result has only been achieved in selected patients treated with the combination of ifosfamide and etoposide. Since ifosfamide with or without etoposide is now incorporated into the therapy of patients with newly diagnosed RMS, this high response rate in patients who have relapsed can be expected to become lower. More important than the response to chemotherapy is the overall best response to multimodality retrieval therapy. At best, less than 50% can be expected to achieve a second complete remission even with aggressive multimodality therapy. Even in this group of complete responders, however, the majority will relapse again.

In order to improve retrieval therapy for children and young adults with recurrent RMS, each of these problems must be overcome. Improved induction regimens utilizing new combinations of agents given at higher dose intensity must be evaluated in order to improve the initial response rate to chemotherapy. New and innovative techniques of radiation therapy and surgery must be developed and incorporated into the treatment regimens in order to be able to eradicate residual metastases or locally recurrent tumor. Finally, new approaches to maintaining the second remission must be explored carefully in the correct experimental setting. Use of high dose therapy followed by bone marrow rescue, the impact of intensified induction therapy on remission maintenance, and the role of newly developed immunologic therapies need to be explored further.

In summary, there has been significant improvement in the results of treatment of recurrent RMS. More than 50% of the patients can now be expected to respond to therapy, over 20% will achieve a complete remission, and more than 10% will have a prolonged disease-free interval in second remission. However, these results are clearly unsatisfactory.

Before the survival of this group of children can be expected to significantly increase, we must better understand the biology of those RMSs that relapse.

REFERENCES

1. **Heyn, R., Holland, R., Newton, W. A., et al.,** The role of combined chemotherapy in the treatment of rhabdomyosarcoma in children, *Cancer,* 34, 2128, 1974.
2. **Maurer, H. M., Beltangady, M., Gehan, E. A., et al.,** The Intergroup Rhabdomyosarcoma Study-I. A final report, *Cancer,* 61, 209, 1988.
3. **Maurer, H. M., Gehan, E. A., Crist, W. M., et al.,** Intergroup Rhabdomyosarcoma Study-III. A preliminary report of overall outcome, *Proc. Am. Soc. Clin. Oncol.,* 8 (Abstr.), 296, 1989.
4. **Maurer, H. M. and Crist, W. M.,** Chemotherapy for previously untreated patients with rhabodomyosarcoma, in *Rhabdomyosarcoma and Related Tumors in Children and Adolescents,* Chap. 11, 1991.
5. **Raney, R. B., Crist, W. M., Maurer, H. M., et al.,** Prognosis of children with soft tissue sarcoma who relapse after achieving a complete response. A report from the Intergroup Rhabdomyosarcoma Study-I, *Cancer,* 52, 44, 1983.
6. **Chan, H. S. L., Thorner, P. S., Haddad, G., et al.,** P-glycoprotein (P170) status predicts outcome of therapy in advanced neuroblastoma (NB) and soft tissue sarcoma (STS), *Proc. Am. Soc. Clin. Oncol.,* 9 (Abstr.), 290, 1990.
7. **Wharam, M., Beltangady, M., Heyn, R., et al.,** Localized orbital rhabdomyosarcoma; a report of the Intergroup Rhabdomyosarcoma Study, *Proc. Am. Soc. Clin. Oncol.,* 4 (Abstr.), 132, 1985.
8. **Wharam, M. D., Foulkes, M. A., Lawrence, W., Jr., et al.,** Soft tissue sarcoma of the head and neck in childhood; non-orbital and parameningeal sites. A report from the Intergroup Rhabdomyosarcoma Study (IRS)-I, *Cancer,* 53, 1016, 1984.
9. **Raney, R. B., Tefft, M., Newton, W. A., et al.,** Improved prognosis with intensive treatment of children with cranial soft tissue sarcomas arising in non-orbital parameningeal sites. A report from the Intergroup Rhabdomyosarcoma Study, *Cancer,* 59, 147, 1987.
10. **Raney, R. B., Ragab, A. H., Ruymann, F. B., et al.,** Soft tissue sarcoma of the trunk in childhood. Results of the Intergroup Rhabdomyosarcoma Study, *Cancer,* 49, 2612, 1982.
11. **Crist, W. M., Raney, R. B., Newton, W., et al.,** Intrathoracic soft tissue sarcomas in children, *Cancer,* 50, 598, 1982.
12. **Ransom, J. L., Pratt, C. B., Hustu, H. O., et al.,** Retroperitoneal rhabdomyosarcoma in children. Results of multimodality therapy, *Cancer,* 45, 845, 1980.
13. **Crist, W. M., Raney, R. B., Tefft, M., et al.,** Soft tissue sarcomas arising in the retroperitoneal space in children. A report from the Intergroup Rhabdomyosarcoma Study (IRS) Committee, *Cancer,* 56, 2125, 1985.
14. **Hays, D. M., Raney, R. B., Lawrence, W., Jr., et al.,** Rhabdomyosarcoma of the female genital tract, *J. Pediatr. Surg.,* 16, 828, 1981.
15. **Hays, D. M., Shimada, H., Raney, R. B., et al.,** Sarcomas of the vagina and uterus. The Intergroup Rhabdomyosarcoma Study, *J. Pediatr. Surg.,* 20, 718, 1985.
16. **Hays, D. M., Raney, R. B., Lawrence, W., Jr., et al.,** Bladder and prostatic tumors in the Intergroup Rhabdomyosarcoma Study (IRS)-I, *Cancer,* 50, 1472, 1982.
17. **Ortega, J. A.,** A therapeutic approach to childhood pelvic rhabdomyosarcoma without pelvic exenteration, *J. Pediatr.,* 94, 205, 1979.
18. **Raney, R. B., Tefft, M., Lawrence, W., et al.,** Paratesticular sarcoma in childhood and adolescence. A report from the Intergroup Rhabdomyosarcoma Studies I and II, 1973—1983, *Cancer,* 60, 2337, 1987.
19. **Hays, D. M., Soule, E. H., Lawrence, W., Jr., et al.,** Extremity lesions in the Intergroup Rhabdomyosarcoma Study (IRS-I). A preliminary report, *Cancer,* 49, 1, 1982.
20. **Heyn, R., Hays, D. M., Lawrence, W., Jr., et al.,** Extremity alveolar rhabdomyosarcoma and lymph node spread. A preliminary report from the Intergroup Rhabdomyosarcoma Study (IRS)-II, *Proc. Am. Soc. Clin. Oncol.,* 3 (Abstr.), 80, 1984.
21. **Nesbit, M. E., Perez, C. A., Tefft, M., et al.,** Multi-modal therapy for the management of primary non-metastatic Ewing's sarcoma of bone. An Intergroup Study, *Natl. Cancer. Inst. Monogr.,* 56, 255, 1981.
22. **Jenkin, R. D. T., Rider, W. D., and Sonley, M. J.,** Ewing's sarcoma; a trial of adjuvant total body irradiation, *Radiology,* 96, 151, 1970.
23. **Jenkin, R. D. T., Rider, W. D., and Sonley, M. J.,** Adjuvant total body irradiation, cyclophosphamide and vincristine, *Int. J. Radiat. Oncol. Biol. Phys.,* 1, 407, 1970.
24. **Bode, U.,** Methotrexate as relapse therapy for rhabdomyosarcoma, *Am. J. Pediatr. Hematol. Oncol.,* 8, 70, 1986.
25. **Houghton, J. A., Code, R. L., Lutz, P. J., et al.,** Melphalan; a potential new agent in the treatment of childhood rhabdomyosarcoma, *Cancer Treat. Rep.,* 69, 91, 1985.
26. **Horowitz, M. E., Etcubanas, E., Christensen, M. L., et al.,** Phase II testing of melphalan in children with newly diagnosed rhabdomyosarcoma; a model for anticancer drug development, *J. Clin. Oncol.,* 6, 308, 1988.

27. **Raney, R. B.,** Inefficacy of cisplatin and etoposide as salvage therapy for children with recurrent or unresponsive soft tissue sarcoma, *Cancer Treat. Rep.,* 71, 407, 1987.
28. **Magrath, I. T., Sandlung, J. T., Raynor, A., et al.,** A phase II study of ifosfamide in the treatment of recurrent sarcomas in young people, *Cancer Chemother. Pharmacol.,* 18 (Suppl.), S25, 1986.
29. **O'Dwyer, P. J., Leyland-Jones, B., Alonso, M. T., et al.,** Etoposide (VP-16-213); current status of an active anticancer drug, *N. Engl. J. Med.,* 312, 692, 1985.
30. **Miser, J. S., Kinsella, T. J., Triche, T. J., et al.,** Ifosfamide with mesna uroprotection and etoposide; an effective retrieval regimen in the treatment of recurrent sarcomas and other tumors of children and young adults, *J. Clin. Oncol.,* 5, 1191, 1987.
31. **Mayo, J. M., Krailo, M. D., Hammond, G. D., et al.,** The toxicity of ifosfamide, etoposide and mesna is exacerbated by prior exposure to cisplatin, *Soc. Pediatr. Res.,* Abstr., 1989.

Chapter 17

LATE EFFECTS OF THERAPY IN RHABDOMYOSARCOMA

Ruth M. Heyn

TABLE OF CONTENTS

I. INTRODUCTION

The past decade has been one in which survival in rhabdomyosarcoma (RMS) has shown continuous improvement.[1] Increased survival has been accomplished through more intensive therapy, together with the use of prognostic factors to define select groups of patients who respond well to a specific therapy. With few exceptions, patients with RMS receive multimodality therapy which includes surgery, chemotherapy, and radiotherapy. The increasing number of long-term survivors has given clinicians the important responsibility of evaluating the quality of life in these children and young adults. Quality of life is dependent not only on the continuing or accruing problems related to individual therapies, but it also depends on the ability of patients to cope with these problems. The long-term sequelae of therapy can be both medical and psychosocial. The medical sequelae are those problems which are either physically evident, such as marked facial asymmetry, or which result in a functional disturbance, such as gonadal failure which may follow cyclophosphamide therapy.

Many of the late effects seen in patients surviving RMS are not particularly different from those seen following treatment of other malignancies in childhood. The rapidly increasing number of reports relating to late effects in children has included several comprehensive monographs. Among these are a symposium comprising an entire volume devoted to late effects,[2] a detailed review within a symposium on pediatric oncology,[3] and a recent monograph on long-term complications of therapy.[4] Limited reviews of late effects seen primarily in RMS have also been published.[5,6]

RMS in children is unique because it arises in anatomic sites that are uncommon in other tumors. The most common sites are the head and neck excluding the brain, which account for about 40% of all cases, and the lower genitourinary tract which accounts for 20%. Other primary sites are the extremities (20%) and the trunk, including retroperitoneal, abdominal, perineal, paraspinal, and thoracic sites (20%).

The initial diagnostic approach for RMS is surgery. Surgery may consist of only a biopsy or it may involve an attempt to achieve gross total removal when feasible. As chemotherapy has become more effective and radiotherapy more refined, there has been a trend to do less extirpative surgery initially, with a plan to reoperate, when practical, following induction chemotherapy and radiotherapy. Children treated from 1970 to the present have received various combinations of chemotherapy, utilizing vincristine, cyclophosphamide, dactinomycin, and doxorubicin. Recently, cisplatin and etoposide (VP-16) have been added to some regimens, and since the mid-1980s ifosfamide has been used in combination with other agents. Radiotherapy has improved since the advent of megavoltage therapy and its effectiveness has been enhanced by computerized tomography, which provides better defined tumor margins for design of treatment ports. Most of these tumors receive total doses between 4000 and 6000 cGy. The additive effect of radiation-enhancing drugs, such as dactinomycin and doxorubicin, may play a role in causing late effects. The majority of treated children has received one or both of these agents in combination with radiotherapy.

The purpose of this chapter is to summarize late effects culled from reports which have either specifically addressed RMS or have discussed problems common to this tumor and other pediatric malignancies. In addition to describing problems encountered within the major primary sites, attention has been directed to second malignant neoplasms in survivors and to psychosocial disturbances. Guidelines for late follow-up and the prevention or treatment of individual problems are included.

II. HEAD AND NECK

RMSs originating in the head and neck can be divided into tumors arising in (1) the lids and orbit, (2) the parameningeal sites, which include the nasopharynx, nasal cavity, middle ear, paranasal sinuses, the infratemporal fossa, and parapharyngeal area, and (3)

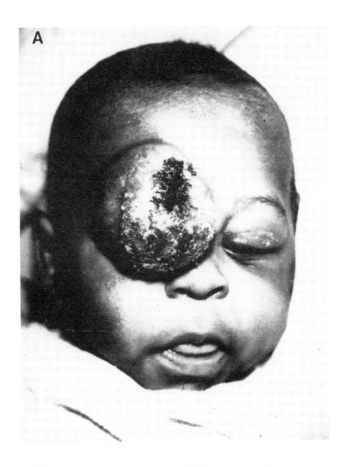

FIGURE 1. (A) Primary embryonal RMS of the upper lid at 3 months of age. (B) Appearance after surgery and the completion of 4000 cGy to the right orbit (5 × 7-cm field) and 4026 cGy to the right face and neck which were the sites of five metastatic lymph nodes (6 × 8-cm field). She received dactinomycin and vincristine for 1 year. (C) Appearance at 5 years of age showing hypoplasia of the right orbit, face, and neck. The right globe is small and has a cataract, resulting in limited vision. (D1) X-ray of the skull at 3 months of age. (D2) X-ray of skull at 5 years showing a hypoplastic right orbit and mandible. (E) Panorex films of the upper and lower bicuspids and first permanent molar. (1,3) The treated right side shows agenesis of the bicuspid teeth, lack of root formation in the primary molars, and malformation of the first permanent molar in the mandible; (2,4) the left mandible shows relatively normal development of the bicuspids and first permanent molar on the untreated side.

other sites. Although there is considerable overlap in occurrence of adverse effects among the various sites, the late problems in the orbit are primarily those affecting the globe and orbital bone, which will be considered separately. The majority of adverse late effects seen in patients with RMS of the head and neck derive from either surgical excision or radiotherapy. Figure 1 shows a patient who illustrates several of the late problems of head and neck tumors which are described below.

Therapy for orbital tumors has changed considerably in the last two decades. Before it was recognized that radiotherapy alone could cure the local tumor, orbital exenteration was the treatment of choice. Exenteration is rarely done now and the tumors are treated *in situ* following surgical biopsy. The few long-term survivors who had orbital exenteration sustain a large cosmetic defect. The lack of orbital contents is usually concealed by wearing a patch

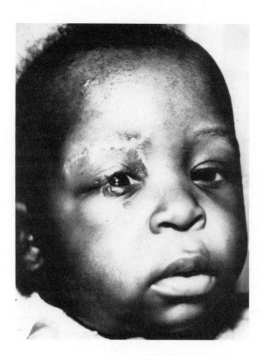

FIGURE 1B.

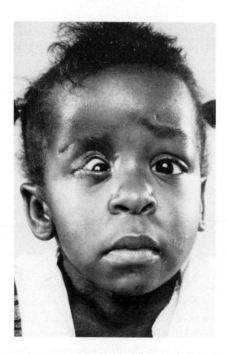

FIGURE 1C.

over the orbit, since prosthetic devices or plastic repair are not very satisfactory. Treating the tumors *in situ* has preserved the global structures even though many well-recognized defects result from radiotherapy. In early reports, nearly all cases developed cataracts within 12 to 18 months following therapy.[7,8] Other recognized problems were photophobia, orbital

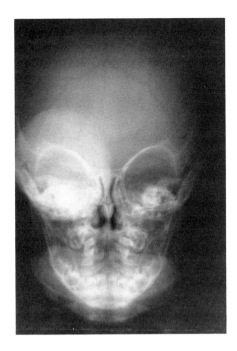

FIGURE 1D-1.

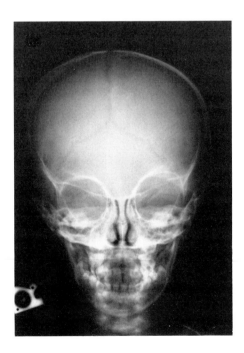

FIGURE 1D-2.

hypoplasia, corneal ulcers, and shrinkage of the globe. Late follow-up of 50 children with orbital tumors treated on the first Intergroup Rhabdomyosarcoma Study (IRS-I) documented decreased vision in the treated eye as the most common functional problem. In most patients this visual impairment was related to cataract formation, which occurred in 90% of the

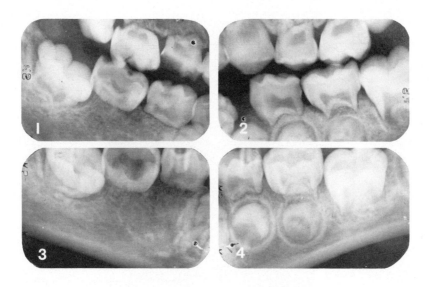

FIGURE 1E.

irradiated eyes.[9] Half of the children had bony hypoplasia or the orbit and surrounding structures resulting in facial asymmetry. Six patients who had orbital exenteration had variable problems with infection at the base of the orbit, chronic otitis requiring frequent myringotomies, and draining sinus tracts.

Other functional problems of the eye included keratoconjunctivitis, photophobia, conjunctivitis, and dryness of the globe. Structural changes in addition to cataracts and bony hypoplasia included corneal abnormalities, enophthalmos, stenosis of the lacrimal duct, and retinal changes. Seventeen children required secondary surgical procedures, including cataract removal, repair of lid ptosis, and repair of a stenosed lacrimal duct. Four secondary enucleations were done for a painful soft globe, chronic cellulitis, keratitis and cataract, and a scarred and opacified cornea associated with a soft globe. An assessment of growth in 44 of these patients showed a deceleration in growth in 61%. These were children whose height had deviated greater than 20 percentile increments downward from their pretreatment height. Radiotherapy damage to the pituitary gland may have been responsible for this finding, since the pituitary lies in the path of the exit dose when a single anterior X-ray portal is used. This effect can be lessened by a more restricted arrangement of portals, such as an anterior and lateral wedge technique.

In another series of six orbital tumors with gross extension to parameningeal sites, there was similar global damage, which consisted of cataract formation in eight eyes, enophthalmos with resultant ptosis and superior sulcus deformity in five, and retinopathy in one.[10] Three patients developed optic atrophy which appeared to be due to optic nerve compression by primary tumor. Prior to treatment, these patients had decreased vision which did not improve after therapy. In a group of six patients with soft tissue sarcomas of the orbit, 9 out of 11 eyes received doses of 2800 to 5500 cGy of radiotherapy to the lens and all but one developed cataracts.[6] Visual acuity was reported to be 20/40 or better in 10 out of 11 eyes. Six eyes developed xerophthalmia which was symptomatic in four, and three eyes had asymptomatic retinopathy.

Clearly, most of the ocular changes occurring during follow-up of patients with orbital lesions demand the attention of an ophthalmologist. These patients warrant concurrent follow-up by both the pediatric oncologist and an ophthalmologist from the time of diagnosis. Growth should be followed annually or semiannually so that children whose growth curve begins to show decreased growth velocity can be studied appropriately, and growth hormone therapy can be initiated early if warranted.

The major problems that children develop as late effects from treatment to parameningeal or other head and neck sites are primarily due to radiotherapy. However, the initial surgical procedure may contribute to a major loss of structural tissues when gross total removal of the primary tumor is carried out. Loss of part of the temporal bone, maxilla, or mandible along with attendant soft tissues is not infrequent. Likewise, some patients with tumors involving only soft tissues, such as the cheek and occasionally the nasopharynx, may have major tissue loss. Secondary tissue damage from radiotherapy makes plastic reconstruction or placement of prostheses difficult in these sites.

When radiotherapy has been used for head and neck tumors, one of the major long-term problems is diminished bone and soft tissue growth within the treated field. Among 43 patients from the IRS-I study who had head and neck tumors, asymmetry of the face or neck was reported in 58%.[5] Muscle atrophy or fibrosis of the subcutaneous tissues occurred in 40% of patients with tumors of the head and in 33% of those with tumors arising in the neck. Bone hypoplasia was documented in one third of the patients with asymmetry. Six children with facial defects had been treated with skin grafts or other reconstructive surgery, but prosthetic devices were rarely used.

In another report, the presence of bone or soft tissue hypoplasia was related to age at treatment.[6] All 16 children who were 9 years of age or younger at diagnosis showed some degree of deformity, whereas 4 who were 11 years or older showed none. In a series of 68 patients with RMSs of the head and neck who were long-term survivors, 45 had received radiotherapy to the maxillofacial region.[11] Most of the latter patients had also received some form of chemotherapy. Among these patients were nine with rhabdomyosarcoma, all of whom had received between 4500 and 6500 cGy to the primary tumor sites. Five of these patients had maxillary or mandibular and facial deformities which were more marked when higher doses of radiotherapy were given.

Dental problems following radiotherapy in head and neck patients can be severe. Dental caries, delayed or absent tooth eruption, absent or missing teeth, absent or rudimentary and malformed roots, and loose teeth were the defects reported in 58% of head and neck patients studied from IRS-I.[5] Several children had lost many teeth and one was edentulous. Several case reports of RMS have described the above findings in detail. One child required radiotherapy to the orbit and neck at 6 months of age.[12] At 7 years of age, she had gross caries and required extraction of seven teeth. At 8, she had further extractions and by 13 years she had short crowns, pitting of incisors, and short and tapering roots of ten teeth. Two other reported cases followed over a 4- to 6-year period had underdeveloped mandibles, and there was either partial development or absence of development of several of the permanent teeth.[13] Another report described a child who had rampant caries and required two extractions and placement of 18 steel crowns within a year of completing therapy.[14] In addition to facial asymmetry from mandibular hypoplasia, there was retarded development of both primary and permanent dentition, premature apical closure of roots, and retardation of developing cementum and dentine. A second patient had gross malocclusion from radiotherapy to the maxillary arch, which requried orthodontic therapy.

A boy who was treated at 2 years of age for a RMS of the middle ear presented at 13 years with marked micrognathia, a thin hypoplastic mandible, and only 18 permanent teeth.[15] The teeth were loose and the premolar crowns were small. Radiographs showed little or no root formation of the remaining teeth. Another boy, treated at 2 years of age for a parameningeal primary tumor in the infratemporal and parapharyngeal region, had erosion of part of the maxilla and partial destruction of the right mandibular ramus at diagnosis.[16] Two years following radiotherapy he had severe caries of primary dentition. Although a program of intensive dental hygiene was introduced, compliance was poor, and at 8 years of age he had absence of some teeth, small crowns, enamel hypoplasia, complete root agenesis, delayed development, and partially erupted and unerupted teeth. The mandible was also atrophic and thin.

It is obvious from the above reports that children treated for tumors in the head and neck during the period of development of both primary and permanent dentition suffer damage not only to the deciduous teeth, but particularly to the developing permanent teeth. The associated retarded bone growth complicates spatial relationships and there is loss of a solid basis for tooth stability. A certain amount of damage appears inevitable when radiotherapy is given, but the single most important preventive measure is meticulous oral hygiene. These children should be examined by a dentist at diagnosis so that any existing need for treatment of caries or other problems can be accomplished before radiotherapy is begun. It is then imperative that they follow the program outlined for dental hygiene and are seen regularly at intervals deemed necessary. As the above reports attest, these problems continue over years of time and demand continued close follow-up.

Problems with diminished hearing occur relatively infrequently in patients treated for tumors of the head and neck. Normal hearing was found in 25 out of 27 middle and inner ears which were situated in the field of radiotherapy for soft tissue sarcomas.[6] Beyond the potential damage from surgery and radiotherapy in tumors of the middle ear, hearing loss may be aggravated by the use of ototoxic chemotherapeutic agents such as cisplatin. Aminoglycoside antibiotics used commonly during periods of fever, neutropenia, and infection may also cause hearing impairment. Children receiving cisplatin as part of chemotherapy should have audiograms performed prior to receiving doses of the drug. The dose and number of courses given correlate well with hearing loss from cisplatin.[17] Probably the most common problem resulting in some degree of sensorineural or conduction hearing loss relates to the degree of fibrosis in the tympanic membrane and middle ear mucosa following radiotherapy. Some patients with parameningeal tumors treated with radiotherapy have chronic otitis media.

There are several other isolated problems due to radiotherapy which occur with some frequency in patients treated for RMSs of the head and neck. A fourth of the children studied from IRS-I had changes in the oral mucosa and showed skin pigmentation in the field of radiotherapy.[5] Dryness of the oral mucosa may be associated with diminished salivary gland secretion. Occasionally children have difficulty swallowing and several have developed trismus due to fibrosis of the temporomandibular joint and surrounding soft tissues. As many as 20% of the children from the IRS-I study reported difficulty with speech which was frequently nasal in quality. This was also reported, along with trismus, in four of a series of nine children.[11] Two children also complained of loss or change of taste perception.

Growth retardation is a potential complication in any child who has had radiotherapy covering a field which included or bordered on the pituitary, hypothalamus, or thyroid. The best measure of early growth deceleration is a change in annual growth velocity from the minimum norm of more than 4.5 cm/year. Children who have entered puberty should show appropriate linear growth acceleration. Annual or semiannual height measurements plotted on standard linear growth curves will identify such children. If a child shows a decrease of 20 percentile increments or more from the pretreatment percentile, assay of growth hormone and thyroid studies are warranted. Hypothyroidism may occur in children receiving neck irradiation[6] and may occur in combination with growth hormone deficiency.[5] Thyroid function studies should be initiated within a year or two after radiotherapy to the neck and these studies should be followed at annual intervals, particularly if growth velocity falls below the norm.

There have been many reports on the adverse consequences of pituitary irradiation in children given cranial radiotherapy for treatment of brain tumors or for prevention or treatment of CNS leukemia. These observations are applicable to children treated for RMS. In general, most patients with this tumor will be getting doses in excess of 3000 cGy either to the whole brain or to specific tumor sites and, therefore, they are more likely to have problems.

Impaired responses of growth hormone to insulin-induced hypoglycemia were shown in a study of 27 children who had been treated with surgery and radiotherapy for intracranial tumors, which did not directly involve the pituitary or hypothalamus.[18] Three months after surgery, none of the patients was growth hormone deficient, although the peak responses of the hormone were blunted when compared to controls. When 16 of these children were studied 1 to 12 years after therapy, 10 were found to be growth hormone deficient as measured by the same tests. Serum levels of thyroid-stimulating hormone in response to thyrotropin-releasing hormone were greater in growth hormone-deficient patients than in those who were not deficient in this hormone. Serum T3 and T4 levels were normal in both groups.

In a subsequent study of 39 brain tumor and 17 acute leukemia patients, a significant inverse correlation was shown between radiation dose to the hypothalamic-pituitary region and the peak growth hormone response to hypoglycemia.[19] Of the total of 56 patients, 37 had an impaired growth hormone response, and 36 of these had received more than 2900 cGy of radiation. Of 5 children who received more than 2900 cGy but showed normal growth hormone responses, 4 were older than 13 years at the time of treatment. These findings were confirmed in a prospective study in 14 children with brain tumors studied before and after receiving radiotherapy and chemotherapy.[20] In another study, nine children treated with cranial irradiation for either medulloblastoma or acute leukemia showed decreased growth velocity.[21] With arginine and l-DOPA stimulation, six of the nine children had normal growth hormone responses, but only two of the nine had normal responses to insulin-induced hypoglycemia. The radiated patients also had lower pulsatile growth hormone secretion and lower somatomedin-C levels than normal. These children were treated with human growth hormone and achieved normalization of growth, although the response measured as absolute growth velocities was less than in children who were growth hormone deficient but who had not been irradiated.

Five prepubertal children with brain tumors who were growth hormone deficient from radiation therapy were treated with human growth hormone for a minimum of 3 years.[22] When compared to a group of five children with brain tumors who had not received radio-therapy, the irradiated patients had diminished annual growth rates relative to the change in chronologic age, and these increments increased after the first year of therapy. It was possible to differentiate whether growth hormone deficiency due to radiation was hypothalamic or pituitary in origin in ten children who had radiation-induced deficiency of this hormone.[23] All ten patients had subnormal growth hormone responses to arginine and insulin, with other pituitary functions being normal. When given hypothalamic growth hormone-releasing factor (GRF), there was no growth hormone response in two patients, and a subnormal response was seen in four. The other four patients showed a significant growth hormone response to GH releasing factor, suggesting that in these patients the damage from radiation was probably to the hypothalamus rather than the pituitary, causing a deficiency of endogenous GRF.

Therapeutically, this differentiation is important since synthetic GRF is available and is capable of stimulating growth hormone secretion and somatomedin production in humans. These findings were confirmed in 22 children with medulloblastoma, all of whom had received craniospinal radiotherapy.[24] Of 19 patients who had not yet completed growth, 14 had retarded growth velocity. Only three out of ten patients studied with the growth hormone stimulation test had evidence of deficiency of this hormone, while seven had normal growth hormone responses to provocative testing. This finding again suggested that there is secretory or regulatory dysfunction of growth hormone in these children, rather than absolute growth hormone deficiency.

The goal of the oncologist when following patients who had head and neck tumors should be close surveillance, looking for evidence of growth deceleration. Therapy with growth hormone can only be effective when given prior to the closure of epiphyses in the midteens. Thus, it is important to have these children examined by a pediatric endocrinologist during the early period of recognition of diminished growth velocity.

In addition to the endocrine disorders resulting from radiation to the cranial vault, children with parameningeal tumors who receive whole brain irradiation, or both irradiation and intrathecal chemotherapy, are vulnerable to disturbances of cortical function and leukoencephalopathy. Poor or deteriorating school performance may be the first sign of damage in children who received cranial radiotherapy for acute leukemia and brain tumors. If there is any indication of difficulty with normal development or learning, children should have psychometric testing done. These tests can help elucidate whether the observed patterns of psychological response are consistent with cortical damage.

Many patients who have parameningeal RMSs are treated with intrathecal chemotherapy when high risk features for meningeal spread are present at diagnosis. In addition to intrathecal chemotherapy which usually includes methotrexate, cytosine arabinoside, and hydrocortisone, most of these children will have radiotherapy to the base of brain or to larger cranial ports, depending on the site and size of primary tumor. Such patients are subject to white matter damage in the form of leukoencephalopathy. Leukoencephalopathy was observed in a child treated for an orbital RMS who developed meningeal involvement by tumor 9 months after initial therapy.[25] Intraventricular chemotherapy via an Ommaya reservoir included methotrexate, cytosine arabinoside, and hydrocortisone. There was a good response with regression of the tumor, but the child began to show deterioration in motor and intellectual function. He showed quick, extraneous movement of his hands, feet, and head, mild clumsiness, and dysmetria. The spinal fluid was normal, but an EEG contained a slow and dysrhythmic background. CT scan showed moderate dilatation of the ventricles, plus irregular areas in the white matter which had a decreased absorption coefficient. After stopping intraventricular chemotherapy, there was some intellectual improvement, as well as improvement in the CT scan. However, meningeal relapse occurred 14 months later. Rare cases of transverse myelitis have been seen in patients with parameningeal tumors treated with radiotherapy plus both systemic and intrathecal chemotherapy.[26]

III. TRUNK

RMSs involving the trunk include those which arise in the thorax as well as those arising in the retroperitoneum or abdomen. The paraspinal tumors can occur either at the thoracic or lumbosacral levels. These sites are uncommon and survival in these patients is relatively poor. Specific problems developing as late effects of therapy for RMS are not unlike those arising in other childhood tumors in these sites and for which therapy is similar.

Primary sites of RMS in the thorax include tumors arising in the chest wall, mediastinum, pleura, and lung, in addition to paraspinal tumors. Surgical deficits in these patients are few since the vast majority of patients have unresectable tumors at diagnosis.[27] Resection of tumors of the chest wall may be an exception. The effect of radiotherapy in treating RMSs of the chest is most evident as localized bone and soft tissue hypoplasia, and the younger the child is at the time of treatment, the more marked the adverse effects. Figure 2 shows the effect of radiotherapy on bone and soft tissue growth following treatment for a primary tumor of the chest, probably arising from the posterior mediastinum. Radiotherapy for paraspinous tumors should include whole vertebral exposure to lessen the risk of developing scoliosis. However, even when radiation is given in this manner, the accompanying effect on adjacent soft tissue growth unilaterally may ultimately be reflected as a mild scoliosis.

Radiotherapy damage to the spinal cord, nerve roots, or brachial plexus is more often due to fibrosis of surrounding structures than to actual damage by radiation to the nerves per se. Patients with paraspinous tumors may have long-term neurologic abnormalities from effects of the tumor itself. Among ten patients with paraspinous tumors who were studied in IRS-I, five had paraparesis at diagnosis, and all of these had findings of spinal cord compression on the myelogram.[28] These patients may not recover complete neurologic function following therapy. If the breast is within the field of radiotherapy, there may be

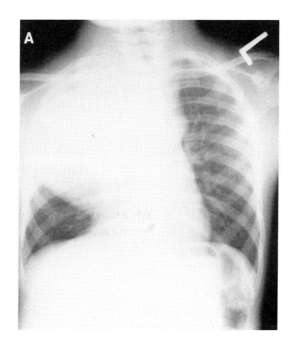

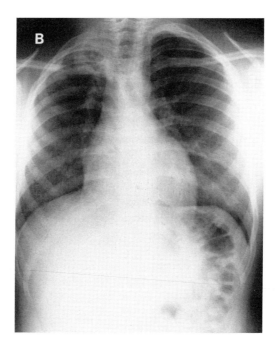

FIGURE 2. (A) Unresectable primary extraosseous Ewing's sarcoma of the right chest at 4 years of age. Treatment consisted of 4500 cGy to a 7 × 11-cm field of the upper anterior and posterior right chest and 2 years of pulse VAC chemotherapy. (B) Chest X-ray 6 years later showing a hypoplastic right thorax with diminished lung volume and apical scarring on the right.

diminished growth of breast tissue on that side. When part of the lung lies within the radiotherapy field, it must be shielded as well as possible since it cannot tolerate the doses used for primary tumor treatment. When the lungs are the site of metastases, they are vulnerable to potential damage from radiotherapy. Long-term effects may include an increased incidence of interstitial pneumonia and the occurrence of pulmonary fibrosis. However, these findings are not common when the dose of radiotherapy to the lungs is limited to less than 1800 cGy. One concern in RMS is whether dactinomycin, doxorubicin, or a combination of the two may enhance pulmonary damage even when the radiotherapy dose is appropriate. Reactivation of latent radiation damage to the lungs has been observed following the administration of these two drugs.[4] In following these patients, attention should be paid to the presence of symptoms such as exercise intolerance or shortness of breath. If these symptoms are present, the patient should have evaluation of pulmonary function.

The potential late cardiac toxicity in RMS is similar to that of other patients being treated with anthracycline drugs. Of particular concern is the small group of patients who were given radiotherapy to the lungs, mediastinum, or some segment of the heart, and who have also received an anthracycline drug either alone or combined with cyclophosphamide. Whether the increase in ventricular wall thickness that has been observed following high doses of cyclophosphamide will be reflected in late cardiac toxicity is not yet known.[4] This possibility is of concern, however, since a related drug, ifosfamide, is being used increasingly for treatment of RMS. Any child who has developed cardiac changes on echocardiogram or MUGA scan during the therapy period should be followed for development of cardiac symptoms, particularly exercise intolerance. Such a child should have repeated assessment with careful physical examination of the heart. Any evidence of pending congestive heart failure warrants immediate attention, since the majority of these patients will survive the acute episode.[29]

Pericardial thickening of undefined significance was seen in 43% of patients between the ages of 5 and 17 years who were treated with mediastinal irradiation for Hodgkin's disease.[30] In the IRS-I, -II, and -III, acute cardiac toxicity of severe, life-threatening, or fatal degree occurred in 21 patients.[31] Two patients died of this complication while still on maintenance therapy. A third patient developed congestive heart failure 7 years after diagnosis. He had had radiotherapy to a chest wall mass, including a segment of the heart, together with doxorubicin. Although he had a diminished shortening fraction on echocardiography while on therapy, he had been well and off therapy for 5 years before heart failure developed. He died of intractable cardiac failure 5 months after the onset of symptoms.

RMSs arising in the abdomen, retroperitoneal space, or lower paraspinous area tend to be large tumors which are frequently unresectable. In IRS-I and -II, only 13 out of 101 patients with retroperitoneal tumors had gross total removal of the tumor and the median tumor diameter was 10 cm.[32] Another group of patients who may have radiotherapy to the abdomen or retroperitoneal space are boys with paratesticular RMSs who have involvement of para-aortic lymph nodes or abdominal extension of tumor. The liver is rarely included in the radiotherapy field in children with RMSs, with the exception of the few cases in which the primary tumor is in the biliary tree. There were only ten such cases in IRS-I and -II, and there were only four survivors.[33] Long-term sequelae of liver irradiation may include fibrosis. If part of the liver can be excluded from the radiotherapy port, hepatic function is usually adequate. Fibrosis of the hepatic duct or common bile duct may cause a picture of chronic cholangitis. The kidneys can usually be protected from radiotherapy by limiting the dose to 1500 cGy and shielding these organs whenever possible. Cisplatin and ifosfamide both have potential for causing damage to the kidney tubules. To prevent late sequelae, kidney function must be followed very closely during the use of these drugs; and for those patients with evidence of acute toxicity, continued monitoring of kidney function and serum electrolytes should extend beyond the therapy period.

Both the large and the small bowel are sensitive to radiotherapy and damage can be enhanced by anthracyclines. Delayed gastrointestinal complications were observed in 16 children treated for retroperitoneal RMSs with combined modality therapy.[34] There was severe enteritis or proctitis in six children, four of whom developed intestinal obstruction. Another child had chronic radiation enteritis with malabsorption and one had hemorrhagic proctitis due to radiation. Three of these children died of complications from small bowel obstruction. In the follow-up of long-term survivors with paratesticular RMSs from IRS-I and -II, eight (9%) developed small bowel obstruction requiring surgery.[35] All of these patients had initial laparotomy for retroperitoneal lymph node dissection, but only four had radiotherapy to the abdomen. All patients who have laparotomies are at risk for adhesions which may result in late obstruction. Three patients from this series, including one who developed obstruction, had chronic diarrhea following abdominal irradiation. In another study of late effects in RMS, five children with either genitourinary primaries or tumors in other abdominal sites had either intestinal malabsorption or bowel obstruction.[36] Four of these patients required parenteral nutrition permanently.

IV. GENITOURINARY

The sites of RMSs addressed in this section are bladder, prostate, paratestis, vagina, vulva, uterus, and pelvis. Unlike tumors in most other primary sites, a high survival rate can be achieved by removing the organs involved. Thus, prior to the introduction of combined modality therapy, pelvic exenteration was the usual treatment. Organ loss in the pelvis, whether bladder, prostate, vagina, uterus, or rectum, results in lifelong major deficits. For tumors in these sites, the initial surgical approach is of great importance and is dependent, in part, on tumor size and extent. For at least the past decade, the initial therapeutic approach to tumors in these sites has been the use of chemotherapy first, followed by radiotherapy. Surgery was reserved for removal of persistent tumor tissue, hoping to limit the degree of normal tissue loss.

In eight surviving patients treated with this sequence, one ultimately required ileal loop diversion without cystectomy; hysterosalpingectomy and partial vaginectomy were carried out in two, and one patient had anterior pelvic exenteration.[37] These losses of affected organs are preferable to pelvic exenteration. In IRS-I and -II, at least one fourth of bladders have been salvaged by using this approach.[38] Similarly, some of the vaginal and vulvar tumors have required only limited resection.[39] Polypoid uterine tumors respond well to limited surgery, while those that are more invasive or disseminated usually require hysterectomy. Of ten patients with primary uterine tumors, six survived and in all of these the bladder and at least one ovary were retained. The uterus was preserved in four patients after polypectomy.

Gonadal function may be salvaged by placing uninvolved testes or ovaries outside the radiotherapy field during treatment. Compounding the potential loss of gonadal tissue from surgery or radiotherapy is the adverse effect of chemotherapy, particularly alkylating agents, on gonadal function. Cyclophosphamide and ifosfamide have been mainstays of the chemotherapy regimens employed for RMSs, and are capable of causing sterility in both the prepubertal and postpubertal ovary and testis. This risk applies to all patients with this tumor and will be discussed later in this section.

Since the peak age incidence for primary genitourinary RMS is the preschool child, some of the patients who had pelvic exenteration in the past are just now becoming young adults. These individuals usually have colostomies and ileal conduits for urinary drainage. Girls may lack the vagina, the uterus, or both of these organs. Since many also had radiotherapy when disease was extensive, they may have damaged ovaries and severe fibrosis of the pelvic organs. These children need a great deal of support, both medically and psychosocially. Since many have grown up with their abnormalities they are not aware of some of their inadequacies until they become prepubertal or pubertal. Managing their problems at school level alone is a distinct challenge for many. Without good parental and physician support they may have serious problems with personal hygiene, difficulty in taking part in sports, and trouble in maintaining friends. They need to be made aware of their differences from normal children and should be given some honest explanations as to the cause. At puberty some will need gonadal hormone replacement in order to develop secondary sexual characteristics. At appropriate ages, some will require secondary surgery which may contribute to becoming a more normal functioning young adult.

Thirteen children with bladder or prostate RMSs were reviewed, with follow-up studies reported on six survivors.[40] All patients had ileal conduit ureterostomies, and three had required a revision of the Bricker loop or ileal stoma for mild to moderate hydronephrosis. In another study, three patients with RMS had radiotherapy to the pelvis in addition to chemotherapy.[41] Among the problems observed in one or more of the three patients were cystitis, proctitis, chronic diarrhea, incontinence, bilateral hydronephrosis, rigid rectum, malabsorption, small bowel obstruction, and perineal fistula with infection. Late effects in 24 patients with genitourinary primaries were summarized from two Children's Cancer Study Group studies.[42] These patients had had partial or total pelvic exenteration initially, followed by radiotherapy and chemotherapy in the majority. A third of these children developed bowel obstruction which necessitated laparotomy. Among other problems were chronic urinary tract infections, chronic diarrhea, hydronephrosis, enuresis, soiling, and chronic bladder problems following hemorrhagic cystitis.

A 26-year-old woman was reported who was treated at 16 months of age by surgical excision for a RMS of the vestibule near the urinary meatus.[43] Following treatment with radiotherapy to the inguinal area and additional surgery for a local recurrence, she developed a vesicovaginal fistula and later had urethral reconstruction. An ileal loop urinary diversion was done 11 years later, leaving the bladder in place. In an attempt to provide her with a functional vagina, her small, stenosed vagina was incorporated with the remaining urethra and bladder and she was started on hormone therapy.

In another report, a case of vaginal RMS was treated at 1 year of age with hysterectomy, total vaginectomy, and transposition of both ovaries. Following surgery, radiotherapy was given to the residual tumor.[44] The child had never been continent of urine and at 7 years became incontinent of stool. Studies showed her to have a small contracted bladder, a hypoplastic sigmoid colon and rectum, and vesicoureteral reflux on the right side. Presence of radiation proctitis was confirmed at sigmoidostomy. She had a two-stage repair of the rectal stenosis by creating a temporary diverting colostomy which was ultimately closed following reanastomosis of the colon.

All patients who have lost bladders and have various urinary diversion procedures must be followed for impairment of kidney function. Besides stomal problems requiring surgical attention, the ureteral insertions into bowel loops may become stenosed or kinked, either from chronic infection or by fibrosis due to scarring. In these patients pyelography, ultrasound examination, or other kidney scans which can detect hydronephrosis and loss of kidney function should be done at intervals of 1 to 2 years. Measurements of blood pressure and blood urea nitrogen or serum creatinine should be done annually. When bladders are intact there may still be strictures of the urethra and chronic urethritis. Occasionally, the ureters may be stenosed following radiotherapy.

One of the most common acute problems affecting patients being treated for RMS with cyclophosphamide is the occurrence of hemorrhagic cystitis from accumulation of acrolein in the bladder due to its excretion in the urine. The initial episode of hemorrhagic cystitis can usually be managed by withholding the drug temporarily, increasing fluid intake, and having the patient void frequently during and after administration of the drug. In spite of good acute management, there are still patients who develop chronic problems with intermittent episodes of hematuria and ultimately develop a small, fibrotic bladder.

Compounding the problem in RMS is the frequent use of radiotherapy in the pelvis. A series of 110 children with either Ewing's sarcoma or Hodgkin's disease received cyclophosphamide with or without pelvic irradiation.[45] Of the 50 children receiving pelvic radiotherapy, 17 (34%) had bladder toxicity which was transient in 8, but chronic or intermittent in 9. In contrast, among the 60 patients whose radiotherapy included areas outside the pelvis, only 5 (8%) had transient hematuria lasting less than 1 month. Radiotherapy doses in the group showing severe toxicity ranged from 2580 to 5300 cGy.

In another study, 28 out of 100 patients who developed hemorrhagic cystitis were children, and 22 of these had received cyclophosphamide for treatment of either Ewing's sarcoma or other sarcomas.[46] When compared to adults, the use of the drug intravenously in children produced cystitis at significantly lower doses and after shorter durations of therapy. In 56 patients symptoms of gross hematuria, irritative voiding complaints, or both persisted after cyclophosphamide was discontinued. In 21 patients, recurrence of gross hematuria occurred between 3 months and 10 years after the initial episode subsided and drug was stopped. An autopsy study of bladders from children treated with cyclophosphamide showed that bladder fibrosis occurred when the total dose of the drug exceeded 6 g/m^2.[47] Out of 40 patients, 10 (25%) had bladder fibrosis, but only 5 had previously had hemorrhagic cystitis.

In an ongoing review of 86 patients with paratesticular RMS from IRS-I and -II, 22 (25%) developed hemorrhagic cystitis while on therapy.[35] Of 22 patients, 16 had also received radiotherapy to the bladder. Five of these patients continued to have episodes of gross hematuria for from 3 to 10 years, and two required transfusion therapy. One or more cystoscopies were necessary in 13 patients for removal of clots, for fulguration of bleeding sites, or other therapy. Currently, the use of mesna may eradicate the prolonged bladder problems previously observed with cyclophosphamide. Mesna is a sodium sulfonate salt of 2-mercaptoethane which provides a free sulfhydryl group that reacts with acrolein, rendering it nontoxic to bladder epithelium. Mesna should be incorporated into all drug regimens containing cyclophosphamide or ifosfamide. For patients who develop hemorrhagic cystitis, urine should be checked intermittently, and if there is persistent microhematuria, gross hematuria, or voiding symptoms, evaluation of bladder size and function should be followed by serial voiding cystourethrograms.

Gonadal dysfunction is one of the prime concerns of children with genitourinary or pelvic RMSs. The initial surgical procedure may result in the loss of a testis, loss of one or both ovaries, and loss of accessory organs such as the prostate, vagina, or uterus. Prostatectomy and retroperitoneal lymph node dissection may interrupt sympathetic innervation necessary for erection and ejaculation. These losses may be compounded by further fibrosis from radiotherapy or gonadal damage from alkylating agents. Much of the data on loss of gonadal function in children treated for cancer has come from studies of leukemia and Hodgkin's disease.[3,4,48] Other extensive reviews on the effects of cancer therapy on gonadal function include sections on children.[49,50] Studies done exclusively in RMS are lacking except for those incorporated in other reports.

Female infants and young girls who had ovaries removed surgically or exposed to radiotherapy may later show primary ovarian failure. In one study, 18 female patients had received abdominal radiotherapy in childhood for treatment of Wilms' tumor or other tumors.[52] Of 13 patients who were 13 years of age or older at the time of evaluation, 12 were not menstruating and had increased levels of serum FSH and LH. Two patients who had menarche before radiation was given became amenorrheic within 2 months of finishing radiotherapy. The serum FSH was markedly increased in the six patients who were less than 13 years of age at the time of evaluation, with the LH being elevated in only three. Only one patient had received cyclophosphamide.

A histopathologic study was done on ovaries from 21 girls with malignant tumors who were given various combinations of chemotherapeutic agents, together with radiation therapy to ports that may have included the gonads.[53] Two of these patients had RMS. The total number of follicles present was normal and the number of follicles was similar whether the patient was less than 10 years or over 10 years of age. However, the majority of these ovaries showed impaired follicular maturation as shown by the presence of reduced numbers of growing and antral follicles as compared to those in controls. In the patients treated prior to puberty, four had received radiotherapy. One of these patients showed a decreased number of follicles and another had small ovaries and nondetectable primary and antral follicles. Among the girls treated during puberty or postpuberty, all but one of the seven treated with chemotherapy alone (without radiotherapy) showed abnormalities. These ovarian abnormalities included cortical fibrosis and hyalinization of the ovarian capsule, and a moderate to severe reduction in the number of follicles. Three girls received both chemotherapy and radiation, and these showed severe changes of neovascularization of the ovarian surface, scattered or diffuse areas of fibrosis, and a moderate to severe reduction in the number of follicles. Similar findings were reported in a study of ovaries from 12 children who died before 7 years of age, following treatment for abdominal tumors.[54] Seven girls had received radiotherapy with doses between 2500 and 3000 cGy and four also received cyclophosphamide. Normal ovaries were found in four patients who had received little or no chemotherapy and no radiotherapy. All of the irradiated children had inhibition of growth of ovarian follicles and varying degrees of small follicle destruction.

Girls who have been treated with pelvic or abdominal radiotherapy should be followed closely for sexual maturation and by 10 years of age should have gonadal hormone studies done. If abnormalities are found, these girls will require hormonal replacement therapy between the ages of 10 and 12 years to assure adequate secondary sexual maturation. For girls who will require corrective surgery, such as vaginal reconstruction, it is best to defer these procedures until they have had hormone therapy and are past puberty. Hormone therapy needs to be continued indefinitely to insure normal bone and vascular integrity.

The problems in boys are somewhat more complex. For those who have primary tumors in the bladder, prostate, or paratesticular areas, the testes may not be included in radiotherapy fields, although scatter irradiation may be a problem. Testicular function was reported in ten adults who as children between 1 and 11 years of age had been treated for Wilms' tumor with orthovoltage radiation to the whole abdomen.[55] In all patients, the penis and scrotum were shielded. It was estimated that scatter doses of irradiation to the testes were between 268 and 983 cGy. Eight of the ten patients had either oligospermia or azoospermia, and seven of these had elevated levels of serum FSH, with only one having an elevated LH level. One patient also showed evidence of Leydig cell dysfunction. A second group of eight boys had been treated prepubertally between 1 and 5 years of age, and were then studied between 8 and 14 years of age. Four received abdominal irradiation for Wilms' tumor with use of a technique similar to that used for the first group, but three received megavoltage radiation. Three patients in this group had paratesticular RMS with one testis being removed surgically, and radiotherapy then being given to the abdomen and scrotum. In four patients the scatter dose of radiation was similar to the first group, whereas four received between 2700 and 3000 cGy directly to the scrotum. The testosterone levels were normal prepubertal levels and only one patient had increased levels of FSH and LH. In the first group, all patients had normal adult genitalia but the testicular volume was significantly reduced, the volume ranging from 5 to 10 ml. In the second group all patients were Tanner stage 1 and testicular volumes were only 1 to 2 ml. These findings confirmed suggestions that spermatogonia were more radiosensitive than Leydig cells. The only chemotherapy received by patients in the second group was vincristine and dactinomycin.

Studies in adults have confirmed the low doses of radiation which can cause temporary or permanent aspermia. When doses of less than 200 cGy are given, there will usually be recovery of aspermia beginning 5 to 13 months post-therapy, but with recovery of normal sperm counts not being complete until 2 to 4 years have elapsed.[56] With doses of radiation between 200 and 300 cGy there will be 100% temporary aspermia, with late recovery of spermatogenesis only after as long as a decade, if at all. In another study, 27 men were treated for soft tissue sarcomas with surgery and radiotherapy, with scatter radiation doses to the testes of up to 2500 cGy.[57] These men were followed prospectively with repeated determinations of FSH, LH, and testosterone levels for 30 months. Sperm counts were not done. All patients developed an increase in FSH levels over baseline and only those receiving radiation doses of less than 50 cGy showed early recovery of normal FSH levels. Patients receiving more than 200 cGy had significantly elevated LH levels, but normal testosterone levels. The observation that an increase in LH levels is dependent on the dose of radiation therapy previously given is consistent with the finding of subtle Leydig cell damage. The peak serum levels of FSH occurred at 6 months following radiation and the levels fell to normal rapidly when less than 50 cGy had been given. When the radiation dose was greater than 50 cGy the FSH levels fell more slowly and were still elevated above baseline at 30 months.

The adverse effects that alkylating agents have on normal gonads may be seen in many children treated for RMSs with cyclophosphamide, chlorambucil, or ifosfamide. Recognition of the adverse effect of cyclophosphamide on the germinal epithelium of the testis was first observed in adults who had received the drug for treatment of various renal diseases.[58] Semen analysis of ten men who had received cyclophosphamide for 2 months or more, but had been off therapy for 3 to 19 months, showed only two who had any mature spermatozoa and in both the sperm counts were very low. Subsequent studies ensued on patients given cyclophosphamide for childhood nephrosis, with a number of reports substantiating the drug's effect on the germinal epithelium in boys.[59-64] Almost all of these reports recognized the relationship between the degree of damage to the germinal epithelium and the dose and duration of chemotherapy. In boys who had germinal epithelium destroyed, testes were apt to be small and show poor growth. Boys who were treated during puberty or postpubertally were most affected. There was some variance in the findings when patients were treated prepubertally, but several studies found persisting spermatogenic dysfunction in this group.[60,61,63] The effects of cyclophosphamide in girls treated for nephrosis were less clear, but overall the adverse effects were usually less damaging than in boys. Among the reports cited, there was a total of 34 girls and none of these had either menstrual dysfunction or ovarian failure.

In another study, 30 boys had received chemotherapy with or without radiotherapy to sites other than the gonads.[65] Most of the patients had lymphoma but three were cases of RMS. Gonadal function tests were done from 1 to 20 years after therapy was completed. Sperm counts were done on 22 patients, testicular biopsies were done in 7, and in 1 patient both assessments were done. Results were normal in 10 cases and abnormal in 20. Seventeen patients were azoospermic by semen analysis and 8 on biopsy had severe changes in the seminiferous tubules, with a marked reduction in the number of germ cells. Of the 20 patients with abnormal testicular function, 9 had assays of serum FSH and LH and all had an increase of FSH over normal levels. Of the 15 patients who received cyclophosphamide in combination with other drugs, treatment had been given prepubertally in 10 patients and testicular function was abnormal in 11. When the dose of cyclophosphamide was measured, 13 had received a total dose greater than 9 g/m^2, and all but 2 had abnormal gonadal function. Of the 25 patients who were prepubertal or intrapubertal at the time of treatment, all had achieved normal puberty and had normal growth.

It is not known whether any of the patients who have sustained germ cell damage from cyclophosphamide will show late recovery. In a study in adults, 26 patients were followed who had been treated with oral cyclophosphamide for periods of 5 to 34 months and were azoospermic.[66] Sperm counts were evaluated at varying periods of time after stopping therapy. A return of spermatogenesis was found in 12 patients within 15 to 49 months after stopping therapy. Recovery occurred in 9 out of 14 patients who had been treated for less than 18 months, but only 3 of 12 recovered who had been treated for a longer period.

Histopathologic examination of the testes in several of the studies on childhood nephrosis and in a study of children treated for extragonadal malignant tumors demonstrated the selective effect of cyclophosphamide on the germinal epithelium, leaving the Sertoli and Leydig cells intact.[67] The latter report showed these changes to be present in prepubertal boys as well as in older males.

Patients with paratesticular tumors may also have disorders of ejaculatory function due to sympathetic nerve damage following retroperitoneal lymph node dissection. Fortunately, some patients who develop retrograde ejaculation may have antegrade ejaculation restored by the use of imipramine.[68] Successful pregnancies have occurred with sperm retrieved from bladder urine which were then used for cervical insemination.[69] Another problem which may occur following surgery or radiotherapy in inguinal and pelvic sites is chronic lymphedema of an extremity. In the follow-up of paratesticular long-term survivors from IRS-I and -II, four patients developed this chronic problem after retroperitoneal lymph node dissection and therapy.[35]

Children who have had pelvic irradiation early in life are subject to the later development of slipped femoral capital epiphyses. This problem was first reported in RMS in children who received radiotherapy to the pelvis.[70,71] There was an incidence of abnormal epiphyseal plates of 9.6% in 50 children under 15 years of age who had had radiotherapy to the pelvis and to one or both capital femoral epiphyseal plates.[72] The abnormal epiphyseal plates occurred in children who received a total dose of more than 2500 cGy of radiation and most were less than 4 years of age when treated. Epiphyseal slippage did not occur until 8 to 10 years of age. If any child who has had pelvic irradiation begins to limp or complain of hip or thigh pain years after therapy, radiographs of the pelvis and hips should be done immediately. This complication can be avoided by better use of blocking systems to provide shaped fields, so that the epiphysis is spared from radiation damage.

All male children with genitourinary RMS and all males who have received an alkylating agent as part of their chemotherapy regimen require precise follow-up for gonadal evaluation. Both Tanner staging and testicular volume should be recorded annually as part of the physical examination. If there has been Leydig cell damage, secondary sexual maturation may be delayed. At the time of early puberty, at 12 to 14 years, gonadal hormone values including FSH, LH, and testosterone levels should be obtained as baseline information for comparison with later studies. There is still some question as to whether FSH may be elevated prepubertally when germinal epithelial damage has occurred. A postpubertal sample at 16 or 17 years of age should give normal adult values. Markedly increased FSH levels at this age are likely to be associated with oligospermia or aspermia. Semen analysis can be done when the patient requests it or when he is receptive to the suggestion that the test be done.

In addition to the previous comments on the follow-up of girls who are likely to have primary ovarian failure, all girls, and particularly those who have received alkylating agents, should have annual examinations for Tanner staging. If there is evidence of delayed development, hormone values for FSH, LH, and estradiol should be measured between 10 and 12 years of age as a baseline, and subsequent values can be obtained serially depending on further sexual development.

V. EXTREMITIES

There are few reports of late effects of therapy occurring in patients with RMSs of the extremities. In one report on acute and late effects in RMS and Ewing's sarcoma, 5 of the 23 RMS patients had primary tumors of the extremities.[41] These patients had received between 4200 and 7000 cGy to the primary tumor, combined with a chemotherapy regimen including dactinomycin, doxorubicin, cyclophosphamide, and vincristine. Two patients showed severe long-term damage. In one the shoulder and chest wall were treated with 7000 cGy and the patient developed a shoulder droop, weakness of the affected extremity, severe fibrosis of the soft tissues, and severe osteolysis of the underlying proximal humerus resulting in a pathologic fracture. A second patient who received a dose of 5000 cGy to the thigh developed severe fibrosis in the treated site. Two other patients developed minimal fibrosis in the treated site and a patient with a primary tumor in the foot showed periosteal and trabecular demineralization. Among 113 patients with RMS evaluated for late effects in another study, 11 patients had primary tumors in an extremity.[36] Six of these were reported to have fibrosis and hypoplasia and one patient each was reported to have gonadal failure, cardiomyopathy, and leukemia.

No systematic study has been made of late effects in patients with extremity tumors included in IRSs. However, a limited flow sheet review of 83 extremity patients surviving longer than 3 years who were included in IRS-II revealed a number of abnormalities.[73] Among the 83 tumors were 40 of the lower extremity, 22 of the upper extremity, 12 of the pelvic girdle, and 9 of the shoulder girdle. There were two amputations for primary tumors of the foot and one amputation for a tumor of the popliteal fossa. Late problems recorded for the upper and lower extremity lesions in 12 patients were shortening of the extremity and atrophy of muscles and subcutaneous tissue at the radiotherapy site. Two of these children had subsequently undergone surgery for limb shortening in the normal leg. Two lower extremity patients had had pathologic fractures, both at the site of radiotherapy. Although slight shortening and atrophy were reported in patients with primary tumors of the forearm and the hand, the upper extremity problems were fewer. In three patients with primary tumors of the buttock, the leg was reported to be shorter on the involved side, and in two of these cases, wasting and atrophy of the buttock were present. Decreased shoulder growth was noted in a shoulder primary. Metaphyseal sclerotic changes or irregularities were identified in two patients. Figure 3 shows X-rays of a patient who had a primary tumor of the calf with metastasis to the popliteal lymph node. Subsequent bone and soft tissue hypoplasia was followed by a limb shortening procedure at 15 years of age.

Children with a primary RMS in an extremity site require follow-up with limb length measurements and evaluation of limb function. If length discrepancies or functional abnormalities occur, orthopedic consultation is necessary. If new complaints of pain or limping occur at a later time, particularly 5 to 10 years after therapy, bone X-rays are warranted to investigate the possibility of a secondary osteogenic sarcoma arising in the previously irradiated site. Since X-rays of bone in previously treated sites may be difficult to interpret, a biopsy is warranted if questionable bony changes are present. When radiographs show bone demineralization or destruction, there is risk of a pathological fracture.

VI. SECOND MALIGNANT NEOPLASMS

The risk of developing a second malignant neoplasm after successfully treating the first is the most ominous of all late complications. During the 1960s, reports of second malignant neoplasms in children were usually of tumors developing in fields of radiotherapy, with a time interval of 10 years or more between the two tumors. As combined modality therapy for cancer in children began to produce increasing numbers of long-term survivors, reports of second malignant neoplasms also increased.[4,74] In this section, reports of second tumors following treatment for RMS and other soft tissue sarcomas will be reviewed. Studies which have helped define the roles of radiotherapy, chemotherapy, and genetic predisposition in the evolution of these second tumors will also be reviewed.

Cases of second malignant neoplasms following an initial RMS in childhood have been included in many reports. In an early attempt to define the incidence of second tumors in children, records of individuals who received radiotherapy as children between 1938 and

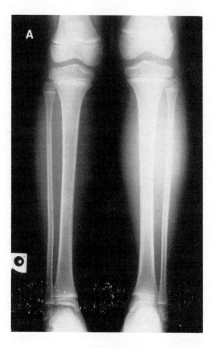

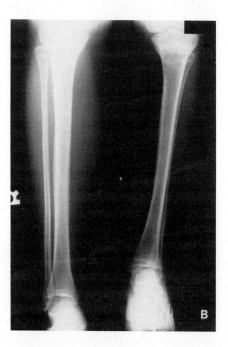

FIGURE 3.   (A) Primary embryonal RMS of the left calf with metastasis to the left popliteal lymph node at 7 years of age. The popliteal node was excised and the calf tumor biopsied. Treatment included 4955 cGy to a 29 × 14-cm field covering the left leg from ankle to above the knee, and 2 years of VAC plus doxorubicin chemotherapy. (B) Appearance of right and left lower legs 6 years later showing demineralization and shortening of the left tibia and fibula narrowing of the epiphyses at the knee, and marked atrophy of the soft tissue and muscles of the left calf.

1963 were reviewed.[75] Seventeen children developed a second malignant tumor, for an incidence of 0.5% in all children seen, or 5.0% among children who received radiotherapy at doses greater than 1000 cGy and had survived at least 2 years. Among the 17 cases was a patient with RMS who developed a chondrosarcoma in the irradiated site 10 years later.

In an epidemiologic study of RMS in children, there were five families with a second child having a soft tissue sarcoma.[76] Among the five patients with primary RMSs, one developed an astrocytoma 5 years after surviving RMS arising at 1 year of age. Other tumors identified in the cancer family syndrome were carcinoma of the breast, as well as other neoplasms such as acute leukemias and carcinomas of the lung, pancreas, and skin. Genetic factors common to these families have been difficult to identify, but for some patients the hereditary factor contributing to their developing a first malignancy may also play a part in developing the second. Many of the second malignant tumors reported following an initial RMS fall into the spectrum of tumors originally described in the early reviews. In an updated report on the cancer family syndrome, 15 patients among 151 cancer patients in 24 kindreds have developed a second tumor and 3 developed a third neoplasm.[77] A soft tissue sarcoma was the first cancer in 55 patients.

In a review of 414 long-term survivors of childhood cancer there were three second malignant tumors among 44 patients with an initial soft tissue sarcoma.[78] Two second tumors were chondrosarcomas occurring in sites radiated 7 and 10 years earlier, and the third secondary malignancy was acute lymphoblastic leukemia. An update on this patient-cohort added another soft tissue sarcoma treated with radiotherapy and chemotherapy who developed an oligodendroglioma 4 years later.[79] An initial report from the Late Effects Study Group culled data on patients treated between 1943 and 1970 from ten participating institutions.[80] There were 102 long-term survivors who had developed second malignant tumors. Six children who had a primary soft tissue sarcoma developed four bone tumors, a brain tumor, and a thyroid cancer. For 47 of the 102 patients, controls were selected within each institution to compare the effects of using dactinomycin with or without radiotherapy. Patients who received both dactinomycin and radiation were seven times less likely to develop a second malignancy in irradiated fields than those who received only radiotherapy. The risk of a second malignancy was not altered in children who received cyclophosphamide, vinca alkaloids, or antifoles.

In a subsequent report from the Late Effects Study Group, patterns of occurrence of second malignant tumors were described.[81] Radiotherapy was associated with 69 cases, a genetic disease was implicated in 27, and both conditions were present in 15 cases of second malignant neoplasms. Among the genetic disorders were retinoblastoma, neurofibromatosis, nevoid basal cell carcinoma syndrome, and xeroderma pigmentosum. The first report of acute nonlymphoblastic leukemia occurring as a second malignant neoplasm following RMS was in a 3-year-old child with RMS of an extremity.[82] This child received 6000 cGy of radiation to the forearm, axilla, and supraclavicular region, plus chemotherapy with vincristine, dactinomycin, and cyclophosphamide. Following the development of a cervical lymph node metastasis, she was treated with doxorubicin and DTIC and subsequently she was given cyclophosphamide and vincristine to complete 2 years of therapy. Three months later she presented with easy bruising and the bone marrow contained 40% Auer-rod positive cells. Karyotype of the leukemic cells was 46XX.

Many of the early reports of second malignant neoplasms occurring in irradiated fields were in the era of orthovoltage radiotherapy, and it was hoped that fewer such problems would be seen with use of megavoltage radiation. Seven second neoplasms were observed among 88 children with cancer who were long-term survivors and who had an average follow-up period of 14 years.[83] Patients were treated with megavoltage therapy using cobalt-60. Only two of the seven neoplasms were malignant and only one was associated with radiation. In another series, 330 children received megavoltage treatment from 1953 to 1970 for both benign (47) and malignant (285) conditions.[84] Only 4 out of 14 second neoplasms were malignant, and this incidence was thought to be lower than most series of cases treated with orthovoltage radiation.

Subsequent reports with use of megavoltage radiation, however, have not supported such a decrease in incidence of second malignancies, but the increasing use of chemotherapy may be compounding the effects of radiation per se. Two patients were reported who developed osteogenic sarcoma following megavoltage radiation and combination chemotherapy given to treat their initial tumors.[85] The second malignancies developed at earlier intervals than previously reported, one at 5 years and one at 7 years, and both patients had cyclophosphamide as part of their chemotherapy. In the continuing study by the Late Effects Study Group, 40 out of 188 cases of second malignant neoplasms were either osteogenic sarcoma or chondrosarcoma.[86] Thirty-two of these occurred in a radiotherapy field and in 23 a genetic susceptibility to cancer was present. Both factors were present in 16, and in this group radiation shortened the time interval to the second tumor to an average of 7 years.

Using the data from the Late Effects Study Group up to 1979, the incidence of second malignancies was estimated according to the initial tumor type.[87] Patient accrual data for each tumor were collected from the participating centers as a base from which to calculate incidence. Survival curves were then generated for each tumor during the calendar period and the annual incidence of second malignant neoplasms by type of first tumor was calculated. For soft tissue sarcomas, the rate was 143.2/100,000/year, which ranked these tumors behind the higher rates of incidence recorded for Hodgkin's disease, neuroblastoma, "other" tumors, Wilms' tumor, and bone tumors. The survival calculated for soft tissue sarcomas was just above 40% in the early 1960s. Thus, the incidence figures may well be different now, in view of the longer survival due to increased use of multimodal therapy.

Recent reports have begun to show a shift in the types of second malignancies seen and the intervals at which they have developed. The relationship of specific therapy to certain second malignancies is becoming increasingly refined. In one report, there were 86 survivors of childhood RMS with a median follow-up period of over 6 years.[88] Three children developed acute nonlymphoid leukemia at intervals of 4, 4.5, and 7 years from diagnosis of the initial malignancy, and all had been treated with radiotherapy and chemotherapy for their primary tumor. Chemotherapy had been either the T2 or T6 protocol, both of which include cyclophosphamide. Among 38 second malignant tumors reported in another series, 7 followed a primary RMS and included 3 bone tumors, a thyroid carcinoma, a fibrosarcoma, a melanoma, and a basal cell carcinoma.[89] In an updated report from the Late Effects Study Group, 292 cases had a total of 308 second malignancies, since 10 patients had 3, and 3 patients had developed 4 malignant neoplasms.[90] Among 40 primary soft tissue sarcomas, second malignancies were represented by 10 bone sarcomas, 9 soft tissue sarcomas, 6 leukemia/lymphomas, 7 brain tumors, 3 skin carcinomas, 2 thyroid carcinomas, and 3 breast carcinomas. Within the total group, those who developed leukemia had been treated with some form of chemotherapy and only one did not receive an alkylating agent. More than half had also received radiotherapy. As many as 87% of the cases of leukemia were acute nonlymphoid leukemia.

A preliminary report of second malignant neoplasms from the first two IRSs was based on follow-up data for patients who had survived 5 years or more from diagnosis and on review of causes of death occurring before 5 years.[91] Of the 426 patients on whom follow-up information was available, 10 second malignancies were observed and 7 occurred before 5 years. All of the study patients received either vincristine and dactinomycin; vincristine, dactinomycin, and cyclophosphamide (VAC); or VAC plus doxorubicin, with or without radiotherapy. The second malignancies included four acute nonlymphoid leukemias (all described as M4 FAB cytology), two osteogenic sarcomas, one optic nerve glioma, one non-Hodgkin's lymphoma, and one squamous cell carcinoma. None of the second malignancies occurred in a patient receiving only vincristine and dactinomycin. Eight of the ten cases had been treated with radiotherapy but only four of ten second malignancies occurred in the radiotherapy field.

With continuing surveillance of the patients from the first two IRSs for occurrence of second malignancies, a current update and new incidence figures are being prepared and will be the subject of a separate report.[92] The current number of known second malignant neoplasms from these two studies is 17. The increasing length of follow-up has shown more bone sarcomas developing with time. Seven osteogenic sarcomas and one chondrosarcoma have developed at a mean time interval of 7.5 years. All but one occurred in the radiotherapy field and all but one had received cyclophosphamide. The latter patient developed the second tumor in the radiotherapy field. Three of the four cases of acute nonlymphoid leukemia occurred before 5 years, and all had been treated with cyclophosphamide and radiotherapy. The fourth case occurred at 10 years and had received cyclophosphamide but no radiotherapy. The remaining five cases include two astrocytomas, a basal cell carcinoma, a squamous cell carcinoma, and an optic nerve glioma. The last patient and one other patient with an astrocytoma had neurofibromatosis. Thirteen of these patients have died.

Further analyses of the Late Effects Study Group data on second malignancies have provided relative risk factors associated with the development of bone sarcomas and leukemia in 9170 patients who had survived 2 or more years from diagnosis. Detailed treatment data from 64 patients who developed a secondary bone tumor were compared to similar data from 209 control patients who had not developed a second malignancy. Assessment of these data showed a 2.7-fold risk of second malignancy in patients who had had radiotherapy, and a sharp dose-response gradient reaching a 40-fold risk after doses of radiation to the bone exceeded 6000 cGy.[93] In this study, equal numbers of patients received orthovoltage and megavoltage radiotherapy. When adjustments were made for radiation therapy, treatment with an alkylating agent was also found to be linked to bone cancer with a relative risk of 4.7, and the risk increased as the cumulative dose of the drug rose. None of the other drugs used increased the risk of bone cancer as a second malignancy. The relative risk of developing bone cancer was greatest in patients whose primary tumor was a retinoblastoma or Ewing's sarcoma, followed by RMS, Wilms' tumor, and Hodgkin's disease. The relative risks increased significantly with the length of the time interval following treatment.

Similar analyses were applied for leukemia in this group of patients.[94] Secondary leukemia occurred in 22 cases, compared to an expected 1.52 cases based on general population rates, giving a 14-fold increase in risk or a relative risk of 14. The case control study was based on 25 cases and 90 matched controls from the total cohort. Most of the excess risk was due to the development of acute nonlymphoid leukemia with 19 cases observed compared to an expected 0.8, increasing the relative risk to 27. The use of alkylating agents was associated with a significantly elevated risk of leukemia, with a relative risk of 4.8. A strong dose-response relationship was noted between leukemia risk and dose of alkylating agents, with the relative risk 23 in the highest dose category. Alkylating agents most commonly used in patients who developed leukemia as a second malignancy were procarbazine and nitrogen mustard, with fewer cases receiving chlorambucil and cyclophosphamide. The interval between the initial drug treatment and leukemia ranged from 2.6 to 12 years, with a median of 3.5 years, whereas the interval between the last drug treatment and leukemia was 0 to 5.7 years with a median of 1.7 years. Radiotherapy was not associated with an increase in risk for leukemia.

It is only by continuing to analyze current and future data on incidence of second malignant neoplasms that one will be able to determine the contributory roles of the complex therapies being used at present in causing these secondary cnacers. The authors have identified groups of patients with RMS who have done well without alkylating agents, and overall there is no patient in whom the radiotherapy dose should exceed 6000 cGy. Eliminating radiotherapy from the treatment of completely resected RMSs has not adversely affected outcome for patients with favorable histology tumors. Future studies to test other therapies which may lessen the need to use alkylating agents and radiotherapy may enable one to reduce the number of second malignant neoplasms now being seen.

VII. PSYCHOSOCIAL DISTURBANCES

During the past decade there has been an increasing number of studies addressing psychosocial consequences of cancer and its therapy in children.[95] The quality of life in children surviving cancer is dependent on the medical and psychological defects present, and how well they are being handled by the patient. No single study of the psychosocial status of children with RMSs has been reported, but these patients have been included in studies along with those on patients with other tumors and leukemias.

It is prudent to remember that the early psychosocial management of the child with cancer may play a role in the ultimate well-being of that child. In one study, 116 patients were interviewed by both a psychologist and a psychiatrist, who assigned adjustment ratings to each patient. These adjustment ratings rated the patient's psychosocial adjustment from the time the patient learned that he or she had cancer.[96] Ten children with RMS were among the total group who had survived more than 5 years and had been off therapy for 1 year or more. Good psychosocial adjustment was associated with patients' early knowledge of the diagnosis. Also, patients, parents, and siblings all felt that early open communication within the family was most desirable. During therapy, attempts to keep children in school as much as possible and to help them keep up with school work are of utmost importance. The period during actual therapy is when the child misses most school and, if not addressed adequately, this loss may cause an ultimate inability to catch up or finish school. A pilot study of 39 long-term survivors of leukemia, lymphomas, and osteosarcomas (consisting of patients of age 16 to 33 years) revealed that there were disruptions in school attendance in 87% of the patients, with 28% having had academic difficulties.[97] As many as 46% indicated that future academic plans were altered, and 38% suggested that they had shifts in career goals as a result of having had cancer.

How physicians, parents, and others handle children who continue to have medical or psychosocial problems after therapy is also important. The family's adaptation to the child's cancer was well illustrated by a case report of a 10-year-old girl with a RMS whose face was significantly disfigured.[98] During the ensuing years, she was given hope for facial reconstruction and her family's expectation was that she stay home to do household chores and help care for younger siblings. At age 21 years a plastic surgeon revealed that less could be done to reconstruct her face than she had come to believe. It was only when she became acutely distressed at this point that she was referred for psychological consultation. Initial interviews revealed her acute depression, her anger toward her family, and a need for guidance and support, to enable her to deal with her family and to accept the reality of her own situation. Children with such problems need to be identified much earlier so that appropriate intervention can be made.

Besides anatomical or physical sequelae, a significant number of children with RMSs of the head and neck get all or part of the brain treated with radiotherapy. This exposure makes them vulnerable to the deleterious effects of cranial radiation, which have been clearly revealed in children treated for leukemia and brain tumors. It behooves physicians to talk about problems in psychosocial adjustment with both patient and family at clinic visits, and to ask about school performance and behavioral problems so that psychologic evaluation and/or therapeutic intervention can be undertaken. In another study, the relationship between physical impairment, based on the visibility of physical changes and any functional limitations they imposed, was evaluated in the group of 116 long-term survivors.[99] The average age at evaluation was 28 years and the average time from diagnosis was 12 years. The patients were given physical impairment ratings based on a scoring system for (1) obviousness of the physical defect, (2) interference by the impairment with activities of daily living, (3) the need for medical attention or equipment, and (4) employability or ability to attend school. Findings revealed no significant relationship between the degree of physical impairment and the current psychological adjustment.

Another study reported on 200 long-term survivors of childhood cancer who were seen in a late-effects clinic designed specifically to evaluate organ systems which might have been affected by therapy.[100] These patients had been diagnosed after 1970, had survived 5 years or longer from diagnosis, and they had had no therapy for 2 years. Disabilities were categorized as mild, moderate, or severe and the study rated physical disabilities as well as school function. A variety of cancers were seen, but leukemia made up 38% of the patients, Wilms' tumor 18%, and the remainder included 6.4% soft tissue sarcomas. It was found that 73% of the patients had some residual effect of disease or treatment and 41% were severely affected. The authors were able to categorize the major concerns found in this group of patients into (1) growth and development problems, (2) oncogenesis, and (3) gonadal failure.

Utilizing the same group of patients as those included in an earlier study,[99] psychosocial adjustment was assessed by measuring intellectual functioning, social maturity, depression, anxiety and death anxiety, and self-esteem. This information was used to determine a combined adjustment rating.[101] Results showed that 59% of the patients fell into the group with adjustment problems compared to the rest in the good adjustment group. More than half of the 59% were only mildly impaired. The differences between the two groups were significant for age at diagnosis and social maturity ratings. The good adjustment group was significantly younger at the time of diagnosis and had significantly higher social maturity ratings. Variability within the separate rating categories showed that residual depression, anxiety, and poor self-esteem were greater in the poor adjustment group. The developmental disruptions caused by cancer treatment were more marked and persistent when occurring in middle childhood or adolescence.

In the previously cited study of 39 long-term survivors, it had been shown that they were not different from their siblings in employment, marital status, living arrangements, or in academic and career attainments.[97] However, 15% reported prior episodes of treated depression, alcoholism, or suicide attempts, a rate higher than that in the general population. About 40% of these patients said they resumed a normal lifestyle within 6 months of diagnosis, but for 15% the time required for psychosocial recovery was more than 2 years.

A total of 185 children with cancer, who were disease-free 5 years from diagnosis and were off therapy for 2 years or more, were evaluated using the Child Behavior Checklist.[102] This checklist was designed to identify children with deficient social competence and excessive behavioral problems. The checklist is filled out by parents or caretakers and has 153 questions. Based on chart review, the most common chronic problems of any severity were scars, visual impairments, learning problems, and obesity. One or more of these were present in 83% of the children. The checklist results showed that the most frequently noted deviations from normal reflected poor school performance and increased somatic complaints. A two- to fourfold greater risk of school-related problems was associated with the presence of a functional impairment, physical disability, prior treatment with cranial irradiation, an age of 12 years or older at evaluation, and living in a single-parent household. Of the total sample, 26% of patients had repeated one or more grades at school and 11% had been placed in special educational programs. It was suggested that such assessments should be done annually after treatment is completed so that efforts at intervention can be made in a timely manner.

Finally, the ability of the long-term childhood cancer survivor to function in the adult world is fraught with still other problems. Difficulties in the patient's ability to obtain health and life insurance, employment problems, and marital disruptions have been noted.[4] A recent study addressed these issues in a telephone interview survey of 95 patients whose diagnosis of cancer was between 1948 and 1975 while the child was less than 16 years of age.[103] Only 28% of these patients had received both chemotherapy and radiotherapy. At the time of the interview, all were over 18 years of age and had been off therapy for at least 5 years. The survey covered educational achievement, occupational status, interpersonal relationships, marital status, pregnancies, employee benefits and insurance, and health status and behavior. Siblings over 18 years of age were used as controls for education and marital status. As many as 45% of these patients had had at least some college courses, and 77% felt that cancer had no effect on their educational achievement. Over half were employed and 25% were classified as professionals. Half of the employed had not told co-workers or employers of their cancer history. None of the responders said that employee benefits were denied them, but 10.6% had had life insurance denied at least once and 2% had had life insurance cancelled. Ninety-five percent of patients had medical insurance. Marital status was similar to that of siblings, with 60% single and 25% married. About half of the patients wanted to have children, but 23% indicated that having had cancer had an effect on their plans for having children. Of 45 female patients, 16 had had one or more pregnancies, and among 50 male patients 10 had sired one or more pregnancies. The median age at which this cohort was informed that they had had cancer was 18 years. The majority of respondents felt their general health was excellent (45%) or good (42%). Sixty-five percent had no obvious physical impairments, and in 58%, the impairments were imperceptible.

There are many problems in interpreting some of the studies reported above and some studies clearly contradict one another. Most of the patients studied had therapy from earlier eras when different therapy was used. Thus, findings may be quite different in patients being treated now. Fewer patients among those treated in earlier times had multiagent chemotherapy, and radiotherapy may actually be used less now than previously. In most of the studies, a variety of diagnoses were lumped together, and this could influence results in several ways. Most leukemia survivors have practically no physical defects. However, of the large group that received cranial irradiation there may be many more patients who would have neuropsychologic sequelae than would occur, for example, in children with Wilms' tumor.

Future studies should be addressed to similar populations with use of similar therapy, to help get better answers to specific questions. With a disease as complex as RMS, it may be well to consider the psychosocial ramifications within precise groups, such as parameningeal tumors or specific genitourinary tumors. The functional status and behavior of a child with leukemia can be measured in the same way as a child without a bladder or uterus. However, the ways in which patients with different types of malignancies need precise follow-up, support, or intervention may be quite different. Future studies may help to give better information than we now have for the evaluation of long-term survivors from childhood RMS. Meanwhile, each patient with RMS is a challenge, and his or her particular needs can only be met with good medical, psychologic, and behavioral follow-up.

VIII. SUMMARY

Among an increasing number of long-term survivors of childhood RMS there are many potential problems which relate to the therapy they received. These adverse effects have been the object of numerous studies during the past two decades. During this period children with RMS have been treated with multimodality therapy including surgery, radiotherapy, and chemotherapy. Late effects related to each of the therapies may be responsible for a diminished quality of life and can be physical, functional, or psychologic in nature. Whether there is major organ loss such as a bladder from surgery, diminished bone growth in a radiotherapy field, or gonadal failure due to alkylating agent chemotherapy, a lasting deficit related to prior therapy must be dealt with. The psychosocial well-being of survivors is dependent on their ability to cope with these problems.

Late effects following therapy for RMS have been reviewed by evaluating problems as they relate to primary tumor sites. Some problems pertain to all sites, but others relate to specific sites. Late effects have been described for tumors in the head and neck, trunk, genitourinary, and extremity sites. Guidelines for following children given certain therapies and suggestions for management of specific problems have been presented.

The ominous problem of developing a second malignant neoplasm is inherent in survivors of RMS as well as in children surviving other malignancies. Second neoplasms may be associated with specific therapies and/or a genetic predisposition such as neurofibromatosis.

Finally, a review of psychosocial studies which have been done in the last decade provides some insight into the handling and follow-up of children with cancer.

Physicians caring for these children need to use the knowledge gained from late effects studies so that future treatment programs may be modified to lessen adverse effects. In addition, these studies provide a plan for follow-up and management of some of the unavoidable problems reported here.

REFERENCES

1. **Maurer, H., Gehan, E., Crist, W., et al.,** Intergroup Rhabdomyosarcoma Study (IRS) III; a preliminary report of overall outcome, *Proc. Am. Soc. Clin. Oncol.,* 8 (Abstr.), 296, 1989.
2. **Nesbit, M. E., et al.,** Late effects in successfully treated children with cancer, *Clin. Oncol.,* 4, 1985.
3. **Byrd, R.,** Late effects of treatment of cancer in children, *Pediatr. Clin. North Am.,* 32, 835, 1985.
4. **Green, D. M.,** *Long-Term Complications of Therapy for Cancer in Childhood and Adolescence,* The Johns Hopkins University Press, Baltimore, 1989.
5. **Heyn, R. M.,** Late effects of therapy in rhabdomyosarcoma, *Clin. Oncol.,* 4, 287, 1985.
6. **Fromm, M., Littman, P., Raney, R. B., et al.,** Late effects after treatment of 20 children with soft tissue sarcomas of the head and neck, *Cancer,* 57, 2070, 1986.
7. **Sagerman, R. H., Tretter, P., and Ellsworth, R. M.,** The treatment of orbital rhabdomyosarcoma of children with primary radiation therapy, *Am. J. Roentgenol. Radium Ther. Nucl. Med.,* 114, 31, 1972.
8. **Sagerman, R. H., Tretter, P., and Ellsworth, R. M.,** Orbital rhabdomyosarcoma in children, *Trans. Am. Acad. Ophthalmol. Otolaryngol.,* 78, 602, 1974.
9. **Heyn, R., Ragab, A., Raney, R. B., et al.,** Late effects of therapy in orbital rhabdomyosarcoma in children, *Cancer,* 57, 1738, 1986.
10. **Jereb, B., Haik, B. G., Ong, R., and Ghavimi, F.,** Parameningeal rhabdomyosarcoma (including the orbit); results of orbital irradiation, *Int. J. Radiat. Oncol. Biol. Phys.,* 11, 2057, 1985.
11. **Jaffe, N., Toth, B. B., Hoar, R. E., et al.,** Dental and maxillofacial abnormalities in long-term survivors of childhood cancer; effects of treatment with chemotherapy and radiation to the head and neck, *Pediatrics,* 73, 816, 1984.
12. **Burke, F. J. T. and Frame, J. W.,** The effect of irradiation on developing teeth, *Oral Surg.,* 47, 11, 1979.
13. **Carl, W. and Wood, R.,** Effects of radiation on the developing dentition and supporting bone, *J. Am. Dent. Assoc.,* 101, 646, 1980.
14. **Hazra, T. and Shipman, B.,** Dental problems in pediatric patients with head and neck tumors undergoing multiple modality therapy, *Med. Pediatr. Oncol.,* 10, 91, 1982.
15. **Dury, D. C., Roberts, M. W., Miser, J. S., and Folio, J.,** Dental root agenesis secondary to irradiation therapy in a case of rhabdomyosarcoma of the middle ear, *Oral Surg.,* 57, 595, 1984.
16. **Helpin, M. L., Krejmas, N. L., and Krolls, S. O.,** Complications following radiation therapy to the head, *Oral Surg. Oral Med. Oral Pathol.,* 61, 209, 1986.
17. **Ruiz, L., Gilden, J., Jaffe, N., et al.,** Auditory function in pediatric osteosarcoma patients treated with multiple doses of cis-diamminedichloroplatinum (II), *Cancer Res.,* 40, 742, 1989.
18. **Shalet, S. M., Beardwell, C. G., Morris Jones, P. H., and Pearson, D.,** Pituitary function after treatment of intracranial tumours in children, *Lancet,* 2, 104, 1975.

19. **Shalet, S. M., Beardwell, C. G., Pearson, D., and Morris Jones, P. H.,** The effect of varying doses of cerebral irradiation on growth hormone production in childhood, *Clin. Endocrinol.,* 5, 287, 1976.
20. **Shalet, S. M., Beardwell, C. G., Aarons, B. M., et al.,** Growth impairment in children treated for brain tumours, *Arch. Dis. Child.,* 53, 491, 1978.
21. **Romshe, C. A., Zipf, W. B., Miser, A., et al.,** Evaluation of growth hormone release and human growth hormone treatment in children with cranial irradiation-associated short stature, *J. Pediatr.,* 104, 177, 1984.
22. **Winter, R. J. and Green, O. C.,** Irradiation-induced growth hormone deficiency; blunted growth response and accelerated skeletal maturation to growth hormone therapy, *J. Pediatr.,* 106, 609, 1985.
23. **Ahmed, S. R. and Shalet, S. M.,** Hypothalamic growth hormone releasing factor deficiency following cranial irradiation, *Clin. Endocrinol.,* 21, 483, 1984.
24. **Oberfield, S. E., Allen, J. C., Pollack, J., et al.,** Long-term endocrine sequelae after treatment of medulloblastoma; prospective study of growth and thyroid function, *J. Pediatr.,* 108, 219, 1986.
25. **Fusner, J. E., Poplack, D. G., Pizzo, P. A., and DiChiro, G.,** Leukoencephalopathy following chemotherapy for rhabdomyosarcoma; reversibility of cerebral changes demonstrated by computed tomography, *J. Pediatr.,* 91, 77, 1977.
26. **Raney, R. B.,** unpublished data, 1990.
27. **Crist, W. M., Raney, R. B., Newton, W., et al.,** Intrathoracic soft tissue sarcomas in children, *Cancer,* 50, 598, 1982.
28. **Raney, R. B., Ragab, A. H., Ruymann, F. B., et al.,** Soft-tissue sarcoma of the trunk in childhood, *Cancer,* 49, 2612, 1982.
29. **Goorin, A. M., Borow, K. M., Goldman, A., et al.,** Congestive heart failure due to adriamycin cardiotoxicity; its natural history in children, *Cancer,* 47, 2810, 1981.
30. **Green, D. M., Gingell, R. L., Pearce, J., et al.,** The effect of mediastinal irradiation on cardiac function of patients treated during childhood and adolescence for Hodgkin's disease, *J. Clin. Oncol.,* 5, 239, 1987.
31. **Pediatric Intergroup Statistical Center,** unpublished data 1989.
32. **Crist, W. M., Raney, R. B., Tefft, M., et al.,** Soft tissue sarcomas arising in the retroperitoneal space in children, *Cancer,* 56, 2125, 1985.
33. **Ruymann, F. B., Raney, R. B., Crist, W. M., et al.,** Rhabdomyosarcoma of the biliary tree in childhood, *Cancer,* 56, 575, 1985.
34. **Ransom, J. L., Novak, R. W., Kumar, A. P. M., et al.,** Delayed gastrointestinal complications after combined modality therapy of childhood rhabdomyosarcoma, *Int. J. Radiat. Oncol. Biol. Phys.,* 5, 1275, 1979.
35. **Heyn, R.,** unpublished data, 1989.
36. **Cacavio, A., Ghavimi, F., Mandell, L., and Exelby, P.,** Late effects of therapy in long-term survivors of rhabdomyosarcoma, *Proc. Am. Soc. Clin. Oncol.,* 8 (Abstr.), 307, 1989.
37. **Ortega, J. A.,** A therapeutic approach to childhood pelvic rhabdomyosarcoma without pelvic exenteration, *J. Pediatr.,* 94, 205, 1979.
38. **Raney, R. B., Gehan, E. A., Hays, D. M., et al.,** Primary chemotherapy and/or irradiation and/or surgery for children with localized sarcoma of the bladder, prostate, vagina, uterus, and cervix; comparison of results in Intergroup Rhabdomyosarcoma Studies (IRS) I and II, *Med. Pediatr. Oncol.,* 16 (Abstr.), 430, 1988.
39. **Hays, D. M., Shimada, H., Raney, R. B., et al.,** Clinical staging and treatment results in rhabdomyosarcoma of the female genital tract among children and adolescents, *Cancer,* 61, 1893, 1988.
40. **Clatworthy, H. W., Braren, V., and Smith, J. P.,** Surgery of bladder and prostatic neoplasms in children, *Cancer,* 32, 1157, 1973.
41. **Tefft, M., Lattin, P. B., Jereb, B., et al.,** Acute and late effects on normal tissues following combined chemo- and radiotherapy for childhood rhabdomyosarcoma and Ewing's sarcoma, *Cancer,* 37, 1201, 1976.
42. **Heyn, R., Holland, R. M., Newton, W. A., et al.,** Late effects following combination therapy with surgery, radiotherapy, and chemotherapy in rhabdomyosarcoma; a follow-up of two studies by Children's Cancer Study Group, in Abstr. 10th Meeting of International Society of Paediatric Oncology, Brussels, 1978, 121.
43. **Silverstone, A. C. and Williams, E. A.,** Long-term urinary and sexual problems with sarcoma botryoides, *J. R. Soc. Med.,* 74, 923, 1981.
44. **Wu, Y., Green, D. M., Duffner, P. K., et al.,** Incontinence of urine and stool following treatment in infancy for embryonal rhabdomyosarcoma, *Oncology,* 40, 90, 1983.
45. **Jayalakshmamma, B. and Pinkel, D.,** Urinary-bladder toxicity following pelvic irradiation and simultaneous cyclophosphamide therapy, *Cancer,* 38, 701, 1976.
46. **Stillwell, T. J. and Benson, R. C.,** Cyclophosphamide-induced hemorrhagic cystitis, *Cancer,* 61, 451, 1988.
47. **Johnson, W. W. and Meadows, D. C.,** Urinary-bladder fibrosis and telangiectasia associated with long-term cyclophosphamide therapy, *N. Engl. J. Med.,* 284, 290, 1971.
48. **Shalet, S. M.,** The effects of cancer treatment on growth and sexual development, *Clin. Oncol.,* 4, 223, 1985.

49. **Schilsky, R. L., Lewis, B. J., Sherins, R. J., and Young, R. C.,** Gonadal dysfunction in patients receiving chemotherapy for cancer, *Ann. Intern. Med.,* 93, 109, 1980.

50. **Damewood, M. D. and Grochow, L. B.,** Prospects for fertility after chemotherapy or radiation for neoplastic disease, *Fertil. Steril.,* 45, 443, 1986.

51. **Gradishar, W. J. and Schilsky, R. L.,** Effects of cancer treatment on the reproductive system, *CRC Crit. Rev. Oncol. Hematol.,* 8, 153, 1988.

52. **Shalet, S. M., Beardwell, C. G., Morris Jones, P. H., et al.,** Ovarian failure following abdominal irradiation in childhood, *Br. J. Cancer,* 33, 655, 1976.

53. **Nicosia, S. V., Matus-Ridley, M., and Meadows, A. T.,** Gonadal effects of cancer therapy in girls, *Cancer,* 55, 2364, 1985.

54. **Himelstein-Braw, R., Peters, H., and Faber, M.,** Influence of irradiation and chemotherapy on the ovaries of children with abdominal tumours, *Br. J. Cancer,* 36, 269, 1977.

55. **Shalet, S. M., Beardwell, C. G., Jacobs, H. S., and Pearson, D.,** Testicular function following irradiation of the human prepubertal testis, *Clin. Endocrinol.,* 9, 483, 1978.

56. **Ash, P.,** The influence of radiation on fertility in man, *Br. J. Radiol.,* 53, 271, 1980.

57. **Shapiro, E., Kinsella, T. J., Makuch, R. W., et al.,** Effects of fractionated irradiation on endocrine aspects of testicular function, *J. Clin. Oncol.,* 3, 1232, 1985.

58. **Fairley, K. F., Barrie, J. U., and Johnson, W.,** Sterility and testicular atrophy related to cyclophosphamide therapy, *Lancet,* 1, 568, 1972.

59. **Rapola, J., Koskimies, O., Huttenen, N. P., et al.,** Cyclophosphamide and the pubertal testis, *Lancet,* 1, 98, 1973.

60. **Penso, J., Lippe, B., Ehrlich, R., and Smith, F. G.,** Testicular function in prepubertal and pubertal male patients treated with cyclophosphamide for nephrotic syndrome, *J. Pediatr.,* 84, 831, 1974.

61. **Pennisi, A. J., Grushkin, C. M., and Lieberman, E.,** Gonadal function in children with nephrosis treated with cyclophosphamide, *Am. J. Dis. Child.,* 129, 315, 1975.

62. **Etteldorf, J. N., West, C. D., Pitcock, J. A., and Williams, D. L.,** Gonadal function, testicular histology, and meiosis following cyclophosphamide therapy in patients with nephrotic syndrome, *J. Pediatr.,* 88, 206, 1976.

63. **Lentz, R. D., Bergstein, J., Steffes, M. W., et al.,** Postpubertal evaluation of gonadal function following cyclophosphamide therapy before and during puberty, *J. Pediatr.,* 91, 385, 1977.

64. **Hsu, A. C., Folami, A. O., Bain, J., and Rance, C. P.,** Gonadal function in males treated with cyclophosphamide for nephrotic syndrome, *Fertil. Steril.,* 31, 173, 1979.

65. **Aubier, F., Flamant, F., Brauner, R., et al.,** Male gonadal function after chemotherapy for solid tumors in childhood, *J. Clin. Oncol.,* 7, 304, 1989.

66. **Buchanan, J. D., Fairley, K. F., and Barrie, J. U.,** Return of spermatogenesis after stopping cyclophosphamide therapy, *Lancet,* 2, 156, 1975.

67. **Matus-Ridley, M., Nicosia, S. V., and Meadows, A. T.,** Gonadal effects of cancer therapy in boys, *Cancer,* 55, 2353, 1985.

68. **Nijman, J. M., Jager, S., Boer, P. W., et al.,** The treatment of ejaculation disorders after retroperitoneal lymph node dissection, *Cancer,* 50, 2967, 1982.

69. **Brassesco, M., Rajmil, O., Viscasillas, P., et al.,** Sperm recuperation and cervical insemination in retrograde ejaculation, *Fertil. Steril.,* 49, 923, 1988.

70. **Wolf, E. L., Berdon, W. E., Cassady, J. R., et al.,** Slipped femoral capital epiphysis as a sequela to childhood irradiation for malignant tumors, *Radiology,* 125, 781, 1977.

71. **Dickerman, J. D., Newberg, A. H., and Moreland, M. D.,** Slipped capital femoral epiphysis (SCFE) following pelvic irradiation for rhabdomyosarcoma, *Cancer,* 44, 480, 1979.

72. **Silverman, C. L., Thomas, P. R. M., McAlister, W. H., et al.,** Slipped femoral capital epiphyses in irradiated children; dose, volume and age relationships, *Int. J. Radiat. Oncol. Biol. Phys.,* 7, 1357, 1981.

73. **Heyn, R.,** unpublished data, 1989.

74. **Meadows, A. T.,** Second malignant neoplasms, *Clin. Oncol.,* 4, 247, 1985.

75. **Tefft, M., Vawter, G. F., and Mitus, A.,** Second primary neoplasms in children, *Am. J. Roentgenol.,* 103, 800, 1968.

76. **Li, F. P. and Fraumeni, J. F.,** Rhabdomyosarcoma in children; epidemiologic study and identification of a familial cancer syndrome, *J. Natl. Cancer Inst.,* 43, 1365, 1969.

77. **Li, F. P., Fraumeni, J. F., Mulvihill, J. J., et al.,** A cancer family syndrome in twenty-four kindreds, *Cancer Res.,* 48, 5358, 1988.

78. **Li, F. P., Cassady, J. R., and Jaffe, N.,** Risk of second tumors in survivors of childhood cancer, *Cancer,* 35, 1230, 1975.

79. **Li, F. P.,** Second malignant tumors after cancer in childhood, *Cancer,* 40, 1899, 1977.

80. **D'Angio, G. J., Meadows, A., Mike, V., et al.,** Decreased risk of radiation-associated second malignant neoplasms in actinomycin-D treated patients, *Cancer,* 37, 1177, 1976.

81. **Meadows, A. T., D'Angio, G. J., Mike, V., et al.,** Patterns of second malignant neoplasms in children, *Cancer,* 40, 1903, 1977.
82. **Hensley, M. F., Cangir, A., Culbert, S. J., and Van Eys, J.,** Acute granulocytic leukemia following successful treatment of rhabdomyosarcoma, *Am. J. Dis. Child.,* 131, 1417, 1977.
83. **Haselow, R. E., Nesbit, M., Dehner, L. P., et al.,** Second neoplasms following megavoltage radiation in a pediatric population, *Cancer,* 42, 1185, 1978.
84. **Potish, R. A., Dehner, L. P., Haselow, R. E., et al.,** The incidence of second neoplasms following megavoltage radiation for pediatric tumors, *Cancer,* 56, 1534, 1985.
85. **Freeman, C. R., Gledhill, R., Chevalier, L. M., et al.,** Osteogenic sarcoma following treatment with megavoltage radiation and chemotherapy for bone tumors in children, *Med. Pediatr. Oncol.,* 8, 375, 1980.
86. **Meadows, A. T., Strong, L. C., Li, F. P., et al.,** Bone sarcoma as a second malignant neoplasm in children; influence of radiation and genetic predisposition, *Cancer,* 46, 2603, 1980.
87. **Mike, V., Meadows, A. T., and D'Angio, G. J.,** Incidence of second malignant neoplasms in children; results of an international study, *Lancet,* 2, 1326, 1982.
88. **Meyers, P. A. and Ghavimi, F.,** Secondary acute non-lymphoblastic leukemia (ANLL) following treatment of childhood rhabodmyosarcoma (RMS), *Proc. Am. Soc. Clin. Oncol.,* Abstr. C-300, 77, 1983.
89. **Oberlin, O., Bernard, A., Flamant, F., et al.,** Les secondes tumeurs malignes de l'enfant, *Arch. Fr. Pediatr.,* 41, 241, 1984.
90. **Meadows, A. T., Baum, E., Fossati-Ballani, F., et al.,** Second malignant neoplasms in children; an update from the Late Effects Study Group, *J. Clin. Oncol.,* 3, 532, 1985.
91. **Heyn, R., Newton, W. A., Ragab, A., et al.,** Second malignant neoplasms in patients treated on the Intergroup Rhabdomyosarcoma Study I-II (IRS I-II), *Proc. Am. Soc. Clin. Oncol.,* 5 (Abstr.), 215, 1986.
92. **Heyn, R.,** unpublished data, 1989.
93. **Tucker, M. A., D'Angio, G. J., Boice, J. D., et al.,** Bone sarcomas linked to radiotherapy and chemotherapy in children, *N. Engl. J. Med.,* 317, 588, 1987.
94. **Tucker, M. A., Meadows, A. T., Boice, J. D., et al.,** Leukemia after therapy with alkylating agents for childhood cancer, *J. Natl. Cancer Inst.,* 78, 459, 1987.
95. **Lansky, S. B., List, M. A., Ritter-Sterr, C., et al.,** Late effects; psychosocial, *Clin. Oncol.,* 4, 239, 1985.
96. **Slavin, L. A., O'Malley, J. E., Koocher, G. P., and Foster, D. J.,** Communication of the cancer diagnosis to pediatric patients; impact on long-term adjustment, *Am. J. Psychiatry,* 139, 179, 1982.
97. **Lansky, S. B., List, M. A., and Ritter-Sterr, C.,** Psychosocial consequences of cure, *Cancer,* 58, 529, 1986.
98. **Copeland, D. R.,** Psychosocial ramifications of childhood malignancy for the child and family, *Head Neck Surg.,* 8, 142, 1986.
99. **O'Malley, J. E., Foster, D., Koocher, G., and Slavin, L.,** Visible physical impairment and psychological adjustment among pediatric cancer survivors, *Am. J. Psychiatry,* 137, 94, 1980.
100. **Meadows, A. T. and Hobbie, W. L.,** The medical consequences of cure, *Cancer,* 58, 524, 1986.
101. **Koocher, G. P., O'Malley, J. E., Gogan, J. L., and Foster, D. J.,** Psychological adjustment among pediatric cancer survivors, *J. Child. Psychol. Psychiatry,* 21, 163, 1980.
102. **Mulhern, R. K., Wasserman, A. L., Friedman, A. G., and Fairclough, D.,** Social competence and behavioral adjustment of children who are long-term survivors of cancer, *Pediatrics,* 83, 18, 1989.
103. **Meadows, A. T., McKee, L., and Kazak, A. E.,** Psychosocial status of young adult survivors of childhood cancer; a survey, *Med. Pediatr. Oncol.,* 17, 466, 1989.

Section IV
Specific Sites of Involvement

Chapter 18

RHABDOMYOSARCOMA AND RELATED TUMORS OF THE HEAD AND NECK IN CHILDHOOD

R. Beverly Raney, Jr.

TABLE OF CONTENTS

I. INTRODUCTION

Rhabdomyosarcoma (RMS), undifferentiated sarcoma, and extraosseous Ewing's sarcoma (Ewing's sarcoma of soft tissue) often occur in the head and neck region in children. In fact, the experience of the Intergroup Rhabdomyosarcoma Study (IRS) shows that approximately 40% of these tumors arise in the head and neck, with the other 60% appearing in the genitourinary tract (20%), extremities (20%), trunk (10%), and other locations (10%).[1,2] Most craniocervical sarcomas are embryonal RMSs. Sarcomas are more frequent in the head and neck in children than are non-Hodgkin's lymphomas, but are somewhat less common than Hodgkin's disease, which usually presents with a cervical and/or supraclavicular mass. By contrast with malignant lymphoma, however, sarcomas of the head and neck can occur in many different anatomical locations because of the wide distribution of mesenchymal tissues in that region of the body. The various locations of these tumors have implications for surgical management, because often these tumors are so situated that complete removal is impossible.

The IRS clinical grouping system, which has been used since 1972, may be summarized as follows: clinical group I contains patients with localized tumors, completely excised, without regional lymph node spread or microscopic residual. Group II includes patients with localized, grossly removed tumors and microscopic residual, regional nodal involvement, or both. Group III contains the largest number of patients with localized head and neck sarcomas, those with visible residual tumor or with unremoved tumors that had undergone incisional biopsy only. Patients in group IV have distant metastases at the time of diagnosis.[1]

Because of the diversity of locations of tumors in the head and neck, the primary sites are separated into three broad categories: nonorbital cranial parameningeal, orbital, and nonorbital nonparameningeal.[3] Table 1 shows the various localizations observed within each category. Tumors arising in the neck with parameningeal extension are quite rare and are discussed elsewhere in this book (see Chapter 21). Because variations in anatomic site and proximity to important structures affect treatment and prognosis, each category will be discussed separately.

II. NONORBITAL CRANIAL PARAMENINGEAL SARCOMAS

A. DIAGNOSIS

As indicated in Table 1, these tumors usually arise in relatively hidden internal places: such as in the nasopharynx, in a paranasal sinus, or in the middle ear and nearby structures. Tumors in the nasopharynx and middle ear usually produce signs of obstruction, with or without discharge of mucopurulent or even bloody fluid. Since upper respiratory infections and otitis media are very common in children, often the diagnosis of sarcoma is delayed until a trial of antibiotics and decongestants has failed to produce relief of the symptoms and signs.

Ominous associated findings are the presence of cranial nerve palsy, usually involving cranial nerves VII (facial), VI (abducens), or VIII (acoustic), along with a mass visible in the nasal cavity, nasopharynx, or ear canal.[4] Tumors arising in the maxillary or ethmoid sinuses often break into the adjacent orbit and produce congestion of the eyelid, simulating proptosis. Although the ocular globe is usually not displaced anteriorly, impaired vision can result from apparent palsy of cranial nerves II (optic), III (oculomotor), IV (trochlear), or VI (abducens) due to nerve compression. More commonly, impaired vision is due to fixation of the globe by the mass. If the tumor has invaded the cranial cavity via one or more neural foramina, or by destroying bone at the cranial base and growing directly onto the meninges, increased intracranial pressure can result. This increased pressure may give rise to headaches, vomiting, papilledema, and visual difficulty.

TABLE 1
Categories of Primary Sites of Soft Tissue Sarcoma in
the Head and Neck

Category	Frequency (approximate, %)	Subgroups
Nonorbital Cranial Parameningeal	50	Nasopharynx-nasal cavity Paranasal sinus Middle ear-mastoid Pterygoid-infratemporal fossa
Orbital	25	Orbital muscle Eyelid
Nonorbital Nonparameningeal	25	Scalp External ear Parotid region Face Buccal mucosa Pharynx-parapharyngeal-tonsil Larynx Neck

As with sarcomas arising elsewhere in the body, precise diagnosis depends upon examination of specimens obtained by biopsy. Usually grossly complete excision of these tumors is impossible, either because of proximity of the tumor to vital structures or because the cosmetic consequences resulting from radical resection would be unacceptable. It is essential to ascertain the size and extent of these tumors using computed tomographic (CT) scans,[5] with or without magnetic resonance imaging (MRI). These imaging studies are needed for several reasons. Scans help the surgeon plan where to obtain the biopsy, and they show whether nearby structures are infiltrated or displaced by the mass. Scans are useful in determining whether any of the cranial neural foramina are enlarged and whether the tumor has destroyed adjacent bone, especially bone next to the meninges at the base of the brain. They also show whether anatomic breakthrough into the cranial cavity has taken place. This information is of critical importance to the radiation oncologist, whose task is to attain local control (in other words, complete disappearance) of the tumor. This is achieved by treating the tumor volume plus a margin of adjacent normal tissue including the nearby meninges.[5] Figures 1, 2, and 3 show the clarity with which a tumor of the nasopharynx and of the middle ear can be demonstrated using modern equipment.

Since these tumors are capable of spreading distantly, other investigations are necessary in order to ascertain whether metastases are present at the time of diagnosis. Presence of metastases is ominous because the likelihood of cure is considerably lower with disseminated as compared to localized sarcomas.[1,2] The most frequent sites of distant involvement are the lungs, bone marrow, other soft tissue sites, and bone.[6] Thus, a CT scan of the chest, a bone marrow aspirate and needle biopsy, plus a total-body bone scan, with or without a skeletal survey, are also needed prior to initiation of therapy. The cerebrospinal fluid (CSF) should be examined for cell count and cytology, and levels of CSF sugar and protein should be determined in order to detect the presence of sarcoma cells in the central nervous system.[7,8]

B. TREATMENT

This includes both irradiation and multiple-agent chemotherapy, usually given intermittently for a period of 2 years. Intrathecal medications are also administered to children who have evidence of meningeal extension. Therapy for children with nonorbital cranial parameningeal sarcoma has become more extensive over the past 15 to 20 years. More aggressive treatment was added as the adverse influence on prognosis of meningeal extension

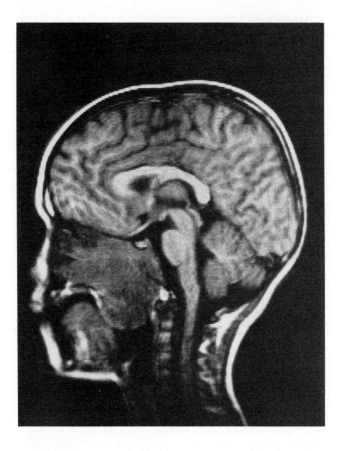

FIGURE 1.   Sagittal MRI showing a massive tumor filling the nasopharynx and deforming the soft palate of a 6-year-old boy. He is currently
free of detectable disease 2.2 years after radiotherapy and chemotherapy
were begun.

from the primary site became more widely appreciated.[8-10] Prior to the availability of CT
scans, the frequency of extension of tumor into the meninges was relatively high, being
approximately 40% according to the initial IRS data.[9] Death was inevitable once intracranial
tumor became established.

It is important to distinguish signs of meningeal impingement, such as cranial nerve
palsy, bony erosion of the base of the cranium, or enlargement of one or more cranial neural
foramina, from meningeal penetration with seeding of tumor cells. This meningeal involvement can take the form of direct intracranial extension, with or without tumor cells in the
CSF, and can produce intraspinal tumor. Patients with definite meningeal involvement require
extensive therapy. However, children with tumors in nonorbital cranial parameningeal sites,
with no sign of meningeal impingement or penetration, have the best outlook.[10] Thus,
meningeal involvement can be classified at the outset as absent, low risk, or high risk.
Treatment is then tailored according both to the status of the tumor regionally and to the
absence or presence of distant metastases. Radiation therapy has also varied with regard to
field size, volume of tissue irradiated, and total dosage, depending on age of the patient
and size (widest diameter) of the primary tumor.

Radiation therapy dosages have been developed by the IRS Committee. These doses
are as follows: none for patients in group I unless the tumor histology is alveolar RMS.
Patients in group II receive 4000 cGy in 4 to 5 weeks. Those in group III receive a dose
tailored to the patient's age and the widest diameter of the tumor. For patients under 6 years

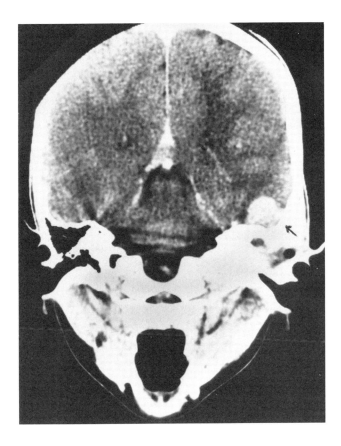

FIGURE 2. Coronal CT scan image showing increased density and loss of air space in the left middle ear region (on the right side of the photograph) plus extension into the left temporal fossa (arrow) of a 6-year-old girl.

of age with tumors less than 5 cm in diameter, 4000 to 4500 cGy of radiation are given in fractions of 180 cGy/d, 5 days/week. For patients under 6 years of age with tumors 5 cm or more in diameter, 4500 to 5000 cGy are given, similarly fractionated. For patients 6 years of age and older with tumors less than 5 cm in diameter, a dose of 4500 to 5000 cGy is prescribed, and 5000 to 5500 cGy is recommended for tumors 5 cm in diameter or larger. A high-energy source of irradiation, such as a 2 to 6 MeV linear accelerator, is used in most instances.

Table 2 shows the IRS experience from 1972 to 1989 in patients with parameningeal sarcomas by treatment era. The findings for cases from IRS-I and -II have been reported.[10] Preliminary data for IRS-III cases were prepared by Drs. Ortega and Gehan in October 1989. It can be seen that the overall results are considerably better now than they were just 12 years ago. Table 3 lists current recommendations of the IRS Committee for children with nonorbital cranial parameningeal sarcomas.

C. TOXICITY

The majority of patients with nonorbital cranial parameningeal sarcomas will have some degree of meningeal extension. Thus, radiation therapy and multiple-agent chemotherapy should be given simultaneously. This is done in order to achieve local control as quickly as possible and to prevent further spread of tumor into the CNS. Such combined therapy is clearly more effective than the earlier approach of starting with chemotherapy and waiting until day 42 to begin irradiation. However, toxicity, especially mucositis, is greatly increased.

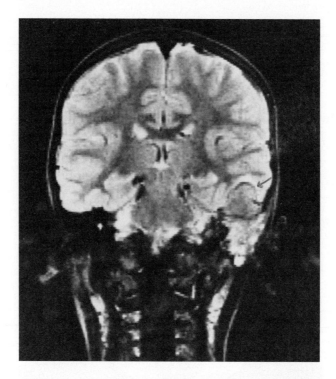

FIGURE 3.   Coronal MRI showing similar findings, with elevation of
the left temporal lobe by encroaching tumor (arrow). This girl is currently
free of detectable disease 3.7 years after radiotherapy and chemotherapy
were initiated.

TABLE 2
Results of IRS Treatment of Children with Nonorbital Cranial Parameningeal Sarcoma[a]

Date	Chemotherapy	Radiotherapy	Intrathecal drugs	Number of patients	% CR at 3 years	% alive at 3 years
1972—1977 (IRS-I)	VA ± C ± ADR	4000—6000 cGy; start on day 42; no whole-brain RT	No	95[b]	33	41
1977—1984 (IRS-I, II)	VA ± C ± ADR (intensified)	4000-5500 cGy; start on day 0 with any sign of meningeal extension using whole-brain RT	Yes, ≥6 doses	68[b]	57	68
1984—1989 (IRS-III)	VA ± C ± ADR ± CPDD ± VP-16	As above, except whole-brain RT only for patients with ICE	Yes, but only 4 doses after 6/87	144[b]	NA	76[c]

[a] CR, complete response (disappearance of all detectable tumor); V, vincristine; A, actinomycin D; C, cyclophosphamide; ADR, adriamycin; CPDD, cisplatinum diammine dichloride; VP-16, etoposide; cGy, centi-Gray; RT, radiotherapy; ICE, intracranial extension; NA, not available.
[b] Five, three, and five patients, respectively, were in clinical group II (grossly complete excision of localized sarcoma). Approximately 80% of the remainder had no metastases at diagnosis.
[c] From an interim analysis prepared by Ortega and Gehan of the IRS Committee, October 1989.

TABLE 3
Current IRS Treatment of Children with Nonorbital Cranial Parameningeal Sarcoma[a]

Amount of meningeal extension	Radiation therapy		Begin radiotherapy	IT drugs	Chemotherapy	
	Dose	Volume			Drugs	Duration
None	4000-5500 cGy depending on age of patient and size of primary (see text)	1° tumor with 5 cm margin + 2 cm of adjacent meninges	Day 42	No	Stage 2 or 3 (TNM): VCR, AMD, CYC (VAC); VA + Ifos (I); or VI + VP-16	
					Stage 4: Ifos + ADR or VP-16, or VCR + MLP, plus VAC	1 year
CNP and/or CBBE	As above	As above	Day 0	Yes, 4 doses	As above	As above
ICE	As above, + 3000[b]	As above, + whole brain	Day 0 Day 0	Yes, 4 doses	As above	As above
Tumor cells in CSF and/or cord block	As above, + 3000[b]	As above, + spinal cord	Day 0 Day 42	Yes, ≥4 doses	As above	As above

[a] CNP, cranial nerve palsy; CBBE, cranial base bony erosion; ICE, intracranial extension; Ifos, ifosfamdide; ADR, adriamycin; MLP, melphalan (phenylalanine mustard).

[b] The dose is 2400 cGy in 3 weeks for patients under 3 years of age.

In the IRS-II experience, moderate to severe mucositis was encountered more than twice as frequently when chemotherapy and radiotherapy were given concomitantly, compared to administering them sequentially.[10] However, in this setting the relative contribution of each modality in effecting severity of mucositis could not be estimated. This is because the antitumor antibiotics actinomycin D and doxorubicin (adriamycin) can cause mucositis even in the absence of local irradiation. The mucositis can be severe enough to require interruption of the planned radiotherapy. Giving radiotherapy and chemotherapy together, especially for treatment of centrally placed tumors such as those in the nasopharynx and ethmoid or sphenoid sinus, nearly always requires prolonged total parenteral nutrition until the mucosa has recovered. This period may last 6 months or longer.

Neutropenia and fever are also frequent as a result of the myelosuppressive chemotherapy. Hospitalization in order to give intravenous broad-spectrum antibiotics is mandatory in this situation in order to anticipate and treat suspected or actual bacterial sepsis. Sepsis is not unusual and is probably related to the amount of mucosal damage caused by biopsy of the tumor, radiotherapy, and chemotherapy. Nausea and vomiting, alopecia, and the neurotoxic effects of vincristine are often observed, especially after several weeks of treatment.

There are many possible long-term side effects of therapy.[11] These include primarily the effects of radiotherapy upon bone growth in the volume of irradiated tissue, occurrence of cataracts, structural growth impairment due to irradiation of the pituitary or thyroid glands, damage to the developing teeth, and development of second malignant neoplasms. Cosmetic reconstruction, careful and prolonged dental care, and growth hormone replacement may be needed as these patients continue to survive.

Whole-brain radiotherapy is not without hazard also, and some degree of intellectual impairment may occur later. This risk is well documented in survivors of childhood leukemia who received whole-brain radiotherapy either alone or with intrathecal methotrexate for CNS prophylaxis.[12,13] Occasionally, leukoencephalopathy has been noted after limited radiotherapy and intrathecal chemotherapy given for treatment of RMS extending into the CNS.[14] Usually the impairment is manifest as diminution in intelligence quotient and learning disabilities. The learning disabilities often include difficulty with memorization of multiplication tables and performance of visual-perceptive tasks such as drawing of shapes.[15] Prior knowledge of these potential hazards may alleviate their severity when special educational programs are provided for affected individuals.

An uncommon but severe complication is ascending transverse myelitis.[16,17] This complication occurred in 5 out of 149 patients (3%) with nonorbital cranial parameningeal sarcoma treated in the IRS since 1977.[18] All five developed flaccid quadriparesis with a high cervical or thoracic sensory level; three died, one after tumor recurrence and the other two from complications of the myelitis. Autopsy in one of the latter showed necrosis of the cervical spinal cord and medulla. Thus, careful attention is mandatory regarding radiation therapy doses and volumes, as well as in administration of radiomimetic and neurotoxic drugs.[18] No additional cases of this syndrome have been seen since 1987, when the number of intrathecal injections was limited to four.

III. ORBITAL TUMORS

A. DIAGNOSIS

By contrast to those arising elsewhere in the head and neck, sarcomas which arise in the orbit are often diagnosed early because they are relatively exposed. The appearance of swelling in an eyelid with or without displacement of the adjacent globe is usually followed soon by consultation with an ophthalmologist. Infection, trauma, and foreign body can usually be ruled out by examination, microbial cultures, and blood counts. Biopsy of the mass is indicated after CT scan and other imaging studies of the orbital contents have been completed. Confusion can arise when the orbit is secondarily involved by a tumor originating in a paranasal sinus. Thus, the scan is critical in determining the exact site of the primary tumor, so that proper treatment may be given. Careful imaging studies are required in order to be as certain as possible that the tumor has not broken through the bony orbit. Examination of the CSF is done at the onset. Other imaging studies such as a chest CT scan and bone scan or radiographic skeletal survey are also obtained, along with a bone marrow aspirate and biopsy.

B. TREATMENT

As with sarcomas in other cranial parameningeal locations, complete removal of orbital sarcomas is usually not undertaken. This limited surgery is appropriate both because removing the eye is not necessary for tumor control[19,20] and because treatment of radiation-related cataracts is relatively successful. Thus, most of these tumors are staged and treated as "gross residual localized sarcomas". Meningeal extension from primary orbital sarcoma is quite uncommon because these lesions nearly always grow outward rather than inward. Nevertheless, meningeal relapse can occur.[21]

After completion of the initial investigations, multiple-agent chemotherapy is then begun, and radiation therapy to the orbit is initiated at week 6. Often the tumor has become undetectable by physical examination and by repeat imaging studies after the first 6 weeks of chemotherapy, even before radiotherapy is started. Intrathecal medications are usually not required, because meningeal extension is very uncommon.

Overall, results of IRS therapy for orbital sarcoma are generally quite good, with 93% of 124 patients treated from 1972 to 1983 being alive at 3 years.[20] The IRS experience in patients with these tumors is listed according to treatment era in Table 4. The IRS-I results (1972 to 1978) were reported in 1988.[1] The IRS-II and IRS-III data come from an interim

TABLE 4
Results of IRS Treatment of Children with Orbital Sarcoma[a]

Including Some with Nonorbital, Nonparameningeal Cranial Tumors from 1978 to the Present

Date	Chemotherapy	Dose	Radiotherapy volume	Begin radiotherapy	Number of patients	% CR[b] at 2 years	% alive[b] at 2 years
1972—1978 (IRS-I)	VA(C), ± ADR (groups III, IV)	See Table 2	1° tumor with 5 cm margin	Day 42	51	76	90
1978—1984 (IRS-II)	VA(C) ± ADR intensified (groups III, IV)	As above except no RT in group I patients with favorable histology			100	76	96
1984—1989 (IRS-III)	V + A for 1 year (favorable histology, groups I, II, III)	As above, except RT begins at day 14 in patients with favorable histology in groups II and III			62	60	96
	VAC ± ADR ± CPDD (unfavorable histology, all group IV)						

[a] The abbreviations are the same as those listed in Table 2. Favorable histology = nonalveolar RMS, undifferentiated sarcoma, and extraosseous Ewing's sarcoma. Unfavorable histology = alveolar RMS.

[b] A few patients were in clinical group II; none were in clinical group IV.

analysis conducted in November 1988. Note that in IRS-II and -III, the data cited include only patients in clinical groups II and III, those with tumors having nonalveolar histology, and those with orbital and other nonparameningeal cranial tumors. These patients were combined because of their relatively favorable prognosis. Note also that the somewhat lower percentage of complete responses at 2 years in IRS-III reflects the fact that some patients have not been treated long enough to achieve a complete response as yet. Nevertheless, the survival rate of these patients is excellent thus far.

C. TOXICITY

Acute toxicity associated with treatment of orbital tumors is similar to that for cranial nonorbital parameningeal tumors. It consists chiefly of nausea and vomiting, hair loss, myelosuppression, and the neurotoxic effects of vincristine. Mucositis is considerably less frequent, however, because with orbital tumors the mucous membranes are usually not included in the radiotherapy field. The late effects of therapy have been reported[22] and are reviewed elsewhere in this book (see Chapter 17). These late effects consist primarily of radiation-associated keratitis, xerophthalmia, and cataracts in most patients, plus orbital and ocular hypoplasia.

Another adverse sequel is diminished linear or statural growth resulting from irradiation of the pituitary area. This can be severe enough to consider giving replacement doses of human growth hormone (HGH) in some patients. Results of careful growth charting, periodic assessment of somatomedin C and thyroid hormone levels, and serial bone age X-rays should enable the clinician to identify these growth-retarded children prior to closure of the long bone epiphyses. If this complication is detected in time, growth hormone can be given with beneficial effects.

IV. NONPARAMENINGEAL SARCOMAS OF THE HEAD AND NECK

A. DIAGNOSIS

This category includes tumors which arise in a variety of locations about the head and neck, some located superficially and others more deeply placed. The superficial tumors can be found in the soft tissues of the scalp, external ear, and face. Many of these are surgically accessible, and complete removal should be attempted in patients where the cosmetic result is expected to be acceptable. Deep tumors may arise in the parotid gland, buccal mucosa, oropharynx, parapharyngeal area, larynx, and neck.

In the neck it is particularly important to assess regional lymph nodes. It should also be ascertained whether the sarcoma tissue is indeed a primary tumor in the neck, or represents metastatic nodal tumor from elsewhere, most likely from a primary tumor located higher in the head. Thus CT and MRI scans should include the tissues above the mandible in order to determine the site of origin of the tumor. Other investigations that should be done to assess the extent of the tumor have already been mentioned.

It should be emphasized that occasionally a sarcoma in one of these "nonparameningeal" sites can expand enough to encroach upon or invade a parameningeal location. As an example, a parotid tumor may grow inward and upward toward the infratemporal fossa. The approach of the IRS to this situation is to treat the patient as for a parameningeal tumor, basing selection of treatment on the meningeal risk categories described above.

B. TREATMENT

Therapy for nonparameningeal tumors of the head and neck is similar to that for orbital tumors, when the primary lesion is above the neck and not causing any sign of meningeal impingement. Based on results of IRS studies, children with nonparameningeal cranial tumors have a moderately favorable outlook.[23,24] Patients with localized sarcomas of the parotid gland, cheek, masseter muscle, oral cavity, oropharynx, larynx, hypopharynx, scalp, face, and pinna had an actuarial survival rate of 83% at 3 years.[24] However, patients with tumors arising in the neck have in the past fared less well.[23] Therefore, chemotherapy for patients with gross residual sarcoma (clinical group III) has remained rather intensive, in contrast to the less aggressive regimens used in the IRS-III study for children with nonalveolar sarcomas of the orbit and head.

If the tumor is small enough and relatively accessible, the radiotherapist may be able to use an interstitial implant.[25] This approach has the advantage of minimizing radiotherapy damage to nearby structures. Results of therapy of these patients according to the IRS-I protocol are outlined in Table 5. Results for IRS-II and IRS-III studies are not listed separately, because tumors of the neck are considered together with those arising in other primary sites within each clinical group, and cranial nonparameningeal tumors are combined with orbital tumors (Table 4).

C. TOXICITY

Acute effects of chemotherapy for nonparameningeal sarcomas of the head and neck are similar to those for tumors in the other locations described. Acute effects of irradiation depend on which tissues are contained in the tissue volume that is radiated. However, in

TABLE 5
Results of IRS-I Treatment of Children with Nonorbital, Nonparameningeal Sarcoma of the Head and Neck

Date	Chemotherapy	Radiotherapy	Number of patients	% CR at 3 years	% alive at 3 years
1972—1978 (IRS-I)	VA(C) ± ADR (groups III, IV)	See Table 4	Head — 37	95	78
			Neck — 27	62	78

general, the acute effects of radiation of tumors in these sites are more severe than for orbital tumors, since the adjacent mucous membranes may receive irradiation, also. Particularly severe mucositis can occur following combined irradiation and chemotherapy of tumors in the pharynx and neck. This includes esophagitis if the esophagus is included in the irradiated volume. Parenteral alimentation may be needed for maintenance of adequate nutrition in some of these patients.

Late sequelae of therapy of sarcomas of the head and neck have been reviewed.[11,26] There is an increased risk of dental caries and tooth malformation in children whose growing teeth, especially the secondary ("permanent") teeth, are present in the field of radiation. Facial asymmetry may require plastic surgical correction.[11] Endocrine effects include suppression of growth and diminution of thyroid function when the pituitary and thyroid glands receive high doses of irradiation.[27]

A second malignant neoplasm is also possible after otherwise successful treatment of a soft tissue sarcoma at any site.[28] The histologic type of the second tumor varies considerably and can include thyroid carcinoma (which usually responds favorably to therapy),[29] another sarcoma of soft tissue or of adjacent bone,[28,30] or even acute myeloblastic leukemia.[30,31] AML and sarcomas of bone and soft tissues are particularly difficult to treat because these patients will often be resistant to vincristine and doxorubicin due to prior treatment with these drugs.

V. CONSIDERATIONS FOR THE FUTURE

It is clear from the foregoing discussion that substantial progress has been made over the last 17 years in curing increasing numbers of young persons with RMS and related tumors of the head and neck. While this progress is gratifying, there is still room for improvement, both in survival rates and in ameliorating acute and long-term consequences of therapy. More and better chemotherapeutic agents, innovative uses of radiotherapy, and advances in supportive care are all needed in order to increase tumor control in these patients and to produce better cosmetic results. At the same time, one needs to anticipate, and hopefully to avoid, serious sequelae such as intellectual, neurologic, and endocrinologic damage, as well as the development of second malignant neoplasms resulting from combined modality therapy.

REFERENCES

1. **Maurer, H. M., Beltangady, M., Gehan, E. A., et al.,** The Intergroup Rhabdomyosarcoma Study-I; a final report, *Cancer,* 61, 209, 1988.
2. **Maurer, H. M., Gehan, E. A., Beltangady, M., et al.,** The Intergroup Rhabdomyosarcoma Study-II, *Cancer,* in press.
3. **Sutow, W. W., Lindberg, R. D., Gehan, E. A., et al.,** Three-year relapse-free survival rates in childhood rhabdomyosarcoma of the head and neck, *Cancer,* 49, 2217, 1982.
4. **Pratt, C. B., Smith, J. W., Woerner, S., et al.,** Factors leading to delay in the diagnosis and affecting survival of children with head and neck rhabdomyosarcoma, *Pediatrics,* 61, 30, 1978.
5. **Raney, R. B., Jr., Zimmerman, R. A., Bilaniuk, L. T., et al.,** Management of craniofacial sarcoma in childhood assisted by computed tomography, *Int. J. Radiat. Oncol. Biol. Phys.,* 5, 529, 1979.
6. **Raney, R. B., Tefft, M., Maurer, H. M., et al.,** Disease patterns and survival rate in children with metastatic soft-tissue sarcoma. A report from the Intergroup Rhabdomyosarcoma Study (IRS)-I, *Cancer,* 62, 1257, 1988.
7. **Hutchinson, R. J., Raney, R. B., and Littman, P.,** Meningeal extension of head and neck rhabdomyosarcoma, *J. Pediatr.,* 91, 516, 1977.
8. **Gerson, J. M., Jaffe, N., Donaldson, M. H., and Tefft, M.,** Meningeal seeding from rhabdomyosarcoma of the head and neck with base of the skull invasion; recognition of the clinical evolution and suggestions for management, *Med. Pediatr. Oncol.,* 5, 137, 1978.
9. **Tefft, M., Fernandez, C., Donaldson, M., et al.,** Incidence of meningeal involvement by rhabdomyosarcoma of the head and neck in children. A report of the Intergroup Rhabdomyosarcoma Study (IRS), *Cancer,* 42, 253, 1978.
10. **Raney, R. B., Jr., Tefft, M., Newton, W. A., et al.,** Improved prognosis with intensive treatment of children with cranial soft tissue sarcomas arising in nonorbital parameningeal sites, *Cancer,* 59, 147, 1987.
11. **Fromm, M., Littman, P., Raney, R. B., et al.,** Late effects after treatment of 20 children with soft tissue sarcomas of the head and neck. Experience at a single institution with a review of the literature, *Cancer,* 57, 2070, 1986.
12. **Meadows, A. T. and Evans, A. E.,** Effects of chemotherapy on the central nervous system. A study of parenteral methotrexate in long-term survivors of leukemia and lymphoma in childhood, *Cancer,* 37, 1079, 1976.
13. **Bleyer, W. A.,** Neurologic sequelae of methotrexate and ionizing radiation; a new classification, *Cancer Treat. Rep.,* 65 (Suppl. 1), 89, 1981.
14. **Fusner, J. E., Poplack, D. G., Pizzo, P. A., and DiChiro, G.,** Leukoencephalopathy following chemotherapy for rhabdomyosarcoma; reversibility of cerebral changes demonstrated by computed tomography, *J. Pediatr.,* 91, 77, 1977.
15. **Meadows, A. T., Massari, D. J., Fergusson, J., et al.,** Declines in IQ scores and cognitive dysfunctions in children with acute lymphocytic leukaemia treated with cranial irradiation, *Lancet,* 2, 1015, 1981.
16. **Goldwein, J. W.,** Radiation myelopathy; a review, *Med. Pediatr. Oncol.,* 15, 89, 1987.
17. **Sundaresan, N., Gutierrez, F. A., and Larsen, M. B.,** Radiation myelopathy in children, *Ann. Neurol.,* 4, 47, 1978.
18. **Raney, R. B., Tefft, M., Newton, W. A., et al.,** Ascending transverse myelitis in patients with parameningeal sarcoma treated intensively on Intergroup Rhabdomyosarcoma Studies (IRS), *Proc. Am. Soc. Clin. Oncol.,* 9 (Abstr. 1129), 291, 1990.
19. **Sagerman, R. H., Tretter, P., and Ellsworth, R. M.,** Orbital rhabdomyosarcoma in children, *Trans. Am. Acad. Ophthalmol. Otol.,* 78, 602, 1974.
20. **Wharam, M., Beltangady, M., Hays, D., et al.,** Localized orbital rhabdomyosarcoma. An interim report of the Intergroup Rhabdomyosarcoma Study Committee, *Ophthalmology,* 94, 251, 1987.
21. **Fusner, J. E., Pizzo, P. A., Poplack, D. G., and Freeman, C.,** Meningeal relapse of orbital rhabdomyosarcoma, *Med. Pediatr. Oncol.,* 4, 247, 1978.
22. **Heyn, R., Ragab, A., Raney, R. B., Jr., et al.,** Late effects of therapy in orbital rhabdomyosarcoma in children; a report from the Intergroup Rhabdomyosarcoma Study, *Cancer,* 57, 1738, 1986.
23. **Wharam, M. D., Jr., Foulkes, M. A., Lawrence, W., Jr., et al.,** Soft tissue sarcoma of the head and neck in childhood; nonorbital and nonparameningeal sites. A report of the Intergroup Rhabdomyosarcoma Study (IRS)-I, *Cancer,* 53, 1016, 1984.
24. **Wharam, M. D., Beltangady, M. S., Heyn, R. M., et al.,** Pediatric orofacial and laryngopharyngeal rhabdomyosarcoma. An Intergroup Rhabdomyosarcoma Study report, *Arch. Otolaryngol. Head Neck Surg.,* 113, 1225, 1987.
25. **Curran, W. J., Jr., Littman, P., and Raney, R. B.,** Interstitial radiation therapy in the treatment of childhood soft-tissue sarcomas, *Int. J. Radiat. Oncol. Biol. Phys.,* 14, 169, 1988.

26. **Jaffe, N., Toth, B. B., Hoan, R. E., et al.,** Dental and maxillofacial abnormalities in long-term survivors of childhood cancer; effects of treatment with chemotherapy and radiation to the head and neck, *Pediatrics,* 73, 816, 1984.
27. **Bajornus, D. R., Ghavimi, F., Jereb, B., and Sonenberg, M.,** Endocrine sequelae of antineoplastic therapy in childhood head and neck malignancies, *J. Clin. Endocrinol. Metab.,* 50, 329, 1980.
28. **Meadows, A. T., D'Angio, G. J., Mike, V., et al.,** Patterns of second malignant neoplasms in children, *Cancer,* 40, 1903, 1977.
29. **Bell, R. M.,** Thyroid carcinoma, *Surg. Clin. North Am.,* 66, 13, 1986.
30. **Heyn, R. M.,** Late effects of therapy in rhabdomyosarcoma, *Clin. Oncol.,* 4, 287, 1985.
31. **Youness, E., Dosik, G., Benjamin, R. S., and Trujillo, J. M.,** Acute myelomonocytic leukemia following a chemotherapeutic regimen for metastatic sarcoma, *Cancer Treat. Rep.,* 62, 1513, 1978.

Chapter 19

RHABDOMYOSARCOMA OF THE GASTROINTESTINAL TRACT

Jorge A. Ortega and Marcio Malogolowkin

TABLE OF CONTENTS

I. INTRODUCTION

Rhabdomyosarcoma (RMS) connotes a tumor originating from tissue that imitates normal striated muscle;[1,2] however, it often arises in sites where striated muscle is not ordinarily found. Within the gastrointestinal (GI) tract and its related structures, RMS arising as a primary malignant neoplasm is rather unusual. Nevertheless, it is of interest that this tumor was first recognized and identified as a separate entity by Weber in 1854 in a report of a man with a recurrent growth of the tongue.[3] Because of the rarity of RMS in the GI tract, very limited information is presently available on the biology, natural history, and therapy of the tumor in this location. Due to its extreme rarity in the GI tract, the correct diagnosis of RMS is often not made until late in the course of disease or even at the time of autopsy.

The purpose of this chapter is to provide comprehensive guidelines of the most common characteristics of RMS in the GI tract, which will facilitate the establishment of an early diagnosis and implementation of appropriate therapy.

II. EPIDEMIOLOGY

Knowledge of the biological characteristics and behavior of RMS of the GI tract is limited by its relative infrequency. This tumor, which constitutes the most common soft tissue sarcoma in the pediatric age group,[4,5] is most frequently seen arising from the extremities, the head and neck region, and the genitourinary system. Primary RMS of the GI tract accounted for only 2.6% of the total number of patients registered in three consecutive Intergroup Rhabdomyosarcoma Studies (IRSs).[6] Primary tumors of the oral cavity and oropharynx, usually included in the head and neck group, constitute the most frequent location within the GI tract. Those arising from the gallbladder and biliary tree constitute the second most common site in order of frequency. A review of 73 patients with RMS of the GI tract entered in IRS-I, -II, and -III revealed the following distribution by primary site: oropharynx, 34; oral cavity, 9; gallbladder and biliary tree, 19; peritoneum, 4; small intestine, 3; colon, 3; and pancreas, 1. Table 1 lists the distribution by clinical group and primary site of RMSs in this patient population.

In general, the bimodal peak age distribution demonstrated in childhood RMS is observed among patients with primary tumors of the GI tract.[7] In contrast to other GI sites, however, RMS of the biliary tree is virtually confined to the early childhood age, and the older age peak is less conspicuously observed, except for those originating in the oral cavity and oropharynx. This latter group tends to be older, frequently over 15 years of age,[8] suggesting a role for environmental factors in its etiology. The general predominance of boys with RMS is also observed in those with tumors originating in the GI tract. However, one study reported a female predilection in the group of patients with RMS of the gallbladder.[9] It is also of interest that among adults, sarcoma of the gallbladder is more prevalent among females.[10] Preliminary information from a case-control study of 33 children with RMS in North Carolina showed a significant association between the occurrence of this tumor in children and cigarette smoking of fathers.[8] At present the Children Cancer Study Group and the Pediatric Oncology Group are collaborating in a case control study.

III. CLINICAL FEATURES

Tumors originating in the GI tract and its annexes accounted for 2.6% of all RMSs registered in three successive IRS studies.[6] This tumor has been observed to originate from almost every possible site along the GI tract: from the oral cavity to the colon, including the biliary tract, liver, and pancreas.

Approximately 30% of all head and neck RMSs have their origin in intraoral and

TABLE 1
Rhabdomyosarcoma of the Gastrointestinal Tract; Distribution of Patients by Primary Site and Clinical Group (IRS-I, -II, and -III)

Primary site	Clinical group				
	I	II	III	IV	Total
Oral cavity		6	3		9
Oropharynx	4	9	19	2	34
Peritoneum		1	2	1	4
Gallbladder/biliary tree		4	11	4	19
Small intestine		1	2		3
Colon		1	2		3
Pancreas			1		1
Total	4	22	40	7	73

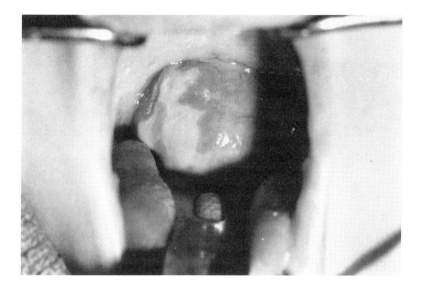

FIGURE 1.   RMS of the soft palate in a 5-year-old female.

pharyngeal structures.[11] Although this tumor was first reported in the tongue,[3] this anatomic location constitutes a rare primary site for RMS, with only a few reported cases.[12] The soft palate,[13,14] and uvula,[11] and rarely the salivary glands[15] can also be involved by this tumor. The clinical presentation of these tumors depends on the location of the primary mass. Findings may vary from the presence of a nontender mass (Figure 1) to the presence of intraoral bleeding, abnormal phonation, dysphagia, and sometimes dyspnea that may evolve to acute airway obstruction requiring tracheostomy.

These tumors frequently are not completely resectable, either because the surgical procedure would be highly mutilating or because of technical difficulty in performing an operative procedure. In a recent review of 73 patients with RMS of the GI tract entered through the IRS-I, -II, and -III studies,[6] only 4 out of 43 patients with oropharyngeal lesions were rendered free of disease (clinical group I) by the initial surgical procedure.

Malignant neoplasms constitute 25% of childhood salivary gland tumors,[24] with mucoepidermoid carcinoma and adenocarcinoma being the most common malignant varieties. Very few cases have been reported in which RMS has involved the salivary glands or occurred in paraglandular tissue involving or compressing the gland itself. Recently, 15 patients with RMS of the salivary gland were reported.[15] The presence of a nontender mass with a variable rate of growth was the most common clinical finding in these patients.

Primary sarcomas of the esophagus are extremely unusual at all ages, whereas carcinoma at this site is more frequent.[17-19] Of the sarcomas, fibrosarcoma is the most common. Up to 1980, only 12 cases of RMS of the esophagus had been reported, and some of them were not pure forms of this tumor, but contained the sarcomatous elements of carcinosarcomas.[18] None of the reported cases of RMS of the esophagus was in the pediatric age group, the youngest patient being a 27-year-old male. Of the 12 reported patients, 9 were males and 3 females. This tumor is often found in the central or distal parts of the esophagus.[18] Epigastric pain, difficulty in swallowing, and vomiting are the most common symptoms associated with tumor in this location.

RMS of the biliary tree is virtually confined to patients of childhood age and probably constitutes the most common neoplasm of the biliary tree in the young.[19] In children, the common bile duct is the most frequent site of location and differs from adults, where it is most commonly seen in the gallbladder. Furthermore, there are reports of this tumor occurring in the liver,[20] hepatic ducts,[21] and in the ampulla of vater.[22] The biliary tract accounted for 26% of all patients with RMSs of the GI tract entered into IRS-I, -II, and -III.[6]

Obstructive jaundice is the most common symptom; however, it occurs relatively late in the course of the disease because bile flow continues between the ductal wall and the intraluminal tumor. Malaise, fever, nonspecific abdominal pain, hepatomegaly, poor general condition, and the presence of a palpable tumor in the right upper quadrant are other symptoms frequently seen in these patients. In a report from the IRS, it was noted that patients were commonly diagnosed as having hepatitis, which delayed performance of definitive diagnostic procedures from 2 weeks to 6 months.[20] However, all laboratory findings supported the diagnosis of an obstructive form of jaundice, with elevated serum alkaline phosphatase, normal to moderate elevation of SGOT, and presence of direct hyperbilirubinemia. The recognition of the obstructive nature of the jaundice is the most important observation leading to definitive diagnostic studies. Spread of this tumor usually occurs by local invasion of surrounding structures or by extension to regional lymph nodes rather than by distant metastases.

Malignant neoplasms of the pancreas may be classified into two general clinical groups: functioning and nonfunctioning. Nonfunctional pancreatic malignancies in children are usually carcinomas;[23,24] however, a few cases of RMSs arising in the pancreas have been described. In two reported cases, the tumor originated in the wall of a recurrent pancreatic cystadenoma.[23]

Few cases of RMS originating in the stomach[25] or in the small bowel[26,27] have been observed in adults. Of the 73 patients with GI tract RMSs entered to the IRS-I, -II, and -III studies, 3 were in the small intestine and another 3 were in the colon.[6] Abdominal pain, distention, constipation, fever, loss of appetite, and weight loss are common features associated with this tumor.

IV. HISTOLOGY

The rare GI sarcoma presents a unique challenge, not only to the pediatric surgeon and oncologist but also to the pathologist. With the exception of those originating from the oral cavity, oropharynx, and biliary tree, the most common mesenchymal tumors of the GI tract are leiomyosarcomas. Earlier series reporting a higher incidence of RMSs in the upper GI tract most likely represent bias due to misdiagnoses.[28] Before the beginning of this decade, only three histologically undisputed cases of RMS of the esophagus had been reported. In the esophagus, this tumor most likely originates from undifferentiated mesenchymal cells which, during embryonal evolution, become localized in the foregut. In 1953, two cases of

TABLE 2
Rhabdomyosarcoma of the Gastrointestinal
Tract; Frequency of Histologic Type
(IRS-I, -II, and -III)

Histology	I	II	III	Total
Botryoides	1	3	2	6
Embryonal	19	14	15	48
Alveolar	1	2	3	6
Other	4	2	2	8

RMS of the stomach were reported,[29] and several years later a 3-year-old black child was described in whom a large gastric sarcoma was first detected from a cervical lymph node metastasis.[25] The differentiation of RMS from spindling sarcomas, such as leiomyosarcoma, can occasionally constitute a serious problem, since RMSs with leiomyosarcomatous areas and presence of cross-striations have been reported.[30]

The development of effective ultrastructural and immunohistochemical techniques obviously will facilitate accurate identification of this malignancy in these unique locations. In other locations of the GI tract, such as the oropharynx, oral cavity, and biliary tract where RMSs are seen with higher frequency, the diagnosis is usually less difficult. In these areas, the well-known embryonal histological type is diagnosed most commonly. The pleomorphic or so-called adult type of RMS has, in general, not been identified in children with this tumor originating in the GI tract.

RMS of the biliary tree usually arises from the common bile duct, from other bile ducts, or hepatic ducts. However, the tumor has been reported arising in the vicinity of the ampulla of vater and projecting into the lumen of the duodenum.[22]

Results from the three IRSs indicated that embryonal histology accounts for 75% of the patients entered with primary tumors of the GI tract (Table 2). This incidence of embryonal RMS is higher than that observed in any other location.[31] The botryoid type, a tumor of young children which is considered a variation of the embryonal type, was seen almost exclusively in those tumors arising from the biliary tree. Four of the six patients with botryoid histology entered in the IRS-I, -II, and -III studies had tumors which originated from this primary location.

V. DIAGNOSTIC EVALUATION

The purposes of diagnostic evaluation of children with this tumor are to (1) define the extent of disease for staging and treatment planning, and (2) to provide objective criteria (baseline data) for measuring response to therapy. Definitive diagnosis always requires histopathological examination of the tumor.

With the advent of new imaging modalities, conventional radiography with its intrinsic limitations has lost its importance as a diagnostic tool in clinical oncology. However, conventional radiography continues to be used for the initial screening, to provide information as to the location of the mass as well as to detect the presence of calcifications. Cholangiography continues to be a useful technique for the detection of tumors in the gallbladder and the biliary tree (Figure 2).

Ultrasonography (US) is particularly suited to use in children since it does not utilize ionizing radiation. At the same time, it provides anatomic and morphologic information, such as distinguishing between solid and cystic masses, which may be difficult or impossible to accomplish by conventional radiographic techniques. For RMSs of the GI tract, US is important in identifying abnormalities within the liver, distinguishing generalized hepato-

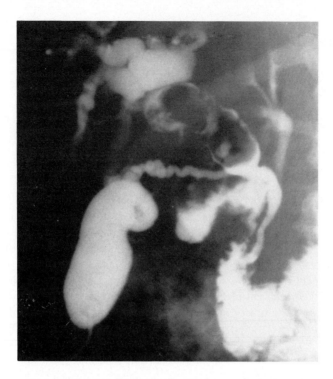

FIGURE 2.   RMS of the biliary tree in an 8-year-old male. Patient presented with jaundice and fullness in the right upper quadrant. The cholangiogram shows a mass inside the common hepatic duct with marked dilatation of the hepatic radicals proximal to the mass.

megaly from solitary or multifocal lesions. It can also clarify the relationship of the mass to the portal vessels and biliary ducts.[32] According to one observer, the finding by US of a tumor in the hilum hepaticus with fluid collection in the margins is pathognomonic for sarcoma botryoides. However, this finding has not been confirmed by other authors.[34] Computed tomography (CT) is now the most frequently used imaging procedure in the diagnosis of pediatric cancers. The use of CT combined with both intravenous and enteric contrast permits good anatomical visualization despite overlying gas and bones. CT is used to determine the location and extent to the tumor, and has also been used to guide percutaneous biopsy of hepatic tumors.

Magnetic resonance imaging (MRI) is increasingly employed as part of the diagnostic evaluation. It is capable of producing vivid anatomic sections of excellent diagnostic quality.[35] Potential advantages of MRI include lack of ionizing radiation, large field display, and greater contrast sensitivity. For RMSs of the oral cavity and oropharynx, MRI can be of considerable help in determining the submucosal extent of the lesion and in showing whether there is meningeal involvement.[14]

Nuclear medicine has a limited but important role in evaluating RMSs of the GI tract. Skeletal scintigraphy can be used to identify osseous involvement resulting from direct extension of the tumor or due to metastases to bone. Gallium scan can help in the detection of metastatic involvement of lymph nodes. If US and CT are not available, hepatobiliary scintigraphy is still a useful procedure for the demonstration of intrahepatic masses and to detect the presence of bile duct obstruction.

VI. PROGNOSTIC FACTORS

The relative influence of many prognostic variables has been extensively investigated

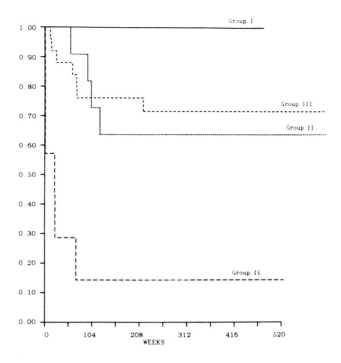

FIGURE 3.   Survival by clinical group for patients with tumors in various
sites in the gastrointestinal tract who were entered into the IRS-I and IRS-
II studies.

in children with RMS.[31] Among the prognostically significant variables, the clinical group
or extent of disease at diagnosis, the primary site, and the histopathologic type have been
identified as being the most important factors in assessing prognosis in children with this
tumor.[31,36] The rarity of RMSs arising from the GI tract has made it rather difficult to validate
the relative importance of these multiple prognostic variables in this group of patients.
Nevertheless, the limited available information appears to confirm the importance of the
clinical group and primary site for determining the likelihood of prolonged survival for
children with RMSs originating in the GI tract.

Figure 3 shows survival by clinical group for patients with tumors in various GI sites
entered into the IRS-I and IRS-II studies. It is shown that patients with no detectable residual
tumor at the time of diagnosis fare much better than those with widespread metastasis.
However, possibly because of the small number of patients involved, the analysis failed to
significantly separate patients with gross residual tumor from those with minimal residual
tumor after the initial surgery. The prognostic implication of findings at the primary site
was demonstrated in the same IRS patient population.

Figure 4 represents survival by primary site, indicating the more favorable prognosis
for patients with tumor arising from the oral cavity and oropharynx. The worst prognosis
is conferred by the more deeply situated tumors within the GI tract, such as those in the
intestine, peritoneum, and gallbladder. This finding is of no surprise since, in general, these
tumors were larger and more extensive at the time they were discovered, suggesting late
diagnosis. On the other hand, those arising from the oral cavity and oropharynx were
generally small lesions (less than 5 cm in size), indicating early detection. The preponderance
of embryonal histology associated with the infrequency of this primary site makes it impossible to determine the influence of histopathologic type on the outcome of this group of
children with RMSs of the GI tract.

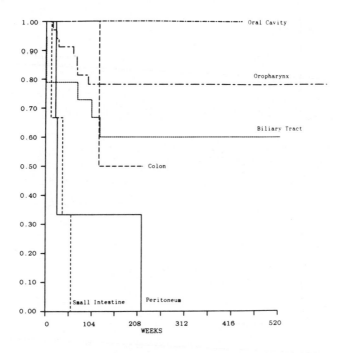

FIGURE 4.   Survival rates of RMSs by primary site, indicating the more favorable prognosis for patients with tumors arising from the oral cavity and oropharynx. The worst prognosis is conferred by tumors of the intestines, peritoneum, and gallbladder.

VII. CLINICAL MANAGEMENT AND RESULTS OF THERAPY

The rather low incidence of primary RMSs of the GI tract has obviously limited the number of patients entered into therapeutic trials, thereby making it difficult to define meaningful therapeutic guidelines. At the present time, most of the available information on results of therapy is derived from sporadic published reports. The IRS constitutes the major source of information, especially for the management of those tumors originating in the oral cavity, oropharynx, gallbladder, and biliary tree.

A. TONGUE

One third of all head and neck RMSs have their origin in the intraoral and pharyngeal structures. In this region, however, the tongue is an uncommon site for this tumor. In one report, a 3-month-old infant with RMS of the base of the tongue was successfully treated with implantation radiotherapy (^{192}Ir seeds) and infusion of actinomycin D into the external carotid artery, followed by a long course of injections of vincristine.[12] Although radical surgery was avoided in this child, other reports suggest that wide surgical excision when possible, following by chemotherapy and radiotherapy, offers the greatest likelihood for long-term survival.[37,38]

B. ORAL CAVITY AND OROPHARYNX

RMS of the soft palate accounts for 7 to 10% of tumors of this type occurring in the head and neck region.[16] Results of the IRS-I and -II studies showed that, of children whose tumors arose within the GI tract, those with RMS of the oral cavity have the best survival. As with other primary locations, treatment depends not only on the site, but more importantly on the extent of disease. The basic principle of complete surgical resection of the tumor, if this is feasible without undue functional or severe cosmetic defects or serious risk to life,

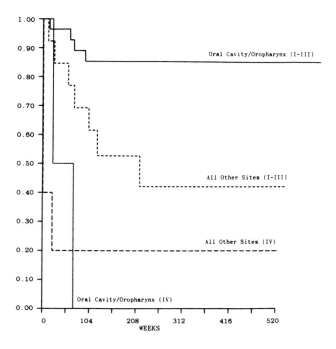

FIGURE 5. Survival rates for patients who had RMSs originating in different sites within the GI tract, but had the same extent of tumor. Patients with widespread tumor at the time of diagnosis had an equally poor outcome regardless of the anatomic site of the primary tumor.

applies to treatment of RMSs of the oral cavity.[39,40] Debulking procedures may be necessary in some of these patients to restore a safe, normal transnasal airway.[14] In general, radical neck dissection is not indicated because of the low incidence of cervical lymph node involvement.[41]

Children with RMS of the oral cavity and oropharynx treated according to the IRS-I and -II studies received chemotherapy with vincristine, dactinomycin, and cyclophosphamide. Adriamycin was added for patients who had more extensive metastases. Radiotherapy to achieve local control of the primary lesion was employed in both IRS studies, including half of the patients with clinical group I treated in the IRS-I study. Results of these two studies showed an 85% survival rate at 10 years in patients with localized tumors (that is, those classified as clinical group I, II, and III) of the oral cavity and oropharynx. This survival rate compares favorably to the 42% survival rate reported (Figure 5) for patients who had different primary sites within the GI tract, but had the same extent of disease. Patients with widespread disease at diagnosis had an equally poor outcome regardless of the anatomical site of the primary tumor.

C. SALIVARY GLANDS

One study reported five cases of RMS in the salivary gland region[16] and two more cases were noted in a literature review of malignant salivary gland tumors,[42] but neither report provided specific treatment details and results. RMS occurring in the submandibular gland has been reported rarely.[15] A therapeutic approach combining surgery, chemotherapy, and radiation therapy results in the best outcome, and eliminates the need for mutilating surgery.

D. ESOPHAGUS, STOMACH, AND INTESTINES

RMS of the esophagus is extremely rare[17,28] and little is written about therapy and outcome. It is of interest that pediatric patients have conspicuously been absent from these reports.

Only a few instances of involvement of the stomach[29] and small bowel[26,27] have been documented, all of them occurring in adults. Of the six patients entered onto IRS studies with primary intestinal lesions, all but one died of progressive disease. These patients had large tumors, being more than 5 cm in diameter, suggesting long intervals between inception of the tumor and its diagnosis. None of these six patients had complete surgical excision of the mass.

E. GALLBLADDER AND BILIARY TREE

Of all RMSs of the GI tract, those arising from the gallbladder and biliary tree have received the most attention. There have been several case reports and a review article.[19,20,43] This information has made it possible to better understand the nature and behavior of RMS in this anatomical location and to improve therapy, as is reflected by an increasingly better survival since the early 1970s.

Until the early 1970s, RMS of the biliary tree was almost invariably fatal.[19,44] The advent of modern chemotherapy and a more aggressive surgical approach led to long-term survival in an increasingly number of children with RMSs in this location. In 1982, it was suggested that the traditional criteria of resectability in biliary cancer, requiring that the tumor be limited to its site of origin without metastases to lymph nodes or invasion of surrounding organs, may not apply to RMSs of the biliary tree.[21] In a report of three patients, it was claimed that children with embryonal RMSs of the biliary tree invariably presented with extensive tumors requiring an aggressive surgical approach.[21]

A study in 1980 reported results obtained with ten cases of RMS of the biliary tree treated on IRS-I and -II.[20] Resection of the tumor with only microscopic or minimal gross residual tumor was achieved in six of the ten patients. Included in this group were four patients surviving free of tumor at the time of their report.

It is expected that the introduction of advanced multimodality therapy will continue to improve the disease-free survival rate for children with RMS of the biliary tree. Furthermore, the increasing number of patients receiving "second-look" surgery to confirm their disease-free status will help to identify those patients who require a modification of their therapy.

RMS of the gallbladder in a child was first described in 1981[45] in a 6-year-old girl. When there is extension of the tumor into the duct, often appearing as polypoid masses, the treatment should consist of cholecystectomy with exposure of the common bile duct. Following the initial surgery, adjuvant chemotherapy plus radiation therapy to the tumor in patients with residual disease offers the best possibility for long-term surgery.

Subsequent to the implementation of the IRS in November 1972, there has been significant improvement in the results of treatment obtained in children with RMS, including those with primary tumors originating from the GI tract. This improvement in outcome is demonstrated in Figure 6, which reveals better survival with each subsequent study.

VIII. PATTERN OF RELAPSE AND RETRIEVAL

There is little information on the pattern of relapse of children with RMSs of the GI tract. The IRS experience constitutes the major, if not the only, source of information. Of the 73 patients entered in the IRS-I, -II, and -III studies, 55 achieved a complete remission (CR) and 6 a partial remission (PR). Of these 64 patients, 19 (35%) have developed recurrent disease. The time of recurrent disease after achieving a CR or a PR ranged from 6 days to 27 months, with a median of 8 months. Local, regional, and distant recurrences were observed with equal frequency, suggesting a need for improvement in both local and systemic treatment. One patient with primary tumor in the oropharynx developed extension into the CNS.

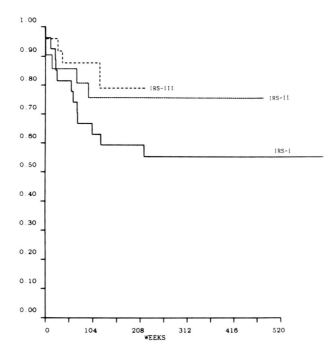

FIGURE 6. Survival curves for RMSs in children treated in sequential studies by the IRS showing better survival with each subsequent study.

Of the 19 patients who developed recurrent tumors, 5 are surviving; of these 5 patients, 4 had primary tumor in the oropharynx and one tumor originated in the oral cavity. All but one of the patients who survived following a relapse of their disease had local recurrences. The salvage therapy given to these patients varied considerably, but all had surgical excision of locally recurrent tumor. The lungs and liver (in that order) were the most frequent sites of distant metastases. The small bowel was a site of distant metastases in one adult patient.[46]

IX. LATE EFFECTS

As the survival of children with RMSs, including those with primary tumors in the GI tract, improves it is expected that the frequency of late effects both from the tumor itself and its therapy will increase. Late effects of therapy in these children varies according to the anatomical location of the primary tumor in the GI tract, as well as with the nature and extent of therapy. In general, these late effects can be classified into two major groups: functional and structural.

Patients with tumors of the oral cavity and oropharynx receiving radiation therapy are at risk for development of dental abnormalities, asymmetry of face and neck, muscle atrophy and fibrosis of the subcutaneous tissues, bone hypoplasia in the treated site, changes in oral mucosa, and skin pigmentation.[47]

Children surviving primary RMS of the gallbladder and biliary tree, who had received radiotherapy as part of their treatment, should be closely monitored for evidence of liver fibrosis and cirrhosis, and occurrence of hepatocellular carcinoma.

The actual incidence of secondary malignancies among survivors from RMS has not been established, but 17 episodes among children treated in the IRS-I and -II studies have been documented.[48] None of the 17 children had primary tumors of the GI tract. Obviously, it is imperative to determine and to identify the long-term effects of the therapy received by these children, so that future therapeutic regimens can be designed to minimize these effects without compromising survival. Furthermore, long-term survivors are most appropriately managed in clinics with capability for providing surveillance for late complications and to manage these when they occur. Guidelines for follow-up must be implemented to properly identify and establish the magnitude of the problems so that early and proper management can be instituted.

X. SUMMARY

RMSs rising as a primary malignant neoplasm within the GI target and its related structures is rather unusual. Of the patients registered in three consecutive IRSs, only 2.6% presented with primary RMS from the GI tract. The most common site was the oral cavity/ oropharynx, followed by the gallbladder and biliary tree. The clinical presentation of these tumors depends on the location of the primary mass. Due to its rarity, the correct diagnosis of RMS is often not made until late in the course of the disease or even at time of autopsy. Embryonal histology accounts for 75% of the patients with primary RMS of the GI tract. Despite the limited information, clinical group and primary site remain as important prognostic factors, with tumor from the oral cavity and oropharynx having the most favorable outcome. Most of the available information on therapy is derived from sporadic published reports or from the IRSs.

Since 1972, there has been significant improvement in the results of treatment obtained in children with RMS. More than 75% of the children with GI tract RMS will respond to the treatment with an overall survival greater than 70%.

As the survival of these children improves, it is expected that the frequency of late effects both from the tumor itself and its therapy will also increase.

REFERENCES

1. **Stout, A. P.,** Rhabdomyosarcoma of the skeletal muscles, *Ann. Surg.,* 123, 447, 1946.
2. **Pack, G. T. and Ariel, I. M.,** Sarcoma of the soft somatic tissue in infants and children, *Surg. Gynecol. Obstet.,* 98, 675, 1954.
3. **Weber, C. O.,** Anatomische Untersuchung einer hypertophische Zunge hebst Bemerkungen veber die Neubildung querquestrifter Musckeltasem, *Virchows Arch. A,* 7, 114, 1854.
4. **Breslow, N. E. and Longholz, B.,** Childhood cancer incidence; geographical and temporal variations, *Int. J. Cancer,* 32, 703, 1983.
5. **Kramer, S., Meadows, A. T., Jarrett, P., and Evans, A. E.,** Incidence of childhood cancer; experience of a decade in a population-based registry, *J. Natl. Cancer Inst.,* 70, 49, 1983.
6. **Malogolowkin, M. and Ortega, J. A.,** Rhabdomyosarcoma of the gastrointestinal tract. The Intergroup Rhabdomyosarcoma Study experience, unpublished observations, 1989.
7. **Miller, R. W. and Dalager, N. A.,** Fatal rhabdomyosarcoma among children in the United States, 1960—1969, *Cancer,* 34, 1897, 1974.
8. **Grufferman, S., Wang, H. H., DeLong, E. R., et al.,** Environmental factors in the etiology of rhabdomyosarcoma in childhood, *J. Natl. Cancer Inst.,* 68, 107, 1982.
9. **Taira, Y., Nakayama, I., Noriuchi, A., et al.,** Sarcoma botryoides arising from the biliary tract of children; a case report with review of the literature, *Acta Pathol. Jpn.,* 26, 709, 1976.
10. **Yasuma, T. and Yanaka, M.,** Primary sarcoma of the gallbladder; report of three cases, *Acta Pathol. Jpn.,* 21(2), 285, 1971.
11. **Dito, N. R. and Batsakis, J. G.,** Intraoral, pharyngeal and nasopharyngeal rhabdomyosarcomas, *Arch. Otolaryngol.,* 77, 123, 1963.
12. **Liebert, P. S. and Stool, S. C.,** Rhabdomyosarcoma of the tongue in an infant; results of combined radiation and chemotherapy, *Ann. Surg.,* 178, 621, 1973.
13. **Wel, W.,** Rhabdomyosarcoma of soft palate; a case of late relapse, *J. Laryngol. Otol.,* 99, 1029, 1985.
14. **Dal Maso, M., Kushner, J. H., and Dedo, H. H.,** Rhabdomyosarcoma of the soft palate in three patients with follow-up longer than 10 years, *Head Neck Surg.,* 9, 46, 1966.

15. **Daou, R. A. and Schloss, M. D.,** Childhood rhabdomyosarcoma of the head and neck; two case reports on salivary glandular and paraglandular involvement, *J. Otolaryngol.,* 44, 52, 1982.

16. **Batsakis, J. G.,** Neoplastic and non-neoplastic tumors of skeletal muscle, in *Tumors of the Head and Neck,* Batsakis, J. G., Ed., Williams & Wilkins, Baltimore, 1979, 280.

17. **Sumiyoshi, A., Sannoe, Y., Tanaka, K.,** Rhabdomyosarcoma of the esophagus; a case report with sarcoid-like lesions in its draining lymph nodes and the spleen, *Acta Pathol. Jpn.,* 22, 581, 1972.

18. **Stout, A. P. and Lattes, R.,** Tumor of the esophagus, in *Atlas of Tumor Pathology,* Vol. 20, Armed Forces Institute of Pathology, Washington, D.C., 1957.

19. **Davis, G. L., Kissane, J. M., and Ishak, K. G.,** Embryonal rhabdomyosarcoma (sarcoma botryoides) of the biliary tree; report of 5 cases and a review of the literature, *Cancer,* 24, 333, 1969.

20. **Ruymann, F. B., Raney, B., Crist, W. M., et al.,** Rhabdomyosarcoma of the biliary tree in childhood, a report from the Intergroup Rhabdomyosarcoma Study, *Cancer,* 56, 575, 1985.

21. **Martinez, F. L. A., Haase, G. M., Koop, L. J., and Akers, D. R.,** Rhabdomyosarcoma of the biliary tree; the case for aggressive surgery, *J. Pediatr. Surg.,* 17, 508, 1982.

22. **Isaacson, C. I.,** Embryonal rhabdomyosarcoma of the ampulla of Vater, *Cancer,* 41, 365, 1978.

23. **Grosfeld, J. L., Clatworthy, H. W., and Hamoudi, A. B.,** Pancreatic malignancy in children, *Arch. Surg.,* 101, 370, 1970.

24. **Welch, K. J.,** *Pediatric Surgery,* 2nd ed., Mustard, W., Ravitch, M. D., Welch, K. J., et al., Eds., Year Book Medical Publishers, Chicago, 1969, 758.

25. **Templeton, A. W. and Heslin, D. J.,** Primary rhabdomyosarcoma of the stomach and esophagus, *Am. J. Roentgenol.,* 86, 896, 1961.

26. **Yamada, K., Douglass, H. O., and Holyoke, D.,** Rhabdomyosarcoma of the duodenum with sinus tract formation into the gastric wall, visualized by gastroduodenoscopy, *Dig. Dis.,* 20, 871, 1975.

27. **Moses, I. and Coudley, E. L.,** Rhabdomyosarcoma of duodenum, *Am. J. Gastroenterol.,* 51, 48, 1969.

28. **Ming, S. C.,** Tumor of the esophagus and stomach, in *Atlas of Tumor Pathology, Second Series. Fascile 7,* Armed Forces Institute of Pathology, Washington, D.C., 1973.

29. **Stout, A. P.,** *Tumors of the Stomach, Section VI, Fascile 21,* Armed Forces Institute of Pathology, Washington, D.C., 1953.

30. **Finegold, M.,** Pathology of neoplasia in children and adolescents, in *Major Problems in Pathology,* W.B. Saunders, Philadelphia, 1986, 196.

31. **Gehan, E. A., Glover, F. N., Maurer, H. M., et al.,** Prognostic factors in children with rhabdomyosarcoma, *Natl. Cancer Inst. Monogr.,* 56, 83, 1981.

32. **Geoffrey, A., Covanet, D., Montagne, J. P., et al.,** Ultrasonography and computed tomography for diagnosis and follow up of biliary duct rhabdomyosarcomas in children, *Pediatr. Radiol.,* 17, 127, 1987.

33. **Friedburg, H., Kauffman, G. W., Bohm, N., et al.,** Sonographic and computed tomographic features of embryonal rhabdomyosarcomas of the biliary tract, *Pediatr. Radiol.,* 14, 436, 1984.

34. **Kaude, J. V., Felman, A. H., and Hawkin, I. F.,** Ultrasonography in primary hepatic tumors in early childhood, *Pediatr. Radiol.,* 9, 77, 1980.

35. **Smith, F. W.,** The value of NMR imaging in pediatric practice; a preliminary report, *Pediatr. Radiol.,* 13, 141, 1983.

36. **Maurer, H., Gehan, E., Beltangady, M., Crist, W., et al.,** Intergroup Rhabdomyosarcoma Study (IRS) II, *Cancer,* in press.

37. **Grosfeld, J. L., Clatworthy, W. W., and Newton, W. A.,** Combined therapy in childhood rhabdomyosarcoma; an analysis of 42 cases, *J. Pediatr. Surg.,* 4, 637, 1969.

38. **Koop, C. E. and Tewerson, I. P.,** Rhabdomyosarcoma of the head and neck in children, *Ann. Surg.,* 160, 95, 1964.

39. **Exelby, P.,** Surgery of the soft tissue sarcomas in children, *Natl. Cancer Inst. Monogr.,* 56, 153, 1981.

40. **Lawrence, W. and Hays, D. H.,** Surgical lesson from the Intergroup Rhabdomyosarcoma Study, *Natl. Cancer Inst. Monogr.,* 56, 159, 1981.

41. **Perry, M. C. and Nasrollah, H.,** Rhabdomyosarcoma of the head and neck, *Ear Nose Throat J.,* 59, 155, 1980.

42. **Schuller, D. E., Lawrence, T., and Newton, W. A., Jr.,** Childhood rhabdomyosarcoma of the head and neck, *Arch. Otolaryngol.,* 105, 689, 1979.

43. **Lack, E. E., Perez-Atayde, A. R., and Schuster, S. R.,** Botryoid rhabdomyosarcoma of the biliary tract, *Am. J. Surg. Pathol.,* 5, 643, 1981.

44. **Akers, D. R. and Needham, M. E.,** Sarcoma botryoides (rhabdomyosarcoma) of the bile ducts with survival, *J. Pediatr. Surg.,* 6, 474, 1971.

45. **Mihara, S., Matsumoto, H., Tokunaga, F., et al.,** Botryoid rhabdomyosarcoma in a child, *Cancer,* 49, 812, 1982.

46. **Avagnina, A., Elsner, B., DeMarco, L., et al.,** Pulmonary rhabdomyosarcoma with isolated small bowel metastasis; a report of a case with immunohistochemical and ultrastructural studies, *Cancer,* 53, 1948, 1984.

47. **Heyn, R. M.,** Late effects of therapy in rhabdomyosarcoma, *Clin. Oncol.,* 4(2), 287, 1985.
48. **Heyn, R., Newton, W. A., Ragab, A., Teft, M., Maurer, H. M., and Beltangady, M.,** Second malignant neoplasms in patients treated on the Intergroup Rhabdomyosarcoma Study I-II (IRS I-II), *ASCO,* 5 (Abstr. 842), 215, 1986.

Chapter 20

GENITOURINARY RHABDOMYOSARCOMA

Fereshteh Ghavimi

TABLE OF CONTENTS

I. INTRODUCTION

Rhabdomyosarcomas (RMS) are among the most common cancers occurring in children under 15 years of age in the U.S. and comprise 6% of all malignancies in children.[1]

These tumors arise from embryonic mesenchymal tissues. Originally four histological subtypes were recognized: embryonal, botryoid, alveolar, and pleomorphic.[2] In addition to these classical forms, other categories such as extraosseous Ewing's tumor, small round cell sarcoma (type indeterminate), and undifferentiated sarcomas have been identified.[3] There has been close agreement among pathologists in the diagnosis of RMSs, but not in certain subtypes, particularly the alveolar type and small round cell sarcoma, indeterminate type.[3] Immunohistochemical, cytohistologic, and electron microscopic methods have been successfully applied to differentiate the various subtypes.

Considerable controversy exists, but it is hoped that a unanimous international classification for soft tissue sarcomas in childhood will be developed.[4] The relation of histologic subtypes to prognosis has been demonstrated,[3] but a uniform, reproducible international classification may validate this variable as a significant prognostic factor. The molecular genetic identification of the embryonal type is based on loss of heterozygosity at loci on chromosome 11,[5-8] and in alveolar RMSs there is an abnormality in chromosome t(2;13) (q35;q14). These findings are very important in diagnosis and may become useful in the study of oncogenesis in this tumor.[9]

Twenty-one percent of RMSs are located in the pelvic portion of the genitourinary tract.[3] The most common sites in this region among 1626 patients enrolled in Intergroup Rhabdomyosarcoma Studies (IRS) I and II were paratesticular, bladder, prostate, and female genital tract. In 6% of patients the tumor was located in the pelvis but its exact site of origin was undeterminable.

The age distribution was bimodal among those dying from this tumor that were reported between 1960 and 1969.[10] An early peak was observed due to primary tumors located in the genitourinary tract or in the head and neck area, and a late peak was seen due to tumors of the male genital tract.

II. PARATESTICULAR

The tumor arises in the distal area of the spermatic cord and may invade the testis or surrounding tissues. Among primary genitourinary tumors, 7% are located in the paratesticular area.[3,11] Rare cases of RMSs originating in the spermatic cord have also been observed.[3] The majority of paratesticular cases, almost 97%, are the embryonal type, in contrast to an incidence of 53% with this type in the overall group.[11] The median age of patients is 11 years.

A. SIGNS AND SYMPTOMS

Paratesticular RMSs often present with a unilateral painless scrotal swelling or mass above the testis and rarely arise in the inguinal area. The common age at diagnosis is prepubertal or pubertal. Thus, the uncertain knowledge of pubertal development and shyness of adolescents contribute to delay in seeking medical attention before the tumor grows to a considerable size. The differential diagnosis includes irreducible hernia, hydrocele of the spermatic cord, and epididymal cyst.

At the time of initial diagnosis it is of utmost importance to determine the extent of spread of the tumor beyond the primary site and its spread through lymphatics or bloodstream. Complete physical examination, sonogram of the primary tumor site, pelvic and abdominal computed tomogram (CT), and pedal lymphangiogram (LAG) to detect the involvement of regional lymph nodes in the retroperitoneal or inguinea areas are mandatory. Chest X-ray,

TABLE 1
Staging Systems for Childhood Rhabdomyosarcoma

Intergroup Rhabdomyosarcoma Study

Group I	Localized disease, completely resected (regional nodes not involved); confined to muscle or organ of origin; contiguous involvement with infiltration outside the muscle or organ of origin, as through fascial planes
Group II	Grossly resected tumor with microscopic residual disease; no evidence of gross residual tumor; no evidence of regional node involvement
	Regional disease, completely resected (regional nodes involved and/or extension of tumor into an adjacent organ); all tumor completely resected with no microscopic residual tumor; regional disease with involved nodes grossly resected but with evidence of microscopic residual
Group III	Incomplete resection or biopsy with gross residual disease
Group IV	Distant metastatic disease present at onset (lung, liver, bones, bone marrow, brain, and distant muscle and nodes)

Memorial Sloan-Kettering Cancer Center

Stage I	Tumor localized, completely resected, regional nodes not involved; IA — margins clear microscopically; IB — margins not clear microscopically
Stage II	Tumor extends to adjacent structures, incompletely resected, regional nodes not involved
Stage III	Tumor extends to adjacent structures, incompletely resected, regional nodes involved
Stage IV	Distant metastases present

St. Jude Children's Research Hospital

Stage I	Localized; recognized tumor completely resected
Stage II	Regional; adjacent structure, or local or regional lymph nodes involved; e.g., vagina and bladder or vagina and pelvic lymph nodes: A, recognized tumor completely resectable
Stage III	Generalized; A, distant metastases with normal bone marrow; B, distant metastases with bone marrow infiltration

CT of lungs, ^{99m}Tc phosphate bone scan, bone marrow aspiration and biopsy, ^{67}Ga scan, and MRI are necessary to detect distant or hematogenous metastases. Some of the tests may be overlapping but the results are needed for accurate determination of extent of disease.[12,13]

B. STAGING

Staging of the tumor at diagnosis is necessary for planning treatment and determining prognosis. Various staging systems have been used in different centers[14-16] (Table 1). The most frequently used staging system is that of the IRS which divides patients into prognostic or treatment groups according to the extent of spread of the tumor. However, in these staging systems, except in patients with metastatic disease, the allocation of a patient to earlier stages is heavily dependent on the extent of surgical intervention. A pretreatment staging system was developed by the Union International Contra Cancrum (UICC) which uses local invasiveness of tumor (T), the presence or absence of regional nodal involvement (N), and distant metastases (M) (Table 2). The UICC staging system may allow accurate and uniform grouping of patients and may facilitate study of all three modalities of treatment: surgery, radiotherapy, and chemotherapy.[17,18]

In the largest reported group of 95 patients with paratesticular RMSs, 60% had early stage (IRS group I) localized disease.[11]

Institution of a multidisciplinary approach by surgery, radiotherapy, and multiple cycles of chemotherapy for the treatment of childhood RMSs has resulted in marked improvement in outcome. Until the late 1960s, only 20 to 30% of children with early stage operable tumors survived.[14,19-22] Now, more than 60% of children treated with multidisciplinary therapy remain alive and disease-free.[16,19,20,23-26]

TABLE 2
Categories in Pretreatment TNM Clinical Staging System for Childhood
Rhabdomyosarcoma (UICC)[a]

T1	Tumor confined to organ or tissue of origin
	5 cm or less in size
	More than 5 cm in size
T2	Tumor involves contiguous organs or structures
	5 cm or less in size
	More than 5 cm in size
N0	No clinical or radiographic evidence of involvement of regional lymph nodes (no histologic determination)
N1	Clinical or radiographic evidence of regional lymph node involvement
M0	No distant metastases on clinical, radiographic, or bone marrow assessment
M1	Evidence of distant metastasis

TNM Staging System for Childhood Soft Tissue Sarcomas (UICC)

Clinical stage	Invasiveness	Size	Status of node	Status of metastasis
I	T1	a or b	N0	M0
II	T2	a or b	N0	M0
III	T1 or T2	a or b	N1	M0
IV	T1 or T2	a or b	N0 or N1	M1

[a] UICC: Union International Contra Cancrum.

C. TREATMENT: SURGERY

Appropriate surgery in a patient with a solid testicular or paratesticular mass is radical orchiectomy through an inguinal incision, with high ligation of the spermatic cord at the level of the inguinal ring. This provides excellent local control of tumor. Hemiscrotectomy is indicated when there is involvement of scrotum by the tumor, or the scrotum has been contaminated due to using a transscrotal approach for biopsy or resection of the intrascrotal mass.[27] Scrotal biopsy and orchiectomy are not uncommon procedures due to mistaken diagnosis. In these cases, a secondary wide local excision of surrounding soft tissue and remaining spermatic cord are indicated because inadequate local excision will lead to local recurrence.[28] Among 28 patients with paratesticular RMS who had radical inguinal orchiectomy, 16 (57%) underwent ipsilateral scrotal resection. Hemiscrotectomy was performed in 87.5% due to scrotal violation and was done because of a residual scrotal mass in 12.5%.[29] Residual tumor was detected in the hemiscrotectomy specimens in 30% of these cases.[29]

Retroperitoneal lymph nodes are usually the first site of metastasis for paratesticular RMSs. The pattern of the lymphatic drainage of the testis and paratesticular area is similar in adults and children. Information about the presence of these nodes is used in the staging and treatment of the tumor. Ability to assess the status of regional nodes prior to surgery is relatively limited. LAG and CT scans are utilized to detect gross involvement of retroperitoneal nodes. However, biopsy of regional lymph nodes and regional node dissections have clearly demonstrated the prevalence of histologically documented lymphatic spread in paratesticular RMS. The incidence of lymph node involvement varies from 28 to 70%.[11,29-33] This high incidence supports the present recommendation that radical orchiectomy should be followed by unilateral nerve-sparing retroperitoneal lymph node dissection.

The recommended surgical approach is transabdominal unilateral resection of the spermatic vessels and node-bearing tissues along the iliac and spermatic vessels, as well as excision of nodes along the aorta or vena cava from the internal ring to the level of the renal vein.[34] An ipsilateral lymph node dissection is generally sufficient and contralateral nodes should be sampled only if they are grossly involved. In studies where retroperitoneal node dissections were performed in 80% of the cases,[11,29] para-aortic and interaortic caval nodes were involved much more commonly than iliac nodes. Contralateral nodes were involved in only one case in these combined studies.[11] The pattern of ipsilateral nodal involvement is similar to that of testicular germ cell tumors in adults.[29,34] In adults with right-sided tumors, nodal metastases were to ipsilateral lymph nodes in 85%, to both sides in 13%, and to the contralateral side alone in 1.6%. However, in left-sided tumors, 80% of nodal metastases were to the ipsilateral lymph nodes and 20% were to both sides. Therefore, bilateral lymph node dissection and its attendant subsequent morbidity, including failure of ejaculation in 75% of patients, should be avoided.

Inguinal nodal involvement is noted in 16% of cases who had lymph node biopsy or nodal dissection.[11] This low frequency of inguinal node involvement suggests that inguinal node dissection is not necessary unless the scrotum is involved by tumor or the scrotum is inappropriately contaminated by surgical intervention.

It was found that routine retroperitoneal lymph node dissection could be avoided in selected patients whose primary tumor was completely resected by high ligation of the spermatic cord and inguinal orchiectomy. These patients did not require node dissection if the distal cord section showed no microscopic residual tumor and the abdominal CT and LAG were normal. Under these conditions, the majority of patients who received adjuvant postoperative chemotherapy survived.[30] However, there is difficulty in detecting occult lymph nodal involvement, there is uncertainty about efficacy of chemotherapy in eradicating micrometastases in regional nodes, and patients who develop recurrent disease have a very poor prognosis.[35] Because of these considerations, surgical-histologic exploration of the regional lymph nodes for presence of tumor remains a reliable, precise method of diagnosis.

D. RADIOTHERAPY

Prior to 1960, surgery was the only modality capable of eradicating localized tumor in anatomic sites accessible to surgery. During the 1960s, the palliative effect of irradiation was demonstrated and it was established that a dose of 6000 cGy delivered in 6 weeks was curative.[36,37] However, this dose was more effective in eradicating micrometastases than in achieving permanent control of large tumors with extensive local invasion.[22] With the introduction of chemotherapy in late 1960s and the discovery that these drugs enhanced the effects of irradiation on both tumor and normal tissues,[38] increased rates of local tumor control, more complete response to therapy, as well as delayed morbidity in normal tissues were noted.[39,40] Recognition of this interaction between irradiation and chemotherapy necessitated reduction of the dose of irradiation and the volume of tissue irradiated. In patients receiving adjuvant chemotherapy following complete resection of their tumor, who have no microscopic evidence of residual tumor, it was clearly shown that radiotherapy was not necessary[16] and its omission had no adverse effect on survival.

The optimal dose of radiation for patients with microscopic local residual disease has not yet been determined. However, when given with effective chemotherapy, a radiation dose of less than 4000 cGy may be adequate.[41] In patients with histologic evidence of regional lymph node involvement, 3500 cGy of irradiation given to the region from which the positive nodes were obtained seems sufficient.[41,42] Until there is reliable information that irradiation is not needed for treating the histologically involved regional lymph nodes, as well as sites from which involved nodes were resected, use of radiotherapy should continue. In patients with gross residual tumor, radiotherapy at a dose of 4500 to 5000 cGy should be given, with adjustment in dose according to the site and size of the tumor and age of the patients.[43] Intensive systemic chemotherapy and use of hyperfractionated radiotherapy may improve local control without causing injury to normal tissues.[44]

E. CHEMOTHERAPY

In patients with recurrent RMSs, objective tumor regression is seen following treatment with dactinomycin, vincristine, intermittent high doses of cyclophosphamide, or adriamycin. The combined use of two or three of these drugs increases the response rate. Also, prophylactic chemotherapy is useful in preventing metastases in patients with localized, completely resected tumors.[45]

Multimodal therapy, using combinations of these drugs, plus surgery and radiotherapy improved both the rate and duration of survival in children with RMSs.[14,19-21,26,46-49] Since the establishment of multicenter, cooperative trials by the IRS, methods of therapy, relation of treatment outcome to prognostic factors, and the potential side effects of therapy among large numbers of patients have been intensively investigated.[16,23,24]

The overall survival rate of patients with RMS is strongly related to primary site. In the favorable genitourinary site, the estimated overall survival rate at 3 years was 89% for the entire group of 95 patients with paratesticular tumors treated according to IRS-I and IRS-II protocols. There was a significant correlation between survival and extent of disease at diagnosis.[11,32] In 57 group I patients (those with localized disease, completely resected), the 3-year survival rate was 93%. For 20 group II patients (those with grossly resected tumor with or without microscopic residual tumor and regional node involvement) the survival rate was 90%. Only four patients were classified as group III (gross residual tumor). In group IV patients with distant metastases, the estimated 3-year survival rate was 64%. The overall survival of patients treated with multimodal therapy in other centers varies from 64 to 88%.[29,30,33,50-52]

The influence of stage of disease at diagnosis on survival is perhaps better demonstrated by the TNM (tumors, nodes, metastases) staging system, which will be used in prospective trials. In the author's experience, when patients' pretreatment staging according to the TNM system was related to survival, overall survival was 65% at 5 years, survival for stage I being 87%; stage III, 64%; and stage IV, 40%. The overall probability of survival was 68%. The presence of distant metastases at diagnosis and presence of large retroperitoneal tumors were the two interrelated variables which indicated high risk for fatal outcome.[29] Histopathologic subtypes also influence survival. The majority of genitourinary tumors are embryonal or botryoid type, which are types with favorable effect on survival.

F. COMPLICATIONS OF THERAPY

Children treated for soft tissue sarcomas of the genitourinary tract with combined modality therapy show a variety of delayed treatment-related effects. As a result of retroperitoneal lymph node dissection, there may be loss of seminal emission and consequent infertility.[53] Spermatogenesis in the remaining testicle may be adversely affected either by scatter irradiation from radiotherapy given to the contralateral tumor site or pelvis, or by administration of cyclophosphamide. Significant intestinal complications such as obstruction and malabsorption can occur after chemotherapy combined with irradiation to pelvic and paraaortic regions. In a series of 27 patients with paratesticular RMS, 2 developed severe chronic bowel obstruction, fibrosis, and malabsorption necessitating total parenteral nutrition. One patient died 14 years after diagnosis.[50] Combined administration of radiotherapy and cyclophosphamide may increase the incidence of hemorrhagic cystitis.[55]

III. TUMORS OF THE PROSTATE-BLADDER AND OF THE BLADDER

Among genitourinary RMSs, the prostate and bladder are equally frequent primary sites.[3] Tumors of the bladder are more common in boys.

The mean ages for occurrence of bladder and prostate-bladder tumors are 4.5 and 5.1 years, respectively.[56] Bladder tumors are commonly located at the base and trigone and spread superficially beneath the mucosa. They produce intravesical pearly grape-like clusters of tissue and may infiltrate the urethra, perivesical tissues, vagina, and cervix. Prostate tumors are usually massive, infiltrating deeply into adjacent structures and compress the membranous urethra. They can extend upward toward the pelvis or downward to the perineum. Frequently, the anatomic distinction as to whether the primary site is in the bladder or in the prostate is arbitrary. The majority of tumors in these areas are the embryonal (71%) or botryoid (20%) subtypes. Only 2% are alveolar.

A. SIGNS AND SYMPTOMS

The bladder and prostate-bladder tumors commonly grow near the trigone and produce symptoms due to mechanical obstruction of the internal urethral orifice. In one third of cases, the tumor is located in the dome of the bladder. Presenting symptoms in bladder tumors are frequency, recurrent urinary infection, and gross hematuria due to mucosal ulceration. Diffuse submucosal tumor infiltration or polypoid masses may encroach upon the urethra or the ureters causing hydroureter or stranguria. In girls the protrusion of tumor from the urethra may have an appearance similar to sarcoma botryoides of the vagina.

Prostate tumors produce symptoms similar to those of bladder tumors. The tumor compresses the base of the bladder and infiltrates the bladder neck and urethra. Symptoms of bladder outlet obstruction, complete urinary obstruction, tenesmus due to pressure on the rectum, and flank pain due to hydronephrosis and hydroureters are common.[28,57,58] In prostatic primaries, rectal examination reveals a smooth, firm mass filling the pelvis. The tumor may be discovered as a palpable lower abdominal mass. In bladder tumors, diagnosis is made by cystoendoscopic visualization and biopsy of the tumor. Prior to biopsy, an intravenous pyelogram (IVP) and voiding cystoureterogram are routinely obtained. These studies will reveal widening of the gap between the lower ends of the ureters and presence of negative filling defects in the bladder. In prostatic tumors, extrinsic deformity of the base of the bladder, compression of the posterior urethra, and elevation of bladder floor may be seen. CT scans may reveal invasion of tumor into adjacent structures.

In addition to biopsies of the tumor, biopsies of the bladder, bladder neck, prostate, and prostatic urethra are required in bladder tumors for accurate determination of extent of tumor. In tumors of the prostate, transrectal biopsy of the prostate, bladder base, and perivesical tissues is needed. Suprapubic biopsy is avoided because of the chance of incisional contamination. After histologic diagnosis of the tumor, additional tests are necessary to detect lymphatic or hematogenous spread of the tumor. These tests include chest X-ray, chest CT, sonogram, and CT of the abdomen to detect enlarged lymph nodes, ^{99m}Tc phosphate bone scan, bone marrow aspiration and biopsy, ^{67}Ga scan, and MRI.

B. STAGING

The preferred plan of treatment is affected by the stage of disease at diagnosis. Of the various staging systems, the most commonly used is that of the IRS (Table 1).[14-16] The Uniform adoption of the staging criteria of the UICC based on the TNM system will allow staging of the tumor prior to therapy.[17] Growth patterns of tumor in the prostate and bladder are infiltrative and invasive along tissue planes; therefore, most primary prostate tumors are classified at stage T2.[50,59] The incidence of regional nodal involvement is not accurately known, since routine sampling and lymph node dissections have not been performed in primary RMSs of the bladder and prostate. However, in IRS-I and -II, the rate of lymph node involvement was 30% in group I, II, and III patients with primary bladder tumors who had regional nodal dissection at the time of initial surgery.[60] Careful studies are necessary to accurately determine the extent of the primary tumor and to provide a baseline for subsequent evaluation of response to therapy.

C. TREATMENT

Before 1970, children with RMS of the bladder or prostate-bladder were treated by radical cystectomy and anterior or total pelvic exenteration. However, the survival rate remained low.[61] When radical surgery was followed by adjuvant chemotherapy, the survival rate increased.[61] With the advent of multidisciplinary therapies consisting of extirpative surgery, followed by radiotherapy and multiagent chemotherapy, marked improvement in disease-free survival was observed.[21,62,63] As cure in these children became an attainable goal and the delayed effects of combined therapies began to be appreciated, there was need for refinement of the treatment to reduce morbidity and still obtain a high rate of survival. Thus, modifications in the intensity and sequence of the three modalities of treatment were made.[56,62,64-66]

D. SURGERY

The surgical management of bladder and prostate-bladder RMSs is still complex and unsettled. Initially, the role of surgery may be limited to biopsy of the tumor for diagnosis and for determination of the local extent of disease. Thereafter, and in general throughout the course of combined therapy, a wide excision of the primary tumor is the preferred surgical approach, if it can be accomplished without sacrificing the bladder or bowel and without seriously affecting their normal functions. For lesions arising at the bladder dome, partial cystectomy is feasible. In tumors of the prostate, simple prostatectomy or excision of the prostatic nodule is occasionally possible.[27,28,67]

Every effort is made to obtain maximum benefit from multiagent chemotherapy and radiotherapy, in order to reduce the size of the tumor and consequently to diminish the extent of radical surgery. Careful histological evaluation and monitoring of tumor response to chemotherapy, given alone or combined with radiotherapy, requires laparotomy, tissue sampling, and examination of the tumor site, as well as biopsy of intra-abdominal structures and regional nodes. Assessment of clinical response can often be changed by second-look operations and evaluation of gross and histological findings.[68] Microscopic residual tumor following tumor resection can be eradicated by subsequent surgery.[69] In the absence of an adequate response to therapy by the tumor, exenteration and urinary diversion may be performed.

E. RADIOTHERAPY

Radiotherapy remains an integral part of multimodal therapy. In patients without microscopic residual tumor at the primary site, radiotherapy is not necessary.[16] In patients with localized residual disease, radiotherapy at a dose less than 4000 cGy, given in combination with effective chemotherapy, may be sufficient.[41,42] A similar dose of radiotherapy may be adequate for sites where histologically involved regional lymph nodes were resected.[41] For gross residual tumor, a radiation dose of 4500 to 5000 cGy is necessary.[43] Intensive chemotherapy and hyperfractionated radiotherapy may improve local control without increasing the morbidity of combined therapy.[44]

F. CHEMOTHERAPY

The usefulness of chemotherapeutic agents in prevention of metastases in patients with localized, completely resected tumors has been clearly demonstrated.[45] The observation that RMSs would regress[39,61] following the administration of combination chemotherapy led to the development of treatment plans in which chemotherapy is given before definitive surgery or radiotherapy.[16,40]

Radical surgery followed by radiotherapy and multiagent chemotherapy resulted in survival rates of 64 to 86%.[35,56,58,62,70,71] In the largest reported group, this scheme of therapy resulted in a survival rate of 81% in primary localized bladder tumors and a survival rate of 92% in primary prostatic tumors.[56] Partial cystectomy produced prolonged disease-free survival in 80% of patients with localized tumor.[72] Primary chemotherapy, including at least three drugs (dactinomycin, vincristine, and cyclophosphamide), followed by surgical resection and radiotherapy if necessary, was tried in IRS-II and several studies.[33,50,59,65] It was noted that chemotherapy alone could eradicate the tumor in fewer than 10% of the patients;[62,67] the other 90% required radiotherapy or needed major surgery to excise the tumor.[62,67,71-73] Although therapy according to the IRS-II study did not compromise the 3-year survival rate seen in IRS-I (68%), it actually worsened the disease-free survival rate. The bladder preservation rate at 3 years was only 25%,[50,52,71] which was similar to that observed in other studies.

The application of intensive initial chemotherapy which included dactinomycin, vincristine, and cyclophosphamide, and the more recently introduced drugs such as cisplatin, melphalan, ifosfamide, etoposide,[74-76] together with earlier definitive local therapy with radiation and surgery, may increase the rate of complete tumor response, bladder salvage, and survival.

G. PROGNOSIS

The most important factors in determination of prognosis is the extent of disease at presentation and primary site of tumor. Among primary sites, the genitourinary site is associated with good prognosis, but the prostate is the least favorable site. Presurgical use of the TNM staging system may allow stage assignment without interfering with therapy. In one study, using the TNM system revealed that tumor invasiveness is a significant predictor of outcome.[59] Histology and age were not significant in assessing prognosis.

H. COMPLICATIONS OF THERAPY

Surgery, radiotherapy, and chemotherapy are all associated with delayed complications. Exenteration, retroperitoneal node dissection, and urinary and fecal diversion are associated with disfigurement, impotence, ureteral or ureteroileal obstruction, and stomal stenosis in 28 to 81% of patients.[27,77-79] Renal complications leading to diminished function or even renal failure occur in the same proportions.[27] Colon carcinoma may develop at the site of ureteral implantation if the implanted ureter is directly exposed to the fecal stream. Radiotherapy is associated with decreased growth of pelvic bones and gonadal dysfunction, as well as induction of secondary malignant tumors in irradiated areas.[80] Chemotherapeutic agents, specifically alkylating agents, can cause cystitis, particularly in an irradiated bladder. Adriamycin may cause cardiac dysfunction. When intestines are exposed to irradiation, the radio-enhancing effect of chemotherapy may cause further damage in normal bowel, leading to chronic obstruction and malabsorption.[77-79] Alkylating agents can also cause gonadal dysfunction and sterility. The combination of chemotherapy and radiotherapy increases the risk of later development of acute myeloblastic leukemia.[80]

IV. FEMALE GENITAL TRACT

RMSs of the vagina, uterus, cervix, and vulva are less frequent sites for genitourinary primaries, and comprise only 3% of cases.[3,81-83] Among 47 patients, in 28 the primary site was the vagina, in 10 the uterus, and in 9 the tumor originated in the vulva.[83] Vaginal tumors originate mainly from the anterior vaginal wall; they may invade the vesicovaginal septum or bladder wall due to its proximity.[84] Uterine tumors may be confined and may present as pedunculated polyps, or they may have diffuse intramural involvement. Determination of primary site of tumor at initial diagnosis in adolescent girls is usually not difficult; but in infants and young children determining the site of the primary tumor may be possible only after chemotherapy has reduced the size of the tumor or when surgical exploration is done.[83]

The mean age for patients at diagnosis varies considerably according to the primary site of the tumor. The mean age is 14 years for patients with uterine tumors; the mean age is 1.8 years for those with vaginal tumors,[83 85] with 90% of cases being under 5 years of age.[84,85] The mean age of girls with vulvar tumors is 8 years.[27,83] Cervical and uterine tumors are also reported in young women.[86,87] All of the vaginal tumors and most of the cervical or uterine tumors are embryonal in type.[82] Vulvar tumors are often the alveolar type.[88]

A. SIGNS AND SYMPTOMS

The presenting symptom is vaginal bleeding, often accompanied by protrusion of a tumor mass from the introitus or by expulsion of tumor fragments.[27] Other symptoms may occur when the tumor extends beyond the vagina. Anterior extension produces symptoms of urinary obstruction and posterior extension produces lower bowel obstruction.[84] A pelvic or abdominal mass is present in 25% of cases.[82] A small botryoid (polypoid) formation may be visible at the introitus. Enlarged inguinal nodes are rarely present.

The differential diagnosis of RMSs in these sites is limited to endodermal sinus tumor or, in older patients, clear cell vaginal carcinoma. Diagnosis is made by direct or endoscopic biopsy of the tumor. For accurate determination of the local extent of tumor, additional procedures are needed. Thus, cystoscopy and proctoscopy may be done to rule out bladder wall or rectal invasion; and multiple biopsies of the vagina and surrounding structures may be needed to determine the extent of the tumor. To determine the extent of tumor beyond the primary site prior to any therapy, chest X-ray, bone scan, CT scan, and pelvic sonogram are obtained. Periodic pelvic examinations and vaginoscopy under anesthesia are performed in patients who are initially given chemotherapy or radiotherapy prior to definitive surgery.

B. STAGING

The various staging systems, of which the IRS system is the most commonly used, have depended on surgical intervention to determine the stage of disease. A uniformly applicable staging system, which is independent of the findings at initial surgery but based on clinical evaluation of the tumor as to its extension or presence of metastases, was proposed by the UICC.[17] Metastases to regional nodes are rare but metastases to distant sites may be present at the time of diagnosis.

C. TREATMENT

In the past, the principle therapy for RMSs of the female genital tract was radical surgery. The transition from use of radical surgery alone in the 1960s to use of multidisciplinary therapy in the 1970s dramatically increased the survival rate of patients with these tumors. As experience with combined modality therapy developed, attempts have been made to improve the quality of survival by performing less radical surgery, to achieve greater preservation of useful organs.

Total pelvic exenteration or anterior exenteration with urinary diversion was considered the best therapy for vaginal RMSs. Due to the multicentric nature of vaginal tumors, vaginectomy and hysterectomy comprised the minimum extent of surgery and resulted in a survival rate of 15 to 30%.[85,89] Pelvic exenteration for localized RMSs resulted in a survival rate of 70%, but this rate fell to 40% for tumors extending beyond the vagina.[85]

The addition of adjuvant chemotherapy (using dactinomycin, cyclophosphamide, and vincristine and, in some cases, adriamycin) with or without radiotherapy to extirpative surgery led to survival rates of 63 to 80%.[21,33,52,62,83,90,91] As survival rates improved, it became clear that effective chemotherapy, given alone or combined with radiotherapy, might decrease the need for radical surgery and lead to preservation of the bladder and rectum.[64,66,92] This program of therapy was subsequently carried out in IRS studies where, following biopsy, patients with unresectable vaginal tumors (group III) received chemotherapy. The response to this chemotherapy was rapid but incomplete, and the local recurrence rate was high (18%). Only 25% of patients who had chemotherapy alone survived. Surgery, consisting of total or partial vaginectomy and hysterectomy, was required in 80% of the patients. As many as 76% remained continuously disease-free and the rate of overall survival was 89%, with 84% of patients retaining an intact bladder. Pelvic exenteration was thus eliminated in this group of patients.

In uterine tumors the results were distinctly different. In patients who presented with localized polypoid tumors, polypectomy and adjuvant chemotherapy resulted in a high rate of prolonged survival. In patients with nonpolypoid, infiltrative tumors, the survival rate was only 58%. This indicated that hysterectomy, pelvic lymphadenectomy, and chemotherapy plus radiotherapy are necessary to improve the survival rate in this group.[83,87]

Vulvar tumors are usually localized. Wide excision of the tumor including hemivulvectomy, followed by chemotherapy either alone or combined with radiotherapy, produced a survival rate of 75%.

Radiotherapy has been a major component of multidisciplinary therapy. To decrease the adverse effects of external beam radiotherapy without compromising local control and cure, several centers use brachytherapy for treatment of RMSs at all sites, particularly for tumors in the pelvis and vagina.[93-95] Chemotherapy, followed by brachytherapy, has been successfully used in selected cases.[96,97] Newer techniques minimize the dose of scatter radiation to the ovaries, either when in their normal location or transposed to the upper abdomen, and reduce radiation exposure of the hips and pelvic organs. Thus, brachytherapy may further decrease the delayed adverse effects of therapy and should be used in selected patients with localized tumors.[98,99]

D. COMPLICATIONS OF THERAPY

Radical surgery and urinary diversion are associated with disfigurement, stomal stenosis, and hydronephrosis.[77-79] External beam radiotherapy is associated with decreased bone growth, infantile hypoplastic genitalia, and rectal stricture.[92]

V. NONGENITOURINARY PELVIC RHABDOMYOSARCOMAS

RMSs arising in the soft tissues of the pelvis but outside genitourinary site are rare. The exact origin of these tumors often cannot be determined. Among patients enrolled in IRS-I and IRS-II, 6% of the tumors were located in the soft tissues of the pelvis. This group, and those with tumors originating in the retroperitoneal sites, together comprised 11% of the patients.[3,100] The median age of the patients was 6.5 years. Embryonal RMSs were noted in 58% of the patients, but alveolar, undifferentiated, and unspecified types accounted for nearly 35% of the patients. In one study, 14 (7%) of 190 patients had nongenitourinary pelvic tumors.[101] The tumor was generally large at the time of diagnosis.[100,101]

A. SIGNS AND SYMPTOMS

The symptoms are usually vague and related to the anatomical site affected by the tumor. The majority of the patients present with abdominal pain, or referred pain in the back or extremity. Urinary symptoms are rare. The most common finding is an abdominal mass. Determination of extent of disease at diagnosis is accomplished by the following studies: sonogram, CT and MRI of pelvis and abdomen, chest X-ray, CT of lungs, ^{99m}Tc bone scan, ^{67}Ga scan, and bone marrow aspiration and biopsy.

B. STAGING

In the largest series reported by the IRS, 87% of the patients had advanced disease at diagnosis, including 50% with unresectable tumor and 37% with distant metastases.[100] The incidence of metastases at diagnosis was significantly higher than the 17% observed among 1271 patients in IRS-I and IRS-II. In studies at individual centers, the same high incidence of advanced disease at diagnosis was noted.[50,102] When the TNM staging system was retrospectively applied, 21% of patients had stage II (invasive tumor), 14% had stage III (nodal involvement), and 64% had stage IV disease.[50]

C. TREATMENT

Extension of tumor to major organs and the size of the tumor generally preclude complete surgical resection. Only 7% of the patients were cured by surgery.[103]

Delivery of radiotherapy to the tumor site at curative doses has been difficult and usually must be interrupted by occurrence of acute toxic effects and myelosuppression.[100,101] Addition of chemotherapy to radiotherapy may enhance the tumoricidal effect, but such combined therapy also increases the side effects, such as hemorrhagic cystitis, myelosuppression, diarrhea, and malnutrition.[100] However, combined therapy has increased the survival rate to from 19 to 42%.[50,100-102] Evaluation of the effectiveness of combined therapy by surgical exploration and second-look operations should be considered to provide information on which to base plans for further therapy.[68]

VI. SUMMARY

RMS comprises 6% of all malignancies in children and 21% of RMSs are located in the pelvic portion of the genitourinary tract. Assessment of the extent of spread of the tumor at diagnosis is of the utmost importance for planning treatment and determining prognosis.

The multidisciplinary approach, using surgery, radiotherapy, and multiple cycles of chemotherapy, has resulted in marked improvement in the survival rate, currently at 60%. Among the primary sites of tumor, paratesticular RMSs have the highest survival rate, particularly in patients with early stage tumor. The lowest survival rate is seen among nongenitourinary pelvic RMSs, which frequently present with the advanced stage of the disease.

However, with the improvement in the survival rate has come the realization of delayed side effects of therapy on normal tissues and organs. Attempts to diminish these ontoward effects without compromising the survival rate has not been fully successful, particularly in the preservation of the bladder in patients with prostate-bladder tumor. New methods of effective treatment programs are needed for patients for whom the outlook is still poor.

REFERENCES

1. **Young, J. L. and Miller, R. W.,** Incidence of malignant tumors in U.S. children, *J. Pediatr.,* 86, 254, 1975.
2. **Horn, R. C. and Enterline, H. T.,** Rhabdomyosarcoma: a clinicopathological study and classification of 39 cases, *Cancer,* 11, 181, 1958.
3. **Newton, W. A., Jr., Soule, E. H., Hamoudi, A. B., et al.,** Histopathology of childhood sarcomas, Intergroup Rhabdomyosarcoma Studies I and II; clinicopathologic correlation, *J. Clin. Oncol.,* 6, 67, 1988.
4. **Newton, W., Triche, T., Marsden, H., et al.,** For the IRS committees of POG, CCSG, and UKCCSG, *Med. Pediatr. Oncol.,* 17, 308, 1989.
5. **Koufos, A., Hansen, M. F., Copeland, N. G., et al.,** Loss of heterozygosity in three embryonal tumours suggests a common pathogenetic mechanism, *Nature,* 316, 330, 1985.
6. **Scrable, H., Witte, D., Shimada, H., et al.,** Molecular differential pathology of rhabdomyosarcoma, *Genes Chromosome and Cancer,* 1, 23, 1989.
7. **Scrable, H., Cavenee, W., Ghavimi, F., et al.,** A model for embryonal rhabdomyosarcoma tumorigenesis that involved genome imprinting, *Proc. Natl. Acad. Sci. U.S.A.,* 86, 7480, 1989.

8. **Scrable, H. J., Witte, D. P., Lampkin, B. C., and Cavenee, W.,** Chromosomal localization of the human rhabdomyosarcoma locus by mitotic recombination mapping, *Nature,* 329, 645, 1987.
9. **Douglass, E. C., Valentine, M., Etcubanas, E., et al.,** A specific chromosomal abnormality in rhabdomyosarcoma, *Cytogenet. Cell Genet.,* 45, 148, 1987.
10. **Miller, R. W. and Dalager, N. A.,** Fatal rhabdomyosarcoma among children in the United States, 1960—69, *Cancer,* 34, 1897, 1974.
11. **Raney, R. B., Jr., Tefft, M., Lawrence, W., Jr., et al.,** Paratesticular sarcoma in childhood and adolescence; a report from the Intergroup Rhabdomyosarcoma Studies I and II, 1973—1983, *Cancer,* 60, 2337, 1987.
12. **Quddus, F. F., Espinola, D., Kramer, S. S., and Leventhal, B. G.,** Comparison between X-ray and bone scan detection of bone metastases in patients with rhabdomyosarcoma, *Med. Pediatr. Oncol.,* 11, 125, 1983.
13. **Weinblatt, M. E. and Miller, J. H.,** Radionuclide scanning in children with rhabdomyosarcoma, *Med. Pediatr. Oncol.,* 9, 293, 1981.
14. **Ghavimi, F., Exelby, P. R., D'Angio, G. J., et al.,** Multidisciplinary treatment of embryonal rhabdomyosarcoma in children, *Cancer,* 35, 677, 1975.
15. **Pratt, C. B., Hustu, H. O., Fleming, I. D., and Pinkel, D.,** Coordinated treatment of childhood rhabdomyosarcoma with surgery, radiotherapy and combination chemotherapy, *Cancer Res.,* 32, 606, 1972.
16. **Maurer, H. M., Beltangady, M., Gehan, E. A., et al.,** The Intergroup Rhabdomyosarcoma Study-I; a final report, *Cancer,* 61, 209, 1988.
17. **Harmer, M., Ed.,** *TNM Classification of Pediatric Tumours,* UICC International Union Against Cancer, Geneva, 1982.
18. **Lawrence, W., Jr., Gehan, E. A., Hays, D. M., et al.,** Prognostic significance of staging factors of the UICC staging system in childhood rhabdomyosarcoma; a report from the Intergroup Rhabdomyosarcoma Study (IRS), *J. Clin. Oncol.,* 5, 46, 1987.
19. **Ghavimi, F., Exelby, P. R., D'Angio, G. J., et al.,** Combination therapy of urogenital rhabdomyosarcoma in children, *Cancer,* 32, 1178, 1973.
20. **Ghavimi, F., Exelby, P. R., Lieberman, P. H., et al.,** Multidisciplinary treatment of embryonal rhabdomyosarcoma in children; a progress report, *Natl. Cancer Inst. Monogr.,* 56, 111, 1981.
21. **Grosfeld, J. L., Weber, T. R., Weetman, R. M., and Baehner, R. L.,** Rhabdomyosarcoma in childhood; analysis of survival in 98 cases, *J. Pediatr. Surg.,* 18, 141, 1983.
22. **Jenkin, D. and Sonley, M.,** Soft-tissue sarcomas in the young; medical treatment advances in perspective, *Cancer,* 46, 621, 1980.
23. **Maurer, H., Gehan, E., Hays, D., et al.,** For the IRS committee of CCSG, POG, and UKCCSG. Intergroup Rhabdomyosarcoma Study (IRS)-II, *Proc. Am. Soc. Clin. Oncol.,* 7, 255, 1988.
24. **Maurer, H., Gehan, E., Crist, W., et al.,** For the IRS committee of CCSG, POG, and UKCCSG. Intergroup Rhabdomyosarcoma Study (IRS)-III; a preliminary report of overall outcome, *Med. Pediatr. Oncol.,* 17, 310, 1989.
25. **Flamant, F. and Hill, C.,** The improvement in survival associated with combined chemotherapy in childhood rhabdomyosarcoma; a historical comparison of 345 patients in the same center, *Cancer,* 53, 2417, 1984.
26. **Ghavimi, F., Exelby, P. R., Jereb, B., et al.,** Multidisciplinary treatment of advanced stages of embryonal rhabdomyosarcoma in children, *Natl. Cancer Inst. Monogr.,* 56, 103, 1981.
27. **Lawrence, W., Jr. and Broecker, B. H.,** Rhabdomyosarcoma: surgical aspects, in *Pediatric Tumors of the Genitourinary Tract,* Broecker, B. H. and Klein, F. A., Eds., Alan R. Liss, New York, 1988, 153.
28. **Herr, H. W.,** Sarcomas of the urinary tract, in *Genitourinary Cancer Management,* de Kernion, J. B., Ed., Lea & Febiger, Philadelphia, 1987, 259.
29. **LaQuaglia, M. P., Ghavimi, F., Heller, G., et al.,** Mortality in pediatric paratesticular rhabdomyosarcoma; a multivariate analysis, *J. Urol.,* 142, 473, 1989.
30. **Olive, D., Flamant, F., Zucker, J. M., et al.,** Paraaortic lymphadenectomy is not necessary in the treatment of the localized paratesticular rhabdomyosarcoma, *Cancer,* 54, 1283, 1984.
31. **Lawrence, W., Jr., Hays, D. M., Heyn, R., et al.,** Lymphatic metastases with childhood rhabdomyosarcoma, *Cancer,* 60, 910, 1987.
32. **Raney, R. B., Jr., Hays, D. M., Lawrence, W., Jr., et al.,** Paratesticular rhabdomyosarcoma in childhood, *Cancer,* 42, 729, 1978.
33. **Fleming, I. D., Etcubanas, E., Patterson, R., et al.,** The role of surgical resection when combined with chemotherapy and radiation in the management of pelvic rhabdomyosarcoma, *Ann. Surg.,* 199, 509, 1984.
34. **Ray, B., Hajdu, S. I., and Whitmore, W. F., Jr.,** Distribution of retroperitoneal lymph node metastases in testicular germinal tumors, *Cancer,* 33, 340, 1974.
35. **Raney, R. B., Jr., Crist, W. M., Maurer, H. M., and Foulkes, M. A.,** Prognosis of children with soft tissue sarcoma who relapse after achieving a complete response; a report from the Intergroup Rhabdomyosarcoma Study I, *Cancer,* 52, 44, 1983.

36. **Perry, H. and Chu, F. C. H.,** Radiation therapy in the palliative management of soft tissue sarcomas, *Cancer,* 15, 179, 1962.

37. **Edland, R.,** Embryonal rhabdomyosarcoma, *Am. J. Roentgenol. Radium Ther. Nucl. Med.,* 93, 671, 1965.

38. **Phillips, T. L. and Fu, K. K.,** Quantification of combined radiation therapy and chemotherapy effects on critical normal tissues, *Cancer,* 37, 1186, 1976.

39. **Tefft, M., Lattin, P. B., Jereb, B., et al.,** Acute and late effects on normal tissues following combined chemo- and radiotherapy for childhood rhabdomyosarcoma and Ewing's sarcoma, *Cancer,* 37, 1213, 1976.

40. **Tefft, M., Fernandez, C. H., and Moon, T. E.,** Rhabdomyosarcoma: response with chemotherapy prior to radiation in patients with gross residual disease, *Cancer,* 39, 665, 1977.

41. **Mandell, L., Ghavimi, F., Peretz, T., et al.,** Radiocurability of microscopic disease in childhood rhabdomyosarcoma with less than 4000 cGy, *J. Clin. Oncol.,* 8, 1536, 1990.

42. **Tefft, M., Hays, D. M., Raney, R. B., Jr., et al.,** Radiation to regional nodes for rhabdomyosarcoma of the genitourinary tract in children: is it necessary? A report for the Intergroup Rhabdomyosarcoma Study I (IRS-I), *Cancer,* 45, 3065, 1980.

43. **Tefft, M., Wharam, M., and Gehan, E.,** Local and regional control by radiation of rhabdomyosarcoma in IRS II, *Med. Pediatr. Oncol.,* 16, 415, 1988.

44. **Mandell, L., Ghavimi, F., Exelby, P., and Fuks, Z.,** Preliminary results of alternating combination chemotherapy (CT) and hyperfractionated radiotherapy (HART) in advanced rhabdomyosarcoma (RMS), *Int. J. Radiat. Oncol. Biol. Phys.,* 15, 197, 1988.

45. **Heyn, R. M., Holland, R., Newton, W. A., Jr., et al.,** The role of combined chemotherapy in the treatment of rhabdomyosarcoma in children, *Cancer,* 34, 2128, 1974.

46. **Green, D. M. and Jaffe, N.,** Progress and controversy in the treatment of childhood rhabdomyosarcoma, *Cancer Treat. Rev.,* 5, 7, 1978.

47. **Okamura, J., Sutow, W. W., and Moon, T. E.,** Prognosis in children with metastatic rhabdomyosarcoma, *Med. Pediatr. Oncol.,* 3, 243, 1977.

48. **Raney, R. B., Jr., Hays, D. M., Tefft, M., and Triche, T. J.,** Rhabdomyosarcoma and the undifferentiated sarcomas, in *Principles and Practice of Pediatric Oncology,* Pizzo, P. A. and Poplack, D. G., Eds., Lippincott, Philadelphia, 1988, 635.

49. **Ruymann, F. B.,** Rhabdomyosarcoma in children and adolescents; a review, *Hematol. Oncol. Clin. North Am.,* 1, 621, 1987.

50. **Ghavimi, F., Mandell, L., Heller, G., et al.,** Genitourinary rhabdomyosarcoma (RMS) in children; Memorial Sloan-Kettering Cancer Center experience, *Med. Pediatr. Oncol.,* 17, 308, 1989.

51. **Cecchetto, G., Grotto, P., De Bernardi, B., et al.,** Paratesticular rhabdomyosarcoma in childhood; experience of the Italian Cooperative Study, *Tumori,* 74, 645, 1988.

52. **Loughlin, K. R., Retik, A. B., Weinstein, H. J., et al.,** Genitourinary rhabdomyosarcoma in children, *Cancer,* 63, 1600, 1989.

53. **Herr, H. W.,** Strategies for the management of recurrent and advanced urologic cancers; quality of life, *Cancer,* 60, 623, 1987.

54. **Ransom, J. L., Novak, R. W., Kumar, M., et al.,** Delayed gastrointestinal complications after combined modality therapy of childhood rhabdomyosarcoma, *Radiol. Oncol. Biol. Phys.,* 5, 1275, 1979.

55. **Jayalakshmamma, B. and Pinkel, D.,** Urinary bladder toxicity following pelvic irradiation and simultaneous cyclophosphamide therapy, *Cancer,* 38, 701, 1976.

56. **Hays, D. M., Raney, R. B., Jr., Lawrence, W., Jr., et al.,** Bladder and prostatic tumors in the Intergroup Rhabdomyosarcoma Study (IRS-I), *Cancer,* 50, 1472, 1982.

57. **Hays, D. M.,** Pelvic rhabdomyosarcomas in children; diagnosis and concept of management results, *Cancer,* 45, 1810, 1980.

58. **Parrott, T.,** Genitourinary rhabdomyosarcomas in children, in *Urologic Oncology,* Graham, S. D., Jr., Ed., Raven Press, New York, 1986, 423.

59. **LaQuaglia, M. P., Ghavimi, F., Herr, H., et al.,** Prognostic factors in bladder and bladder-prostate rhabdomyosarcoma, *J. Pediatr. Surg.,* 25, 1, 1990.

60. **Maurer, H. M., Lawrence, W., Hays, D., et al.,** Lymphatic metastases with childhood rhabdomyosarcoma; a report from the Intergroup Rhabdomyosarcoma Study (IRS), *Proc. Soc. Int. Oncol. Pediatr.,* 1987.

61. **Tefft, M. and Jaffe, N.,** Sarcoma of the bladder and prostate in children; rationale for the role of radiation therapy based on a review of the literature and a report of fourteen additional patients, *Cancer,* 32, 1161, 1973.

62. **Ghavimi, F., Herr, H., Jereb, B., and Exelby, P. R.,** Treatment of genitourinary rhabdomyosarcoma in children, *J. Urol.,* 132, 313, 1984.

63. **McDougal, W. S. and Persky, L.,** Rhabdomyosarcoma of the bladder and prostate in children, *J. Urol.,* 124, 882, 1980.

64. **Rivard, G., Ortega, H., Hittle, R., et al.,** Intensive chemotherapy as primary treatment for rhabdomyosarcoma of the pelvis, *Cancer,* 36, 1593, 1975.

65. **Hays, D. M., Raney, R. B., Jr., Lawrence, W., Jr., et al.,** Primary chemotherapy in the treatment of children with bladder-prostate tumors in the Intergroup Rhabdomyosarcoma Study (IRS-II), *J. Pediatr. Surg.,* 17, 812, 1982.

66. **Kumar, M. A. P., Wrenn, E. L., Jr., Fleming, I. D., et al.,** Combined therapy to prevent complete pelvic exenteration for rhabdomyosarcoma of the vagina or uterus, *Cancer,* 37, 118, 1976.

67. **Hays, D. M.,** Rhabdomyosarcoma and other soft tissue sarcomas, in *Pediatric Surgical Oncology,* Hays, D. M., Ed., Harcourt Brace and Jovanovich, New York, 1986, 95.

68. **Wiener, E., Hays, D., Lawrence, W., et al.,** For the IRS committee of CCSG, POG, and UKCCSG. Second look operations are important for children in groups III and IV rhabdomyosarcoma (RMS), *Proc. Am. Soc. Clin. Oncol.,* 8, 304, 1989.

69. **Hays, D. M., Lawrence, W., Jr., Wharam, M., et al.,** Primary reexcision for patients with "microscopic residual" tumor following initial excision of sarcomas of trunk and extremity sites, *J. Pediatr. Surg.,* 24, 5, 1989.

70. **Broecker, B. H., Plowman, N., Pritchard, J., and Ransley, P. G.,** Pelvic rhabdomyosarcoma in children, *Eur. J. Urol.,* 61, 427, 1988.

71. **Raney, R. B., Jr., Gehan, E. A., Hays, D. M., et al.,** Primary chemotherapy and/or irradiation and/or surgery for children with localized sarcoma of the bladder, prostate, vagina, and uterus and cervix; comparison of results in Intergroup Rhabdomyosarcoma Studies (IRS) I and II, *Med. Pediatr. Oncol.,* 16, 430, 1988.

72. **Hays, D. M., Wiener, E., Lawrence, W., Jr., et al.,** Partial cystectomy for rhabdomyosarcoma (RMS) of the bladder; a report from the Intergroup Rhabdomyosarcoma Study (IRS), *Proc. Am. Soc. Clin. Oncol.,* 8, 298, 1989.

73. **Flamant, F., Rodary, C., Vôute, P. A., and Otten, J.,** Primary chemotherapy in the treatment of rhabdomyosarcoma in children: trial of the international society of pediatric oncology (SIOP) preliminary results, *Radiother. Oncol.,* 3, 227, 1985.

74. **Horowitz, M. E., Etcubanas, E., Christensen, M. L., et al.,** Phase II testing of melphalan in children with newly diagnosed rhabdomyosarcoma; a model for anticancer drug development, *J. Clin. Oncol.,* 6, 308, 1988.

75. **Houghton, J. A., Cook, R. L., Lutz, P. J., and Houghton, P. J.,** Melphalan; a potential new agent in the treatment of childhood rhabdomyosarcoma, *Cancer Treat. Rep.,* 69, 91, 1985.

76. **Miser, J., Kinsella, T., Triche, T., et al.,** Treatment of recurrent sarcomas in children and young adults; the use of a multimodality approach including ifosfamide (IFF) and etoposide (VP-16), *Proc. Am. Soc. Clin. Oncol.,* 7, 258, 1988.

77. **Jaffe, N., McNeese, M., Mayfield, J. K., and Riseborough, E. J.,** Childhood urologic cancer therapy related sequelae and their impact on management, *Cancer,* 45, 1815, 1980.

78. **Cacavio, A., Ghavimi, F., Mandell, L., and Exelby, P.,** Late effects of therapy in long term survivors of rhabdomyosarcoma, *Proc. Am. Soc. Clin. Oncol.,* 8, 307, 1989.

79. **Heyn, R. M.,** Late effects of therapy in rhabdomyosarcoma, *Clin. Oncol.,* 4, 287, 1985.

80. **Meyers, P. A. and Ghavimi, F.,** Secondary acute non-lymphoblastic leukemia (ANLL) following treatment of childhood rhabdomyosarcoma (RMS), *Proc. Am. Soc. Clin. Oncol.,* 2, 77, 1983.

81. **Hays, D. M., Raney, R. B., Jr., Lawrence, W., Jr., et al.,** Rhabdomyosarcoma of the female urogenital tract, *J. Pediatr. Surg.,* 16, 828, 1981.

82. **Hays, D. M., Shimada, H., Raney, R. B., Jr., et al.,** Sarcomas of the vagina and uterus; the Intergroup Rhabdomyosarcoma Study, *J. Pediatr. Surg.,* 20, 718, 1985.

83. **Hays, D. M., Shimada, H., Raney, R. B., Jr., et al.,** Clinical staging and treatment results in rhabdomyosarcoma of the female genital tract among children and adolescents, *Cancer,* 61, 1893, 1988.

84. **Hilgers, R. D., Malkasian, G. D., Jr., and Soule, E. H.,** Embryonal rhabdomyosarcoma (botryoid type) of the vagina; a clinicopathologic review, *Am. J. Obstet. Gynecol.,* 107, 484, 1970.

85. **Hilgers, R. D.,** Pelvic exenteration for vaginal embryonal rhabdomyosarcoma; a review, *Obstet. Gynecol.,* 45, 175, 1975.

86. **Daya, D. A. and Scully, R. E.,** Sarcoma botryoides of the uterine cervix in young women; a clinico-pathological study of 13 cases, *Gynecol. Oncol.,* 29, 290, 1988.

87. **Montag, T. W., D'Ablaing, G., Schlaerth, J. B., et al.,** Embryonal rhabdomyosarcoma of the uterine corpus and cervix, *Gynecol. Oncol.,* 25, 171, 1986.

88. **Copeland, L. J., Sneige, N., Stringer, A., et al.,** Alveolar rhabdomyosarcoma of the female genitalia, *Cancer,* 56, 849, 1985.

89. **Daniel, W. W., Koss, L. G., and Brunschwig, A.,** Sarcoma botryoides of the vagina, *Cancer,* 12, 74, 1959.

90. **Copeland, L. J., Gershenson, D. M., Saul, P. B., et al.,** Sarcoma botryoides of the female genital tract, *Obstet. Gynecol.,* 66, 262, 1985.

91. **Brand, E., Berek, J. S., Nieberg, R. K., and Hacker, N. F.,** Rhabdomyosarcoma of the uterine cervix; sarcoma botryoides, *Cancer,* 60, 1552, 1987.

92. **Piver, S. M. and Rose, P.,** Long-term follow-up and complication of infants with vulvovaginal embryonal rhabdomyosarcoma treated with surgery, radiation therapy, and chemotherapy, *Obstet. Gynecol.,* 71, 435, 1988.

93. **Novaes, P. E.,** Interstitial therapy in the management of soft tissue sarcomas in childhood, *Med. Pediatr. Oncol.,* 13, 221, 1985.

94. **Goffinet, D. R., Martinez, A., Pooles, D., et al.,** Pediatric brachytherapy, in *Modern Interstitial and Intracavitary Radiation Cancer Management,* Vol. 6, George, F. W., III, Ed., Masson, New York, 1981, 57.

95. **Gerbaulet, A., Panis, X., Flamant, F., and Chassagne, D.,** Iridium afterloading curietherapy in the treatment of pediatric malignancies; the Institut Gustave Roussy experience, *Cancer,* 56, 1274, 1985.

96. **Flamant, F., Chassagne, D., Cosset, J. M., et al.,** Embryonal rhabdomyosarcoma of the vagina in children; conservative treatment with curietherapy and chemotherapy, *Eur. J. Cancer,* 15, 527, 1979.

97. **Curran, W. J., Jr., Littman, P., and Raney, R. B., Jr.,** Interstitial radiation therapy in the treatment of childhood soft-tissue sarcomas, *Int. J. Radium Oncol. Biol. Phys.,* 14, 169, 1988.

98. **Nori, D., Peretz, T., Exelby, P., et al.,** Sarcoma botryoides of the vagina; multimodal treatment with limited surgery, brachytherapy, and chemotherapy, *Endocuriether. Hyperthermia Oncol.,* 5, 147, 1989.

99. **Plowman, P. N., Doughty, D., and Harnett, A. N.,** Paediatric brachytherapy. I. The role of brachytherapy in the multidisciplinary therapy of localized cancers, *Br. J. Radiol.,* 62, 218, 1989.

100. **Crist, W. M., Raney, B. R., Tefft, M., et al.,** Soft tissue sarcomas arising in the retroperitoneal space in children; a report from the Intergroup Rhabdomyosarcoma Study (IRS) Committee, *Cancer,* 56, 2125, 1985.

101. **Raney, R. B., Jr., Carey, A., McSnyder, H., et al.,** Primary site as a prognostic variable for children with pelvic soft tissue sarcomas, *J. Urol.,* 136, 874, 1986.

102. **Ransom, J. L., Pratt, C. B., Hustu, H. O., et al.,** Retroperitoneal rhabdomyosarcoma in children: result of multimodality therapy, *Cancer,* 45, 845, 1980.

103. **Lawrence, W., Jr., Jegge, G., and Foote, F. W., Jr.,** Embryonal rhabdomyosarcoma; a clinicopathological study, *Cancer,* 17, 361, 1964.

Chapter 21

RHABDOMYOSARCOMA IN EXTREMITY AND TRUNK SITES

Eugene S. Wiener and Daniel M. Hays

TABLE OF CONTENTS

I. RHABDOMYOSARCOMA IN EXTREMITY SITES

Approximately 20% of all children with rhabdomyosarcoma (RMS) have tumors in extremity sites. In Intergroup Rhabdomyosarcoma Study I (IRS-I),[1] among 686 eligible patients there were 137 with extremity tumors, while in IRS-II,[2] among 1002 eligible patients, 170 had extremity primaries. The extremities, therefore, are the site of a large number of cases of RMS. Extremity tumors occur in a relatively homogeneous group of anatomic settings with very little variation in prognosis between specific sites.

A. HISTORICAL NOTES

The early published studies of RMS of the extremities are not limited to the childhood age group. However, in a review of the available reports from 1946 to 1969, there were 73 children among the 431 patients with extremity RMSs.[3] In these collected patients in which surgery, frequently quite radical, was the predominant mode of therapy, survival was in the range of 20%. Radiation therapy was used when tumors recurred locally. Chemotherapy, which was used infrequently, was reserved for patients with disseminated tumors. In retrospect, however, distant metastases undoubtedly were present at the time of initial diagnosis in a large number of these children who had failed excisional therapy.

During this era, the particularly lethal nature of the alveolar subtype was established.[3-6] Among 110 patients with median age of 15 years who had alveolar RMS, more than 50% had extremity tumors; 94% of these patients died within 4 years of diagnosis. Also noted during this time period was the lower survival rate following primary amputation when compared to local excision. The more advanced stage of the disease at diagnosis, which precluded local excision, may have been responsible for the difference in outcome.[3]

From 1969 to 1976, there were several studies on the early use of multimodality therapy for RMS of the extremities in children. Survival of 28% of patients from M. D. Anderson,[7] survival in 4 out of 7 children from Columbus Children's Hospital,[8] in 5 out of 7 children from Children's Hospital of Pittsburgh,[9] and in 2 out of 15 children from Boston Children's Hospital[10] were reported for patients treated with local excision, irradiation, and multiagent chemotherapy (usually vincristine, actinomycin D, and cyclophosphamide — VAC). With use of such therapy, amputation could frequently be avoided.

In 1967, a prospective study of adjuvant chemotherapy and local radiation therapy for childhood RMS was undertaken by the Children's Cancer Study Group.[3,10] This study demonstrated the efficacy of excision and radiotherapy in achieving local control. It also showed the value of multiagent chemotherapy in eliminating microscopically disseminated disease, with only 1 fatality among 11 patients who presented with localized tumors. Similar results were achieved in another study, with seven out of seven such extremity patients surviving without recurrence.[11]

B. SURGICAL PATHOLOGIC GROUPING

The distribution of extremity patients by surgical pathologic group, the staging system employed in the IRS, is shown in Table 1. In this study, 56% of patients with extremity tumors underwent total gross removal of the tumor (group I or II) compared to total gross excision in 33% at all site categories. This difference is presumably due to the tumor's greater accessibility when present in an extremity. Among patients who did not have metastasis at the time of presentation, total gross removal was accomplished at operation in 78% of those with extremity lesions, compared to only 41% of patients achieving total gross removal with nonmetastatic tumors located at all sites. Unfortunately, 27% of patients with extremity tumors presented with metastases at the time of diagnosis, compared to the presence of metastases in only 18% in the overall series.[12]

In all surgical pathologic groups, the proportion of patients with the alveolar histologic

TABLE 1

Distribution by Surgical Pathologic Group of Patients with Extremity Primary Sites Compared with Those with Tumors in All Other Sites: For Patients Enrolled in IRS-I and II

Clinical group	Extremity (%)	All other sites (%)
I	24	13
II	32	20
III[a]	16	47
IV[a]	27	18

[a] $p < 0.001$.

Modified from Lawrence, W., Hays, D. M., Heyn, R., et al., *World J. Surg.*, 12, 676, 1988.

TABLE 2

Frequency of Alveolar Histology among Patients in Each Clinical Group: Extremity Compared to All Other Sites[a]

Clinical group	Extremity (%)	Nonextremity (%)
I	45	8
II	50	22
III	45	9
IV	54	24

[a] p all < 0.001.

Modified from Lawrence, W., Hays, D. M., Heyn, R., et al., *World J. Surg.*, 12, 676, 1988.

type of RMS is significantly greater at extremity sites than for all other major site categories in IRS-I and II.[6] This difference is most notable in group I, 45% of tumors in extremity sites vs. 8% of tumors in nonextremity sites and group II, 45% vs. 9%[12] (Table 2).

RMSs arise in lower extremity sites more commonly than in upper extremity sites, with the distal portion of the affected extremity being most often involved. The male/female ratio is essentially equal. Primary extremity tumors are less common in infancy, but otherwise there is no age predilection.[3]

A total of 593 patients in IRS-I and II had histologic evaluation of regional lymph nodes. Of these patients, 12% of extremity patients had positive nodes, compared to the presence of positive nodes in 24% of patients with genitourinary primaries and in 14% of all patients.[12-14] Nodal involvement was not influenced by histology, that is, the alveolar subtype was not associated with a higher incidence of nodal involvement. Involvement of regional lymph nodes, whether detected by clinical examination or pathologically confirmed, is a significant prognostic factor for patients with RMS of an extremity. The adverse impact of nodal involvement on the survival of patients with extremity RMS in the IRS is shown in Figure 1. When nodes were proven to be negative, the 3-year survival was 80%, as opposed to a 46% rate of survival in patients with positive nodes.[12-14]

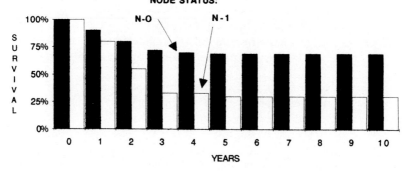

FIGURE 1.   Comparison of survival of 217 children with nonmetastic extremity RMS in IRS-I and -II relative to clinical regional lymph node involvement. (N-0 = no clinical involvement; N-1 = nodes clinically involved.) (Modified from Lawrence, W., Hays, D. M., Heyn, R., et al., *World J. Surg.*, 12, 676, 1988 and *Cancer*, 60, 910, 1987.)

Recently, the results of re-excision of the primary tumor site in selected IRS patients with extremity and trunk tumors were retrospectively studied. This review raised concerns regarding the clinical interpretation of the term "microscopic residual".[15] Among those patients in whom re-excision was performed specifically because of the microscopic residual, many had gross residual in the second specimen, including some with sizable masses. Eleven patients had microscopic residual after the first excision and, after a second wider local excision, still had microscopic residual in the margins of the specimen. This group of patients presumably had gross (not microscopic) residual after the first procedure. Examination of these specimens also demonstrated that when there was microscopic residual at one site in the margin of the specimen, it was also frequently present in other sites, which were unrecognized in the initial examination. A small group of patients in clinical group I, who did not have microscopic residual, but had re-excision on the basis of clinical judgment alone, was also found to have tumor in the second specimen.

Thus, a pathology report regarding the presence or absence of microscopic residual at the margins of the tumor in a patient with grossly removed extremity or trunk RMS must be evaluated based on the following criteria: (1) if histopathologic findings are negative, there may have been unevaluated sites in the margins which are involved; (2) if histopathologic findings are positive, the result may indicate that gross residual tumor rather than microscopic residual remains; and (3) when residual tumor is found at one site on a tumor margin, this is presumptive evidence that it probably also exists at other unrecognized sites. This and other studies[16] suggest that when the initial resection is performed without preoperative suspicion that the lesion is malignant, re-excision should be performed even if the margins are apparently "negative". Re-excision is recommended because microscopic examination of margins would probably be retrospective if not perfunctory in these situations.

C. THE INFLUENCE OF SURGICAL MANAGEMENT ON SURVIVAL

Complete resection of extremity RMS results in significantly increased survival (Figure 2). Group I patients have a 5-year survival rate of 80%, and group II patients have a 5-year survival of 70%. This is compared to group III patients who have a 5-year survival rate of only 30%. However, group III included patients with tumors that were truly unresectable even by radical local resection or amputation, as well as patients in whom lesser procedures had been chosen even when complete resection might have been performed.[12]

In a review of 55 group III extremity patients in IRS-I and -II, it was concluded that in

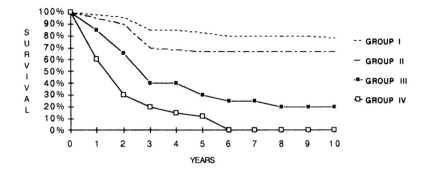

FIGURE 2. Survival curves by clinical group for 309 IRS-I and -II patients with extremity RMS. (Modified from Lawrence, W., Hays, D. M., Heyn, R., et al., *World J. Surg.*, 12, 676, 1988.)

35 total gross resection could have been accomplished.[12] When these 35 potentially resectable patients were compared to the 20 "truly" nonresectable patients, a 3-year survival of 48% (for potentially resectable patients) vs. 28% (nonresectable patients) was noted ($p > 0.001$). When the potentially resectable group was compared to group II patients treated during the same interval, a survival benefit of gross resection was shown: there was a 48% 3-year survival rate for group III vs. 70% 3-year survival in group II ($p > 0.001$).

The importance of pathological evaluation of regional lymph nodes in patients with extremity RMSs is also suggested by IRS data.[1,2,12-14] Proven microscopic involvement in regional nodes occurred in 12% of patients with tumors of the extremities. The 3-year survival in completely resected patients was 80% when nodes were pathologically negative, as compared to a survival rate of 46% when the nodes were positive. In these IRS protocols, when nodes were positive, radiotherapy, generally at a dose of more than 400 cGy, was delivered to the nodal basin. Fourteen patients who had localized RMSs of an extremity with microscopic nodal involvement were evaluated to have been given appropriate radiotherapy. In these 14 patients there was only one regional node relapse.[17]

D. CHEMOTHERAPY AND RADIOTHERAPY

In IRS-I, patients in group I with extremity tumors had a 2-year disease-free survival rate of 62%, compared to a rate of survival of 83% for all patients in group I.[1,17] Among patients in group II, the survival rate was 63% for extremity sites compared to a rate of 72% for all site categories. Following this analysis, it was decided during IRS-II that all group I and group II patients with alveolar RMS at extremity sites would receive chemotherapy for 2 years. Chemotherapy consisted of repetitive pulses of vincristine, dactinomycin, and cyclophosphamide (a regimen designated as intensive "pulse" VAC). In addition, group II patients received 4500 cGy of irradiation to the primary site and to any identifiably involved nodes.

The outcome of these intensively treated patients (13 group I and 31 group II, identified as "B") were compared to a control group of IRS-I patients (14 group I and 16 group II, identified as "A").[17] The 3-year survival difference was 77% for B and 57% for A, while the rate of 3-year disease-free survival was 69% for B and 43% for A (Figure 3). Both assessments clearly favor the intensive treatment. A reduction in the relapse rate was also shown, although retrieval after relapse remained poor in patients in both groups A and B.

E. CURRENT TREATMENT

New chemotherapy regimens in children with RMS are currently being evaluated using different drug combinations, which are discussed elsewhere in this book. (See Chapters 11

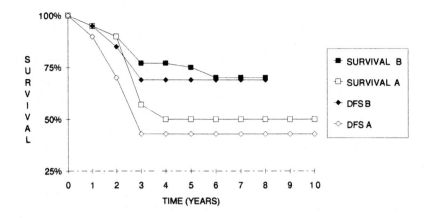

FIGURE 3.   Survival and disease-free survival (DFS) of patients with alveolar extremity RMS in IRS-I and -II. Group A patients received standard VAC (regimens A, B, D), n = 20, or sequential VA (regimen C), n = 10. Group B (n = 44) patients received more intensive, repetitive pulse VAC (regimen 25). (Modified from Heyn, R., Beltangady, M., Hays, D. M., et al., *J. Clin. Oncol.*, 7, 200, 1989.)

and 16.) Modifications in giving radiation therapy, including use of fractionation and brachytherapy techniques, are also being investigated.

Currently available data suggest three conclusions regarding surgical management of patients with extremity RMS. First, total gross resection should be attempted wherever possible even if microscopically clear margins cannot be achieved. This appears to be true even if amputation is required, especially for sites in distal extremities. However, when margins are microscopically involved, re-excision of margins should be performed where possible (see Section III). Second, those patients with unplanned removal of an extremity lesion should have a formal re-excision of the operative site to achieve adequate margins, whether the initial margins were found to be involved or not, that is classifiable as group I or group II A (see Section III). Finally, it is noted that regional lymph node spread has a negative impact on prognosis and also affects management. Thus, evaluation of regional lymph nodes by multiple biopsies or by modified node dissection is justified for all patients with extremity lesions, even though there is a relatively low incidence of nodal involvement.

II. RHABDOMYOSARCOMA IN TRUNK SITES

The scapular and buttocks areas of the trunk are ordinarily classified as extensions of the extremity; and retroperitoneal and perineal tumors are placed in separate anatomic categories in the IRS and other studies.[1,2] Therefore, this section will be confined to the three remaining trunk areas: the chest wall, paraspinal area, and the abdominal wall.[18-20]

The trunk, when defined in this way, includes RMSs with a high incidence of the alveolar histologic subtype, comprising more than 40% of these cases.[18] Survival rates for patients with tumors in the trunk category have been lowest among those with either the alveolar or the undifferentiated histologic subtype. Relapse was less common among those patients with trunk primary tumors, in whom complete or gross initial tumor removal was possible. In comparison with patients with tumors in extremity sites, children with tumors in trunk sites have a higher incidence of local recurrence and a lower incidence of nodal and distant metastases.

However, many of the characteristics of extremity RMS are shared by tumors originating in the trunk. In particular, trunk tumors show a lack of consistent and durable response to standard chemotherapy regimens, which have been so effective in the management of patients with RMS primary in paratesticular, orbital, vaginal, and other sites. The ability of the surgeon to achieve complete gross tumor resection has a greater influence on outcome among children with primary tumors of the trunk and extremities as opposed to other sites.

Combining all trunk sites, the survival rate has been approximately 50%, with initial local or local and regional relapse occurring with almost twice the frequency of initial distant relapse.[18]

A. CHEST WALL TUMORS

Approximately 50% of these patients have tumors of an alveolar histologic subtype. Extraosseous Ewing's sarcoma and undifferentiated sarcomas also occur frequently in this site; while embryonal RMS, which is recognized as the predominate subtype in most sites, is seen infrequently among chest wall tumors.[19]

Patients with chest wall tumors present the most difficult problems in histologic diagnosis among children with sarcomas of the trunk or extremities. The nature of a group of chest wall sarcomas, which histologically consist of small, round cells and are seen primarily in adolescent patients, is currently of major interest to pediatric pathologists worldwide. One report in 1979 described a group of patients (primarily female) with neoplasms of this general type as a distinct tumor entity.[21] At the same time a previously obscure tumor, the primitive neuroectodermal tumor (PNET), was recognized as a neoplasm occurring in chest wall sites among pediatric patients with a frequency not previously appreciated.[22] These studies have raised many questions regarding the histologic diagnosis in all adolescent patients with chest wall sarcomas or sarcoma-like tumors. It is probable that in most prior studies, a number of the tumors classified as extraosseous Ewings' sarcomas or undifferentiated RMS are in retrospect histologically similar to those described by Askin et al.,[21] or have the features of PNET.[22]

In the IRS, patients with chest wall tumors have been predominantly females with a median age of 12.5 years at diagnosis, making this one of the oldest groups of patients in the study when divided by site category. The operative approach to these tumors, irrespective of the precise microscopic diagnosis, is similar. Wide local excision is the procedure of choice, performed either primarily or following intensive chemotherapy or a combination of chemotherapy and radiotherapy.[18,19] If "microscopic" residual tumor remains following primary excision, a re-excision of the area is indicated, if this is feasible.[15] Patients with microscopic or gross residual tumor following operation receive irradiation at a total dose of more than 4000 cGy using tangential fields as indicated. Pneumothorax may be employed to minimize irradiation effects on the lungs.

The early response to therapy in this group of patients has been impressive. All of the initial ten IRS patients with nonmetastatic disease achieved a complete response. However, only approximately one third of these patients have remained disease-free. Like tumors of the extremities, tumors of the chest wall carry a major threat of late relapse. In some cases relapse may occur as long as 4 years after the time of diagnosis, and more than 2 years following the end of therapy.[18]

With respect to patients with either Askin's tumors or PNETs in chest wall sites, similar or more intensive therapy regimens than those used in the treatment of RMS are employed because of the uncertain prognosis associated with these tumors.[18-22]

B. PARASPINAL TUMORS

A recent review of IRS-I and -II patients included 56 children with primary paraspinal RMS.[20] Distribution by age, sex, and clinical group was similar to that of the overall IRS study population, of which this group accounted for 3.5%. Among patients in whom data were available, presenting signs and symptoms consisted of a mass in 22, pain in 21, paresis in 6, sensory loss in 1, and scoliosis in 1. Diagnosis was often delayed so that the median duration of symptoms prior to the establishment of a diagnosis was 6 weeks, but was as long as 3 years in some patients. By the time of initiation of therapy, 31 patients (55%) had developed clinical evidence of neurologic dysfunction and one third had tumor cells or elevated protein in the cerebrospinal fluid.[18,20]

Paraspinal tumors were confined to lumbar and lumbosacral sites in 21 patients, to thorax and thoracolumbar area in 17, and to cervical and cervicothoracic sites in 9. Initial decompressive laminectomy was performed in 26 patients. Tumor resection was performed in 12 and the remainder had only biopsies. Except in patients who had disseminated tumors, irradiation fields consisted of the immediate spinal segments involved with a margin of one or two vertebral bodies above and below the limits of the tumor. Neither the tumor site nor the type or completeness of the operative procedure influenced survival among patients in this study.[20]

Extraosseous Ewing's sarcoma and undifferentiated sarcoma accounted for 55% of paraspinal tumors, in contrast to the relatively low incidence of these histologic subtypes in the overall population of the IRS. There was a relatively lower incidence (18%) of the embryonal subtype. Also of note was the relatively larger size of paraspinal tumors: 61% had tumors more than 5.0 cm in maximum diameter.

Among the 56 patients with paraspinal tumors, 46 (82%) achieved complete remission (CR), which is similar to the rate of CR among all patients in IRS-I and -II. However, in the group of paraspinal tumors CRs were not durable, as 26 patients (46%) subsequently relapsed — 17 at either distant sites or local plus distant sites.

Among IRS patients with paraspinal tumors, there were surprisingly similar survival rates in each of the four clinical groups. This finding is in contrast to significant differences in survival in each group when all sites are combined. The 5-year survival by clinical group was group I, 50%; group II, 50%; group III, 57%; and group IV, 33%. The 5-year disease-free survival among children with paraspinal tumors was significantly lower than the rate for children with tumors in all other sites. Despite more aggressive treatment in IRS-II the survival among these patients was similar to that seen in IRS-I.

C. ABDOMINAL WALL TUMORS

This rare category of RMSs had an equal sex distribution and a median age at diagnosis of 9.5 years in children entered in the IRS. Two of the six children in IRS-I had alveolar and three had undifferentiated histologic subtypes. A complete response to therapy was achieved in six out of six, but in two of these patients, relapse occurred within 2 years, one at the primary site and one in the ipsilateral thigh.[18]

III. PRIMARY RE-EXCISION

In some children with extremity or trunk RMS, initial tumor resection is considered by the surgeon to be complete, but histopathological examination reveals it to be incomplete. It is found that the margins of the specimen contain tumor, a status termed "microscopic residual" disease. In many patients, it is possible to re-excise the entire tumor bed, creating wider margins prior to any intervening therapy. This type of excisional procedure performed prior to adjunctive therapy has been termed "primary re-excision" (PRE).[15] This approach may be applicable to RMSs in other sites, but its use has been concentrated in patients with tumors in extremity and trunk sites.

In IRS-I and -II, PRE was carried out in 41 patients with tumors in extremity or trunk sites. The mean interval between the two excisional procedures was 14 days. In 60% of these children, the second procedure followed transfer of the patient to a second institution for continuing care. The secondary procedures ordinarily consisted of wider excision of the entire tumor bed, that is, excision in all directions irrespective of the apparent site of residual tumor. The 3-year survival estimate (Kaplan-Meier) in this group of patients was 91% (SE, 4%).

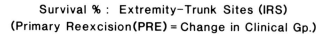

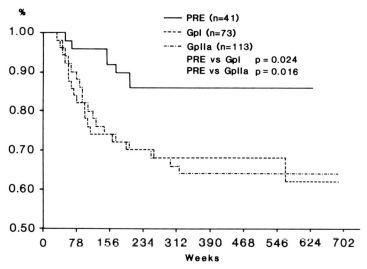

FIGURE 4. Kaplan-Meier survival estimates for (1) 41 PRE patients; (2) 73 clinical group I patients without PRE; and (3) 113 clinical group IIa patients without PRE. The 3-year survival estimate was 91% for the PRE group, 73% for group I, and 74% for group IIa. The 5-year survival estimate was 86% for the PRE group, 68% for group I, and 67% for group IIa. (From Hays, D. M., Lawrence, W., Wharam, M., et al., *J. Pediatr. Surg.*, 24, 5, 1989.)

In a comparative group of 113 patients in clinical group IIA, that is, with microscopic residual tumor, in whom PRE was *not* performed, the 3-year survival estimate was 74% (SE, 4%) (Figure 4). All recognized prognostic factors, including histologic subgroup, specific sites, and patient age among those patients who did or did not undergo re-excision, were similar. Chemotherapy was more intensive and radiotherapy was more frequently employed in the patients remaining in group IIA, that is, those who did not undergo PRE, as those in the PRE group were upgraded to clinical group I by the second operation. This comparison demonstrated that PRE, when feasible, probably increases survival duration and significantly reduces the chemotherapy/radiotherapy requirements for this group of patients in whom it is employed.[15]

It was also of interest that during the same interval, 73 patients with tumors in the same sites who were in clinical group I, having complete excision by a single procedure, had an estimated 3-year survival rate of 74% (Figure 4). This finding suggests that two independent attempts at excision are more effective than one, even when both achieve "negative" margins, a result also suggested by studies of adults with soft tissue sarcomas.[16]

IV. SUMMARY

Children and young adults with RMSs located in extremity and trunk sites are unique in several respects: (1) they include a high proportion of patients with the alveolar and undifferentiated subtypes and relatively few patients have tumors of embryonal histology; (2) their responsiveness to chemotherapy regimens has been more limited and less durable than that of patients with primary tumors in most other anatomic sites; (3) disease-free survival is more clearly related to relative completeness of initial excision of the primary tumor than is the case among patients with tumors in many other locations; and (4) relapse may occur late in the course.

REFERENCES

1. **Maurer, H. M., et al.,** The Intergroup Rhabdomyosarcoma Study I, *Cancer,* 61, 209, 1988.
2. **Maurer, H. M., et al.,** The Intergroup Rhabdomyosarcoma Study II, *Cancer,* in press.
3. **Hays, D. M., Sutow, W. W., Lawrence, W., Jr., et al.,** Rhabdomyosarcoma; surgical therapy in extremity lesions in children, *Orthop. Clin. North Am.,* 4:883—901, 1977.
4. **Enzinger, F. M. and Shiraki, M.,** Alveolar rhabdomyosarcoma, *Cancer,* 24, 18, 1969.
5. **Hays, D. M., Newton, W., Soule, E. H., et al.,** Mortality among children with rhabdomyosarcomas of the alveolar histologic subtype, *J. Pediatr. Surg.,* 18, 412, 1983.
6. **Gaiger, A. M., Soule, E. H., and Newton, W. A.,** Pathology of rhabdomyosarcoma; experience of the Intergroup Rhabdomyosarcoma Study, 1972—1978, *Natl. Cancer Inst. Monogr.,* 56, 19, 1981.
7. **Fernandez, C. H., Sutow, W. W., Merino, O. R., and George, S. L.,** Childhood rhabdomyosarcoma; analysis of coordinated therapy and results, *Am. J. Roentgenol. Radium Ther. Nucl. Med.,* 123, 588, 1975.
8. **Grosfeld, J. L., Clatworthy, H. W., and Newton, W. A.,** Combined therapy in childhood rhabdomyosarcoma, *J. Pediatr. Surg.,* 4, 637, 1969.
9. **Ehrlich, F. E., Haas, J. E., and Kiesewetter, W. B.,** Rhabdomyosarcoma in infants and children; factors affecting long-term survival, *J. Pediatr. Surg.,* 6, 571, 1971.
10. **Jaffe, N., Filler, R. M., Farber, S., et al.,** Rhabdomyosarcoma in children, *Am. J. Surg.,* 125, 482, 1973.
11. **Ghavimi, F., Exelby, P. R., D'Angio, G., et al.,** Multidisciplinary treatment of embryonal rhabdomyosarcoma in children, *Cancer,* 35, 677, 1975.
12. **Lawrence, W., Hays, D. M., Heyn, R., et al.,** Surgical lessons from the Intergroup Rhabdomyosarcoma Study (IRS) pertaining to extremity tumors, *World J. Surg.,* 12, 676, 1988.
13. **Lawrence, W., Hays, D. M., Heyn, R., et al.,** Lymphatic metastasis with childhood rhabdomyosarcoma; a report from the IRS, *Cancer,* 60, 910, 1987.
14. **Lawrence, W., Hays, D. M., and Moon, T. E.,** Lymphatic metastasis with childhood rhabdomyosarcoma, *Cancer,* 39, 556, 1977.
15. **Hays, D. M., Lawrence, W., Wharam, M., et al.,** Primary re-excision for patients with ''microscopic residual'' tumor following initial excision of sarcomas of trunk and extremity sites, *J. Pediatr. Surg.,* 24, 5, 1989.
16. **Giulian, A. E. and Eilber, F. R.,** The rationale for planned reoperation after unplanned local excision of soft tissue sarcomas, *J. Clin. Oncol.,* 3, 1344, 1985.
17. **Heyn, R., Beltangady, M., Hays, D. M., et al.,** Results of intensive therapy in children with localized alveolar extremity rhabdomyosarcoma; a report from the Intergroup Rhabdomyosarcoma Study, *J. Clin. Oncol.,* 7, 200, 1989.
18. **Raney, R. B., Abdelsalam, H., Ragab, A., et al.,** Soft tissue sarcoma of the trunk in childhood; results of the Intergroup Rhabdomyosarcoma Study, *Cancer,* 49, 2612, 1982.
19. **Shamberger, R. C., Grier, H. E., Weinstein, H. J., et al.,** Chest wall tumors in infancy and childhood, *Cancer,* 63, 774, 1989.
20. **Ortega, J. A., Wharam, M., Gehan, E. A., et al.,** Clinical features and end results of therapy for children with paraspinal rhabdomyosarcoma; a report of the Intergroup Rhabdomyosarcoma Study, submitted for publication.
21. **Askin, F. B., Rosai, J., Sibley, R. K., et al.,** Malignant small cell tumor of the thoracopulmonary region in childhood, *Cancer,* 43, 2438, 1979.
22. **Gonzalez-Crussi, F., Wolfson, S. L., Misugi, K., and Nakajima, T.,** Peripheral neuroectodermal tumors of the chest wall in childhood, *Cancer,* 54, 2519, 1984.

Chapter 22

RHABDOMYOSARCOMAS IN INFANCY

Ray C. Pais and Abdelsalam H. Ragab

TABLE OF CONTENTS

I. INTRODUCTION

The occurrence of malignancy during infancy (defined as the first 12 months of life) is relatively uncommon. In the U.S., the overall incidence of malignancy in infants is 183.4 per million live births per year, with at least one fifth of the cases representing congenital malignancies (defined as cases diagnosed before the first month of life). Information from the Intergroup Rhabdomyosarcoma Study (IRS),[1] the German Soft Tissue Sarcoma Study (CWS-81),[2] and the Institut Gustavy-Roussy[3] represents the only published systematic analyses of rhabdomyosarcoma (RMS) occurring during infancy. RMS in infancy has some characteristics which deserve special attention, and represents a challenging treatment problem.

II. CHARACTERISTICS

A. EPIDEMIOLOGY

The pattern of malignancies in infants differs from that of older children. The most common pediatric malignancies in the U.S. (in descending order of frequency) are leukemia, central nervous system tumors, and lymphomas. Together, these malignancies account for nearly two thirds of all neoplasms occurring in children less than 15 years of age.[4] In contrast, for children less than 1 year old, the most common malignancies are neuroblastoma, leukemia, and renal tumors (mostly Wilms' tumors).[5] The frequencies of various tumors that occur during infancy are shown in Table 1. RMSs represent only about 2% of all malignancies occurring in infants.[5]

As shown in Tables 2 and 3, 4 to 5% of all North American children with RMS are less than 12 months old when they are first diagnosed.[1,6] In other countries, the percentage of infants may be higher (Table 3). If the information from the underdeveloped nations listed in Table 3 (China,[7] Malaysia,[8] Nigeria,[9] and Thailand[10]) is combined, infants account for 18% of cases (11 out of 62) of childhood RMS. In Germany[2] and the U.K.,[11] the percentages of cases occurring in infants are 5.0 and 6.8%, respectively, similar to the situation in the U.S. and Canada. In France about 11% of all cases of RMS occur during infancy.[3] However, in small series of cases from the Netherlands,[12] Germany (formerly East Germany),[13] and Australia,[14] infants represent 16 to 29% of cases of childhood RMS. The higher proportion of cases in infants in some countries may be an artifact due to small numbers, referral bias, or differences in birth rates.

In IRS-I and IRS-II, the male/female ratio was not different for infants (of whom 58% were male), compared to the older children (where 57% were male).[1]

B. CONGENITAL RHABDOMYOSARCOMA

The authors define congenital RMS as any case diagnosed before the age of 1 month. Occasional cases of congenital RMS have been reported as originating at a variety of sites, including the bladder,[15,16] extremity,[17,18] head and neck,[19] eyelid,[20] orbit,[21-23] pararectal area,[24] and trunk.[25] In IRS-I and -II, 0.9% (14 out of 1561 cases) met our definition for congenital RMS.[1] Congenital RMSs represent 1.7 and 2.9% of the cases in the German and French series, respectively.[2,3] Outcome in cases of congenital RMS was not analyzed separately from the rest of the cases who were less than 12 months old at diagnosis in any of the three largest series.[1-3] As shown in Table 4, congenital RMS represents about 18% of cases (14 out of 78) occurring during the first year of life.

Congenital anomalies were discovered in 37 out of 115 children and adolescents (32%) with RMS who were examined at autopsy.[26] A more detailed description and analysis of congenital anomalies associated with RMS are given in Chapter 1, Section V.A by Ruymann.

TABLE 1
Incidence of Malignancy in U.S. in Children during the First Year of Life

Malignancy	Number per million live births/year	Infants with malignancies (%)
Neuroblastoma	62.7	34.2
Leukemia	31.8	17.3
Renal tumors	19.7	10.7
Sarcomas[a]	17.8[a]	9.7
Retinoblastoma	15.9	8.7
CNS tumors	14.0	7.6
Hepatic tumors	7.5	4.1
Carcinomas	5.6	3.1
Teratomas	2.8	1.5
Other	5.6	3.1
Total	183.4	100.0

[a] If only confirmed RMSs are included, the incidence is 3.7 per million live births per year.

Derived from data in Reference 5, Third National Cancer Survey.

TABLE 2
Age Distribution of Children with Rhabdomyosarcomas Studied in IRS-I

Age (years)	Total (%)
Less than 1 year	4
1—4	34
5—9	25
10—14	22
15	15

From Maurer, H. M., Beltangady, M., Gehan, E. A., et al., *Cancer*, 61, 209, 1988. With permission.

C. PRIMARY SITES

Table 5 compares the distribution of primary tumor sites in infants to the location of primary tumors in the older children. For most tumor sites, there is no statistically significant difference between the two age groups. The exception may be the incidence rate of tumors originating in the bladder, prostate, and vagina, which was higher in infants (26%) than in older children (10%) in the IRS series.[1] However, this difference was not apparent in the smaller French and German studies.[2,3]

D. CLINICAL GROUPING

The clinical groups as defined by the IRS were listed in an earlie⁻ chapter. In Table 6 the clinical groupings of infants are compared to those observed in older children. In the IRS series, a slightly higher percentage of the older children (19%) had tumors classified as group IV than was seen in infants (12%). However, this difference was not statistically

TABLE 3
Rhabdomyosarcoma and Related Soft Tissue Sarcomas in Infancy

Country	Years	Total number of children	Younger than 1 year		Under 1 month		
			Number	%	Number	%	Ref.
U.S. and Canada	1978—1983	1561	78	5.0	14	0.9	1
Germany	1981—1986	357	21	5.8	6	1.7	2
France	1955—1984	383	43	11.2	11	2.9	3
U.K.	1974—1981	73	5	6.8	NA	NA	11
Netherlands	1970—1980	18[a]	3	16.7	0	0	12
Germany[b]	1974—1984	28	8	28.6	0	0	13
Australia	NA	95	15	15.8	3	3.2	14
China	1955—1981	17[a]	2	11.8	0	0	7
Malaysia	1967—1980	11	4	36.4	0	0	8
Nigeria	1976—1982	8	1	12.5	0	0	9
Thailand	1970—1982	26	4	15.4	0	0	10

Note: NA = not available.

[a] Only includes urogenital cases.
[b] Formerly GDR (East Germany).

TABLE 4
Age Distribution of Infants
Studied in IRS-I/II

Age in months	Number of patients
1	14
2	2
3	12
4	2
5	1
6	6
7	8
8	7
9	8
10	6
11	12

From Ragab, A. H., Heyn, R., Tefft, M., et al., *Cancer,* 58, 2606, 1986. With permission.

significant.[1] There was also no statistically significant difference in the distribution of clinical stages in the French and German series.[2,3] Thus, the size and extent of spread of RMSs at the time of initial diagnosis are essentially the same in infants as they are in older children.

E. PATHOLOGY

The pathologic subtypes used to classify tumors for the IRS are listed in Table 7. There are differences in the frequency of certain pathological types between infants and older children. In the IRS series, infants had a higher proportion of cases of undifferentiated sarcoma (18% vs. 7%);[1] however, the CWS-81 protocol results failed to support this finding.[2] In the IRS series botryoid histology was more common in infants (10% vs. 4%);[1] however, in the series from the Institut Gustavy-Roussy botyroid histology was more common in older children rather than in infants.[3] The alveolar type of RMS has been associated with a poor

TABLE 5
Primary Site of Tumor by Age Group

	Percent under 1 year old			Percent over 1 year old		
Primary site	**IRS** **(N = 78)**	**CWS-81** **(N = 21)**	**IGR** **(N = 43)**	**IRS** **(N = 1483)**	**CWS-81** **(N = 331)**	**IGR** **(N = 340)**
Extremity	23	33	23	18	26	18
Bladder/prostate/vagina	26[a]	24	12	10[a]	17	19
Pelvis/retroperitoneum	14	NS	NS	10	NS	NS
Head/neck	10	10	28	12	28	37
Orbit	6	9	7	8	6	7
Trunk	10	NS	NS	9	NS	NS
Others	11	24	30	32	23	19

Note: IRS = Intergroup Rhabdomyosarcoma Study I and II;[1] CWS-81 = German Cooperative Soft Tissue Sarcoma Study;[2] IGR = Institut Gustavy-Roussy;[3] NS = not specified.

[a] $p < 0.05$, comparing infants to older children.

TABLE 6
Clinical Group by Age

	Percent under 1 year old			Percent over 1 year old		
Clinical group	**IRS** **(N = 78)**	**CWS-81** **(N = 21)**	**IGR** **(N = 43)**	**IRS** **(N = 1483)**	**CWS-81** **(N = 325)**	**IGR** **(N = 340)**
I	13	28	30	15	20	31
II	28	14	30	21	14	39
III	47	48	28	44	51	18
IV	12	10	12	19	15	2

Note: IRS = Intergroup Rhabdomyosarcoma Study I and II;[1] CWS-81 = German Cooperative Soft Tissue Sarcoma Study;[2] IGR = Institut Gustavy-Roussy.[3]

TABLE 7
Pathologic Subgroups by Age

	Percent under 1 year old			Percent over 1 year old		
Pathologic type of tumor	**IRS** **(N = 78)**	**CWS-81** **(N = 21)**	**IGR** **(N = 43)**	**IRS** **(N = 1483)**	**CWS-81** **(N = 331)**	**IGR** **(N = 340)**
Embryonal	44	57	53	49	44	44
Botryoid	10[a]	NS	12[b]	4[a]	NS	29[b]
Alveolar	13	10	35[c]	18	15	21[c]
Extraosseous Ewing's	6	NS	EX	5	NS	EX
Undifferentiated sarcoma	18[d]	5	EX	7[d]	5	EX
Others	9	28	0	17	36	6

Note: EX = excluded from study; NS = not specified; IRS = Intergroup Rhabdomyosarcoma Study;[1] CWS-81 = German Cooperative Soft Tissue Sarcoma Study;[2] IGR = Institut Gustavy-Roussy.[3]

[a] $p < 0.005$, comparing infants to older children.
[b] $p < 0.02$, comparing infants to older children.
[c] $p = 0.05$, comparing infants to older children.
[d] $p < 0.0005$, comparing infants to older children.

TABLE 8
Palmer Cytopathologic Classification
by Age Group in IRS-I/II

Pathologic type	Percent under 1 year (N-78)	Percent 1—20 years (N-1483)
Undifferentiated	12	9
Mixed	54	44
Monomorphous	4	4
Anaplastic	5	7
Unclassified	25	36

From Ragab, A. H., Heyn, R., Tefft, M., et al.,
Cancer, 58, 2606, 1986. With permission.

prognosis.[27,28] According to data derived from the IRS and CWS-81 protocols, there is no statistically significant difference between the proportion of cases with the alveolar type in infants and in older children,[1,2] although a higher proportion of cases of alveolar histology was noted in infants treated at the Institut Gustavy-Roussy.[3]

An alternative classification of RMSs has been proposed by Palmer et al. Cytologic features are used to categorize the tumors as monomorphous (unfavorable prognosis), anaplastic (also unfavorable), or mixed.[28] In Table 8, the frequencies of the proposed cytopathologic types of RMSs in infants are compared with the frequencies seen in older children. As shown in this table, there is no difference in the distribution of the monomorphous or anaplastic varieties in the two age groups.

III. DIAGNOSIS

In older children, the presenting signs and symptoms of RMS depend on the site of the primary tumor. This is also true in infants. Orbital tumors may present with proptosis,[21-23] bladder tumors may present with anuria or hydronephrosis,[16] perianal tumors may present with rectal bleeding,[29] and tumors compressing nerves may present with paralysis and irritability.[30] Like older children, infants may present with apparently painless masses. These masses are sometimes even noted immediately at birth.[17,19,20,22,23,25] One newborn presented with respiratory failure due to hypoplastic lungs. This finding was related to *in utero* urine outflow obstruction and massive enlargement of the bladder due to a congenital RMS of the bladder.[15]

When a mass is discovered in an infant, the differential diagnosis may include many of the malignant tumors listed in Table 1. There are also many benign conditions of infancy which may present as a mass, such as benign teratomas, ganglioneuromas, hemangiomas, hematomas, and congenital cysts. Imaging studies may help rule out some of these conditions. When malignancy is suspected, imaging studies to define the size and extent of the tumor are just as important in infants as in older children. Complete workup should include computerized axial tomography or magnetic resonance imaging study of the primary tumor, as well as the pelvis, abdomen, and chest. A skeletal survey (or bone scan) and bone marrow biopsy should be done in cases of suspected RMS. Complete blood count and routine serum chemistry panel (including renal and liver function tests) should be done. Since neuroblastoma is a more common tumor in infants than RMS, the preoperative workup should include catecholamine levels in the urine, in the plasma, or both.

As in the case with older children, obtaining an adequate biopsy specimen for histologic examination is the most essential diagnostic test in infants. Some tumors of infancy, such as stage IV-S neuroblastoma and stage I Wilms' tumor, do not always require the intensive cytotoxic chemotherapy, radiotherapy, or both which are used to treat RMSs.[31,32] In its clinical presentation, a RMS may mimic a neuroblastoma.[30] Because of the increased risks for toxicity when treating infants,[1,33-35] the clinician should make every effort to confirm the diagnosis histologically before committing an infant to chemotherapy or radiation therapy.

IV. TREATMENT

The principles for treating RMSs and related tumors were discussed extensively in an earlier chapter. Only those treatment considerations of particular importance during infancy are reviewed here.

A. SURGERY

The importance of an adequate tissue specimen for diagnosis was previously emphasized. As with older children, complete gross resection of the tumor should be done, when this is technically feasible without incurring excessive risk or causing severe disfigurement. The surgeon and the anesthesiologist should have experience with managing children in this age group, especially in cases of congenital and neonatal tumors.[36]

B. RADIATION THERAPY

Infants are more susceptible to certain adverse effects of radiation therapy than older children.[33] Infants are especially at risk for developing defects related to radiation-induced abnormalities in skeletal growth as compared to older children.[33-37] The human brain is still developing and growing rapidly during infancy; it reaches 90% of the adult brain weight by the end of the first year. Thus, infants who receive central nervous system radiation are at a very high risk to develop mental retardation.[33] Underdevelopment of the aortic arch has been associated with radiation therapy to the thorax.[33] During the first few weeks of life, the kidneys, liver, and lungs may be more sensitive to radiation than they are later in childhood.[33]

In reviewing findings associated with radiation therapy from data generated by IRS-I and IRS-II, it was noted that the dose of radiation therapy delivered to the primary tumor was lower in infants (who were given a dose of 4000 cGy) as compared to the older children (who received 5000 to 6000 cGy).[1] The reasons for withholding radiation therapy in individual cases were not analyzed. However, these observations suggest that infants may have an increased incidence of short-term radiation-induced sequelae, in addition to their higher risk for occurrence of delayed or long-term sequelae previously mentioned.

C. CHEMOTHERAPY

In general, infants do not tolerate chemotherapy as well as older children.[35] Excessive neurotoxicity due to vincristine has been described in infants.[38] Myelosuppression was found to be more profound in infants than in older children who received chemotherapy as part of the National Wilms' Tumor Study (NWTS). This finding prompted the NWTS coordinators to reduce by 50% the chemotherapy dosages for infants.[34] Renal and hepatic metabolism of chemotherapeutic agents is especially undeveloped in neonates;[35] therefore, particular caution should be exercised when treating newborns with congenital malignancies.

As shown in Table 9, infants enrolled in IRS-I and IRS-II did not tolerate chemotherapy as well as older children. Thus, infants did not receive the prescribed full doses of drugs as often as older children.[1] Analysis of findings from IRS-I revealed that there were more deaths attributable to chemotherapy-related toxicity in infants than in older children. This finding resulted in an amendment to the IRS-II protocol in January 1980 in which the initial chemotherapy dosage for infants was reduced by 50%. Prior to the amendment, 4 out of 44

TABLE 9
Percentage of Children Receiving 75—100% of
Chemotherapy Dosage, IRS-I/II

Drug	Percent receiving 100% of dosage		Percent receiving 75—99% of dosage	
	Infants	Older children	Infants	Older children
Doxorubicin	35	55	24	30
Cyclophosphamide	31	32	39	48
Dactinomycin	47	60	28	31
Vincristine	24	37	34	35

From Ragab, A. H., Heyn, R., Tefft, M., et al., *Cancer*, 58, 2606, 1986. With permission.

infants (9.1%) who were treated died due to chemotherapy-related toxicity, and 8 more infants experienced life-threatening toxicity. After the chemotherapy dose was reduced, only 1 out of 34 infants (2.9%) died of toxicity-related complications, and only 3 infants showed life-threatening toxicity. The 9.1% rate of toxic deaths for infants observed prior to this amendment compares unfavorably with the rate of only 1.3% (17 out of 1309) observed in older children.[1]

Infants treated as part of the German CWS-81 protocol had chemotherapy dosages calculated using body weight rather than body surface area. This resulted in dosages 20 to 50% less than dosages based on surface area. No fatal or life-threatening chemotherapy-related toxicities were observed in the 21 infants treated.[2]

V. OUTCOME

For certain tumors, such as Wilms' tumor and neuroblastoma, infants have a better overall prognosis than older children. On the other hand, infants with leukemia have a worse prognosis than older children. Studies done on patients treated prior to the modern era of chemotherapy suggested that infants with RMS had a worse prognosis than older children.[39] However, more recent studies have failed to show any major prognostic significance of young age in RMS.[1-3,11,40-43]

Figure 1 shows the estimated survival rates for 78 infants as compared with 1483 older children who were treated as part of IRS-I and -II. There was no statistically significant difference in the overall survival rates for the two groups (log-rank test).[1] Table 10 gives 3-year Kaplan-Meier survival estimates for each separate clinical group. For group III patients, the infants' 3-year survival rate of 41% was significantly lower than the 62% 3-year survival rate of the older children.[1] There were no statistically significant differences among the other clinical groups. The data in Table 11 suggest that the worse survival in group III patients may be related to a higher risk for local recurrence of tumor. Only 11% of at-risk children who were classified in group III and who were older than 1 year at the time of diagnosis experienced a local recurrence. On the other hand, as many as 29% of the at-risk infants experienced a local recurrence ($p = 0.02$).[1]

Table 11 shows that infants achieve a complete response following initial chemotherapy as often as older children. Table 12, derived from data obtained in IRS-I and IRS-II, shows that chemotherapy-related toxicity can be reduced in infants without compromising the rate of complete responses.[1] This finding was confirmed in the German CWS.[2] Longer follow-up will be needed to determine whether reducing the chemotherapy will eventually result in more tumor recurrences.

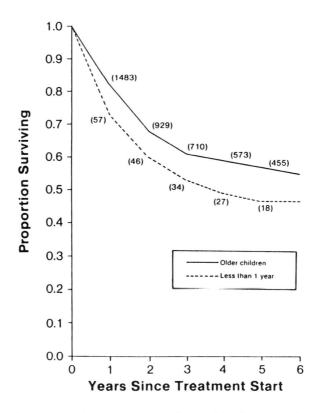

FIGURE 1.   Kaplan-Meier estimates of survival function for 78 infants and 1483 older children studied in IRS-I/II. Numbers in parentheses indicate patients alive at each anniversary. There was no significant difference between the two curves (log-rank test). (From Ragab, A. H., Heyn, R., Tefft, M., et al., *Cancer*, 58, 2606, 1986. With permission.)

TABLE 10
Kaplan-Meier 3-Year Survival Estimates by Age Group, IRS-I/II

Clinical group	Infants		Older children		
	Number	Percent alive at 3 years	Number	Percent alive at 3 years	*p* value[a]
I	10	90	221	88	0.69
II	22	66	314	76	0.48
III	37	41	659	62	0.0002
IV	9	33	289	23	0.66

[a]   Log-rank test, comparing infants to older children.

From Ragab, A. H., Heyn, R., Tefft, M., et al., *Cancer*, 58, 2606, 1986. With permission.

VI. CONCLUSIONS

Treating infants with RMS presents a challenging problem. In general, infants do not have larger or more widespread tumors than older children when they are diagnosed. Other than a possible slightly increased incidence of tumors originating in the urogenital tract,

TABLE 11

**Rate of Complete Response and Local Recurrence by Age
Group in Infants and Children Studied in IRS-I/II**

Clinical group	Infants		Older children	
	Percent CR	Percent LR[a]	Percent CR	Percent LR[a]
I	100	20	100	8
II	100	9	100	7
III	57	29	66	11[b]
IV	44	25	46	13

Note: CR = complete response; LR = local recurrence.

[a] % LR computed among patients who achieved CR.
[b] $p = 0.02$, comparing infants to older children.

From Ragab, A. H., Heyn, R., Tefft, M., et al., *Cancer,* 58, 2606, 1986. With
permission.

TABLE 12

**Rate of Complete Response and Local Recurrence in Infants Studied in
IRS-I/II, before and after Amendment of the Chemotherapy Regimen**

Group	Preamendment			Postamendment		
	Number	Percent CR	Percent LR	Number	Percent CR	Percent LR
I	6	100	17	4	100	25
II	15	100	7	7	100	14
III	18	50	22	19	63	38
IV	5	40	50	4	50	0

Note: CR = complete response; LR = local recurrence; preamendment = prior to January 1980;
postamendment = after January 1980, chemotherapy dosage reduced by 50%.

From Ragab, A. H., Heyn, R., Tefft, M., et al., *Cancer,* 58, 2606, 1986. With permission.

infants do not differ significantly from older children in the distribution of primary tumor
sites. Botryoid histology and undifferentiated sarcoma may occur more frequently in infants,
although this finding was not consistently observed in all studies.

Infants tolerate both chemotherapy and radiation therapy poorly compared to older
children. Initial chemotherapy for infants should be started at 50% of the dosage used for
older children. The dose can then be gradually increased if the drugs are tolerated. The
clinician must give special consideration to therapy-related toxicity in congenital or neonatal
RMS. In contrast to certain other malignancies, the age of less than 1 year is not a significant
overall prognostic factor in RMS. Only with further follow-up of infants treated for RMS
as part of multiinstitutional cooperative studies will we learn whether these children are at
a higher risk for long-term sequelae as compared to older children.

ACKNOWLEDGMENTS

This work was supported in part by NIH Grant CA20549, Cure Foundation of Georgia,
and the Emory University Research Fund. Dr. Ragab is an American Cancer Society Professor
of Clinical Oncology.

REFERENCES

1. **Ragab, A. H., Heyn, R., Tefft, M., et al.,** Infants younger than 1 year of age with rhabdomyosarcoma, *Cancer,* 58, 2606, 1986.
2. **Koscielniak, E., Harms, D., Schmidt, D., et al.,** Soft tissue sarcomas in infants younger than 1 year of age: a report of two German Soft Tissue Sarcoma Study Group (CWS-81), *Med. Pediatr. Oncol.,* 17, 105, 1989.
3. **Salloum, E., Flamant, F., Rey, A., et al.,** Rhabdomyosarcoma in infants under one year of age: experience of the Institut Gustavy-Roussy, *Med. Pediatr. Oncol.,* 17, 424, 1989.
4. **Silverberg, E. and Lubera, J.,** Cancer statistics, 1986, *Ca-A Cancer J. Clin.,* 36, 9, 1986.
5. **Bader, J. L. and Miller, R. W.,** U.S. cancer incidence and mortality in the first year of life, *Am. J. Dis. Child.,* 133, 157, 1979.
6. **Maurer, H. M., Beltangady, M., Gehan, E. A., et al.,** The Intergroup Rhabdomyosarcoma Study-1; a final report, *Cancer,* 61, 209, 1988.
7. **Huang, C.,** Rhabdomyosarcoma involving the genitourinary organs, retroperitoneum and pelvis, *J. Pediatr. Surg.,* 21, 101, 1986.
8. **Sinniah, D., Tan, H. M., Lin, H. P., and Looi, L. M.,** Rhabdomyosarcoma in childhood; a 13-year review from the University Hospital Kuala Lumpur 1967—1980, *Singapore Med. J.,* 22, 158, 1981.
9. **Umar, B. A. and Cederquist, R. A.,** Rhabdomyosarcoma in Nigerian children, *Trop. Geogr. Med.,* 37, 51, 1985.
10. **Hathirat, P., Pipatanakul, S., Pochanugool, L., et al.,** Rhabdomyosarcoma in Thai children, *Southeast Asian J. Trop. Med. Public Health,* 16, 688, 1985.
11. **Kingston, J. E., McElwain, T. J., and Malpas, J. S.,** Childhood rhabdomyosarcoma; experience of the Children's Solid Tumor Group, *Br. J. Cancer,* 48, 195, 1983.
12. **Scholtmeijer, R. J., Tromp, C. G., and Hazebroek, F. W. J.,** Embryonal rhabdomyosarcoma of the urogenital tract in childhood, *Eur. Urol.,* 9, 69, 1983.
13. **Willnow, V. U., Lindner, H., Rothe, K., and Kamprad, F.,** Ergebnisse einer prospektiven studie zur behandlung von rhabdomyosarkomen im kindesalter, *Kinderaerztl. Prax.,* 54, 661, 1986.
14. **Bale, P. M., Parsons, R. E., and Stevens, M.,** Pathology and behavior of juvenile rhabdomyosarcoma, in *Major Problems in Pathology,* Vol. 18, Finegold, M., Ed., W.B. Saunders, Philadelphia, 1986, 196.
15. **Harvey, J. M. and Scott, J. M.,** Neonatal embryonal rhabdomyosarcoma of the bladder, *Scot. Med. J.,* 27, 52, 1982.
16. **Trigueiro, W. S., Chandao, M. M., et al.,** Rhabdomiossarcoma congenito da bexiga-relato de um caso, *Rev. Bras. Circ.,* 69, 261, 1979.
17. **Cohen, M., Ghosh, L., and Schafer, M. E.,** Congenital embryonal rhabdomyosarcoma of the hand and Apert's syndrome, *J. Hand Surg.,* 12A, 614, 1987.
18. **Khan, A., Hoy, G., and Sinks, L. F.,** Unexpected favorable outcome of congenital stage III rhabdomyosarcoma, *Ca-A Cancer J. Clin.,* 30, 189, 1980.
19. **Foet, K. and Prott, W.,** Seltener fall eines angeborenen rhabtomyosarkoms, *Laryng. Rhinol.,* 56, 528, 1977.
20. **Hayashi, Y., Inaba, T., Hanada, R., and Yamanato, K.,** Translocation 2;8 in a congenital rhabdomyosarcoma, *Cancer Genet. Cytogenet.,* 30, 343, 1988.
21. **Basta, L. L., DePersio, E. J., and Brown, R. E.,** Orbital rhabdomyosarcoma in a three week old infant, *J.C.U.,* 4, 205, 1976.
22. **Kubistova, V., Otradovec, J., Koutecky, R., and Kodet, R.,** Rhabdomyosarkom orbity U novorozence, *Cs Oftal.,* 39, 119, 1983.
23. **Ramos-Perea, C., Fernandez-Sein, A., Bonet, N., et al.,** Congenital orbital alveolar rhabdomyosarcoma, *Bol. Asoc. Med. P.R.,* 75, 481, 1983.
24. **Fleischmann, J., Perinetti, E. P., and Catalova, W. J.,** Embryonal rhabdomyosarcoma of the genitourinary organs, *J. Urol.,* 126, 389, 1981.
25. **Zuniga, S., Las Heras, J., and Benveniste, S.,** Rhabdomyosarcoma arising in a congenital giant nevus associated with neurocutaneous melanosis in a neonate, *J. Pediatr. Surg.,* 22, 1036, 1987.
26. **Ruymann, F. B., Maddux, H. R., Ragab, A., et al.,** Congenital anomalies associated with rhabdomyosarcoma; an autopsy study of 115 cases, *Med. Pediatr. Oncol.,* 16, 33, 1988.
27. **Hays, D. M., Newton, W., Soule, E. H., et al.,** Mortality among children with rhabdomyosarcoma of the alveolar histologic subtype, *J. Pediatr. Surg.,* 18, 411, 1983.
28. **Palmer, N. F., Foulkes, M. A., Sachs, N., and Newton, W. A.,** Rhabdomyosarcoma; a cytologic classification of prognostic significance, *Proc. Am. Soc. Clin. Oncol.,* 2, 229, 1983.
29. **Moir, C. R., Dimmick, J. E., and Fraser, G. C.,** Perianal rhabdomyosarcoma; report of a case in an infant, *J. Pediatr. Surg.,* 21, 180, 1986.
30. **Watanabe, I., Ohtomo, S., and Kimura, N.,** Dumbbell type rhabdomyosarcoma in an infant, *J. Pediatr. Surg.,* 9, 407, 1974.

31. **Finklestein, J. Z.,** Neuroblastoma; the challenge and frustration, *Hematol. Oncol. Clin. North Am.,* 1, 675, 1987.
32. **Ganick, D. J.,** Wilms' tumor, *Hematol. Oncol. Clin. North Am.,* 1, 695, 1987.
33. **Littman, P. and D'Angio, G. J.,** Radiation therapy in the neonate, *Am. J. Pediatr. Hematol. Oncol.,* 3, 279, 1981.
34. **Morgan, E., Baum, E., Breslow, N., et al.,** Chemotherapy related toxicity in infants treated according to the 2nd National Wilms' Tumor Study, *J. Clin. Oncol.,* 6, 51, 1988.
35. **Siegal, S. E. and Moran, R. G.,** Problems in the chemotherapy of cancer in the neonate, *Am. J. Pediatr. Hematol. Oncol.,* 3, 287, 1981.
36. **DeLorimier, A. A. and Harrison, M. R.,** Surgical treatment of tumors in the newborn, *Am. J. Pediatr. Hematol. Oncol.,* 3, 271, 1981.
37. **Neuhauser, E. B. D., Wittenborg, M., Berman, L., et al.,** Irradiation effects of roentgen therapy on the growing spine, *Radiology,* 59, 637, 1952.
38. **Allen, J. C.,** The effects of cancer therapy on the nervous system, *J. Pediatr.,* 93, 903, 1978.
39. **Grosfeld, J. L., Clatworthy, H. W., and Newton, W. A.** Combined therapy in childhood rhabdomyosarcoma; an analysis of 42 cases, *J. Pediatr. Surg.,* 4, 637, 1969.
40. **Flamant, F. and Hill, C.,** The improvement in survival associated with combined therapy in childhood rhabdomyosarcoma, *Cancer,* 53, 2417 and 2421, 1984.
41. **Grosfeld, J. L., Weber, T. R., Weetman, R. M., and Baehner, R. L.,** Rhabdomyosarcoma in childhood; analysis of survival of 98 cases, *J. Pediatr. Surg.,* 18, 141, 1983.
42. **Harms, D., Schmidt, D., and Treuner, J.,** Soft tissue sarcomas in childhood; a study of 262 cases including 169 cases of rhabdomyosarcoma, *Z. Kinderchir.,* 40, 140, 1985.
43. **Pedrick, T. J., Donaldson, S. S., and Cox, R. S.,** Rhabdomyosarcoma; the Stanford experience using a TNM staging system, *J. Clin. Oncol.,* 4, 370, 1986.

Chapter 23

PATHOLOGY OF SOFT TISSUE SARCOMAS IN CHILDREN AND ADOLESCENTS

Paul E. Swanson and Louis P. Dehner

TABLE OF CONTENTS

I. INTRODUCTION

Rhabdomyosarcoma represents the most common and important of the soft tissue malignancies that afflict children. However, nonrhabdomyomatous sarcomas occurring in the young constitute a histologic spectrum no less diverse than that seen in adults, and, when considered together, these tumors represent nearly half of all pediatric sarcomas.[1-6] Of course, no one tumor within this spectrum is as common as rhabdomyosarcoma. Nevertheless, accurate recognition and management of these tumors in children may not only benefit the patients, but may also provide insights into the pathogenesis and treatment of similar tumors in adults. Hence, a summary of their salient pathological and clinical features is warranted here. This overview will emphasize the application of electron microscopy and immuno-histochemistry as adjuncts in the diagnosis of these soft tissue sarcomas. The expected immunohistochemical findings are summarized in Table 1.

As in adults, younger children and adolescents may occasionally have a soft tissue lesion that simulates a malignancy in its histologic features. There are also soft tissue tumors that represent a bona fide neoplasm whose benign clinical behavior belies its degree of cellularity and mitotic activity. Examples of such malignant-appearing, benign-behaving neoplasms include congenital-infantile fibrosarcoma and hemangiopericytoma.

The major histogenetic or phenotypic categories of soft tissue sarcomas in adults are malignant fibrous histiocytoma, liposarcoma, fibrosarcoma, and malignant peripheral nerve sheath tumor (neurofibrosarcoma). Together, these clinical entities comprise less than 1% of all cancers in adults.[7,8] In contrast, soft tissue sarcomas account for about 6 to 10% of all malignancies in children.[1-6,8-12]

The lower extremity is the primary site for 40 to 45% of soft tissue sarcomas in adults. The remaining tumors occur in the retroperitoneum (30 to 35% of cases), upper extremity (12 to 15%), and the head and neck (8 to 10%).[8] Except for Ewing's sarcoma and the primitive neuroectodermal tumors, the regional distribution of "adult-type" sarcomas in childhood is similar to the occurrence of these tumors in adults.[4,5,9,12-14]

Finally, the clinical behavior of these neoplasms is comparable in adults and children, when tumor size, histologic grade, and degree of resectability are commensurate.[4,11] As noted previously, fibrosarcoma in infancy is an exception to this generalization. Similarly, certain pathologic variants or subtypes of the more common sarcomas in adults, malignant fibrous histiocytoma and liposarcoma in particular, may show both a predilection to younger patients and a more favorable prognosis.[2-4]

II. FIBROHISTIOCYTIC NEOPLASMS

There is usually little difficulty in the histologic recognition of most fibrous-appearing tumors in children.[4,13,15,16] However, considerable debate continues concerning the histogenesis of these predominantly spindle cell neoplasms. By convention, tumors with spindled or epithelioid cell features that are accompanied by histiocyte-like elements are regarded as "fibrous histiocytomas", even though the spindled cells show the ultrastructural and immunohistochemical attributes of fibroblasts or myofibroblasts.[17-22] The presence of proteolytic enzymes, such as α-1-antichymotrypsin, characterizes the histiocytic elements in these tumors, but immunoreactivity for these substances clearly is not specific for such lesions.[20,23] Fibrous histiocytomas of skin (dermatofibroma) or superficial soft tissues, and certain so-called "epithelioid" histiocytomas are generally allied with various fibrohistiocytic malignancies of superficial and deep soft tissues. These include malignant fibrous histiocytoma, atypical fibroxanthoma, and dermatofibrosarcoma protuberans.

Benign fibrous histiocytomas, although usually cytologically bland, may occasionally infiltrate adjacent soft tissues, and thus may recur after excision. Furthermore, exceptional

TABLE 1
Idealized[a] Immunophenotypes in Childhood Sarcomas

Tumor	Vim	Des	Act	CK	EMA	HMB	S100	L7	NSE	Snp	UEA	F8
Spindled-pleomorphic tumors												
Fibrosarcoma	+	0	0	0	0	0	0	0	0	0	0	0
Malignant fibrous histiocytoma	+	0	+/−	0	0	0	0	0	0	0	0	0
Leiomyosarcoma	+	+	+	0	0	0	0	0	0	0	0	0
Angiosarcoma	+	0	0	0	0	0	0	0	0	0	+/−	+/−
Epithelioid sarcoma	+	0	0	+	+	0	0	0	0	0	+/−	0
Synovial sarcoma	+	0	0	+	+	0	+	+/−	0	0	0	0
Chordoma	+	0	0	+	+	0	+	+/−	0	0	0	0
Malignant peripheral nerve sheath tumor	+	0	0	0	0	0	+	+	+/−	0	0	0
Clear cell sarcoma	+	0	0	0	0	+	+	+/−	+/−	0	0	0
Small cell neoplasms												
Rhabdomyosarcoma	+	+	+	0	0	0	0	+/−	0	0	0	0
Peripheral neuroectodermal tumor	+	0	0	0	0	0	0	+/−	+	+	0	0
Ewing's sarcoma	+	0	0	0	0	0	0	0	+/−	0	0	0
Mesenchymal chondrosarcoma	+	0	0	0	0	0	+[b]	+	+	0	0	0

Abbreviations: Vim = vimentin; Des = Desmin; Act = muscle-specific actin; CK = cytokeratin; EMA = epithelial membrane antigen; S100 = S100 protein; L7 = Leu-7 antigen; HMB = HMB45 antigen; NSE = neuron-specific enolase; UEA = *Ulex europaeus I* agglutinin; F8 = factor VIII-related antigen.

[a] Minor patterns of reactivity, for instance, S100 protein, Leu-7 antigen, cytokeratin, or epithelial membrane antigen in leiomyosarcoma, are excluded from the table, unless they are sufficiently common or worrisome to merit comment. Important patterns present in less than 30% of cases are reported as "+/−". Reactivity in 30% or more cases are "+", while those reactive in fewer than 10% (unless vital to the immunophenotypic separation) are labeled "0".

[b] S100 protein in chondroid foci only.

instances occur in which cytologic atypia provokes concern about the prognosis, but abundance of mitotic activity does not usually characterize these lesions.[8] It is important to note that it is the latter cytological feature, increased mitotic activity, which more accurately predicts clinical behavior in most instances. The storiform and plexiform variants of fibrous histiocytoma are of some interest in this context. The storiform variant, because of the histologic pattern which gives its name to the lesion, may be mistaken for architecturally and histologically similar malignant fibrous histiocytomas. Plexiform fibrohistiocytic tumors, in contrast, bear some resemblance to plexiform neurofibromas.[24] Misinterpretation may thus result in a diagnosis with unwarranted implications for neurofibromatosis, which carries an attendant risk for malignant degeneration.

The upper and lower extremities are the principal sites for plexiform fibrohistiocytic tumors, and most such lesions are diagnosed in the first two decades of life. A superficial location in the deeper dermis or subcutis, and a tumoral size of 3 cm or less account in part for the favorable prognosis usually associated with this tumor. Plexiform nodules of spindled cells, occasionally admixed with multinucleated cells, are the characteristic histological features. Local recurrence is reported in 35 to 40% of cases of plexiform fibrohistiocytic tumors, but their metastatic potential is very low.[24]

Aggressive or overtly malignant fibrohistiocytic neoplasms are comparatively uncommon in childhood. The prototypic lesion in this class is malignant fibrous histiocytoma (MFH), a tumor usually occurring in the deep soft tissues or retroperitoneum of adults.[8,25-27] Fewer than 5% of all cases occur in children, and these are most likely to arise in the second decade of life.[3,4,12,25,28,29] In contrast to MFHs in adults, these lesions in children more often affect the soft tissues of the head and neck. In exceptional cases, this tumor presents as the second malignancy in children who have survived their first tumor.[4] The gross pathologic appearance of MFH is that of a firm, fibrous mass that is either sharply circumscribed but nonencapsulated, or is poorly demarcated from adjacent tissues. Areas of tumoral hemorrhage may be prominent, and some lesions have a predominantly myxoid appearance on cut sections.[8,25,27]

Histologically, five distinct patterns of MFH are recognized,[8,25,27] each of which may occur in children.[4,28-30] These histologic patterns of MFH are storiform-pleomorphic, myxoid (in which a loose myxoid matrix supports spindled or pleomorphic cells) (Figure 1), giant cell (wherein multinucleated cells are admixed with pleomorphic elements), inflammatory (with numerous intratumoral inflammatory cells, principally neutrophils, obscuring the typical storiform-pleomorphic pattern), and angiomatoid. Some MFHs display more than one pattern,[8,25] but generally a neoplasm can be characterized by its dominant pattern. Tumors with a prominent storiform or myxoid pattern, of relatively small size (less than 2.5 cm), and which contain elements of inflammation are usually cured by complete excision.[8,25,27] However, even in children, distant metastases to the lung, liver, and lymph nodes and tumor-related deaths may sometimes occur.[4]

The angiomatoid variant of MFH is peculiar in that it typically presents in children, nearly three fourths of cases being diagnosed in the first decade of life, and most tumors arise in the upper extremities.[4,8,31,32] There is a tendency for the patients to present with constitutional symptoms of weight loss and fever. Lymphadenopathy, together with systemic manifestations similar to Castleman's disease (fever, anemia, and lymphoid hyperplasia), has also been observed.[33] Similar constitutional symptoms have been encountered in children with an inflammatory myofibroblastic tumor (see below).

The distinguishing pathological features of the angiomatoid type of MFH are the conspicuous cystic or cleft-like blood-filled spaces. These blood lakes are not lined by endothelium, hence the term "angiomatoid", but rather the lakes abut cellular neoplastic foci composed of spindled and histiocytoid cells. A reactive lymphoid infiltrate and hemosiderin are usually prominent at the periphery, which occasionally causes the mass to be confused

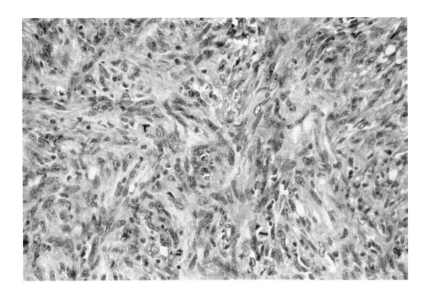

FIGURE 1. MFH. Spindled cells interweave haphazardly in a storiform pattern. Atypical mitotic figures are present.

with a partially effaced lymph node.[8,31] These tumors may recur locally, but they only rarely metastasize. Thus, the designation of "malignant" is overstated in a sense. The differential diagnosis of the angiomatoid MFH includes a variety of vascular neoplasms. However, it also has certain histologic features in common with another variant of benign fibrous histiocytoma, the so-called angiomatoid fibrous histiocytoma.[34] The latter tumor lacks the prominent lymphoid infiltrate typical of the angiomatoid variant of MFH, and is cytologically bland. Nevertheless, the gross appearances of the two tumors may be remarkably similar. In turn, angiomatoid fibrous histiocytoma, due to its location in the dermis, has been mistaken for Kaposi's sarcoma.[8,34,35]

Although each variant of MFH may be found in superficial soft tissues, there are two distinct fibrohistiocytic "malignancies" that characteristically involve these tissues primarily. The first, the atypical fibroxanthoma, is histologically similar in most respects to MFH, except that it is centered on the dermis and only secondarily infiltrates superficial soft tissues.[8,18,36] Despite their marked cytologic atypia and mitotic activity, these lesions generally remain confined to dermal tissues. They may recur locally after excision, but usually do not metastasize.

Similarly, the dermatofibrosarcoma protuberans is a cytologically bland but mitotically active lesion that shows only locally aggressive behavior.[4,8,37] Unlike both atypical fibroxanthoma and MFH, dermatofibrosarcoma protuberans is composed of a relatively uniform spindle cell population that is arranged in densely cellular fascicles. These fascicles interweave haphazardly, forming the classic storiform pattern. Unlike most benign fibrohistiocytic lesions, dermatofibrosarcoma protuberans shows an irregular or ragged infiltration of adjacent dermis and may invade underlying subcutis. This tumor infrequently presents in late childhood or adolescence, and usually arises on the trunk.[8,37] Atypical fibroxanthoma very rarely occurs in children, but like its adult counterpart is seen in the head and neck region.

III. FIBROUS-MYOFIBROBLASTIC NEOPLASMS

The clinical and pathologic diversity of the various entities included in the category of (myo)fibroblastic tumors or fibromatoses is the source of confusion. There is uncertainty with regard to the appropriate treatment as well as prognosis after therapy, since the natural history of these tumors is often unpredictable.[4,8,15] Such lesions evoke considerable alarm because of their presence in infancy, their occasional multifocality, and their tendency to present as large, often hypercellular and mitotically active lesions.[4,8]

The common feature in these lesions is the presence of spindle cells with the ultrastructural and immunohistochemical features of myofibroblasts. These cells contain abundant rough endoplasmic reticulum, cytoplasmic microfilaments which are interrupted occasionally by dense bodies, plasmalemmal plaques, and pinocytotic vesicles.[8] The degree of myogenous differentiation varies, and some lesions are dominated by cells with fibroblastic qualities. As a result, these lesions are strongly immunoreactive for vimentin,[20,38] while the intensity and extent of reactivity for muscle-specific actins are dependent upon the degree of myofibroblastic differentiation.[20] Compared to normal myofibroblasts and smooth muscle cells, they are less likely to contain detectable amounts of desmin, although focal reactivity may be observed. In further distinction to the smooth muscle tumors to be discussed, markers often associated with neural neoplasms, such as S100 protein and Leu-7 antigen, are also lacking.[20,21]

Although clinically and pathologically worrisome, there are several tumors consisting of myofibroblastic proliferations that are reactive or inflammatory in nature. These tumors may regress without surgery. Examples of such reactive proliferations are nodular fascitis, proliferative myositis, and cranial and intravascular fascitis.[8,39-46] Lesions that are inflammatory in nature are represented by somatic and visceral mesenchymal lesions collectively known as inflammatory myofibroblastic tumors. The fascitides are similar in histologic appearance. They are formed of loosely woven or whorled fascicles of spindled cells which have infiltrated adjacent structures, including soft tissues, lung, or bowel wall.[4,8,39,42] Erosion into underlying bone, as in the case of cranial fascitis, is a worrisome feature, but it does not imply malignant potential.

The inflammatory myofibroblastic tumor may develop rapidly, sometimes with a history of antecedent trauma. However, more often this tumor evolves insidiously, with constitutional symptoms of several weeks or months duration.[4,8,47] Most tumors present as a circumscribed fibrous or fibromyxoid mass measuring 3 to 4 cm in diameter, or in some cases the tumor may be considerably larger, being in excess of 10 to 12 cm in size, arising in visceral or abdominal sites. Microscopically, spindle cells predominate, and a storiform or fascicular pattern is often present. In focal areas, stromal myxoid changes impart a nodular fasciitis-like appearance. A lymphoplasmacytic infiltrate is especially prominent; single cells or clusters may be intimately admixed with the spindled elements. Inflammatory cells may also be present in myxoid areas, accompanied by extravasated erythrocytes. Fibrogenic foci are more or less conspicuous; these areas are hypocellular and show minimal inflammation.[4,47] Dystrophic calcification and even metaplastic bone are present in a minority of cases.[8] Mitotic activity, as in the other fascitides,[8,39] may be seen, particularly in cellular foci. However, atypical mitotic figures are lacking.[8,47]

The differential diagnosis from the perspective of these histologic findings includes MFH and leiomyosarcoma. The amelioration or disappearance of constitutional abnormalities, such as anemia, fever, weight loss, and hypergammaglobulinemia (when present), following resection of the tumor serves as an important clue to the diagnosis. It is strongly suspected that inflammatory cells in such cases are elaborating cytokines, such as IL-1 or IL-6, each of which may induce the characteristic symptoms and signs.[47]

The (myo)fibromatoses, as a group, are generally benign lesions. Nonetheless, certain examples, either because of their anatomic location or their histologic features, may be difficult to separate in some cases from overtly malignant neoplasms. The tumors of infancy, referred to as "generalized congenital fibromatosis" and "infantile (diffuse) myofibromatosis", are two such examples.[4,40,48-50] Each of these lesions shares the typical histology of the other forms of fibromatoses, including relatively uniform spindle cells forming broad bands and irregularly intersecting fascicles. However, these lesions occasionally show variable mitotic activity and divergent chondro-osseous differentiation.[4,8,49,50]

Despite these features, the long-term outcome of solitary lesions is benign.[40,48-50] The prognosis is less favorable for patients who have generalized congenital fibromatoses, especially when there is major visceral involvement. A less indolent lesion, the so-called aggressive or musculoaponeurotic fibromatosis (desmoid tumor), may uncommonly arise in children, often in association with Gardner's syndrome.[4,8,51] Unlike other fibromatoses, desmoid tumors actively infiltrate soft tissues and show a relatively high rate of recurrence.

Two entities that are unique to skin or superficial soft tissue have certain features which overlap those of the myofibromatoses. Both of these lesions may be confused with a non-myofibroblastic malignancy.

The first of these, the so-called infantile or congenital hemangiopericytoma, is a multinodular lesion in the subcutis which is usually diagnosed at birth or shortly thereafter.[4,8,52,53] Typically, this tumor is comprised mainly of spindled cells. The most recognizable feature is the presence of anastomosing and "staghorn" vascular spaces, otherwise indistinguishable from the adult-type hemangiopericytoma, that separate groups of neoplastic cells. Ultrastructural findings suggest that most such lesions in the subcutis, unlike true hemangiopericytomas of deep soft tissues, are composed of myofibroblast-like elements.[4,53] Most congenital hemangiopericytomas are relatively cellular, exhibit nuclear pleomorphism, and have several mitoses. They irregularly infiltrate adjacent soft tissue and may undergo spontaneous necrosis and regression.[52] Because of the vascular pattern which in part characterizes them, these lesions are potentially misdiagnosed as synovial sarcoma, leiomyosarcoma, and even mesenchymal chondrosarcoma. Nonetheless, these tumors behave in a uniformly benign fashion.

The second lesion is the giant cell fibroblastoma.[54,55] Over half of the cases occur in children less than 5 years of age. Giant cell fibroblastomas usually present as a slow-growing, small nodular subcuticular or deep dermal nodule that is often fixed to overlying skin. Histologically, this tumor is typified by the presence of richly cellular foci that alternate with less cellular sclerotic areas, as well as foci in which dissection of collagen by infiltrating cells imparts a sinusoidal appearance. The cells are elongate, slender, and spindled in shape, and the nuclei are uniformly fusiform or ovoid. The cells are either arranged in loose fascicles or they haphazardly permeate stromal collagen. In myxoid areas, tumor cells may show a more irregular or stellate appearance.

Finally, giant cell fibroblastoma, as its name implies, contains variable numbers of large pleomorphic spindled or multinucleated cells.[55] The stellate and pleomorphic cells may resemble those seen in atypical fibroxanthoma, and myxoid changes may be similar to those of MFH or liposarcoma. However, it is the dissection of collagen that evokes the greatest concern, since Kaposi's sarcoma and other vascular neoplasms may occasionally exhibit such behavior. Nonetheless, giant cell fibroblastoma is uniformly benign.[54,55] The ultrastructural or immunohistochemical demonstration of myofibroblastic or fibroblastic features in some instances qualifies the inclusion of this tumor with other childhood fibromatoses.

Myofibroblastic tumors of indeterminant biologic behavior exist only by convention. Indeed, the tumor most often cited in this context is a lesion that the authors regard as a very low grade myofibroblastic malignancy. This tumor is variously referred to as infantile/congenital fibrosarcoma and congenital fibrosarcoma-like fibromatosis.[4,56-60] This lesion usually presents as a solitary deeply situated soft tissue mass in the trunk, extremity, or abdomen of a child less than 1 year of age. Involvement of viscera or mucosal surfaces has also been noted.[4] Moreover, it has been questioned whether the low grade (myo)fibroblastic neoplasms of the tracheobronchial tree in children represent a similar or identical neoplastic process.[61]

These tumors may attain considerable size (Figure 2A), measuring 10 to 15 cm and essentially occupying an entire extremity or a major portion of the limb.[4,56] The macroscopic appearance is similar to the fibromatoses already described, although cystic or myxoid stromal changes may be evident, and tumoral necrosis may occur.[4] The histologic features differ substantially from other fibromatoses in terms of cellularity, mitotic activity, and paucity of a collagenous stroma. The cells are compact, ovoid or spindle-shaped, and are often arranged in tightly interweaving fascicles, or they may have a herringbone pattern which is typical of the adult-type fibrosarcoma (Figure 2B). Conspicuous cytologic atypia is almost never present, but nuclear pleomorphism, increased mitotic activity, and focal tumoral necrosis indicate the potential malignant nature of this neoplasm.[4]

Classification of these tumors as being of indeterminate malignancy is based on their indolent behavior, exclusive of their large size. There are isolated instances of spontaneous regression, but in most cases infantile fibrosarcoma has the potential for local recurrence, and rarely for pulmonary or other distant metastases.[4,62] There are no reliable markers to identify with consistency those lesions with the potential for aggressive behavior.[4]

Occasionally, adult-type fibrosarcomas occur in children, usually in children over 5 years of age.[4,8,59,60] These tumors behave in a manner analogous to the same neoplasms in adults. Thus, prognostic indices of size, histologic grade, and resectability are applicable in these cases. However, because of the close histologic resemblance between the adult fibrosarcoma and congenital fibrosarcoma, distinguishing between the two tumors may be particularly difficult in very young children, those less than 5 years of age. The lack of metastases in the overwhelming majority of young patients with "fibrosarcoma" raises the question of whether they are in fact truly different from fibrosarcoma of adults. However, in older children the distinction is immediately evident, since as many as half of the patients who are 10 years or older develop metastases.[4,59]

IV. SMOOTH MUSCLE NEOPLASMS

Benign smooth muscle tumors are especially rare in children. Leiomyosarcomas are nearly as uncommon, particularly when lesions associated with visceral are excluded.[4,63] In a series of 12 leiomyosarcomas in children, only one tumor arose in soft tissues.[64] Fewer than 30 other cases have been reported.[1,4,63-65] Even in adults, soft tissue leiomyosarcomas are quite uncommon. The tumors tend to occur in major arteries or veins and have a poor prognosis.[8,65]

The authors recently observed six primary soft tissue leiomyosarcomas whose histologic, immunophenotypic, and ultrastructural features closely paralleled those of the tumor in adults.[66] Most of the tumors are firm, lobulated masses located in deep soft tissues, and have a soft consistency. They have a whorled or fibrous appearance on cut section. The histologic features vary somewhat, since mildly pleomorphic spindle cells (Figure 3A) may be admixed with or completely replaced by epithelioid cells (Figure 3B). Myxoid changes may be prominent in some areas, and tumoral necrosis is relatively common. Cytologic atypia alone does not imply malignancy, since marked atypia may occur in benign leiomyosarcomas undergoing degeneration. On the other hand, the presence of more than two mitoses per ten high power fields usually predicts aggressive behavior.[63-66]

The separation of leiomyosarcoma from other spindle cell sarcomas may be difficult at times, but ancillary diagnostic techniques are generally quite helpful. Compared to myofibroblastic proliferations, smooth muscle tumors have appreciably less rough endoplasmic reticulum, whereas contractile elements (microfilaments interrupted by dense bodies) and plasmalemmal plaques are more conspicuous. Pinocytosis is present, as in other contractile cells, and a partial basal lamina may be elaborated[21,66-68] (Figure 3D). Immunohistochemically, most leiomyosarcomas are positive for vimentin and muscle-specific actin, and unlike the myofibromatoses, this tumor generally stains for desmin as well[19-21,38,66-69] (Figure 3C).

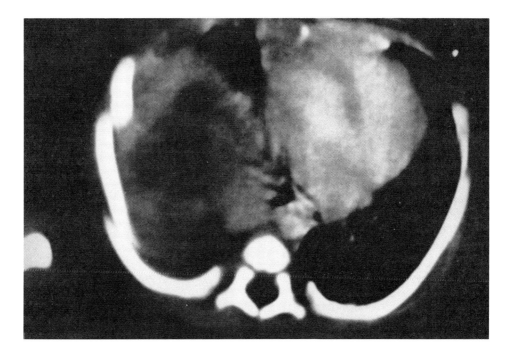

A

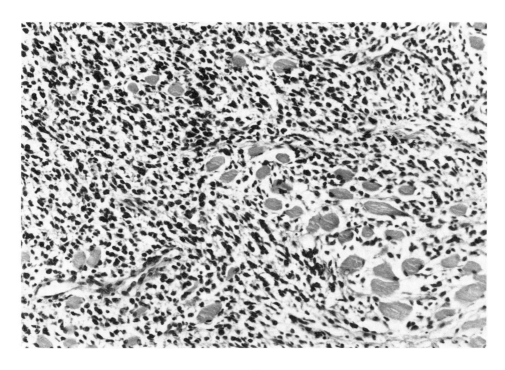

B

FIGURE 2. Congenital fibrosarcoma. These tumors may attain considerable size, as shown by computed tomography of a massive chest wall and intrathoracic lesions (A). The neoplastic cells are compact, ovoid, forming clusters that diffusely infiltrate adjacent soft tissues (B).

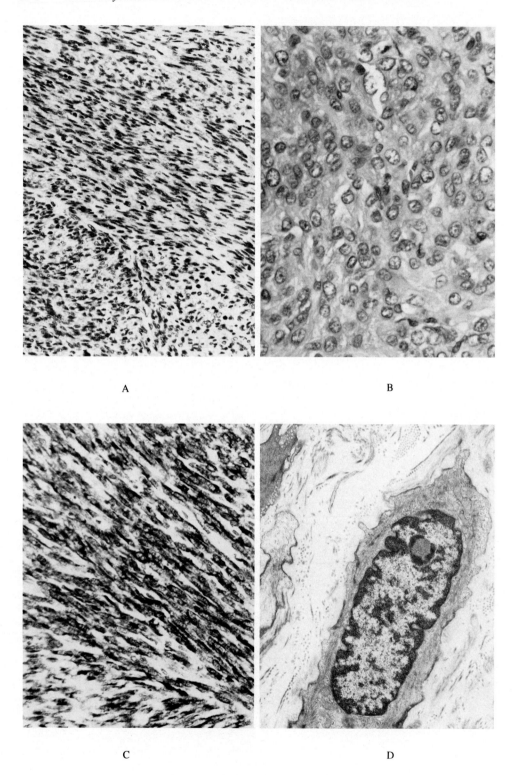

FIGURE 3.   Leiomyosarcoma. Spindle cells in interweaving fascicles are typical (A), although occasional examples are dominated by plump epithelioid cells (B). Immunoreactivity for desmin is usually demonstrable (C). Electron microscopy reveals cells with abundant cytoplasmic filaments interrupted by dense bodies, plasmalemmal plaques, pinocytosis, and an incomplete basal lamina (D).

Occasional cases of embryonal rhabdomyosarcoma may have a striking spindle cell pattern reminiscent of leiomyosarcoma. Tumors with this atypical appearance are especially notable in the paratesticular region. A myxoid background, the presence of scattered polygonal cells with eosinophilic cytoplasm, together with the patient's symptoms and clinical findings should suggest the correct diagnosis. As mentioned earlier in this book (see Chapter 2 on histopathology of rhabdomyosarcoma), presence of organized thick and thin filaments in the cytoplasm and the demonstration of myoglobin are ultrastructural and immunohistochemical findings which help to confirm the rhabdomyogenic nature of such atypical tumors.[70]

The invasive behavior of childhood leiomyosarcoma is intermediate, compared to malignant nerve sheath tumors, synovial sarcoma, and MFH.[4,8] In contrast, leiomyosarcomas of superficial soft tissues and skin are relatively indolent neoplasms.[8,65,68] Such tumors are especially rare in children; fewer than ten cases have been reported.[65,66] As in adults, cutaneous leiomyosarcomas may be primarily dermal or subcuticular proliferations. Varying degrees of pleomorphism, mitotic activity, and tumoral necrosis may be seen in such tumors. However, the single most important predictor of behavior is the presence of subcuticular involvement. Among these deeper lesions, there is an increased risk of recurrence of metastasis. In contrast, tumors confined to the dermis rarely if ever show local or regional extension.[8,65,68]

One peculiar aspect of smooth muscle tumors in children is their association with immunodeficient states. The authors observed a mesenteric leiomyosarcoma in a young child who was immunosuppressed for maintenance of a renal allograft.[66] Another leiomyosarcoma was seen in a child recovering from leukemia.[71] Another study described the occurrence of smooth muscle tumors in three children infected with human immunodeficiency virus (HIV); two patients had leiomyosarcomas and the third had multiple leiomyomas of the lung.[72] Kaposi's sarcoma is also known to arise in association with HIV infection, but whether other sarcomas may be more common in these patients remains to be shown.

V. ALVEOLAR SOFT PART SARCOMA

Alveolar soft part sarcoma (ASPS) is a tumor whose phenotype remains an enigma. However, recent studies suggest that this tumor is in fact a skeletal muscle-like neoplasm.[8,20,73,74] Clinically, ASPS is a peculiar lesion because of (1) its tendency to occur in children, most patients being in their first two decades of life, and (2) because of its female preponderance. Usually this tumor arises in the extremities or head and neck region,[8,75] the orbit being a well-documented site in the latter area.[76] Perhaps because of its location in extremity sites, a size greater than 5 cm is often attained before detection. This fact is important, since larger lesions tend to behave in a more aggressive fashion. Overall, ASPS is an indolent, but relentlessly progressive tumor that recurs over a period of 10 to 20 years before metastases to the lung, bone, or brain become apparent.[4,8,75,76]

The macroscopic appearance is that of a well-circumscribed, but nonencapsulated, gray or yellow mass that involves muscle or deep soft tissues. Histologically, the tumor is composed of large, remarkably bland, polygonal cells that are arranged in loosely cohesive spaces or alveoli, supported by a richly vascular matrix.[8,73,75,76] Abundant clear or granular eosinophilic cytoplasm is punctuated by numerous crystals. These crystals are reactive with the periodic acid-Schiff stain[8,73] and show a consistent periodicity when studied by electron microscopy.[21,73,74] The presence of these crystals is characteristic of ASPS, but they are not always readily identified. Otherwise, electron microscopy is not particularly helpful since neither neuroectodermal features nor elements of a contractile apparatus are evident.[73,74] Nevertheless, immunohistochemical findings support the myogenic nature of ASPS by revealing desmin intermediate filaments, as well as actin isoforms and other contractile-related moieties.[20,73,74]

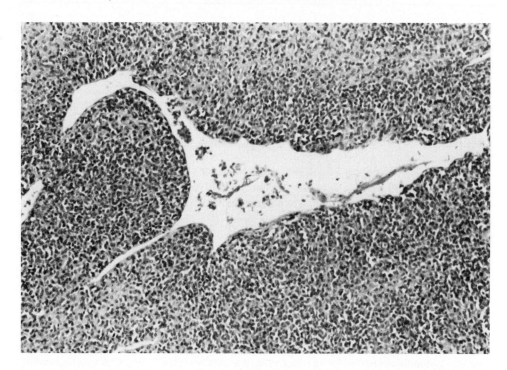

FIGURE 4. Hemangiopericytoma. Large, branching "staghorn" vessels compartmentalize relatively uniform ovoid-spindle cells.

Because of its alveolar pattern, ASPS may be confused with alveolar rhabdomyosarcoma. Both tumors affect the same age group in children and have primary sites in common. Several important histologic features differentiate alveolar rhabdomyosarcoma from ASPS. Alveolar-like structures are less well developed in alveolar rhabdomyosarcoma, cellular atypia is more pronounced, a diffuse growth pattern is more apparent, and multinucleated cells are characteristic.

VI. HEMANGIOPERICYTOMA

The last category of neoplasms considered "myogenic" is the hemangiopericytoma. These tumors often appear to be more closely allied with vascular neoplasms than they are to lesions of pericytes or smooth muscle. Nevertheless, both the histologic pattern and ultrastructural appearances of the hemangiopericytoma suggest pericytic differentiation.[8,77,78]

Benign and malignant forms of this tumor have been observed in children, although each form is only anecdotal in frequency. The histologic features of hemangiopericytoma are relatively uniform and, as a result, do not accurately predict clinical behavior.[78-80] Most cases are composed of a monotonous pattern of spindled or epithelioid cells that are intimately associated with, and are separated into compartments by, nonneoplastic capillaries and small venules. These venules are often larger, irregularly branched, and show the characteristic "staghorn" configuration[8,78] (Figure 4). Actually, the vascular component itself is not regarded as the neoplastic constituent. Even so, the term "hemangiopericytoma-like" has been applied to a similar vascular pattern in such diverse tumors as synovial sarcoma, MFH, leiomyosarcoma, and mesenchymal chondrosarcoma.[81]

Cytologic atypia and mitotic activity are generally sparse in hemangiopericytomas. Tumoral necrosis may be evident, even in clinically benign lesions, and divergent mesenchymal differentiation may also be observed. In some cases, malignant behavior may be predicted from the presence of overt cytologic atypia or the appearance of atypical mitoses.

However, the most reliable indicators of malignancy are locally infiltrative growth of the tumor and the presence of metastasis.[78,79]

VII. PERIPHERAL NEUROGENIC NEOPLASMS

Peripheral nerve sheath tumors are a diverse group of neoplasms that exhibit perineurial, Schwann cell-like, or complex mesenchymal patterns of differentiation.[4,8] The malignant transformation of a benign form of this tumor is thought to be a fairly common phenomenon in patients with neurofibromatosis. However, such transformation may also occur very rarely as a sporadic event in both children and adults.[4,82] The classic soft tissue neoplasm of neurofibromatosis is the plexiform neurofibroma,[8] but apart from its transformation to a malignancy in 10 to 15% of cases, the histologic and clinical features of most such tumors are unequivocally benign. Two other peripheral nerve sheath tumors, each apparently quite benign in behavior, are nonetheless difficult to separate histologically from malignant neoplasms. These will be briefly discussed.

The first of these tumors is the so-called dermal nerve sheath myxoma or neurothekeoma.[8,83] This neoplasm is usually found in the superficial soft tissues and dermis, but it is also occasionally encountered in submucosal locations. It is seen most commonly during childhood or early adulthood. The tumor presents as a multinodular mass in the upper trunk or head and neck region.[83] Typically, a neurothekeoma is formed of discrete cell clusters separated by loose, cellular fibrous septae. The neoplastic cells may be spindled or epithelioid, but in general they are arranged in fascicles or whorls in a myxoid stroma. When the myxoid stroma is inconspicuous, or when epithelioid cells predominate, neurothekeoma may be confused with epithelioid fibrohistiocytic tumors. In most cases, however, the overall pattern is more similar to that of a myxoid plexiform neurofibroma.

Perhaps the most ominous aspect of neurothekeoma is the presence of mitotic activity. Although cellular atypia is not usually seen, proliferative activity may impose a resemblance to low grade myxoid sarcomas of the nerve sheath.[8,83] However the circumscription of neurothekeoma, its lack of association with large nerves, and the infrequency of malignant peripheral nerve sheath tumors in skin and subcutis are features which suggest the proper diagnosis.

Another distinct variant of peripheral nerve sheath tumors consists of cellular foci of compact fusiform cells arranged in a neurotactoid, fascicular, herringbone, or storiform pattern (Figure 5). This tumor has been called "cellular schwannoma" when observed in adult patients,[84,85] or "cellular peripheral neural tumor" in pediatric cases.[86] However, these neoplasms lack the characteristic Antoni A and Antoni B areas of a typical schwannoma. Cellular peripheral neural tumors may exhibit pronounced cytologic atypia and even a limited degree of mitotic activity.[84-86] The cells have the ultrastructural features of Schwann cells, consisting of spindle cells with multiple interdigitating cell processes and with cell junctions at points of apposition. However, there is some disagreement as to whether this tumor shows immunoreactivity for S100 protein or Leu-7 antigen as frequently as other benign peripheral nerve sheath tumors.[84,85]

Cellular peripheral neural tumors are most often encountered in the mediastinum and retroperitoneum, as well as in paravertebral areas. Thus, they may grow to a relatively large size. Despite initial concerns that they were in fact low grade malignancies of the peripheral nerve sheath, subsequent clinicopathologic studies have shown their indolent behavior in the majority of cases.[84,86]

Malignant peripheral nerve sheath tumors are relatively common in adults, and occur in four major settings. They may occur in patients with neurofibromatosis (which represents less than half of all such lesions),[4,8,87] they may occur in patients who do not have the stigmata of neurofibromatosis,[87] they may occur following exposure to ionizing radiation,[87,88]

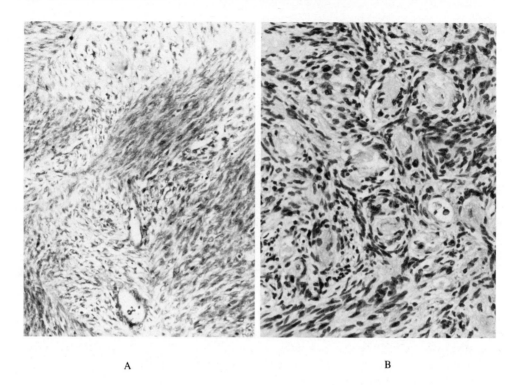

A   B

FIGURE 5.   Cellular peripheral neural tumor. Compactly cellular bundles of spindle cells distinguish this lesion from ordinary peripheral nerve sheath tumors (A). In areas, neurotactoid differentiation may be seen (B).

and they may occur in association with tumors of the adrenal medulla.[87] Lesions occurring in association with neurofibromatosis are more likely to occur in younger individuals. Nonetheless, such tumors are relatively uncommon in childhood.[4,87,89]

Often, a malignant peripheral nerve sheath tumor appears to arise in a large nerve or nerve trunk. Not all lesions share this attribute. Thus, without a clinical history of neurofibromatosis, diagnosis of this tumor in such cases may be difficult.[4,8,87] Ancillary studies are generally required because there is often little in the histologic appearance of these tumors that is typical of the more readily recognizable benign peripheral nerve sheath tumor. Indeed, many cases may be dominated by a spindled or pleomorphic cell population arranged in a storiform or herringbone pattern, not unlike that of MFH or fibrosarcoma[4,8,87] (Figure 6A). Fewer than one third of malignant peripheral nerve sheath tumors show nuclear palisades, Verocay bodies, or attempts at neurotactoid differentiation.[4,8,87,89] The diagnosis of this tumor may be further complicated by the presence of melanin pigment or presence of a dominant cell population that exhibits epithelioid features.[8,87,90] In each of the latter instances, the alternative diagnosis of malignant melanoma may be mistakenly considered.

Perhaps the greatest difficulty, apart from accurately diagnosing these lesions, is establishing with certainty the difference between atypical (but benign) neurofibromas and low grade malignant peripheral nerve sheath tumors. Careful attention to mitotic activity, cellularity, and tumoral necrosis is a useful indication that a benign diagnosis is inappropriate, but the distinction is not always clear. Instead, distinction between benign and malignant forms relies on clinical follow-up to establish the true nature of the lesion.[4,8,87,89]

In 12 to 20% of malignant peripheral nerve sheath tumors, divergent mesenchymal or epithelial elements may be present and may include evidence of rhabdomyoblastic, angiosarcomatous, chondro-osseous, and glandular differentiation[8,87,91-93] (Figures 7A and 7C). Rather than complicating the diagnosis in these instances, presence of such divergent elements

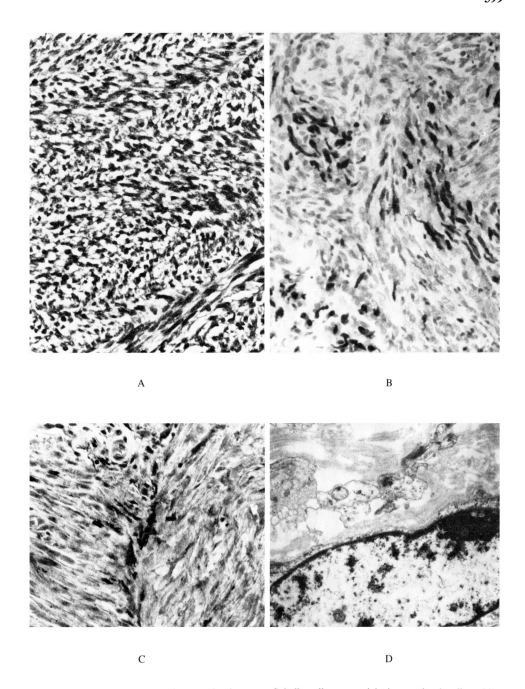

A

B

C

D

FIGURE 6. Malignant peripheral nerve sheath tumor. Spindle cells arranged in intersecting bundles with a herringbone-like pattern (A) may be immunoreactive for S100 protein (B) and Leu-7 antigen (C). Although light microscopic features may not always resemble benign nerve sheath neoplasms, ultrastructural evidence of neurilemmal differentiation, including interdigitating cell processes with well-formed junctions, and long-spaced collagen bundles (D) may be observed.

often favors the diagnosis of malignant peripheral nerve sheath tumor, since these findings are infrequent in other sarcomas.[8,87,92]

These heterologous elements may express immunoprofiles typical of skeletal muscle, endothelium, cartilage, and epithelium (Figures 7B and 7D). However, the diagnostically useful staining pattern is that exhibited by the predominant spindled/pleomorphic or epithe-

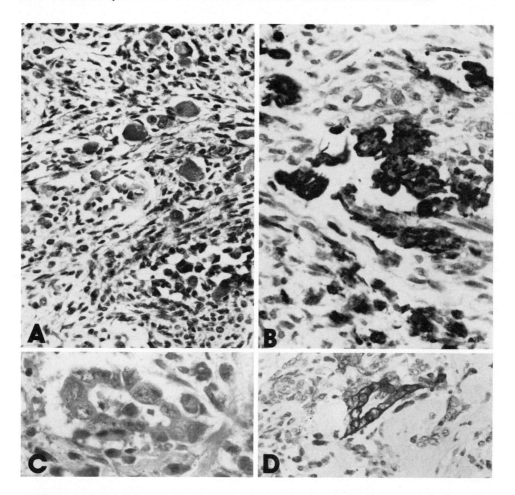

FIGURE 7.   Divergent differentiation in malignant peripheral nerve sheath tumor. Rhabdomyoblastic differentiation (A) is a feature of the so-called ''malignant triton tumor'' that is confirmed by immunostaining for desmin (B). Unusual examples may exhibit glandular differentiation (C), in which epithelial determinants such as cytokeratin (D) may be detected.

lioid cell.[20,21,94] Regardless of the histologic pattern, malignant peripheral nerve sheath tumors will stain for S100 protein or Leu-7 antigen in one half to two thirds of cases[69,94-96] (Figures 6B and 6C). The occasional detection of myogenic markers, including desmin or muscle-specific actin,[20,84,94] and the spurious detection of cytokeratins[97] may complicate the diagnosis of a malignant peripheral nerve sheath tumor. In such cases, the detection of rudimentary neurilemmal features by electron microscopy may be of assistance.[21,69,87,98,99]

The overall survival for malignant peripheral nerve sheath tumors is poor and is adversely affected by an association with neurofibromatosis. The adverse effect of this association is due in part to the nature of this tumor when it occurs in such patients. However, the adverse effect also reflects the relatively large size and the surgically inapparent intraneural spread of such lesions, since both large size and intraneural spread complicate attempts at surgical resection. Not unexpectedly, incomplete excision usually heralds a poorer outcome. The presence of divergent differentiation does not affect survival.[4,8,87,89]

VIII. PRIMITIVE NEUROECTODERMAL NEOPLASMS

It would be naive to expect that primitive neuroectodermal tumors (PNET) can be summarized briefly without mentioning points of controversy. Even the nomenclature of these tumors is not universally accepted. Moreover, the lack of agreement on nomenclature often reflects the various opinions about the histogenesis of these usually monotonous small cell neoplasms, which alone can result in irreparable differences in perspective.[100] The authors' inclination is to consider all primitive mesenchymal or ''neurocristal'' lesions of bone and soft tissue that show neuroectodermal features as being variations on a theme, to which the appellation ''PNET'' is applied.

PNET is an uncommon malignancy that usually involves the deep soft tissues or large nerves in the trunk and lower extremity.[101-103] In the thoracopulmonary region, an essentially similar neoplasm has been observed that is perhaps better known as the ''Askin tumor''.[104,105] More than half of these patients are less than 20 years of age. However, unlike the classic adrenal and extra-adrenal neuroblastic neoplasms, primitive neuroectodermal tumor tends not to occur in very young children.[4,101,104] The macroscopic features of PNET are not distinctive. They may be circumscribed, or they may infiltrate adjacent soft tissues as an irregular or multilobular mass. Varying degrees of tumoral necrosis, stromal degeneration, and hemorrhage are present on cut surfaces, which produce a variable solid or cystic appearance.[102-104]

Histologically, a PNET is more uniform. It is composed of small, round, primitive-appearing cells that form sheets, organoid clusters, or occasional Homer-Wright pseudo-rosettes. Unlike neuroblastoma, PNET rarely exhibits a well-defined neurofibrillary matrix, and ganglion cells are not seen.[4,101,104] Ultrastructurally, cells elaborate rudimentary cell processes, in which occasional microtubules and dense core ''neurosecretory'' granules are found. Collections of intermediate filaments are unusual and glycogen is typically sparse, but primitive macula adherens may be seen at points of cell apposition.[4,21,101,103,104,106] These ultrastructural features may help to distinguish PNET from other round cell tumors, including rhabdomyosarcoma.

However, the most consistently helpful approach for diagnosis is through the application of immunohistochemistry (Table 1). Using this technique, most PNETs are reactive for the following neural markers in different combinations: neuron specific enolase, Leu-7 antigen, synaptophysin, and (to a lesser extent) chromogranin.[4,8,20,103,105,107-109] The presence of neuron specific enolase and Leu-7 in occasional examples of rhabdomyosarcoma is of limited concern, since muscle specific actin or desmin intermediate filaments are usually detected in such instances.[21,38] Separation of PNET from the poorly differentiated neuroblastoma is also based on other clinical features, including presence of urinary catecholamines by neuroblastoma, and the preferential expression of class I histocompatibility antigens[110] as well as the MB2 antigen[111] by PNET. A number of other antibodies specific to or selective for PNET and neuroblastoma have been described, but they are not of practical importance in most routine laboratory diagnosis.

PNET is a very aggressive neoplasm, regardless of its primary site, when its behavior is compared to the other small round cell tumors of childhood. Although complete surgical excision may occasionally effect a cure, many such neoplasms are inoperable, particularly those in the chest wall or thoracic cavity. Hence, local recurrence is common and dissemination often ensues.[4,101,104]

The final diagnostic group among the small cell tumors of soft tissue, other than rhabdomyosarcoma, is the so-called extraskeletal Ewing's sarcoma.[8,112,115,115a] The name reflects the basic morphologic similarities that exist between this neoplasm and the osseous Ewing's sarcoma. Extraskeletal Ewing's sarcoma usually occurs in the extremities, paravertebral region, and chest wall. The median age is somewhat older than that of rhabdomyosarcoma and PNET, but the majority of cases are discovered in childhood. Like some cases of PNET, extraskeletal Ewing's sarcoma may be a rapidly growing lesion that may attain considerable size before diagnosis. The behavior of this tumor is similar to that of osseous Ewing's sarcoma. Thus, bone and pulmonary metastases may develop early. Nonetheless, the prognosis for extraskeletal Ewing's sarcoma is favorable compared to PNET; as many as 70% of patients may respond to a combination of radiation and chemotherapy.[8,115]

As if to impose symmetry on these small cell tumors, there is considerable overlap in light microscopic and immunohistochemical findings between extraskeletal Ewing's sarcoma and PNET.[4,21,116-118] Ultrastructurally, extraskeletal Ewing's sarcoma is typically composed of primitive round cells with abundant glycogen and primitive cell junctions, but occasional cases also contain blunt processes and rare neurosecretory granules.[8,21,113,114] Moreover, there is compelling evidence of a more fundamental similarity between extraskeletal Ewing's sarcoma and PNET, as evidenced by their shared karyotypic abnormality [translocation t(11;22)][119] and similar patterns of proto-oncogene expression.[120-122] That osseous Ewing's sarcoma may be induced *in vivo* to express a neural phenotype also suggests a possible similarity between the two tumors.[123] Whether osseous Ewing's sarcoma, extraskeletal Ewing's sarcoma, and PNET all represent merely different manifestations of a common neoplastic process remains to be proven. However, the differences in their clinical behavior and response to therapy still indicate the need to classify them separately for prognostic purposes.

Occasional examples of pediatric small round cell tumors may show either microscopic or immunophenotypic evidence of divergent epithelial or myogenic differentiation.[124-126] Some of these tumors have been classified as aberrant forms of PNET and extraskeletal Ewing's sarcoma. However, the authors feel that these lesions, variously designated "polyhistioma",[127] "primitive multipotential primary sarcoma of bone",[128] "ectomesenchymoma",[129] "intraabdominal desmoplastic small roundcell tumor",[130,131] and "polyphenotypic small cell tumor",[132] are more properly considered as primitive mesenchymal neoplasms with the capacity for multilineage expression or differentiation. These tumors may share ultrastructural, biochemical, and immunophenotypic qualities with PNET, but stand apart in all other respects.[132]

IX. SYNOVIAL SARCOMA

Based on composite surveys, synovial sarcoma constitutes approximately 15% of nonrhabdomyomatous pediatric soft tissue malignancies.[4,133] Most children with this tumor are in their second decade of life. The most common sites of involvement are the lower extremity (adjacent to major joints) and the head and neck region (in nasopharyngeal, occipital, and cervical soft tissues).[4,134] With rare exceptions, neither the retroperitoneum nor the mediastinum harbor these tumors.[8,135]

The clinical diagnosis is generally precipitated by signs or symptoms of a mass or altered function of an affected joint. Nonetheless, the tumor may attain considerable size, even in small children.[4,134,136] The tumor grossly infiltrates adjacent soft tissues and may exhibit focal or widely distributed fine or coarse calcifications.[4,8,137] This latter feature provides provocative radiographic evidence of synovial sarcoma in some instances. When calcifications dominate the cellular elements of the neoplasm, the term "calcifying synovial sarcoma" has been applied.[8,138] Recognition of this tumor is of clinical significance since diffuse tumoral calcifications have been correlated with improved survival. Children with calcifying synovial sarcoma have a 5-year survival rate of 85%, compared to an overall tumor mortality in excess of 50%.[4,8,138]

Grossly, these tumors appear cystic or may exhibit striking intratumoral hemorrhage or necrosis.[8,136] Histologically, synovial sarcoma is characteristically a biphasic neoplasm. It is composed of compact fusiform or spindle cells, interrupted by clefts or angiomatoid spaces that are lined by plump epithelial cells (Figure 8A). These clefts may also form well-defined glandular spaces, a pattern which may dominate in some instances to the extent that the

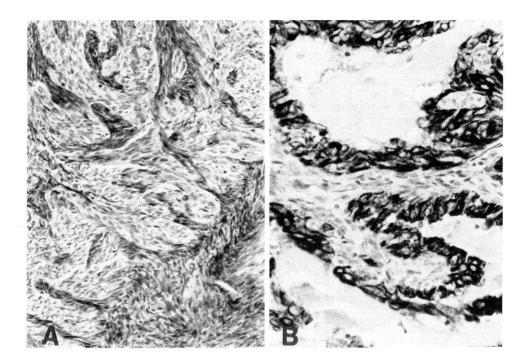

FIGURE 8. Synovial sarcoma. A biphasic pattern of spindle cells admixed with plum, ovoid, or polygonal elements is characteristic (A). Of these cell populations, those with epithelial features are more strongly immunoreactive for cytokeratin (B).

neoplasm resembles an adenocarcinoma.[4,8,134] Indeed, the epithelial nature of these cells has been shown by both ultrastructural and immunohistochemical studies.[20,21,134,139,139a] Immunohistochemistry reveals either cytokeratin or epithelial membrane antigen-like determinants in most tumors[20,38,134,139,139a] (Figure 8B). As a general rule, the spindle cells are less strongly reactive for these markers, and ultrastructural features of epithelial differentiation are rudimentary.[21,139,139a] As a result, a monophasic spindled synovial sarcoma may be difficult to separate from other sarcomas, including hemangiopericytoma, leiomyosarcoma, and malignant peripheral nerve sheath tumor,[8] unless immunohistochemical features are unequivocal.

In difficult cases, attention to certain histologic features may facilitate the diagnosis of synovial sarcoma. Small angulated and anastomosing vascular spaces, similar to those of hemangiopericytoma, may be conspicuous, particularly at the periphery of these tumors or between adjacent lobular condensations of spindled cells. In addition, as noted previously, small calcospherules may interrupt cellular foci. Less characteristically, large keloid-like bundles of collagen, areas of stromal myxoid degeneration, and intratumoral mast cells may be seen.[8] The latter two features may assist in the separation of synovial sarcoma from most fibrous or fibrohistiocytic tumors, but they do not provide sufficient contrast from malignant peripheral nerve sheath tumor. This latter differential consideration is often the most difficult to exclude, even when a clear biphasic pattern is manifest.

Indeed, the unusual glandular variant of malignant peripheral nerve sheath tumor may be quite similar in appearance to synovial sarcoma, and may share with synovial sarcoma the capacity to express epithelial markers.[20,93,134] Similarly, the spindle cells of synovial sarcoma may contain the ''neural'' markers S100 protein and the Leu-7 antigen.[20,69] Finally, the juxtaposition of synovial sarcoma to major joint spaces may place the tumor in proximity to larger nerve bundles. Nonetheless, the intimate association of neoplastic elements with such nerves typifies only malignant peripheral nerve sheath tumor.

X. LIPOMATOUS NEOPLASMS

The recognition of benign lipomatous neoplasms in children is usually not complicated.[4,8] However, three aspects of lipomas in children may present considerable problems to the uninitiated observer. First, they may arise in mediastinal and retroperitoneal spaces, where the latter is a well-known site for liposarcomas in adults.[4,8,140] Deep soft tissue lesions of the sacrococcygeal region and tumors within or between major muscle groups are also encountered.[4] Second, even in deeply situated lesions, infiltrative growth, cellular pleomorphism, and nuclear atypia may be associated with a benign clinical course.[4,141] Finally, benign lipomatous neoplasms may harbor immature elements, including collections of lipoblasts.[4,8]

The presence of lipoblasts characterizes one of the more typical benign tumors in children younger than 3 years of age. Lipoblastomas are usually superficial lesions of the extremities, although they may also involve the mediastinum, retroperitoneum, and chest wall.[4,8,142,143] Grossly, superficial lesions are often well-circumscribed lobular masses, whereas deeper tumors may infiltrate adjacent soft tissue, giving rise to so-called "lipoblastomatosis".[4,8,143,144] Patients with lipoblastomatosis have local recurrences or persistence of disease in 10 to 15% of cases, due largely to difficulties in complete excision.[4,8,143]

Histologically, a lipoblastoma is composed of lobules, separated by fibrous septae. In the lobules, lipoblasts and immature cellular elements appear to be in transition to mature adipose tissue, the latter being most prominent centrally.[4,142,143] In older lesions, the mature elements may predominate. This finding supports the impression that lipomas with atypical or immature lipoblasts that occur in older children are in fact maturing or partially mature lipoblastomas.[4] Notably, the stroma in a lipoblastoma is often myxoid in character and may be associated with an anastomotic network of small capillaries.[4,8,143] These features impart a resemblance to myxoid liposarcoma.

Liposarcomas are rare, but their occurrence is well documented in children. They account for fewer than 1% of soft tissue malignancies in the young. The anatomical location of liposarcoma overlaps with lipoblastoma. Moreover, the myxoid variant of liposarcoma is the most common among such lesions in children[4,142,145,146] (Figure 9), which fosters its histopathologic confusion with lipoblastoma. Nonetheless, the two neoplasms should rarely be confused in clinical practice. The benign lesion (lipoblastoma) typically occurs in children less than 3 years of age, whereas liposarcoma is generally detected in the second decade of life.

Since the clinically aggressive types of liposarcoma are virtually never encountered in children, metastases are rarely, if ever, seen.[4,145-147] Immunohistochemistry offers little in the evaluation of these tumors, since lipoblastic elements are characterized by the presence of vimentin[20,38] and S100 protein,[20] a phenotype shared with malignant peripheral nerve sheath tumor. On the other hand, electron microscopy may support a diagnosis of liposarcoma, by revealing the presence of lipid vacuoles that impinge upon nuclear contours.[21,142]

XI. VASCULAR NEOPLASMS

Benign vascular tumors are not often mistaken for malignancy, but they may occasionally present as part of a complex disease that is not readily ameliorated by conservative management. Of particular importance are cases of diffuse angiomatosis (Figure 10). Because of their large volume, these tumors cause aberrations in cardiodynamics or, more dramatically, they may be associated with a consumptive coagulopathy.[148] The angiotic proliferations encountered in the Klippel-Trenaunay-Weber and the Kasabach-Merritt syndromes are illustrative examples.[149-151]

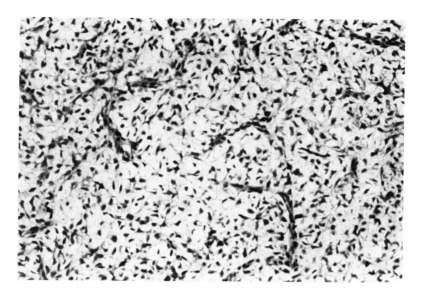

FIGURE 9. Myxoid liposarcoma. In most instances of childhood liposarcoma, the myxoid pattern predominates. Vacuolated lipoblasts are supported by a loose myxoid matrix in which small capillaries are conspicuous.

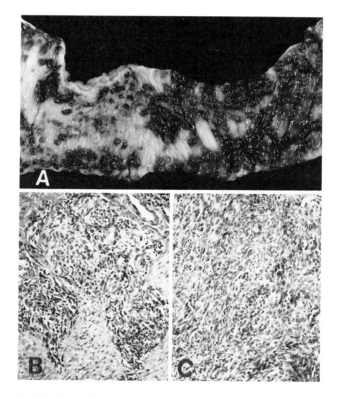

FIGURE 10. Diffuse angiomatosis in Kasabach-Merritt syndrome. In this example, multiple small angiomatous lesions are noted in the bowel mucosa (A) of a profoundly thrombocytopenic infant with diffuse intra-abdominal and subcutaneous capillary proliferations. In these lesions, densely cellular clusters of plump (B) or spindled (C) endothelial cells are encountered. These histologic changes have also been described in localized endothelial lesions of infancy; such tumors have been referred to as "cellular angiomas". (See reference 152.)

Localized benign endothelial lesions may occasionally create complications in surgical management because of their infiltrative nature. Cystic hygroma, lymphangiomyomatosis, and infiltrating hemangioma (intramuscular hemangioma) are tumors with these growth characteristics.[4,8,153] Some benign endothelial proliferations may morphologically mimic angiosarcoma. One example is Masson's vegetant intravascular hemangioendothelioma, a tumor which probably represents an organizing thrombus.[154] Nonetheless, complex intravascular papillary structures in this lesion are lined by hyperchromatic reactive endothelial cells. This histological pattern closely simulates angiosarcoma, except that angiosarcomas form vascular spaces rather than proliferating as an intravascular growth. In occasional cases of pyogenic granuloma, similar papillary structures may provoke some concern of possible angiosarcoma on microscopic examination.[4,8]

Endothelial tumors of low grade malignancy are uncommon in children.[4,8,155,164] Only one such tumor preferentially affects this age group: this is the so-called "malignant" endovascular papillary angioendothelioma.[156-158] This rare tumor usually arises in the skin or subcutis. It is characterized by complex anastomosing vascular spaces in which atypical-appearing endothelial cells line endovascular papillary structures. Reactive lymphoid infiltrates are conspicuous within and adjacent to the papillary profiles.[156] As in other endothelial tumors, the neoplastic cells are avidly decorated by the *Ulex europaeus I* agglutinin (UEA), and are often immunoreactive for Factor VIII-related antigen (von Willebrand factor).[157] The purported malignant nature of endovascular papillary angioendothelioma is based on its locally infiltrative growth and its tendency to recur after resection. Cases with regional lymph nodal metastasis have been reported. However, the intimate association with lymphoid cells that typifies this tumor has led to speculation that nodal lesions, instead of being metastases, are primary proliferations in that site. Because of clinical uncertainty regarding this lesion, its designation as having borderline or low grade malignant potential must be accepted with caution.[157]

Even less common in children are the epithelioid and spindle cell hemangioendotheliomas. Epithelioid hemangioendothelioma is typically a well-circumscribed mass in the soft tissues of the extremities.[8,159,160] However, similar-appearing tumors are identified in a variety of soft tissue sites, as well as in the lung (intravascular bronchioalveolar tumor) and liver.[8] Epithelioid hemangioendothelioma consists of round to oval cells that form inconspicuous vascular or intracytoplasmic lumina (Figure 11A). The endothelial nature of these cells is confirmed by both detection of pinocytosis and Weibel-Palade bodies on electron microscopy and presence of histochemical reactivity with *Ulex europaeus I* lectin[20,21,160] (Figure 11B). Mitotic activity is generally not pronounced in this tumor, and neither nuclear pleomorphism nor tumoral necrosis is apparent. The presence of the latter features is more characteristic of the overtly malignant epithelioid angiosarcoma. Epithelioid hemangioendothelioma generally follows an indolent clinical course, although most cases may recur locally. The documentation of metastasis in 20% of cases is compelling evidence of its malignant potential.[8,160]

The second of these lesions, the spindle cell hemangioendothelioma, more commonly involves the skin of extremities.[161,162] Only one case has been reported in the first two decades of life. The distinctive feature of this lesion is the juxtaposition of solid areas of spindle cells (resembling Kaposi's sarcoma) with cavernous vascular spaces (simulating cavernous hemangioma).[161,162] This tumor, like epithelioid hemangioendothelioma, can be distinguished from overtly malignant neoplasms by its lack of significant atypia and mitotic activity. The endothelial nature of the spindle cells is often difficult to establish by histochemical or ultrastructural evaluation. However, the transition from spindled to epithelioid elements and the presence of cavernous vascular spaces are sufficient evidence of angiogenesis.[161]

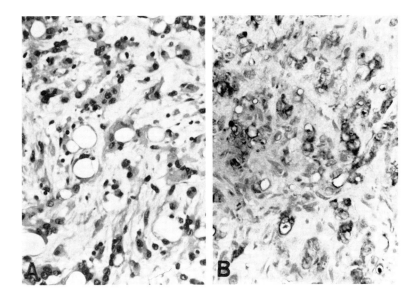

FIGURE 11. Epithelioid hemangioendothelioma. Clusters of plump epithelioid cells are arranged around rudimentary vascular spaces. Intracytoplasmic lumens are also apparent (A). The cells are labeled with UEA (B).

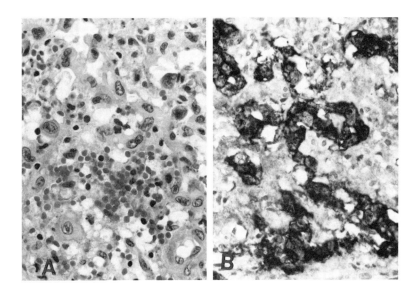

FIGURE 12. Epithelioid angiosarcoma. Although rare in children, epithelioid angiosarcomas may occur, and can be distinguished from epithelioid hemangioendothelioma by their cellularity and nuclear pleomorphism (A). Although unusual, this example is immunoreactive for Factor VIII-related antigen (B).

Angiosarcomas are rarely observed in the superficial soft tissues in children.[4,163,164] Occasional cases may be composed predominantly of pleomorphic, spindled, or epithelioid cells (Figure 12A), which obscure their distinction from other histologically similar sarcomas. Diagnosis in such cases is facilitated by the binding of *Ulex europaeus I* lectin,[20,165,166] but as one will see, this finding alone may not exclude the diagnosis of other epithelioid malignancies. Reactivity for Factor VIII-related antigen is less helpful, since only 20% of angiosarcomas may express this substance[21,165] (Figure 12B). Similarly, the characteristic ultrastructural features of endothelium may be lacking.[8,21]

Malignant tumors of lymphatic vessels may also occur in children. They almost always occur as a complication of congenital or acquired lymphedema.[167,168]

Kaposi's sarcoma is rare in children outside of endemic areas, but has been reported occasionally in children infected with HIV. When this tumor occurs in children, cutaneous lesions are usually not seen, but lymph nodal involvement is a characteristic finding.[169-171]

XII. OTHER SARCOMAS AND SARCOMATOUS NEOPLASMS

A. EPITHELIOID SARCOMA

Although epithelioid sarcoma is most common in young male adults, the occasional occurrence of this neoplasm in children and adolescents is well established.[4,8,172,173] The site most commonly involved is the upper extremity, particularly the hand and flexor surfaces. Superficial soft tissues are often compressed or distorted by the tumor. Skin lesions are not uncommon, but ulceration of overlying epidermis is unusual.[8,172]

Histologically, epithelioid sarcoma is a tumor of large, polygonal cells with densely eosinophilic cytoplasm. Binucleate and multinucleated tumor cells may be present in varying numbers. Ultrastructurally, these cells are dominated by perinuclear intermediate filaments that are immunoreactive for both vimentin and cytokeratin. As in synovial sarcoma, cytokeratin is often coexpressed with cytoplasmic and membrane-bound epithelial membrane antigen. Thus, the nature of this "epithelioid" entity, much as with synovial sarcoma, is more aptly considered to be "epithelial".[20,38,123,173,175]

The accurate diagnosis of this lesion is facilitated by its general location and histological features, particularly when large polygonal cells predominate. Unfortunately, in some cases these cells may only be evident in the periphery of tumor lobules, the center being dominated by less cellular or overtly necrotic tissue. Not coincidentally, such areas may exhibit a mantle of multinucleated tumor cells and may thus resemble a granulomatous lesion, such as granuloma annulare.[8,172] Necrosis may also be attended by proliferation of epithelioid neoplastic cells around clefts or angiomatoid spaces, imparting a resemblance to an epithelioid vascular neoplasm.[8,172] Fortunately, epithelioid sarcoma may be distinguished from both granulomatous and vascular lesions by its immunoreactivity for cytokeratin and epithelial membrane antigen. Conversely, this tumor may be identified by its lack of vascular determinants, such as Factor VIII-related antigen.[20,123] It should be noted that reliance on UEA as a means to identify a vascular tumor in this setting is inappropriate, since epithelioid sarcoma, like other epithelial neoplasms, may express substances (including H antigen) that bind this putative "vascular" marker.[20,175]

B. CLEAR CELL SARCOMA (MALIGNANT MELANOMA OF SOFT PARTS)

Clear cell sarcoma of tendons and aponeuroses is a peculiar entity whose true histogenesis has been debated since its original description. Currently, this tumor is thought to be related to malignant melanoma.[8,176-178] Although it is an uncommon tumor at all ages, a substantial proportion of clear cell sarcomas occurs in children; approximately 20% of the cases in one series were diagnosed in patients less than 20 years of age.[8,176]

As in adults, clear cell sarcomas in children usually arise in the soft tissues of the lower extremity, especially near the ankle or in the feet in proximity to the tendons or aponeuroses. Regional lymph node metastases are common, a feature which contrasts sharply with most other soft tissue malignancies in children, except for alveolar rhabdomyosarcoma.[4,8,176,177] Grossly, the tumor may be multilobulated, and it often appears to be sharply circumscribed from adjacent tissues. As its nature would imply, melanotic pigmentation is grossly apparent in 25 to 50% of cases, and almost 75% of tumors will stain with the Fontana-Masson

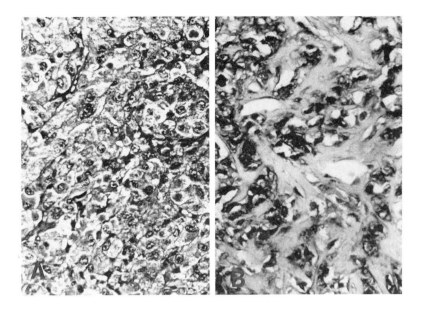

FIGURE 13.   Clear cell sarcoma. Cells are ovoid or spindled, and arranged in tightly packed nests. The resemblance to malignant melanoma is often striking (A). As in melanoma, the neoplastic cells are reactive for the HMB-45 antigen (B).

stain.[8,176,177] Accordingly, ultrastructural examination often reveals melanosomes. Nearly all cases of clear cell sarcoma show immunohistochemical reactivity for vimentin, S100 protein, and HMB45 antigen, the latter two being sensitive markers of melanocytic differentiation.[20,95,178]

The histologic features of this tumor are distinct. In primary neoplasms, alveolar clusters or nodules of pale eosinophilic, fusiform, or spindled cells containing large vesicular nuclei predominate (Figure 13). Unlike malignant melanoma, however, cytologic atypia is not often pronounced and mitotic activity is often sparse. Presence of epithelioid cells does not typify this entity, although such elements may be pronounced in metastatic or recurrent lesions.[8,176,177]

C. MALIGNANT RHABDOID TUMOR

Primary soft tissue neoplasms resembling the malignant rhabdoid tumor of the kidney have been recognized with increasing frequency.[179-182] The nature of this soft tissue neoplasm, as with the tumor in the kidney, is unknown. The complex immunohistochemical features of the cases reported thus far indicate that no one immunophenotype better distinguishes this entity from other soft tissue neoplasms than does its histological appearance. Indeed, the diversity of immunophenotypic expression in this tumor and the presence of "rhabdoid" elements in other soft tissue malignancies[8,20,182,183] suggest that malignant rhabdoid tumor may, like MFH, represent a "final common pathway" in the evolution of mesenchymal (and perhaps even epithelial) malignancies.[183]

Regardless of its true nature, malignant rhabdoid tumor is a unique neoplasm. It is composed predominantly of large polygonal cells containing single or multiple nuclei with abundant eosinophilic cytoplasm, and an eccentrically disposed vesicular nucleus.[8,179] Unlike epithelioid sarcoma, which it may resemble, malignant rhabdoid tumor often exhibits extreme cytologic and nuclear pleomorphism, and mitotic activity may be brisk.[4,8,179] Even so, this tumor may be confused with epithelioid sarcoma, malignant melanoma, and even a high grade carcinoma, particularly in tumors arising in the peripheral soft tissues. One important

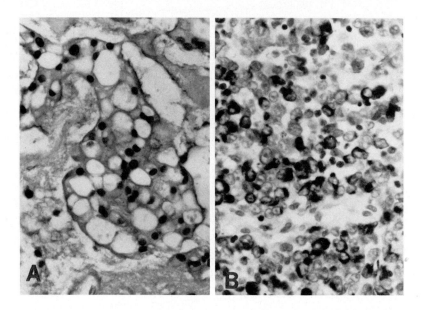

FIGURE 14.   Chordoma. In childhood, the typical physaliferous cells are often lacking, but nests of vacuolated cells may be suspended in a loosely textured mucoid matrix (A). Cytokeratin reactivity is typically pronounced in chordoma (B).

clinical discriminant is the relatively indolent behavior of epithelioid sarcoma, which contrasts with the relatively brief, aggressive course of malignant rhabdoid tumor.[8,179-181,183]

D. CHORDOMA

Chordomas primarily occur in adults in their third or fourth decade of life. Most cases arise in midline osseous structures of sacrococcygeal and basisphenoid regions or in cervicothoracic vertebrae. Nonetheless, rare cases of primary soft tissue chordomas in childhood have been reported.[4,8] Apart from the acknowledgment that chordoma is an aggressive neoplasm in both children and adults, two observations are relevant to this discussion. First, chordomas in children often are not dominated by the characteristic notochord-like cellular elements or by presence of the classic "physaliferous" cell. Indeed, areas in these tumors may be composed of relatively uniform spindled elements or, conversely, made up of sheets of pleomorphic polygonal cells. When the characteristic myxoid stroma of this tumor is manifest, neoplastic cells are arranged in loosely apposed cellular clusters[4] (Figure 14A).

Second, the relationship of neoplastic cells to matrix in a chordoma may, as in adults, impart a resemblance to chondrosarcoma, particularly the myxoid variant (so-called "chordoid sarcoma"). Less commonly, this tumor may resemble a metastatic mucinous carcinoma.[4,8] Immunohistochemistry findings are clearly relevant to this differential diagnosis; these findings usually facilitate the diagnosis of chordoma even in the absence of diagnostic histologic features, since the coexpression of cytokeratin, epithelial membrane antigen, and S100 protein characterizes chordoma (Figure 14B) and excludes the diagnosis of a chondrosarcoma.[20,21] This immunohistochemical profile cannot distinguish chordoma from monophasic synovial sarcoma. However, neither the clinical nor the histologic features of the monophasic synovial sarcoma overlap with chordoma to a degree that is sufficient to warrant diagnostic concern. Obviously, the separation of chordoma from metastatic carcinoma may be quite difficult in some cases, but usually this diagnostic dilemma is more pertinent to diagnosis of chordoma in adults.

411

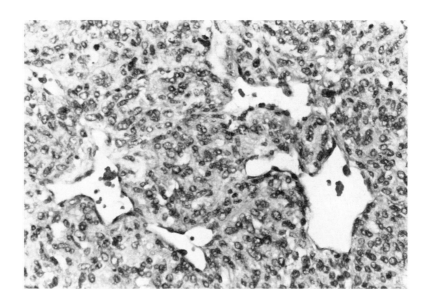

FIGURE 15. Mesenchymal chondrosarcoma. Small round cells are interrupted by irregularly anastomotic capillaries; the resultant pattern may resemble hemangiopericytoma.

XIII. NEOPLASMS RESEMBLING LESIONS OF BONE

A. CARTILAGINOUS TUMORS

Among tumors resembling malignancies in bone, the so-called extraskeletal Ewing's sarcoma has already been discussed. Of those tumors showing features of chondro-osseous differentiation, it is the chondroblastic neoplasms that are more common.[155,184,185]

Nearly 20% of soft tissue chondromas arise in patients younger than 20 years of age. Although myxoid foci in these lesions may simulate malignancy, most such tumors exhibit areas of well-defined mature cartilaginous elements, rendering this potential dilemma of little practical concern.[4,8]

More important in children are the malignant cartilaginous tumors. As in adults, the most common of these unlikely lesions is the mesenchymal chondrosarcoma.[155,186,187] This neoplasm tends to occur in adolescents and young adults. Osseous mesenchymal chondrosarcoma usually arises in the jaw or rib, whereas extraskeletal mesenchymal chondrosarcoma is more common in the head or neck or extremities.[8,186] Involvement of the dura mater or orbital soft tissues is another manifestation of this tumor in adolescents.[188] There is a slight female predilection regardless of age.

The gross appearance of mesenchymal chondrosarcoma is that of a multilobulated, circumscribed mass. In contrast to other forms of chondrosarcoma, this lesion has a soft, fleshy appearance that is only regionally interrupted by areas of cartilaginous or osseous tissue.[8,186,188,189] Histologically, mesenchymal chondrosarcoma consists of sheets or nodules composed of uniform small round or spindled cells admixed with islands of poorly formed cartilage. Within small cell foci, anastomotic plexi of thin-walled vessels impart a hemangiopericytoma-like appearance to the pattern (Figure 15). Although mitotic activity may be conspicuous in areas, the tumor generally does not exhibit significant cytologic pleomorphism.[8,186,187]

The histologic diagnosis of mesenchymal chondrosarcoma is complicated only in the absence of cartilaginous foci. In this circumstance, confusion with other small round cell tumors, particularly rhabdomyosarcoma in orbital sites, may be problematic. Immunohistochemically, mesenchymal chondrosarcoma shares its expression of S100 protein in lacunar

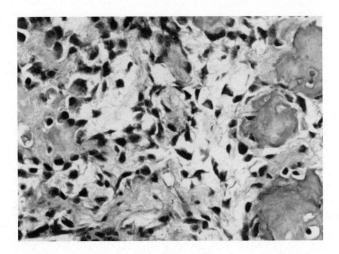

FIGURE 16.   Extraskeletal osteosarcoma. Atypical polygonal and spindle
cell are intimately associated with an osteoid matrix.

chondrocytes with other forms of chondrosarcoma.[20,187,188,190] However, the small cells are
typically negative for this substance. Instead, these small cells may express both neuron-
specific enolase and Leu-7 antigen,[189] both of which may also characterize primitive neuroectodermal tumors and extraskeletal Ewing's sarcoma. The absence of myogenic determinants, particularly muscle-specific actin and desmin, provides a useful contrast to rhabdomyosarcoma.[20,189]

Less common in both adults and children are examples of so-called chordoid sarcoma,
or extraskeletal myxoid chondrosarcoma.[4,8,191] Typically a lesion of deep soft tissue in the
lower extremity, myxoid chondrosarcoma shows a gender predilection more like that of
osseous chondrosarcoma, with a male predominant. Like mesenchymal chondrosarcoma,
chordoid sarcoma is often multilobulated and appears well circumscribed.[8] Areas of hemorrhage and necrosis are more common than in mesenchymal chondrosarcoma. Histologically, tumor lobules are composed of polygonal or elongate epithelioid cells unevenly dispersed in a mucoid matrix. Overt chondroid differentiation may be lacking. Cytologically,
nuclei are small and hyperchromatic, while abundant eosinophilic cytoplasm is present.
Hence, unlike the predominant cell type in mesenchymal chondrosarcoma, the neoplastic
cells of myxoid chondrosarcoma resemble the chondroblast.[8,191] The immunohistochemical
profile of this lesion is typical of chondrosarcomas in general, in that S100 protein is
commonly expressed, while both cellular and matrical components contain a Leu-7-reactive
moiety.[20,191]

Chondrosarcomas otherwise characteristic of osseous lesions, exclusive of the histologic
types already discussed, are extremely rare in soft tissues of children.[4] Four cases arising
in the paranasal sinuses have been reported. A peculiar variant of chondrosarcoma, described
as "embryonal chondrosarcoma", is a nasoethmoid tumor of small round cells in a myxoid
matrix. Unlike other variants of chondrosarcoma, this tumor may occur in the very young.[192]

B. EXTRAOSSEOUS OSTEOSARCOMA

True osteogenic malignancies of somatic soft tissues are extremely rare in all age groups.
However, this diagnostic possibility must still be considered when confronted by a population
of proliferating mesenchymal cells that is associated with an osteoid[8,155] (Figure 16). In some
instances, these lesions may occur as the result of previously administered radiotherapy.[8,193-196] Extraskeletal osteosarcoma may appear relatively well differentiated and may
be virtually indistinguishable from areas of ossification in myositis ossificans. However, the

zonality of the lesions in myositis ossificans, with osseous material peripheral to immature-appearing mesenchymal elements, is sufficient in most instances to separate this entity from the generally haphazard arrangement of cellular elements in extraskeletal osteosarcoma.[8] The loose cellular fibrous proliferation that may characterize this tumor may also impart a resemblance to nodular fasciitis.

Cartilaginous foci may be prominent in these lesions, although essentially all histologic variants of osteosarcoma may be seen in soft tissue.[8,135] Importantly, occasional cases may lack obvious osteoid and may express marked pleomorphism. Such tumors resemble high grade MFH and may be difficult to separate from the latter.

Perhaps the most important aspect of these osseous lesions is their recognition distinct from other soft tissue sarcomas in which metaplastic bone may arise, such as in synovial sarcoma, epithelioid sarcoma, liposarcoma, malignant peripheral nerve sheath tumor, and MFH.[8]

XIV. CONCLUSIONS

The complex diagnostic challenges posed by soft tissue neoplasms in children often obscure the more important aspects of these neoplasms from a clinical point of view. Much of the current clinical practice is directed at treating the tumor by stage and location, as is discussed elsewhere in this book. It remains true today that in both childhood and adult sarcomas, generalizations about tumoral grade, size, and infiltrative or metastatic potential suffice for most approaches to the clinical management of these tumors. However, these practices have been predicated on a historical approach, shared by pathologists, in which accurate separation of the differing histologic types of sarcoma was not emphasized.

In this chapter the authors have attempted to provide, for most pediatric soft tissue malignancies, guidelines by which a clear and unequivocal histological classification can be made. Differences in survival can in several instances be predicted from a tumor's histologic, immunohistochemical, or ultrastructural phenotype. As the precision of one's diagnostic techniques evolve, it is hoped that the options for surgical and nonsurgical management can be modified to illuminate one's growing understanding of the relationship between patterns of tumoral differentiation and biological behavior.

REFERENCES

1. **Anderson, D. H.,** Tumors of infancy and childhood, *Cancer,* 4, 890, 1951.
2. **Coffin, C. M. and Dehner, L. P.,** Soft tissue tumors in first year of life: a report of 190 cases, *Pediatr. Pathol.,* 10, 509, 1990.
3. **Coffin, C. M. and Dehner, L. P.,** Soft tissue neoplasms in childhood. A clinicopathological overview, in *Pathology of Neoplasia in Children and Adolescents,* Finegold, M., Ed., W.B. Saunders, Philadelphia, 1986, 223.
4. **Dehner, L. P.,** *Pediatric Surgical Pathology,* 2nd ed., Williams & Wilkins, Baltimore, 1987.
5. **Pack, G. T. and Ariel, I. M.,** Sarcomas of the somatic soft tissues in infants and children, *Surg. Gynecol. Obstet.,* 98, 675, 1954.
6. **Young, J. L. and Miller, R. W.,** Incidence of malignant tumors in US children, *J. Pediatr.,* 86, 254, 1975.
7. **Chang, A. E., Rosenberg, S. A., Glatskin, E. J., and Antman, K. H.,** Sarcomas of soft tissues, in *Cancer. Principles and Practice of Oncology,* 3rd ed., DeVita, D. E., Jr., Hallman, S., and Rosenberg, S. A., Eds., Lippincott, Philadelphia, 1989, 1345.
8. **Enzinger, F. M. and Weiss, S. W.,** *Soft Tissue Tumors,* 2nd ed., C.V. Mosby, St. Louis, 1988.
9. **Crist, W. M., Raney, B., Tefft, M., et al.,** Soft tissue sarcomas arising in the retroperitoneal space in children, *Cancer,* 56, 2125, 1985.

10. **Miser, J. S., Triche, T. J., Pritchard, D. J., and Kinsella, T.,** Ewing's sarcoma and the nonrhabdomyomatous soft tissue sarcomas of childhood, in *Principles and Practice of Pediatric Oncology,* Pizzo, P. A. and Poplack, D. G., Eds., Lippincott, Philadelphia, 1989, 659.

11. **Niefeld, J. P., Godwin, D., Berg, J. W., and Salzberg, A. M.,** Prognostic features of pediatric soft tissue sarcomas, *Surgery,* 98, 93, 1985.

12. **Wharam, M., Jr., Foulkes, M. A., Lawrence, W., Jr., et al.,** Soft tissue sarcoma of the head and neck in childhood: nonorbital and nonparameningeal sites, *Cancer,* 53, 1016, 1984.

13. **Cozzutto, C., de Bernardi, B., Gaurino, M., et al.,** Retroperitoneal fibrohistiocytic tumors in children: report of five cases, *Cancer,* 42, 1350, 1978.

14. **Littman, P., Raney, B., Zimmerman, R., et al.,** Soft tissue sarcomas of the head and neck in children, *Int. J. Radiol. Oncol. Biol. Phys.,* 9, 1367, 1971.

15. **Dehner, L. P. and Askin, F. B.,** Tumors of fibrous tissue origin in childhood. A clinicopathologic study of cutaneous and soft tissue neoplasms in 66 children, *Cancer,* 38, 888, 1976.

16. **Rice, D. H., Batsakis, J. G., Headington, J. T., and Boles, R.,** Fibrous histiocytomas of the nose and paranasal sinuses, *Arch. Otolaryngol.,* 100, 398, 1974.

17. **Martorelli, M., Calabuig, C., Peydro-Olaya, A., et al.,** Fibroblast and myofibroblast participation in malignant fibrous histiocytoma (MFH) of bone. Ultrastructural study of eight cases with immunohistochemical support, *Pathol. Res. Pract.,* 184, 582, 1989.

18. **Ricci, A., Jr., Cartun, R. W., and Zakowski, M. F.,** Atypical fibroxanthoma. A study of 14 cases emphasizing the presence of Langerhan's histiocytes with implications for differential diagnosis by antibody panels, *Am. J. Surg. Pathol.,* 12, 591, 1988.

19. **Silvis, N. G., Swanson, P. E., Manivel, J. C., et al.,** Spindle cell and pleomorphic neoplasms of the skin: a clinicopathologic and immunohistochemical study of 30 cases, with emphasis on "atypical fibroxanthoma", *Am. J. Dermatopathol.,* 10, 9, 1988.

20. **Wick, M. R., Manivel, J. C., and Swanson, P. E.,** Contributions of immunohistochemical analysis to the diagnosis of soft tissue tumors: a review, *Prog. Surg. Pathol.,* 8, 197, 1988.

21. **Wick, M. R., Swanson, P. E., and Manivel, J. C.,** Immunohistochemical analysis of soft tissue sarcomas. Comparison with electron microscopy, *Appl. Pathol.,* 6, 169, 1988.

22. **Wood, G. S., Beckstead, J. H., Turner, R. R., et al.,** Malignant fibrous histiocytoma tumor cells resemble fibroblasts, *Am. J. Surg. Pathol.,* 10, 323, 1986.

23. **Leader, M., Patel, J., Collins, M., and Henry, K.,** Alpha-1-antichymotrypsin staining of 194 sarcomas, 38 carcinomas, and 17 malignant melanomas, *Am. J. Surg. Pathol.,* 11, 133, 1987.

24. **Enzinger, F. M. and Zhang, R.,** Plexiform fibrohistiocytic tumor presenting in children and young adults. An analysis of 65 cases, *Am. J. Surg. Pathol.,* 12, 818, 1988.

25. **Enjoji, M., Hashimoto, H., Tsuneyoshi, M., and Iwasaki, H.,** Malignant fibrous histiocytoma: a clinicopathologic study of 130 cases, *Acta Pathol. Jpn.,* 30, 727, 1980.

26. **Kearney, M. M., Soule, E. H., and Ivins, J. C.,** Malignant fibrous histiocytoma: a retrospective study of 167 cases, *Cancer,* 45, 167, 1980.

27. **Weiss, S. W.,** Malignant fibrous histiocytoma, *Am. J. Surg. Pathol.,* 6, 773, 1982.

28. **Tracy, T., Jr., Niefeld, J. P., DeMay, R. M., and Salzberg, A. M.,** Malignant fibrous histiocytomas in children, *J. Pediatr. Surg.,* 19, 81, 1984.

29. **Zuppan, C. W., Mierau, G. W., and Wilson, H. L.,** Malignant fibrous histiocytoma in childhood: a report of two cases and review of the literature, *Pediatr. Pathol.,* 7, 303, 1987.

30. **Raney, R. B., Jr., Allen, A., O'Neill, J., et al.,** Malignant fibrous histiocytoma of soft tissue in childhood, *Cancer,* 57, 2198, 1986.

31. **Enzinger, F. M.,** Angiomatoid malignant fibrous histiocytoma. A distinct fibrohistiocytic tumor of children and young adults simulating a vascular neoplasm, *Cancer,* 44, 2147, 1979.

32. **Wegmann, W. and Heitz, P. U.,** Angiomatoid malignant fibrous histiocytoma, *Virchows Arch. A,* 406, 59, 1985.

33. **Seo, I. S., Frizzera, G., Coates, T. D., et al.,** Angiomatoid malignant fibrous histiocytoma with extensive lymphadenopathy simulating Castleman's disease, *Pediatr. Pathol.,* 6, 233, 1986.

34. **Santa Cruz, D. J. and Kyriakos, M.,** Aneurysmal ("angiomatoid") fibrous histiocytoma of the skin, *Cancer,* 47, 2053, 1981.

35. **Blumenfeld, W., Egbert, B. M., and Sagebiel, R. W.,** Differential diagnosis of Kaposi's sarcoma, *Arch. Pathol. Lab. Med.,* 109, 123, 1985.

36. **Dahl, I.,** Atypical fibroxanthoma of the skin. A clinicopathologic study of 57 cases, *Acta Pathol. Microbiol. Scand. Sect. A,* 84, 183, 1976.

37. **Metz, G.,** Dermatofibrosarcoma protuberans in Kindesalter, *Hautarzt,* 39, 435, 1978.

38. **Gown, A. M. and Vogel, A. M.,** Monoclonal antibodies to human intermediate filament proteins. III. Analysis of tumors, *Am. J. Clin. Pathol.,* 84, 413, 1984.

39. **Allen, P. W.,** Nodular fasciitis, *Pathology,* 4, 9, 1972.

40. **Allen, P. W.,** The fibromatoses: a clinicopathologic classification based on 140 cases. I and II, *Am. J. Surg. Pathol.,* 1, 255 and 305, 1977.

41. **Chung, E. B. and Enzinger, F. M.,** Proliferative fasciitis, *Cancer,* 36, 1450, 1975.

42. **Enzinger, F. M. and Dulcey, F.,** Proliferative myositis. Report of thirty-three cases, *Cancer,* 20, 2213, 1967.

43. **Kleinman, G. M., Zelem, J. D., and Sander, F. J.,** Proliferative myositis in a two year old child, *Pediatr. Pathol.,* 7, 71, 1987.

44. **Lauer, D. M. and Enzinger, F. M.,** Cranial fasciitis of childhood, *Cancer,* 45, 401, 1980.

45. **Morgan, K., Aparicio, S., Spicer, R. D., and Marsden, H. B.,** Proliferative fasciitis in childhood: a case report, *Pediatr. Pathol.,* 10, 431, 1990.

46. **Patchevsky, A. S. and Enzinger, F. M.,** Intravascular fasciitis. A report of 17 cases, *Am. J. Surg. Pathol.,* 5, 29, 1981.

47. **Dehner, L. P., Kaye, V., Levitt, C., and Askin, F. B.,** Cellular inflammatory pseudotumor in young individuals: a lesion distinguishable from fibrous histiocytoma or myxosarcoma?, *Lab. Invest.,* 44 (Abstr.), 14A, 1981.

48. **Chung, E. B. and Enzinger, F. M.,** Infantile myofibromatosis, *Cancer,* 48, 1807, 1981.

49. **Kindblom, L.-G., Termen, G., Save-Soderbergh, J., and Angervall, L.,** Congenital fibromatosis of soft tissues, a variant of congenital generalized fibromatosis, *Acta Pathol. Microbiol. Scand. Sect. A,* 85, 640, 1977.

50. **Schmidt, D. and Harms, D.,** Fibromatosis of infancy and childhood. Histology, ultrastructure and clinicopathologic correlation, *Z. Kinderchir.,* 40, 40, 1985.

51. **Griffiths, H. J., Robinson, K., and Bonfiglio, T. A.,** Aggressive fibromatosis, *Skel. Radiol.,* 9, 179, 1983.

52. **Alpers, C. E., Rosenau, W., Finkbeiner, W. E., et al.,** Congenital (infantile) hemangiopericytoma of the tongue and sublingual region, *Am. J. Clin. Pathol.,* 81, 377, 1984.

53. **Eimoto, T.,** Ultrastructure of infantile hemangiopericytoma, *Cancer,* 40, 2161, 1977.

54. **Chou, P., Gonzalez-Crussi, F., and Mangkornkanok, M.,** Giant cell fibroblastoma, *Cancer,* 63, 756, 1989.

55. **Shmookler, B. M., Enzinger, F. M., and Weiss, S. W.,** Giant cell fibroblastoma. A juvenile form of dermatofibrosarcoma protuberans, *Cancer,* 64, 2154, 1989.

56. **Chung, E. B. and Enzinger, F. M.,** Infantile fibrosarcoma, *Cancer,* 38, 729, 1976.

57. **Dahl, T., Save-Soderbergh, J., and Angervall, L.,** Fibrosarcoma in early infancy, *Pathol. Eur.,* 8, 193, 1973.

58. **Gonzalez-Crussi, F., Wiederhold, M. D., and Sotelo-Avila, C.,** Congenital fibrosarcoma. Presence of a histiocytic component, *Cancer,* 46, 77, 1980.

59. **Iwasaki, H. and Enjoji, M.,** Infantile and adult fibrosarcomas of the soft tissue, *Acta Pathol. Jpn.,* 29, 377, 1979.

60. **Soule, E. H. and Pritchard, D. J.,** Fibrosarcoma in infants and children: a review of 110 cases, *Cancer,* 40, 1711, 1977.

61. **Pettinato, G., Manivel, J. C., Saldana, M. J., et al.,** Primary bronchopulmonary fibrosarcoma of childhood and adolescence: reassessment of a low-grade malignancy. Clinicopathologic study of five cases and review of the literature, *Hum. Pathol.,* 20, 463, 1989.

62. **Rootman, J., Carvounis, E. P., Dolman, C. L., and Dimmick, J. E.,** Congenital fibrosarcoma metastatic to the choroid, *Am. J. Ophthalmol.,* 87, 632, 1979.

63. **Yannopoulos, K. and Stout, A. P.,** Smooth muscle tumors in children, *Cancer,* 15, 958, 1962.

64. **Lack, E. E.,** Leiomyosarcomas in childhood: a clinical and pathologic study of 10 cases, *Pediatr. Pathol.,* 6, 181, 1986.

65. **Fields, J. P. and Helwig, E. B.,** Leiomyosarcoma of the skin and subcutaneous tissue, *Cancer,* 47, 156, 1981.

66. **Swanson, P. E., Wick, M. R., and Dehner, L. P.,** Leiomyosarcoma in childhood: an immunohistochemical and ultrastructural study, *Human Pathol.,* in press.

67. **Bures, J. C., Barnes, L., and Mercer, D.,** A comparative study of smooth muscle tumors using light and electron microscopy, immunocytochemical staining, and enzymatic assay, *Cancer,* 48, 2420, 1981.

68. **Swanson, P. E., Stanley, M. W., Scheithauer, B. W., and Wick, M. R.,** Primary cutaneous leiomyosarcoma. A histologic and immunohistochemical study of nine cases, with ultrastructural correlation, *J. Cutan. Pathol.,* 15, 129, 1988.

69. **Swanson, P. E., Manivel, J. C., and Wick, M. R.,** Immunoreactivity for Leu 7 in neurofibrosarcoma and other spindle-cell soft tissue sarcomas, *Am. J. Pathol.,* 126, 546, 1987.

70. **Bale, P. M., Parsons, R. E., and Stevens, M. M.,** Pathology and behavior of juvenile rhabdomyosarcoma, in *Pathology of Neoplasia in Children and Adolescents,* Finegold, M., Ed., W.B. Saunders, Philadelphia, 1986, 186.

71. **Shen, S. C. and Yunis, E. J.,** Leiomyosarcoma developing in a child during remission of leukemia, *J. Pediatr.,* 89, 780, 1976.

72. **Chadwick, E. G., Connor, E. J., Hanson, C. G., et al.,** Tumors of smooth muscle origin in HIV-infected children, *J.A.M.A.,* 263, 3182, 1990.

73. **Mukai, M., Iri, H., Nakajima, T., et al.,** Alveolar soft part sarcoma. A review on its histogenesis and further studies based on electron microscopy, immunocytochemistry, and biochemistry, *Am. J. Surg. Pathol.,* 7, 679, 1983.

74. **Ordonez, N. G., Ro, J. Y., and Mackay, B.,** Alveolar soft part sarcoma. An ultrastructural and immunocytochemical investigation of its histogenesis, *Cancer,* 63, 1721, 1989.

75. **Lieberman, P. H., Brennan, M. F., Kimmel, M., et al.,** Alveolar soft-part sarcoma. A clinico-pathologic study of half a century, *Cancer,* 63, 1, 1989.

76. **Font, R. L., Jurco, S., and Zimmerman, L. E.,** Alveolar soft part sarcoma of the orbit. A clinicopathologic analysis of seventeen cases and a review of the literature, *Hum. Pathol.,* 13, 569, 1982.

77. **Battifora, H.,** Hemangiopericytoma: ultrastructural study of five cases, *Cancer,* 31, 1418, 1973.

78. **Enzinger, F. M. and Smith, B. H.,** Hemangiopericytoma. An analysis of 106 cases, *Hum. Pathol.,* 7, 62, 1976.

79. **McMaster, M. J., Soule, E. H., and Ivins, J. C.,** Hemangiopericytoma. A clinicopathologic study and long term followup of 60 patients, *Cancer,* 36, 2232, 1975.

80. **Ortega, J. A., Finklestein, J. Z., Isaacs, H., Jr., et al.,** Chemotherapy of malignant hemangiopericytoma of childhood. Report of a case and review of the literature, *Cancer,* 27, 730, 1971.

81. **Tsuneyoshi, M., Daimaru, Y., and Enjoji, M.,** Malignant hemangiopericytoma and other sarcomas with hemangiopericytoma-like pattern, *Pathol. Res. Pract.,* 178, 446, 1984.

82. **Schneider, M., Obringer, A. C., Zackai, E., and Meadows, A. T.,** Childhood neurofibromatosis: risk factors for malignant disease, *Cancer Genet. Cytogenet.,* 21, 347, 1986.

83. **Gallager, R. L. and Helwig, E. B.,** Neurothekeoma — a benign cutaneous tumor of neural origin, *Am. J. Clin. Pathol.,* 74, 759, 1980.

84. **Lodding, P., Kindblom, L.-G., Angervall, L., and Stenman, G.,** Cellular schwannoma. A clinico-pathologic study of 29 cases, *Virchows Arch. A,* 416, 237, 1990.

85. **Woodruff, J. M., Goodwin, T. A., Erlandson, R. A., et al.,** Cellular schwannoma. A variety of schwannoma sometimes mistaken for a malignant tumor, *Am. J. Surg. Pathol.,* 5, 733, 1981.

86. **Coffin, C. M. and Dehner, L. P.,** Cellular peripheral neural tumors (neurofibromas) in children and adolescents: a clinicopathologic and immunohistochemical study, *Pediatr. Pathol.,* 10, 351, 1990.

87. **Ducatman, B. S., Scheithauer, B. W., Piepgras, D. G., et al.,** Malignant peripheral nerve sheath tumors. A clinicopathologic study of 120 cases, *Cancer,* 57, 2006, 1986.

88. **Ducatman, B. S. and Scheithauer, B. W.,** Postirradiation neurofibrosarcoma, *Cancer,* 51, 1028, 1983.

89. **Ducatman, B. S., Scheithauer, B. W., Piepgras, D. G., and Reiman, H. M.,** Malignant peripheral nerve sheath tumors in childhood, *Neurol. Oncol.,* 21, 241, 1984.

90. **DiCarlo, E. F., Woodruff, J. M., Bansal, M., and Erlandson, R. A.,** The purely epithelioid malignant peripheral nerve sheath tumor, *Am. J. Surg. Pathol.,* 10, 478, 1986.

91. **Chaudhuri, B., Ronan, S. G., and Manaligod, J. R.,** Angiosarcoma arising in a plexiform neurofibroma: a case report, *Cancer,* 46, 605, 1980.

92. **Ducatman, B. S. and Scheithauer, B. W.,** Malignant peripheral nerve sheath tumors with divergent differentiation, *Cancer,* 54, 1049, 1984.

93. **Woodruff, J. M.,** Peripheral nerve tumors showing glandular differentiation (glandular schwannomas), *Cancer,* 37, 2399, 1976.

94. **Wick, M. R., Swanson, P. E., Scheithauer, B. W., and Manivel, J. C.,** Malignant peripheral nerve sheath tumor. An immunohistochemical analysis of 62 cases, *Am. J. Clin. Pathol.,* 87, 425, 1987.

95. **Stefansson, K., Wollman, R., and Jerkovic, M.,** S-100 protein in soft tissue tumors derived from schwann cells and melanocytes, *Am. J. Pathol.,* 106, 261, 1982.

96. **Weiss, S. W., Langloss, J. M., and Enzinger, F. M.,** Value of S100 protein in the diagnosis of soft tissue tumors with particular reference to benign and malignant Schwann cell tumors, *Lab. Invest.,* 49, 299, 1983.

97. **Miettinen, M.,** Immunohistochemistry of peripheral nerve sheath sarcomas, *Mod. Pathol.,* 3(Abstr.), 67A, 1990.

98. **Chitale, A. R. and Dickersin, G. R.,** Electron microscopy in the diagnosis of malignant schwannomas, *Cancer,* 51, 1448, 1983.

99. **Erlandson, R. A. and Woodruff, J. M.,** Peripheral nerve sheath tumors: an electron microscopic study of 43 cases, *Cancer,* 43, 273, 1982.

100. **Dehner, L. P.,** Peripheral and central primitive neuroectodermal tumors. A nosologic concept seeking a consensus, *Arch. Pathol. Lab. Med.,* 110, 997, 1986.

101. **Gonzalez-Crussi, F., Wolfson, S. L., Misugi, K., and Nakajima, T.,** Peripheral neuroectodermal tumors of the chest wall in childhood, *Cancer,* 54, 2519, 1984.

102. **Jurgens, H., Bier, V., Harms, D., et al.,** Malignant peripheral neuroectodermal tumors. A retrospective analysis of 42 patients, *Cancer,* 61, 349, 1988.

103. **Marina, N. M., Etcubanas, E., Parham, D. M., et al.,** Peripheral primitive neuroectodermal tumor (peripheral neuroepithelioma) in children. A review of the St. Jude experience and controversies in diagnosis and management, *Cancer,* 64, 1952, 1984.

104. **Askin, F. B., Rosai, J., Sibley, R. K., et al.,** Malignant small cell tumor of the thoracopulmonary region in childhood: a distinct clinicopathologic entity of uncertain histogenesis, *Cancer,* 43, 2438, 1979.

105. **Linnoila, R. I., Tsokos, M., Triche, T. J., et al.,** Evidence for neural origin and PAS-positive variants of the malignant small cell tumor of thoracopulmonary region (''Askin tumor''), *Am. J. Surg. Pathol.,* 10, 124, 1986.

106. **Henderson, D. W., Leppard, P. J., Brennan, J. S., et al.,** Primitive neuroepithelial tumours of soft tissue and of bone: further ultrastructural and immunocytochemical clarification of 'Ewing's sarcoma', including freeze fracture analysis, *J. Submicrosc. Cytol. Pathol.,* 21, 35, 1989.

107. **Michels, S., Swanson, P. E., Robb, J. A., and Wick, M. R.,** Leu 7 in small-cell neoplasms. An immunohistochemical study, with ultrastructural correlations, *Cancer,* 60, 2958, 1987.

108. **Schmidt, D., Harms, D., and Burdach, S.,** Malignant peripheral neuroectodermal tumours of childhood and adolescence, *Virchows Arch. A,* 406, 351, 1985.

109. **Swanson, P. E., Wick, M. R., Hagen, K. A., and Dehner, L. P.,** Synaptophysin in small round cell tumors, *Am. J. Clin. Pathol.,* 88(Abstr.), 523, 1987.

110. **Lampson, L. A., Whelan, J. F., and Fisher, C. A.,** HLA-A,B,C and beta-2-microglobulin are expressed weakly by human cells of neuronal origin, but can be induced in neuroblastoma cell lines by interferon. Advances in neuroblastoma research, *Prog. Clin. Biol. Res.,* 175, 379, 1985.

111. **Kahn, H. J. and Thorner, P. S.,** Monoclonal antibody MB2: a potential marker for Ewing's sarcoma and primitive neuroectodermal tumor, *Pediatr. Pathol.,* 9, 153, 1989.

112. **Crist, W. M., Raney, R. B., Newton, W., et al.,** Intrathoracic soft tissue sarcomas in children, *Cancer,* 50, 598, 1982.

113. **Dickman, P. S. and Triche, T. J.,** Extraosseous Ewing's sarcoma versus primitive rhabdomyosarcoma: diagnostic criteria and clinical correlation, *Hum. Pathol.,* 17, 888, 1986.

114. **Hashimoto, H., Tsuneyoshi, M., Daimaru, Y., and Enjoji, M.,** Extraskeletal Ewing's sarcoma. A clinicopathologic and electron microscopic analysis of 8 cases, *Acta Pathol. Jpn.,* 35, 1087, 1985.

115. **Kinsella, T. J., Triche, T. J., Dickman, P. S., et al.,** Extraskeletal Ewing's sarcoma: results of combined modality treatment, *J. Clin. Oncol.,* 1, 489, 1983.

115a. **Rud, N. P., Reiman, H. M., Pritchard, D. J., et al.,** Extraosseous Ewing's sarcoma. A study of 42 cases, *Cancer,* 64, 1548, 1989.

116. **Kawaguchi, K. and Koike, M.,** Neuron-specific enolase and Leu-7 immunoreactive small round cell neoplasms. The relationship of Ewing's sarcoma in bone and soft tissue, *Am. J. Clin. Pathol.,* 86, 79, 1986.

117. **Moll, R., Lee, I., Gould, V., et al.,** Immunocytochemical analysis of Ewing's tumors. Patterns of expression of intermediate filaments and desmosomal proteins indicate cell type heterogeneity and pluripotential differentiation, *Am. J. Pathol.,* 127, 288, 1987.

118. **Navas-Palacios, J., Aparicio-Duque, R., and Valdes, M. D.,** On the histogenesis of Ewing's sarcoma. An ultrastructural, immunohistochemical, and cytochemical study, *Cancer,* 53, 1882, 1984.

119. **Turc-Carel, C., Aurias, A., Mugneret, F., et al.,** Chromosomes in Ewing's sarcoma. I. An evaluation of 85 cases of remarkable consistency of t(11;22) (q24;q12), *Cancer Genet. Cytogenet.,* 32, 229, 1988.

120. **McKeon, C., Thiele, C. J., Ross, M. A., et al.,** Indistinguishable patterns of protooncogene expression in two distinct but closely related tumors: Ewing's sarcoma and neuroepithelioma, *Cancer Res.,* 49, 4307, 1988.

121. **Thiele, C. J., McKeon, C., Triche, T. J., et al.,** Differential protooncogene expression characterizes histopathologically indistinguishable tumors of the peripheral nervous system, *J. Clin. Invest.,* 80, 804, 1987.

122. **Triche, T. J., Cavazzana, A. O., Navarro, S., et al.,** N-myc protein expression in small round cell tumors, *Prog. Clin. Biol. Res.,* 271, 475, 1988.

123. **Cavazanna, A. O., Miser, J. S., Jeffereson, J., and Triche, T. J.,** Experimental evidence for a neural origin of Ewing's sarcoma of bone, *Am. J. Pathol.,* 127, 507, 1987.

124. **Fujii, Y., Hongo, T., Nakagawa, Y., et al.,** Cell culture of small round cell tumor originating in the thoracopulmonary region. Evidence for derivation from a primitive pluripotential cell, *Cancer,* 64, 43, 1989.

125. **Hachitanda, Y., Tsuneyoshi, M., Enjoji, M., et al.,** Congenital primitive neuroectodermal tumor with epithelial and glial differentiation. An ultrastructural and immunohistochemical study, *Arch. Pathol. Lab. Med.,* 114, 101, 1990.

126. **Shinoda, M., Tsutsumi, Y., Hata, J., and Yokoyama, S.,** Peripheral neuroepithelioma in childhood. Immunohistochemical demonstration of epithelial differentiation, *Arch. Pathol. Lab. Med.,* 112, 1155, 1988.

127. **Jacobson, S. A.,** Polyhistioma. A malignant tumor of bone and extraskeletal tissues, *Cancer,* 40, 2116, 1977.

128. **Hutter, R. V. P., Foote, F. W., Francis, K. C., and Sherman, R. S.,** Primitive multipotential primary sarcoma of bone, *Cancer,* 19, 1, 1966.

129. **Karcoglu, Z., Someren, A., and Mathes, S. J.,** Ectomesenchymoma: a malignant tumor of migratory neural crest (ectomesenchyme) remnants showing ganglionic, schwannian, melanocytic, and rhabdomyoblastic differentiation, *Cancer,* 39, 2486, 1977.

130. **Gerald, W. L., Miller, H. K., Battifora, H., et al.,** Intra-abdominal desmoplastic small round-cell tumor: report of 19 cases of a distinctive type of high-grade polyphenotypic malignancy affecting young individuals, *Am. J. Surg. Pathol.,* 15, 499, 1991.

131. **Gonzalez-Crussi, F., Crawford, S. E., and Sun, C.-C. J.,** Intraabdominal desmoplastic small-cell tumors with divergent differentiation. Observations on three cases of childhood, *Am. J. Surg. Pathol.,* 14, 633, 1990.

132. **Swanson, P. E., Dehner, L. P., and Wick, M. R.,** Polyphenotypic small cell tumors of childhood, *Lab. Invest.,* 58(Abstr.), 9P, 1988.

133. **Crocker, D. W. and Stout, A. P.,** Synovial sarcoma in children, *Cancer,* 12, 1123, 1959.

134. **Abenoza, P., Manivel, J. C., Swanson, P. E., and Wick, M. R.,** Synovial sarcoma: ultrastructural study and immunohistochemical analysis by a combined peroxidase-antiperoxidase/avidin-biotin-peroxidase complex procedure, *Hum. Pathol.,* 17, 1107, 1986.

135. **Schmookler, B. M.,** Retroperitoneal synovial sarcoma, *Am. J. Clin. Pathol.,* 77, 686, 1982.

136. **Lee, S. M., Hajdu, S. I., and Exelby, P. R.,** Synovial sarcoma in children, *Surg. Gynecol. Obstet.,* 138, 701, 1974.

137. **Cagle, L. A., Mirra, J. M., Storm, F. K., et al.,** Histologic features relating to prognosis in synovial sarcoma, *Cancer,* 59, 1810, 1987.

138. **Varela-Duran, J. and Enzinger, F. M.,** Calcifying synovial sarcoma, *Cancer,* 50, 345, 1982.

139. **Tsuneyoshi, M., Yokoyama, K., and Enjoji, M.,** Synovial sarcoma: a clinicopathologic and ultrastructural study of 42 cases, *Acta Pathol. Jpn.,* 33, 23, 1983.

139a. **Ordonez, N. G., Mahfouz, S. M., and Mackay, B.,** Synovial sarcoma: an immunohistochemical and ultrastructural study, *Hum. Pathol.,* 21, 733, 1990.

140. **Gonzalez, E. T., Jr. and Anderson, E. E.,** Retroperitoneal lipoblastic tumors in children, *J. Urol.,* 110, 474, 1973.

141. **Schmookler, B. M. and Enzinger, F. M.,** Pleomorphic lipoma: a benign tumor simulating liposarcoma. A clinicopathologic analysis of 48 cases, *Cancer,* 47, 126, 1981.

142. **Bolen, J. W. and Thorning, D.,** Benign lipoblastoma and myxoid liposarcoma. A comparative light- and electron-microscopic study, *Am. J. Surg. Pathol.,* 4, 163, 1980.

143. **Chung, E. B. and Enzinger, F. M.,** Benign lipoblastomatosis: an analysis of 35 cases, *Cancer,* 32, 482, 1973.

144. **Jimenez, J. F.,** Lipoblastoma in infancy and childhood, *J. Surg. Oncol.,* 32, 238, 1986.

145. **Plukker, J. T. M., Joosten, H. J. M., Rensing, J. B. M., and Van Haelst, U. J. G. M.,** Primary liposarcoma of the mediastinum in a child, *J. Surg. Oncol.,* 37, 257, 1988.

146. **Schmookler, B. M. and Enzinger, F. M.,** Liposarcoma occurring in children: an analysis of 17 cases and review of the literature, *Cancer,* 52, 567, 1983.

146. **Chang, H. R., Hajdu, S. I., Collin, C., and Brennan, M. F.,** The prognostic value of histologic subtypes in primary extremity liposarcoma, *Cancer,* 64, 1514, 1989.

148. **Hagerman, L. J., Czapek, E. E., Donnellan, W. L., and Schwartz, A. D.,** Giant hemangioma with consumption coagulopathy, *Pediatrics,* 87, 766, 1975.

149. **Dabashi, Y. and Eisen, R. N.,** Infantile hemangioendothelioma of the pelvis associated with Kasabach-Merritt syndrome, *Pediatr. Pathol.,* 10, 407, 1990.

150. **Kasabach, H. H. and Merritt, K. K.,** Capillary hemangioma with extensive purpura, *Am. J. Dis. Child.,* 59, 1063, 1940.

151. **Kuffer, F. R., Starzynski, T. E., Girolami, A., et al.,** Klippel-Trenaunay syndrome, visceral angiomatosis and thrombocytopenia, *J. Pediatr. Surg.,* 3, 65, 1968.

152. **Taxy, J. C. and Gray, S. R.,** Cellular angiomas in infancy: an ultrastructural study of two cases, *Cancer,* 43, 2322, 1979.

153. **Allen, P. W. and Enzinger, F. M.,** Hemangioma of skeletal muscle. An analysis of 89 cases, *Cancer,* 28, 8, 1972.

154. **Kuo, T. T., Sayers, C. P., and Rosai, J.,** Masson's "vegetant intravascular hemangioendothelioma" — a lesion often mistaken for angiosarcoma, *Cancer,* 38, 1227, 1976.

155. **Kauffman, S. L. and Stout, A. P.,** Extraskeletal osteogenic sarcomas and chondrosarcomas in children, *Cancer,* 16, 432, 1963.
156. **Dabska, M.,** Malignant endovascular papillary angioendothelioma of the skin in childhood, *Cancer,* 24, 503, 1969.
157. **Manivel, J. C., Wick, M. R., Swanson, P. E., Patterson, K., and Dehner, L. P.,** Endovascular papillary angioendothelioma: a vascular lesion showing possible "high" endothelial differentiation, *Hum. Pathol.,* 17, 1240, 1986.
158. **Morgan, J., Robinson, M. J., Rosen, L. B., et al.,** Malignant endovascular papillary angioendothelioma (Dabska tumor). A case report and review of the literature, *Am. J. Dermatopathol.,* 11, 64, 1989.
159. **Rosai, J., Gold, J., and Landy, R.,** The histiocytoid hemangiomas. A unifying concept embracing several previously described entities of skin, soft tissue, large vessels, bone and heart, *Hum. Pathol.,* 10, 707, 1979.
160. **Weiss, S. W. and Enzinger, F. M.,** Epithelioid hemangioendothelioma, *Cancer,* 50, 970, 1982.
161. **Scott, G. A. and Rosai, J.,** Spindle cell hemangioendothelioma. Report of seven additional cases of a recently described vascular neoplasm, *Am. J. Dermatopathol.,* 10, 281, 1988.
162. **Weiss, S. W. and Enzinger, F. M.,** Spindle cell hemangioendothelioma. A low-grade angiosarcoma resembling cavernous hemangioma and Kaposi's sarcoma, *Am. J. Surg. Pathol.,* 10, 521, 1986.
163. **Abratt, R. P., Williams, M., Raff, M., et al.,** Angiosarcoma of the superior vena cava, *Cancer,* 52, 740, 1983.
164. **Kauffman, S. L. and Stout, A. P.,** Malignant hemangioendothelioma in infants and children, *Cancer,* 14, 1186, 1961.
165. **Burgdorf, W. H., Mukai, K., and Rosai, J.,** Immunohistochemical identification of factor VIII-related antigen in endothelial cells of cutaneous lesions of alleged vascular nature, *Am. J. Clin. Pathol.,* 75, 167, 1981.
166. **Miettinen, M., Holthofer, H., Lehto, V.-P., et al.,** *Ulex europaeus* lectin as a marker for tumors derived from endothelial cells, *Am. J. Clin. Pathol.,* 79, 32, 1983.
167. **Dubin, H. V., Creehan, E. P., and Headington, J. T.,** Lymphangiosarcoma and congenital lymphedema of the extremity, *Arch. Dermatol.,* 110, 608, 1974.
168. **Muller, R., Hajdu, S. I., and Brennan, M. F.,** Lymphangiosarcoma associated with chronic filarial lymphedema, *Cancer,* 59, 179, 1987.
169. **Bisceglia, M., Mostafa, A., and Bosman, C.,** Primary Kaposi's sarcoma of the lymph node in children, *Cancer,* 61, 1715, 1988.
170. **Slavin, G., Cameron, H. M., and Singh, H.,** Kaposi's sarcoma in mainland Tanzania: a report of 117 cases, *Br. J. Cancer,* 23, 349, 1969.
171. **Su, I. J., Kuo, T. T., Wu, S. Y., and Hung, I. J.,** Lymphadenopathic type of Kaposi's sarcoma presenting with generalized petechial hemorrhages, *Cancer,* 54, 948, 1984.
172. **Chase, D. R. and Enzinger, F. M.,** Epithelioid sarcoma. Diagnosis, prognostic indicators and treatment, *Am. J. Surg. Pathol.,* 9, 241, 1985.
173. **Schmidt, D. and Harms, D.,** Epithelioid sarcoma in children and adolescents. An immunohistochemical study, *Virchows Arch. A,* 410, 423, 1987.
174. **Daimaru, Y., Hashimoto, H., Tsuneyoshi, M., and Enjoji, M.,** Epithelial profile of epithelioid sarcoma. An immunohistochemical analysis of eight cases, *Cancer,* 59, 134, 1987.
175. **Manivel, J. C., Wick, M. R., Dehner, L. P., and Sibley, R. K.,** Epithelioid sarcoma. An immunohistochemical study, *Am. J. Clin. Pathol.,* 87, 319, 1987.
176. **Chung, E. B. and Enzinger, F. M.,** Malignant melanoma of soft parts: a reassessment of clear cell sarcoma, *Am. J. Surg. Pathol.,* 7, 405, 1983.
177. **Eckardt, J. J., Pritchard, D. J., and Soule, E. H.,** Clear cell sarcoma: a clinicopathologic study of 27 cases, *Cancer,* 52, 1482, 1983.
178. **Swanson, P. E. and Wick, M. R.,** Clear cell sarcoma. An immunohistochemical analysis of six cases, with comparison to other epithelioid neoplasms of soft tissue, *Arch. Pathol. Lab. Med.,* 113, 55, 1989.
179. **Kent, A. L., Mahoney, D. H., Gresik, M. V., et al.,** Malignant rhabdoid tumor of the extremity, *Cancer,* 60, 1056, 1987.
180. **Lynch, H. T., Shurin, S. B., Dahms, B. B., et al.,** paravertebral malignant rhabdoid tumor in infancy. In vitro studies of a familial tumor, *Cancer,* 52, 290, 1983.
181. **Sotelo-Avila, C., Gonzalez-Crussi, F., deMello, D., et al.,** Renal and extrarenal rhabdoid tumors in children: a clinicopathologic study of 14 patients, *Sem. Diagn. Pathol.,* 3, 151, 1986.
182. **Tsuneyoshi, M., Daimaru, Y., Hashimoto, H., and Enjoji, M.,** Malignant soft tissue neoplasms with the histologic features of renal rhabdoid tumors: an ultrastructural and immunohistochemical study, *Hum. Pathol.,* 16, 1235, 1985.
183. **Perrone, T., Swanson, P. E., Twiggs, L., et al.,** Malignant rhabdoid tumor of the vulva: is distinction from epithelioid sarcoma possible? A pathologic and immunohistochemical study, *Am. J. Surg. Pathol.,* 13, 848, 1989.

184. **Dahlin, D. C. and Salvador, A. H.,** Cartilaginous tumors of the soft tissues of the hands and feet, *Mayo Clin. Proc.*, 49, 721, 1974.

185. **Huvos, A. G. and Marcove, R. C.,** Chondrosarcoma in the young. A clinicopathologic analysis of 79 patients younger than 21 years of age, *Am. J. Surg. Pathol.*, 11, 930, 1987.

186. **Huvos, A. G., Rosen, G., Dabska, M., and Marcove, R. C.,** Mesenchymal chondrosarcoma. A clinicopathologic analysis of 35 patients with emphasis on treatment, *Cancer*, 51, 1230, 1983.

187. **Nakashima, Y., Unni, K. K., Shives, T. C., et al.,** Mesenchymal chondrosarcoma of bone and soft tissue. A review of 111 cases, *Cancer*, 57, 2444, 1986.

188. **Scheithauer, B. W. and Rubinstein, L. J.,** Meningeal mesenchymal chondrosarcoma: report of 8 cases with review of the literature, *Cancer*, 42, 2744, 1978.

189. **Swanson, P. E., Manivel, J. C., Lillemoe, T. J., and Wick, M. R.,** Mesenchymal chondrosarcoma. An immunohistochemical analysis, *Arch. Pathol. Lab. Med.*, 114, 943, 1990.

190. **Nakamura, Y., Becker, L. E., and Marks, A.,** S-100 protein in tumors of cartilage and bone. An immunohistochemical study, *Cancer*, 52, 1820, 1983.

191. **Hachitanda, Y., Tsuneyoshi, M., Daimaru, Y., et al.,** Extraskeletal myxoid chondrosarcoma in young children, *Cancer*, 61, 2521, 1988.

192. **Albores-Saavedra, J., Angeles-Angeles, A., Ridaura, C., and Brandt, H.,** Embryonal chondrosarcoma in children, *Patologia*, 15, 153, 1977.

193. **Huvos, A. G., Woodard, H. Q., Cahan, W. G., et al.,** Postradiation osteogenic sarcoma of bone and soft tissues, *Cancer*, 55, 1244, 1985.

194. **Karapurkar, A. P., Pandya, S. K., and Desai, A. P.,** Radiation induced sarcoma, *Surg. Neurol.*, 13, 419, 1980.

195. **Potish, R. A., Dehner, L. P., Haselow, R. E., et al.,** The incidence of second neoplasms following megavoltage radiation for pediatric tumors, *Cancer*, 56, 1534, 1985.

196. **Tucker, M. A., D'Angio, G. J., Boice, J. D., Jr., et al.,** Bone sarcomas linked to radiotherapy and chemotherapy in children, *N. Engl. J. Med.*, 317, 588, 1987.

Chapter 24

CLINICAL MANIFESTATIONS AND TREATMENT OF SOFT TISSUE SARCOMAS OTHER THAN RHABDOMYOSARCOMA

Charles B. Pratt

TABLE OF CONTENTS

I. INTRODUCTION

Nonrhabdomyosarcomatous soft tissue sarcomas may develop anywhere in the body,[1-3] usually presenting as a mass which may be either painless or associated with pain. The mass is usually discovered by the child or his or her parent. The mass may be small if it is located in a subcutaneous region. Masses which involve an extremity or are located in retroperitoneal or intrathoracic areas may become extremely large before they are discovered.

The symptoms produced by these neoplasma are caused by tumor growth or pressure on adjacent structures; symptoms may also be due to hemorrhage, obstruction, or perforation of viscera, or caused by necrosis of the tumors themselves. Sarcomas usually are painless, but pain may develop acutely after spontaneous hemorrhage or following trauma. Patients often date onset of symptoms to an injury that has no causal relationship to the development of sarcoma. Tumor necrosis is associated with the insidious onset of pain, which may be due to direct compression of nerves or due to pressure on a neurovascular bundle. Pain may occur without presence of a palpable mass, or it may be associated with pressure from the mass on surrounding tissues. A schwannoma or a neurogenic sarcoma, arising on a peripheral nerve, may cause pain within the distribution of that nerve.

Cranial nerve dysfunction may occur in patients with soft tissue sarcomas involving the head and neck region. Intrathoracic sarcomas can produce shortness of breath and may be associated with pleural effusion. Retroperitoneal tumors generally present as a large mass which is discovered incidentally, or they may be associated with abdominal enlargement. Soft tissue sarcomas of an extremity can disturb function of the limb, but are rarely associated with pain unless there is direct bony or neurovascular involvement by tumor.

Bone marrow metastases from these tumors are rare, yet direct invasion of bones by primary tumors is not uncommon. Lymph node infiltration and metastases to lymph nodes are also uncommon,[4] in comparison to the occurrence of these findings in rhabdomyosarcoma.

Nonrhabdomyosarcomatous soft tissue sarcomas are rarely associated with paraneoplastic syndromes.[5] Hypoglycemia has been observed to accompany advanced fibrosarcomas, schwannomas, and hemangiopericytomas. The hypoglycemia associated with hemangiopericytoma may be produced by substances with nonsuppressive, insulin-like activity. Altered carbohydrate metabolism and development of diabetes mellitus have been seen in patients with fibrosarcoma of the lung.

High grade sarcomas occasionally produce fever, which may be associated with tumor necrosis.

The histologic diagnosis and grading of soft tissue sarcomas were discussed in Chapter 23. Also discussed previously is the staging of tumors by both the clinical groupings of the Intergroup Rhabdomyosarcoma Study (IRS) Committee and the TNM (tumor, nodes, metastases) groupings of the American Joint Commission. For soft tissue sarcomas of children, the author's personal preference is to use the groupings of the IRS Committee because of the almost universal use of this system, and because of its greater relevance to sarcomas in children. By convention, sarcomas originating in the brain and liver are excluded from the designation of nonrhabdomyosarcomatous soft tissue sarcomas. Also, this discussion focuses on the more common tumors, other than rhabdomyosarcoma, which involve the head, neck, trunk, and extremities.

II. INCIDENCE

Rhabdomyosarcomas and the other soft tissue sarcomas comprise about 10% of all malignant neoplasms seen in childhood and adolescence.[6] Soft tissue sarcomas other than rhabdomyosarcomas represent almost 25% of all soft tissue sarcomas occurring in persons

TABLE 1
Nonrhabdomyosarcomatous Soft Tissue Sarcomas, St. Jude Children's Research Hospital, 1962—1988: Distribution of Patients by Site and Clinical Grouping

Site of tumor	Clinical groupings				All groups
	I	II	III	IV	
Head and neck	6 (30)[a]	4 (20)	8 (40)	2 (10)	20 (17)
Trunk	20 (42)	5 (10)	12 (25)	11 (23)	48 (40)
Extremities	31 (60)	6 (12)	6 (12)	8 (16)	51 (43)
All sites	57 (48)[b]	15 (12)	26 (22)	21 (18)	119 (100)

[a] Number of patients (%) in each group according to site of malignancy.
[b] Percentages for all sites and all groups are based on the total number (119) of patients in this study.

TABLE 2
Nonrhabdomyosarcomatous Soft Tissue Sarcomas of Head and Neck, St. Jude Children's Research Hospital, 1962—1988: Survival by Clinical Grouping

Type of tumor	Clinical groupings (number of patients surviving/treated)			
	I	II	III	IV
Synovial sarcoma			0/1	
Fibrosarcoma, infantile	0/1			0/1
Fibrosarcoma	1/1			
Malignant fibrous histiocytoma			0/1	
Epithelioid sarcoma	1/1			
Schwannoma	0/1	1/1	0/3	
Alveolar soft part sarcoma	1/1			
Myeloid chondrosarcoma	1/1			
Sarcoma, not otherwise specified			1/1	0/1
Hemangiopericytoma		2/2	0/1	
Hemangioendothelioma		0/1[a]	1/1	
Total patients	4/6	3/4	2/8	0/2

[a] Died of accidental causes.

younger than 20 years of age. Because of their rarity and diverse characteristics, information about the frequency of these tumors or their sites of origin is limited. Therefore, the author reviewed the 119 patients with nonrhabdomyosarcomatous soft tissue sarcoma seen at one institution during a 27-year period. These 119 cases represent 28% of the 419 patients with soft tissue sarcomas seen at the hospital during that period of time.

In Table 1, soft tissue sarcomas are listed by site and clinical grouping, using the classification of the IRS Committee. According to site of origin, the greatest number of nonrhabdomyosarcoma soft tissue sarcomas occurred in the extremities, representing 43% of the total number of patients. By clinical grouping, 48% of all patients were classified as group I, 12% had clinical group II, 22% were in clinical group III, and 18% were classified as clinical group IV.

Survival according to clinical grouping for patients with various soft tissue sarcomas located in the head and neck region is depicted in Table 2. These rare soft tissue sarcomas represent a mixture of histologic types, the most frequent of which was schwannoma. Survival

TABLE 3
Nonrhabdomyosarcomatous Soft Tissue Sarcomas of the Trunk, St.
Jude Children's Research Hospital, 1962—1988: Survival by Clinical
Grouping

Type of tumor	Clinical groupings (number of patients surviving/treated)			
	I	II	III	IV
Synovial sarcoma	2/3		0/1	0/2
Fibrosarcoma, infantile	1/1	1/1		
Fibrosarcoma	2/2		1/1[a]	
Malignant fibrous histiocy- toma	2/2	1/1		0/1
Epithelioid sarcoma				0/1
Schwannoma	1/1	0/1	0/3	0/3
Alveolar soft part sarcoma	2/2		1/1	
Sarcoma, not otherwise speci- fied	2/2		0/2	1/1
Leiomyosarcoma	0/2	1/2		0/2
Angiosarcoma			0/1	
Liposarcoma	1/1		1/2	0/1
Mesothelioma			1/1	
Extraosseous Ewing's sarcoma	3/4			
Total patients	16/20	3/5	4/12	1/11

[a]   Died of accidental causes.

was good for patients who had localized tumors, or tumors which were grossly resected leaving only microscopic residual neoplastic tissue.

Survival by clinical grouping of patients with nonrhabdomyosarcomatous soft tissue sarcomas of the trunk is shown in Table 3. Survival was good for individuals with clinical group I or II disease. For the trunk area, the most frequently encountered nonrhabdomyosarcomatous soft tissue sarcomas were those designated ''sarcoma not otherwise specified'' (NOS) and extraosseous Ewing's sarcoma.

The most frequent site of these soft tissue sarcomas was the extremities, and the most common tumor type was synovial sarcoma. In Table 4, the relation of survival to clinical grouping is listed. It is apparent that survival is better for persons with nonrhabdomyosarcomatous soft tissue sarcomas of the extremities classified as clinical groups I or II than for those in clinical groups III or IV.

Table 5 combines Tables 2 through 4 and indicates survival by clinical grouping of patients with tumors at all sites. For all patients, survival was best for individuals with synovial sarcoma, malignant fibrous histiocytoma, infantile fibrosarcoma, fibrosarcoma, alveolar soft part sarcoma, sarcoma NOS, dermatofibrosarcoma protuberans, and extraosseous Ewing's sarcoma.

III. MANAGEMENT

Patients underwent various surgical techniques for biopsy or resection of tumor, and many received chemotherapy, radiotherapy, or both. Details of these procedures have been published in part.[1] More recently, patients have been treated by the Pediatric Oncology Group Protocol 8653/54 entitled ''A Study of Childhood Soft Tissue Sarcomas Other Than Rhabdomyosarcoma and Its Variants''. In this study, patients received follow-up evaluation whether they were given chemotherapy, radiotherapy, or both modalities following diagnosis (Figure 1).

TABLE 4
Nonrhabdomyosarcomatous Soft Tissue Sarcomas of the Extremities, St. Jude Children's Research Hospital, 1962—1988: Survival by Clinical Grouping

Type of tumor	Clinical groupings (number surviving/treated)			
	I	II	III	IV
Synovial sarcoma	13/16	2/2	0/3	1/4[a]
Fibrosarcoma, infantile	2/3			
Fibrosarcoma	1/1			
Malignant fibrous histiocytoma	4/4			0/2
Epithelioid sarcoma	1/1[a]			
Schwannoma	1/1	1/2		
Alveolar soft part sarcoma	0/1[b]			
Myxoid chondrosarcoma				0/1
Sarcoma, not otherwise specified	1/1	1/1		
Hemangiopericytoma	1/1		0/1	0/1
Angiosarcoma			0/1	
Liposarcoma			0/1	
Dermatofibrosarcoma protuberans	1/1	1/1		
Extraosseous Ewing's sarcoma	0/1			
Total patients	25/31	5/6	0/6	1/8

[a] Living with disease.
[b] Died of accidental causes.

TABLE 5
Nonrhabdomyosarcomatous Soft Tissue Sarcomas at All Sites: Survival by Clinical Grouping

Type of tumor	Clinical groupings (number of patients surviving/treated)				All groups
	I	II	III	IV	
Synovial sarcoma	15/19	2/2	0/5	1/6	18/32
Schwannoma	2/3	2/4	0/6	0/3	4/16
Malignant fibrous histiocytoma	6/6	1/1	0/1	0/3	7/11
Fibrosarcoma, infantile	3/5	1/1		0/1	4/7
Fibrosarcoma	4/4		1/1[a]		5/5
Alveolar soft part	3/4[b]		1/1		4/5
Myxoid chondrosarcoma	1/1			0/1	1/2
Epithelioid sarcoma	2/2[a]			0/1	2/3
Sarcoma, not otherwise specified	3/3	1/1	1/3	1/2	6/9
Hemangiopericytoma	1/1	2/2	0/2	0/1	3/6
Leiomyosarcoma	0/2	1/2		0/2	1/6
Angiosarcoma			0/2		0/2
Liposarcoma	1/1		1/3	0/1	2/5
Dermatofibrosarcoma protuberans	1/1	1/1			2/2
Mesothelioma			1/1		1/1
Hemangioendothelioma		0/1[b]	1/1		1/2
Extraosseous Ewing's sarcoma	3/5				3/5
Total patients	45/57	11/15	6/26	2/21	64/119

[a] Living with disease.
[b] Died of accidental causes.

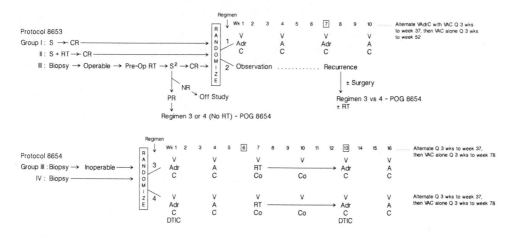

FIGURE 1.   Soft tissue sarcoma study scheme: Pediatric Oncology Group (POG) protocol 8653/8654. Abbreviations: V = vincristine, 1.5 mg/m² i.v. (no dose to exceed 2 mg); Adr = adriamycin (doxorubicin), 60 mg/m² i.v. (cumulative dose = 360 mg/m²); C = cyclophosphamide, 750 mg/m² i.v.; A = actinomycin D (dactinomycin), 1.25 mg/m² i.v. (no top dose); DTIC = imidazole carboxamide, 500 mg/m² (no top dose); S = surgery; S² = second surgery 6 to 12 weeks after completion of radiotherapy; ☐☐☐ = evaluation for response and/or recurrence; Co = omit cyclophosphamide if bladder is in field of radiotherapy.

The approach to management of nonrhabdomyosarcomatous soft tissue sarcomas of children and adolescents[7-11] in many ways resembles that used for treating tumors with similar histologies involving adults, for which there is greater experience in management.[2,3,12-16] Preoperative evaluation assesses the degree of local spread and the location of distant metastases. Tumors are evaluated according to size and number, and for possible presence of lymph node and distant metastases, as well as for potential resectability.[2,3]

IV. SURGERY

Surgical procedures for managing soft tissue sarcomas may include fine needle aspiration, needle biopsy, excisional biopsy, incisional biopsy with or without frozen section, or total resection of the tumor.[2,3] The exact nature of the surgical procedure is influenced by the site and the potential resectability of the lesion. Local control of the tumor may be more difficult to achieve in the retroperitoneal area or in the head and neck area due to the proximity of vital structures. For extremity tumors, local control may be more difficult to obtain because of the proximal location of tumors. The nonrhabdomyosarcomatous soft tissue sarcomas of children and adolescents rarely involve bones except by direct extension, and they almost never involve the bone marrow.

For extremity lesions, appropriate surgical procedures may include intracapsular resection, marginal resection, wide resection, radical resection, muscle compartment excisions, or other limb-sparing procedures.[2,3] Need for amputation depends on the site and extent of the primary tumor and expected natural history of the specific soft tissue sarcoma.

Surgery is the primary treatment for soft tissue sarcomas, but chemotherapy and irradiation may also be needed.[1,7-10] The shelling out of a lesion at surgery is inadequate, since such limited excision is followed by local recurrence in as many as 90% of cases. However, even wide local excision yields a local recurrence rate of as high as 50%.[17,18] Probability of local recurrence may be reduced by giving postoperative radiation therapy after performing conservative surgery. High local failure rates and high overall failure rates for nonrhabdomyosarcomatous soft tissue sarcomas in adults range from 38 to 80%, which indicates the need for effective adjuvant chemotherapy.[2,3]

It is not known whether there is a difference in disease-free or overall survival rates[19-23] between patients treated by amputation and those having limb-sparing procedures,[24] or local excision of tumor followed by radiotherapy and chemotherapy.

V. RADIATION THERAPY

Objective responses to radiotherapy in patients with soft tissue sarcomas have been achieved for many years. Recommended dosages of irradiation have been as high as 6000 cGy for adults when microscopic disease was to be eradicated. However, responses were seen with lower dosages.

Studies are needed of the time-dosage fractionation relationships in children and adults with nonrhabdomyosarcomatous soft tissue sarcomas.[1-3,14,25,26] This would include the use of hyperfractionated irradiation to deliver higher cumulative dosages, with fewer side effects on normal tissues surrounding the tumor.

Also, there have been prospective studies of the efficacy of adjuvant radiotherapy. Amputation and local surgery with radiotherapy for soft tissue sarcomas of the extremities have yielded similar results.[1-3] Uncontrolled studies failed to determine an advantage for pediatric patients with soft tissue sarcomas who received adjuvant chemotherapy either alone or with radiation therapy after limited surgery, or who were given chemotherapy following amputation.

By the scheme shown in Figure 1, patients classified as group I are given no radiation therapy. Patients classified as group II receive radiation as primary treatment and then are randomized to receive or to not receive chemotherapy. Patients with groups III and IV tumors receive radiation to the primary tumor site after determining the initial response following chemotherapy. Those with group IV disease also receive radiation to the sites of metastatic tumor.

The volume encompassed by the radiation should include the primary tumor area plus a 2-cm margin around the tumor. The extent of this margin is determined before the initial surgery for patients classified in groups II, III, and IV. For patients in groups III and IV, a boost to the initial tumor volume is recommended, with special consideration for limiting the dose of irradiation delivered to growing bones and normal tissues.

Megavoltage radiotherapy equipment should be used with parallel opposed portals (which are equally, or unevenly, weighted), or multiple convergent beams plus an electron-beam boost are used.

Dosage schedules are designed with consideration for protecting vital organs such as lungs, liver, kidneys, and bowel and other normal tissues. The recommended dosage is 3500 cGy delivered to the initial tumor volume in children younger than 6 years, with a total dosage of 4500 cGy for the reduced tumor volume. For children older than 6 years, 4500 cGy can be delivered to the initial volume, and up to 5000 cGy can be given to the reduced volume (Figure 1). Occasionally, tumors in younger patients may be given boosts of up to 5500 cGy, and for older children this dose may approach 6500 cGy. Total dosage to the kidneys should not exceed 1500 cGy, given over a period of 2 to 4 weeks. For the liver, dosages of 2400 cGy should not be exceeded, and no more than 1800 cGy should be delivered when both lungs are irradiated.

Brachytherapy may be utilized for large tumors, or for a boost to the primary tumor site after the delivery of standard dosage-volume of irradiation.[27,28]

VI. CHEMOTHERAPY

The use of specific chemotherapy for nonrhabdomyosarcomatous soft tissue sarcomas in children remains ill-defined. The value of chemotherapy after resection of localized tumors is controversial, because the survival rate for these tumors is greater than 75%. To qualify as a candidate for adjuvant chemotherapy, the patient's tumor must have a great potential to metastasize and have a high mortality rate associated with metastases. The tumor must also be one for which there is a reasonable possibility of response to chemotherapy.

Phase I and II chemotherapy trials since 1960 have contributed to the design of present multiagent chemotherapy schemes for treatment of the various soft tissue sarcomas. These studies have indicated that vincristine,[29] cyclophosphamide,[30] dactinomycin,[31] adri; mycin,[14,32,33] imidazole carboxamide,[34] cisplatin,[35] etoposide,[36] and ifosfamide[37,38] given either alone or in combination[39-47] have activity against soft tissue sarcomas. Survival in adults has been influenced by the administration of these agents in combination. The most effective of these agents probably are adriamycin and ifosfamide.[16,32]

Few studies have been designed to determine the effectiveness of adjuvant chemotherapy for the soft tissue sarcomas of young patients,[1] but important studies are now in progress in Europe[9] and in the U.S. (Figure 1).[40] Phase II studies of adults and children helped to demonstrate the effectiveness of single-agent therapy on measurable tumors, either primary or metastatic. Many drug combinations are being used, either alone or in combination with radiotherapy. Several of these studies are randomized, which may result in providing answers to important epidemiologic questions.

The oncologist who treats these rare pediatric sarcomas at the present time has several options for primary treatment. These treatment options are reviewed in the following paragraphs.

The Pediatric Oncology Group Protocols 8653/8654 (Figure 1) are designed to determine whether adjuvant chemotherapy, given either alone or in combination with postoperative radiotherapy, increases the relapse-free survival rate of patients with localized, completely resected soft tissue sarcomas. Chemotherapeutic agents that are used include vincristine, cyclophosphamide, dactinomycin, and adriamycin, with or without imidazole carboxamide (DTIC). This regimen is for patients with metastatic soft tissue sarcomas at diagnosis, for those with previously "untreated" recurrent tumors, or for patients who have localized, persistent, residual tumors after surgery and radiation therapy. Details of the treatment scheme, including dosages of chemotherapeutic agents, are as presented in Figure 1.

A second treatment option is the Malignant Mesenchymal Tumor Protocol '89 of the Societé Internationale Oncologie Pediatrique.[46] This program uses surgery, radiation therapy, and chemotherapy. Chemotherapy consists of ifosfamide (3 g/m^2) plus mesna on days 1 and 2, vincristine (1.5 mg/m^2, maximum 2 mg) intravenously on days 1 and 14, and dactinomycin (0.9 mg/m^2, maximum 1.0 mg) on days 1 and 2, with a 14-day interval between courses. Ten courses of chemotherapy are given without irradiation if a complete response, proved by surgery, is obtained. If a partial remission is achieved, patients are given two to six courses of cisplatin and adriamycin. If a surgically documented complete response is obtained, treatment is stopped and radiotherapy is not given; if a partial response is obtained, further surgery or radiotherapy becomes the option.

A third option is treatment by the protocol of the Pediatric Branch of the National Cancer Institute (U.S.).[40] This protocol includes vincristine (2 mg/m^2, maximum dose 2 mg) on day 1, adriamycin (35 mg/m^2 on days 1 and 2), and cyclophosphamide. Cyclophosphamide is given at a dose of 900 mg/m^2 on days 1 and 2 intravenously over 1 h along with mesna (360 mg/m^2 intravenously) given over 1 h mixed with cyclophosphamide, and followed by mesna (120 mg/m^2) as a continuous infusion during hours 2 to 5, and then at hours 5, 8, 11, 14, 17, and 20 given either intravenously over 15 to 30 min or given orally. Vincristine, adriamycin, and cyclophosphamide are subsequently alternated with ifosfamide (1800 mg/m^2/day) and etoposide (100 mg/m^2/day) for 5 days, with courses given at intervals of 3 weeks. Vincristine is given weekly on weeks 0, 1, 2, 4, 5, 6, 12, 24, 30, 36, and 42. Radiation therapy is given over a period of 6 to 8 weeks, beginning at week 13. Courses of ifosfamide-etoposide-mesna are given every 3 weeks during radiation therapy. Following radiation therapy, the dose of adriamycin is increased to 50 mg/m² and cyclophosphamide is increased to 1200 mg/m², with the drugs given as a single dose once only and not on consecutive days. In all, 18 cycles of chemotherapy are planned for delivery during 51 weeks. Early favorable results of this treatment have been observed.[40]

There are patients who have recurrence of tumors after earlier favorable responses, and those who fail to achieve a complete regression of tumor after surgery, chemotherapy, and radiation therapy. For these patients there remain optional chemotherapy regimens, if remaining disease cannot be resected or retreated with irradiation, which may include brachytherapy. These chemotherapy options include the use of (1) the combination of ifosfamide and etoposide,[42,47] or (2) the combination of cisplatin and etoposide. These drug combinations may be given in conventional dosages,[43] or they may be given in high dosages together with granulocyte-macrophage colony-stimulating factor or granulocyte colony-stimulating factor, with or without autologous bone marrow transplantation.

VII. TREATMENT AND PROGNOSIS

In children, nonrhabdomyosarcomatous soft tissue sarcomas may occur at the same sites as rhabdomyosarcomas.[48-64] Symptoms, signs, and diagnostic evaluations are the same for these tumors as for rhabdomyosarcomas at the same sites. The same principles of surgical and radiotherapeutic management should be used, yet chemotherapy may differ. As experience is gained with chemotherapeutic regimens that are effective for soft tissue sarcomas, more specific recommendations may then be made.

Table 1 presents the experience at a single institution with nonrhabdomyosarcomatous soft tissue sarcomas classified according to site of primary tumor and clinical grouping. The table gives adequate details of these tumors by primary site. It is evident that more of these tumors involve the extremities than the trunk or the head and neck. In most instances for both adults and children, these tumors more frequently involve lower rather than upper extremities.

Overall, it can be stated that the prognosis for patients with soft tissue sarcomas depends upon site and clinical grouping. There is a better outcome for individuals with tumors classified as groups I or II, with survival rates of 79% for group I and 73% for group II patients. Unfortunately, the exact contribution of surgery, radiation, and chemotherapy to these findings cannot be adequately addressed because of the varying treatments given and lack of control groups.

Nonrhabdomyosarcomatous soft tissue sarcomas may occur in adolescents as well as adults. They may also occur as second malignant neoplasms following earlier treatment with radiotherapy, chemotherapy, or both.[65] Four such patients have been treated at the author's institution, and their tumors are not included in the analyses in Tables 1 through 5. Sarcomas of soft tissues and bone only rarely develop following treatment for acute leukemia. Treatment options for these tumors depend upon the site and resectability of the second malignancy. Treatment may also be limited by the type and amount of prior chemotherapy and radiotherapy.

Recently, a series of 53 postirradiation soft tissue sarcomas were reported. The study indicated that these poorly differentiated tumors were detected after a mean latency period of 10 years and that the patients had dismal prognoses.[65] Most of these tumors were identified as malignant fibrous histiocytomas, which was followed in frequency by extraskeletal osteosarcomas, fibrosarcomas, schwannomas, extraskeletal chondrosarcomas, and angiosarcomas.

Because of the rarity of nonrhabdomyosarcomatous soft tissue sarcomas in children and adolescents, patients with these tumors should be admitted to therapeutic protocols which may contribute to the knowledge of natural history, epidemiology, and response to therapy.

Therapeutic modalities must be tailored for the site and extent of disease and the patient's age, as well as for consideration to normal tissues that may be adversely affected by surgery, radiation, and chemotherapy. Tailoring of treatment should be performed within the setting of the multimodality protocol chosen for the patient. The exact influence that the histology of these rare tumors has on ultimate prognosis remains to be determined.

VIII. SUMMARY

The signs and symptoms associated with the soft tissue sarcomas other than rhabdomyosarcoma are in most instances similar to those associated with rhabdomyosarcoma. These signs and symptoms depend on the site and size of the primary tumor and the presence or absence of metastases. Bone marrow involvement in patients with these soft tissue sarcomas is less frequent than with rhabdomyosarcoma. Treatment for children with these soft tissue sarcomas other than rhabdomyosarcoma should evaluate combined modality therapy, including irradiation after surgery for incompletely resected lesions. For completely resected tumors, the value of adjuvant chemotherapy or irradiation is unknown. For metastatic or unresectable tumors at the time of diagnosis, multiagent chemotherapy should use conventional agents in addition to irradiation. Because of the rarity of these soft tissue sarcomas other than rhabdomyosarcoma, treatment at a pediatric oncology center is recommended.

ACKNOWLEDGMENTS

Gratitude is expressed to Mrs. Alvida Cain, Mrs. Laurel Avery, Mrs. Debbie Poe, and Miss Patricia Logan for technical assistance, to Ms. Jessyca Mosby and Ms. Linda Wood for typing the manuscript, and Mrs. Ann Morris for editorial assistance.

This work was supported in part by Childhood Cancer Program Project Grant CA23099, Cancer Center (CORE) Grant CA21765 from the National Cancer Institute, Bethesda, MD, and by the American Lebanese Syrian Associated Charities (ALSAC), Memphis, TN.

REFERENCES

1. **Horowitz, M. E., Pratt, C. B., Webber, B. L., et al.,** Therapy of childhood soft-tissue sarcomas other than rhabdomyosarcoma: a review of 62 cases treated at a single institution, *J. Clin. Oncol.,* 4, 559, 1986.
2. **Chang, A. E. and Rosenberg, S. A.,** Clinical evaluation and treatment of soft tissue sarcomas, in *Soft Tissue Tumors,* 2nd ed., Enzinger, F. M. and Weiss, S. W., Eds., C.V. Mosby, St. Louis, 1988, 19.
3. **Chang, A. E., Rosenberg, S. A., Glatstein, S. A., and Antman, K. H.,** Sarcomas of soft tissues, in *Cancer: Principles and Practice of Oncology,* 3rd ed., DeVita, V. T., Jr., Hellman, S., and Rosenberg, S. A., Eds., Lippincott, Philadelphia, 1989, 1345.
4. **Mazeron, J. J. and Suit, H. D.,** Lymph nodes as sites of metastases from sarcomas of soft tissue, *Cancer,* 60, 1800, 1987.
5. **Bunn, P. A., Jr. and Ridgway, E. C.,** Paraneoplastic syndromes in cancer, in *Cancer: Principles and Practice of Oncology,* 3rd ed., DeVita, V. T., Jr., Hellman, S., and Rosenberg, S. A., Eds., Lippincott, Philadelphia, 1989, 1896.
6. **Young, J. L., Jr. and Miller, R. W.,** Incidence of malignant tumors in U.S. children, *J. Pediatr.,* 86, 254, 1975.
7. **Rao, B. N., Etcubanas, E. E., Horowitz, M., et al.,** The results of conservative management of extremity soft tissue sarcomas in children, *Proc. Annu. Meet. Am. Soc. Clin. Oncol.,* 5, 266, 1986.
8. **Brizel, D. M., Weinstein, H., Hunt, M., et al.,** Failure pattern and survival in childhood soft tissue sarcomas, *Proc. Am. Soc. Ther. Radiat. Oncol.,* 29, 183, 1988.
9. **Carli, M., Perilongo, G. T., Paolucci, P., et al.,** Role of primary chemotherapy in childhood malignant mesenchymal tumors other than rhabdomyosarcoma. Preliminary results, *Proc. Am. Soc. Clin. Oncol.,* 5, 208, 1986.

10. **Olive, D., Famant, F., Rodary, C., et al.,** Responsiveness of non-rhabdomyosarcoma malignant mesenchymal tumors (NRMMT) to primary chemotherapy (CT), in Proc. 20th Meeting SIOP, Trondheim, Norway, 1988, 118.

11. **Mandell, L. R., Ghavini, F., Exelby, P., and Fuks, Z.,** Preliminary results of alternating combination chemotherapy (CT) and hyperfractionated radiotherapy (HART) in advanced rhabdomyosarcoma (RMS), *Int. J. Radiat. Oncol. Biol. Phys.,* 15, 197, 1988.

12. **Rosenberg, S. A., Tepper, J., Glatstein, E., et al.,** Prospective randomized evaluation of adjuvant chemotherapy in adults with soft tissue sarcomas of the extremities, *Cancer,* 52, 424, 1983.

13. **Antman, K., Suit, H., Amato, D., et al.,** Preliminary results of a randomized trial of adjuvant doxorubicin for sarcomas: lack of apparent difference between treatment groups, *J. Clin. Oncol.,* 2, 601, 1984.

14. **Suit, H. D., Manken, H. J., Schiller, A. L., et al.,** Results of treatment of sarcomas of soft tissue by radiation and surgery at Massachusetts General Hospital, *Cancer Treat. Symp.,* 3, 43, 1985.

15. **Bramwell, V. H., Mouridsen, H. T., Santoro, A., et al.,** Cyclophosphamide versus ifosfamide: final report of a randomized phase II trial in adult soft tissue sarcomas, *Eur. J. Cancer Clin. Oncol.,* 23, 311, 1987.

16. **Stuart-Harris, R., Harper, P. G., Kaye, S. B., et al.,** High-dose ifosfamide by infusion with mesna in advanced soft tissue sarcoma, *Cancer Treat. Rev.,* 10(Suppl. A), 93, 1983.

17. **Suit, H. D.,** Patterns of failure after treatment of sarcoma of soft tissue by radical surgery or by conservative surgery and radiation, *Cancer Treat. Symp.,* 2, 241, 1983.

18. **Potter, D. A., Glenn, J., Kinsella, T., et al.,** Patterns of recurrence in patients with high-grade soft-tissue sarcomas, *J. Clin. Oncol.,* 3, 353, 1985.

19. **Collin, C., Godbold, J., Hajdu, S., and Brennan, M.,** Localized extremity soft tissue sarcoma: an analysis of factors affecting survival, *J. Clin. Oncol.,* 5, 601, 1987.

20. **Roth, J. A., Putnam, J. B., Jr., Wesley, M. N., and Rosenberg, S. A.,** Differing determinants of prognosis following resection of pulmonary metastasis from osteogenic and soft tissue sarcomas, *Cancer,* 55, 1361, 1988.

21. **Ueda, T., Aozasa, K., Tsujimoto, M., et al.,** Multivariate analysis for clinical prognostic factors in 163 patients with soft tissue sarcoma, *Cancer,* 62, 1444, 1988.

22. **Mannard, A. M., Petiot, J. F., Marnay, J., et al.,** Prognostic factors in soft tissue sarcomas: a multivariate analysis of 109 cases, *Cancer,* 63, 1437, 1989.

23. **Shiraki, M., Enterline, H. T., Brooks, J. J., et al.,** Pathologic analysis of advanced adult soft tissue sarcomas, bone sarcomas and mesotheliomas. The Eastern Cooperative Oncology Group (ECOG) experience, *Cancer,* 64, 484, 1989.

24. **Eilber, F. R., Morton, D. L., Eckardt, J., et al.,** Limb salvage for skeletal and soft tissue sarcomas: multidisciplinary preoperative therapy, *Cancer,* 53, 2579, 1984.

25. **Slater, J. D., McNeese, M. D., and Peters, L. J.,** Radiation therapy for unresectable soft tissue sarcomas, *Int. J. Radiat. Oncol. Biol. Phys.,* 12, 1729, 1986.

26. **Willett, C. G., Schiller, A. L., Suit, H. D., et al.,** The histologic response of soft tissue sarcoma to radiation therapy, *Cancer,* 60, 1500, 1987.

27. **Curran, W. J., Jr., Littman, P., and Raney, R. B.,** Interstitial radiation therapy in the treatment of childhood soft-tissue sarcomas, *Int. J. Radiat. Oncol. Biol. Phys.,* 14, 169, 1988.

28. **Knight, P. J., Doornbos, J. F., Rosen, D., et al.,** The use of interstitial radiation therapy in the treatment of persistent, localized, and unresectable cancer in children, *Cancer,* 57, 951, 1986.

29. **Pratt, C., James, D. H., Holton, C. P., and Pinkel, D.,** Combination therapy including vincristine for malignant solid tumors in children, *Cancer Chemother. Rep.,* 52, 589, 1968.

30. **Pinkel, D.,** Cyclophosphamide in children with cancer, *Cancer,* 15, 42, 1962.

31. **Pinkel, D.,** Actinomycin D in childhood cancer: a preliminary report, *Pediatrics,* 23, 342, 1959.

32. **Gottleib, J. A., Baker, L. H., O'Bryan, R. M., et al.,** Adriamycin (NSC-123127) used alone and in combination for soft tissue and bony sarcomas, *Cancer Chemother. Rep.,* 6, 271, 1975.

33. **Tan, C., Rosen, G., Ghavimi, F., et al.,** Adriamycin (NSC-123127) in pediatric malignancies, *Cancer Chemother. Rep.,* 6(Part 3), 259, 1975.

34. **Gottleib, J. A., Benjamin, R. S., Baker, L. M., et al.,** Role of DTIC (NSC-45388) in the chemotherapy of sarcomas, *Cancer Treat. Rep.,* 60, 199, 1976.

35. **Pratt, C. B., Hayes, F. A., Green, A. A., et al.,** Pharmacokinetic evaluation of cisplatin in children with malignant solid tumors. A phase II study, *Cancer Treat. Rep.,* 65, 1021, 1981.

36. **O'Dwyer, P. J., Leyland-Jones, B., Alonso, M. T., et al.,** Etoposide (VP-16,213): current status of an active anticancer drug, *N. Engl. J. Med.,* 312, 692, 1985.

37. **Magrath, I., Sandlund, J., Raynor, A., et al.,** A phase II study of ifosfamide in the treatment of recurrent sarcomas in young people, *Cancer Chemother. Pharmacol.,* 15, 258, 1985.

38. **Pratt, C. B., Douglass, E. C., Goren, M. P., et al.,** Clinical studies of Ifosfamide/Mesna at St. Jude Children's Research Hospital, 1983—1988, *Semin. Oncol.,* 16(Suppl. 3), 51, 1989.

39. **Grier, H. E., Perez-Atayde, A. R., and Weinstein, H. J.**, Chemotherapy for inoperable infantile fibro-sarcoma, *Cancer,* 56, 1507, 1985.

40. **Horowitz, M., Balis, F., Pastakia, B., et al.**, Integration of Ifosfamide and VP-16 (IE) into the frontline therapy of pediatric sarcomas (PS), *Proc. Annu. Meet. Am. Soc. Clin. Oncol.,* 7, 260, 1988.

41. **Castello, M. A., Clerico, A., Jenkner, A., and Dominici, C.**, High-dose carboplatin and etoposide in children with malignant solid tumors, *Proc. SIOP,* p. 195, 1988.

42. **Miser, J. S., Kinsella, T. J., Triche, T. J., et al.**, Ifosfamide with Mesna uroprotection and etoposide: an effective regimen in the treatment of recurrent sarcomas and other tumors of children and young adults, *J. Clin. Oncol.,* 5, 1191, 1987.

43. **Crist, W. M., Raney, R. B. Ragab, A., et al.**, Intensive chemotherapy including cisplatin with and without etoposide for children with soft tissue sarcomas, *Med. Pediatr. Oncol.,* 15, 51, 1987.

44. **Edmonson, J. H., Fleming, T. R., Ivans, J. C., et al.**, Randomized study of systemic chemotherapy following complete excision of non-osseous sarcoma, *J. Clin. Oncol.,* 2, 1390, 1984.

45. **de Paula, U., Suit, H. D., and Harmon, D.**, Adjuvant chemotherapy in clinical stage M_0 sarcoma of soft tissue, *Cancer,* 62, 1907, 1988.

46. **Flamant, F., Rodary, C., Rey, A., and Praquin, M. T.**, Preliminary report on the SIOP protocol for malignant mesenchymal tumors, in Proc. 17th Meeting SIOP, Venice, Italy, 1985, 81.

47. **Kung, F. H., Pratt, C. D., and Krischer, J. P.**, Ifosfamide and VP-16 in the treatment of recurrent malignant solid tumors of childhood, *Proc. Annu. Meet. Am. Soc. Clin. Oncol.,* 8, 301, 1989.

48. **Stout, A. P.**, Fibrosarcoma in infants and children, *Cancer,* 5, 1028, 1962.

49. **Soule, E. H. and Pritchard, D. J.**, Fibrosarcoma of infants and children: a review of 110 cases, *Cancer,* 40, 1711, 1977.

50. **Ninane, J., Gosseye, S., Panteon, E., et al.**, Congenital fibrosarcoma: preoperative chemotherapy and conservative surgery, *Cancer,* 58, 1400, 1986.

51. **Blockner, S., Koenig, J., and Ternberg, J.**, Congenital fibrosarcoma, *J. Pediatr. Surg.,* 22, 665, 1987.

52. **Gausar, G. F. and Kremetz, E. T.**, Desmoid tumors: experience with new modes of therapy, *South. Med. J.,* 81, 794, 1988.

53. **Raney, R. B.**, Synovial sarcoma, *Med. Pediatr. Oncol.,* 9, 41, 1981.

54. **Kauffman, S. L. and Stout, A. P.**, Hemangiopericytoma in children, *Cancer,* 13, 695, 1960.

55. **Shmookler, B. M. and Enzinger, F. M.**, Liposarcoma occurring in children: analysis of 17 cases and review of the literature, *Cancer,* 52, 567, 1983.

56. **Weiss, S. W. and Enzinger, F. M.**, Malignant fibrous histiocytoma: an analysis of 200 cases, *Cancer,* 41, 2250, 1978.

57. **Raney, R. B., Allen, A., O'Neill, J., et al.**, Malignant fibrous histiocytoma of soft tissue in childhood, *Cancer,* 57, 2198, 1986.

58. **Mayer, C. M. H., Favara, B. E., Holton, C. P., and Rainer, G.**, Malignant mesenchymoma in infants, *Am. J. Dis. Child.,* 128, 847, 1974.

59. **Ducatman, B. S., Scheithauer, B. W., Piepgras, D. G., et al.**, Malignant peripheral nerve sheath tumors: a clinicopathologic study of 120 cases, *Cancer,* 57, 2006, 1986.

60. **Raney, R. B., Schnaufer, L., Zeigler, M., et al.**, Treatment of children with neurogenic sarcoma, *Cancer,* 59, 1, 1987.

61. **Enzinger, F. M. and Weiss, S. W.**, Malignant tumors of uncertain histogenesis, in *Soft Tissue Tumors,* 2nd ed., Enzinger, F. M. and Weiss, S. W., Eds., C.V. Mosby, St. Louis, 1988, 929.

62. **Nakashima, Y., Unni, K. K., Shives, T. C., et al.**, Mesenchymal chondrosarcoma of bone and soft tissue: a review of 111 cases, *Cancer,* 57, 2444, 1986.

63. **Chase, D. R. and Enzinger, F. M.**, Epithelioid sarcoma: diagnosis, prognostic indications and treatment, *Am. J. Surg. Pathol.,* 9, 241, 1985.

64. **Kawamoto, E. H., Weidner, N., Agostini, R. M., Jr., and Jaffe, R.**, Malignant ectomesenchymoma of soft tissue: report of 2 cases and review of the literature, *Cancer,* 59, 1791, 1987.

65. **Laskin, W. B., Silverman, T. A., and Enzinger, F. M.**, Postradiation soft tissue sarcomas: an analysis of 53 cases, *Cancer,* 62, 2330, 1988.

Index

INDEX

Nongenitourinary pelvic, 357—358
Non-Hodgkin's lymphoma, hypercalcemia and
    hyperuricemia in, 223
Nonorbital cranial parameningeal sarcoma, 321—
    326
Nonparameningeal sarcomas, head and neck, 328—
    329
Nonrhabdomyosarcomatous soft tissue sarcomas, see
    Soft tissue sarcomas, nonrhabdomyo-
    sarcomatous
Normalization induction, application of animal
    models of RMS in, 54—55
NSE, see Neurone specific enolase
Nuclear medicine, 338
Nuclear oncogenes, 62—63

O

Oncogenes, 62—64
Oncogenesis, susceptibility to, 61
Onkoloski Institut, 248—249
    assessment of chemotherapy in, 257
    chemotherapy results in, 251
Oophorectomy, 178
Operative resection, general principles of in
    children, 173—174
Oral cavity rhabdomyosarcoma, 109—110, 334,
    340—341, 344
Orbit
    RMS of, 94—96
        diagnostic imaging of, 127—129
        late therapy effects in, 289—292
        operative procedure for in children, 175
        prognosis of with radiation therapy, 184—185
        relapse rate in, 265, 276
    tumors of
        diagnosis of, 326
        extension of to parameningeal sites, 292
        toxicity with treatment of, 327—328
        treatment of, 326—327
Organ meats, ingestion of, 11
Oropharyngeal rhabdomyosarcoma, 109—111,
    334—335, 340—341, 344
Orthovoltage radiotherapy, risk of second
    malignancy with, 307
Osteosarcoma
    with breast cancers, 10—11
    extraosseous, 411—413, 429
    treatment of, 244
Ovaries, 299—302
Ovoid-spindle cells, 396

P

p53 gene, 68—69
Palate, soft, rhabdomyosarcoma of, 110, 335
Palmer cytopathologic classification, 377
Pancreas, malignant neoplasms of, 336
Paracardiac rhabdomyosarcoma, 118
Parameningeal rhabdomyosarcoma, 33—34
    diagnosis of, 95

diagnostic imaging of, 129
operative procedure for in children, 175
radiation therapy for, 183—185
relapse in, 276
spread to, 111
Parameningeal sarcomas, nonorbital cranial,
    320—326
Parameningeal tumors, late treatment effects of, 293
Paranasal rhabdomyosarcoma
    CT scan of, 104—105
    involving orbit, 101
    superior, lateral, and inferior extension of, 102
Paranasal sinus rhabdomyosarcoma, 129, 131
Paraspinal tumors, 369—370
Paratesticular rhabdomyosarcoma, 35, 348, 358
    histological study of, 114
    hypercalcemia with, 219—222
    imaging and diagnosis of, 114—115
    operative procedure for in children, 176—177
    relapse with, 277
    signs and symptoms of, 348—349
    staging of, 349—350
    treatment of
        chemotherapy, 352
        complications of, 352
        radiotherapy, 351
        surgical, 350—351
Parathyroid hormone, serum levels of in hypercal-
    cemia and RMS, 222—223
Paravertebral tumor, morphology of, 5
Parenteral alimentation, 329
Parotid gland, 107—109
Partial thromboplastin time (PTT), 218—219
Pathologists, classification of childhood soft tissue
    sarcomas by, 4
Patient characteristics and prognosis, 140—144,
    148—151
Pedal lymphangiography, 348
Pediatric oncologists, interest of in soft tissue
    sarcomas, 4
Pediatric Oncology Group Protocol, 424, 426
Pelvic bone growth retardation, with radiotherapy,
    355
Pelvic exenteration, 178, 356
Pelvic wall rhabdomyosarcoma, 119
Pelvis
    effects of radiotherapy in, 301, 304
    RMS of
        CT scan of, 136
        nongenitourinary, 357—358
        operative procedure for in children, 177—178
        radiation therapy for, 185
        relapse with, 277
        spread of through, 133—137
Pericardial rhabdomyosarcoma, 118
Pericardial thickening, with mediastinal irradiation,
    298
Perineal rhabdomyosarcoma, 121
Peripheral nerve sheath tumors, 397—400, 403
Peripheral neural tumors, cellular, 397—398

S